Handbook of Practical
Psychopharmacology

Handbook of Practical
Psychopharmacology

Matthew Macaluso, D.O.
Calley H. Johnston, M.D.

AMERICAN
PSYCHIATRIC
ASSOCIATION
PUBLISHING

Note: The authors have worked to ensure that all information in this book is accurate at the time of publication and consistent with general psychiatric and medical standards, and that information concerning drug dosages, schedules, and routes of administration is accurate at the time of publication and consistent with standards set by the U.S. Food and Drug Administration and the general medical community. As medical research and practice continue to advance, however, therapeutic standards may change. Moreover, specific situations may require a specific therapeutic response not included in this book. For these reasons and because human and mechanical errors sometimes occur, we recommend that readers follow the advice of physicians directly involved in their care or the care of a member of their family.

Books published by American Psychiatric Association Publishing represent the findings, conclusions, and views of the individual authors and do not necessarily represent the policies and opinions of American Psychiatric Association Publishing or the American Psychiatric Association.

If you wish to buy 50 or more copies of the same title, please go to www.appi.org/specialdiscounts for more information.

First Edition

Manufactured in the United States of America on acid-free paper
28 27 26 25 24 5 4 3 2 1

American Psychiatric Association Publishing
800 Maine Avenue SW, Suite 900
Washington, DC 20024-2812
www.appi.org

Library of Congress Cataloging-in-Publication Data
Names: Macaluso, Matthew, editor. | Johnston, Calley, editor. | American Psychiatric Association Publishing, publisher.
Title: Handbook of practical psychopharmacology / editors, Matthew Macaluso, Calley Johnston.
Description: First edition. | Washington, DC : American Psychiatric Association Publishing, [2025] | Includes bibliographical references and index.
Identifiers: LCCN 2024011077 (print) | LCCN 2024011078 (ebook) | ISBN 9781615374878 (paperback : alk. paper) | ISBN 9781615374885 (ebook)
Subjects: MESH: Psychotropic Drugs | Handbook
Classification: LCC RC483 (print) | LCC RC483 (ebook) | NLM QV 39 | DDC 616.89/18—dc23/eng/20240401
LC record available at https://lccn.loc.gov/2024011077
LC ebook record available at https://lccn.loc.gov/2024011078

British Library Cataloguing in Publication Data
A CIP record is available from the British Library.

To our patients,
for whom we do this work with the hope that we can improve lives
and alleviate suffering.

M.M. and C.J.

To my wife, Katharine,
and my children, Matthew Jr. (Matty) and William:
You are the most important people in my life
and the inspiration for everything that I do.

To my mentor and dear friend, Sheldon Preskorn,
who taught me important lessons about academic medicine and life:
Your teachings made me a better person and professional.

M.M.

To my husband, Ryan,
for his abiding encouragement, love, and patience.

To my mom, Kathy, my dad, Dan, and my sister, Karah,
for a lifetime of unconditional love.

To my patients,
from whom, and for, I continually learn.

And finally to God,
for the ability and privilege to do this work.

C.J.

Contents

PART III
Medications Used to Treat Specific Disorders/Conditions

PART IV
Other Agents/Treatments

PART V
Treatment of Special Populations

List of Tables

Contributors

Advisory Board Members

Great efforts were made to ensure that this Handbook contains up-to-date and factually correct evidence-based information. Essential to these efforts was the review by the members of our Advisory Board, who ascertained that the content was factually correct and based on the most reliable and current information available at the time it was written.

Kimberly A. Smith, Ph.D. (Lead)
Assistant Professor, Department of Family and Community Medicine, Heersink School of Medicine, University of Alabama at Birmingham

Theadia L. Carey, M.D., M.S.
Professor, Department of Psychiatry, Michigan State University College of Osteopathic Medicine, East Lansing, Michigan; Director, Psychiatry Residency Program, Detroit Wayne County Authority—General Medical Education, Detroit, Michigan

Lawrence J. Cohen, Pharm.D., BCPP, FASHP, FCCP, FCP, FNAP
Distinguished Professor of Pharmacotherapy (Retired) and Adjunct Professor of Pharmacotherapy, University of North Texas System College of Pharmacy, and Adjunct Professor of Medical Education, Texas College of Osteopathic Medicine, University of North Texas Health Science Center, Fort Worth, Texas; Emeritus Professor of Pharmacotherapy, Washington State University College of Pharmacy, Spokane, Washington

L. Joy Houston, M.D.
Associate Professor and Vice Chair of Education, Southern Illinois University School of Medicine, Springfield, Illinois

Abhishek Wadhwa, M.D.
Assistant Professor, Department of Psychiatry—Child & Adolescent, Heersink School of Medicine, The University of Alabama at Birmingham

Daniel Warren, M.D.
Assistant Professor, Department of Family and Community Medicine, University of Kansas School of Medicine, Wichita, Kansas

Authors

Patricia Aguayo, M.D., M.P.H.
Assistant Professor, Department of Psychiatry, University of Utah School of Medicine, Huntsman Mental Health Institute, Salt Lake City, Utah

Shanon E. Astley, M.D., PMH-C
Chief Resident, Family Medicine and Psychiatry, University of California Davis School of Medicine, Volunteer Clinical Faculty, Sacramento, California

Sahand Babapoor-Farrokhran, M.D., Ph.D.
Chief, Division of Neuropsychiatry and Neuromodulation; Director, Laboratory for Circuit Neuroscience & Neuromodulation; Director, Transcranial Magnetic Stimulation (TMS) clinical service, Massachusetts General Hospital; Associate Professor of Psychiatry and Neurology, Harvard Medical School, Boston, Massachusetts

Gabrielle Bleich, M.D.
PGY2 Resident, Obstetrics/Gynecology, New Jersey Medical School, Rutgers Newark Campus, Newark, New Jersey

Bradley G. Burk, Pharm.D., BCPP
Clinical Pharmacist, Acute Psychiatry and Addiction Recovery, and Assistant Professor, Department of Psychiatry & Behavioral Neurobiology, Heersink School of Medicine, The University of Alabama at Birmingham

Erick Calvario-Sanchez, M.D.
Research Fellow, Department of Psychiatry, University of Utah School of Medicine, Huntsman Mental Health Institute, Salt Lake City, Utah

Austin Campbell, Pharm.D., BCPP
Clinical Associate Professor, University of Missouri–Kansas City School of Pharmacy; Adjunct Assistant Professor, Department of Psychiatry, University of Missouri Medical School, Columbia, Missouri

Joan A. Camprodon, M.D., M.P.H., Ph.D.
Director, Laboratory for Neuropsychiatry & Neuromodulation, Massachusetts General Hospital, and Associate Professor of Psychiatry, Harvard Medical School, Boston, Massachusetts

Tammy Duong, M.D.
Clinical Associate Professor, Department of Psychiatry and Behavioral Sciences, UCSF Weill Institute for Neurosciences, University of California San Francisco

Matthew J. Ehrlich, M.D.
Assistant Professor, Department of Psychiatry & Behavioral Neurobiology, The University of Alabama at Birmingham

Cheryl Graber, M.D.
Associate Professor of Psychiatry, Rutgers Robert Wood Johnson Medical School, Rutgers University, New Brunswick, New Jersey

John Grissom, B.A.
Medical Student, Heersink School of Medicine, The University of Alabama at Birmingham

Shailesh (Bobby) Jain, M.D.
Director, Psychiatry Residency Program, Department of Psychiatry, School of Medicine, Texas Tech University Health Sciences Center, Midland, Texas

Calley Johnston, M.D.
Assistant Professor and Quality Medical Director for Inpatient Psychiatry, Department of Psychiatry & Behavioral Neurobiology, Heersink School of Medicine, The University of Alabama at Birmingham

Linda Kang, M.D.
Associate Physician, University of California Davis School of Medicine, Department of Psychiatry and Behavioral Medicine, Sacramento, California

Laura Kenkel, M.D.
Psychiatrist, Telecare Corporation, Placerville, California

Becky Kinkead, Ph.D.
Research Professor, Department of Psychiatry, University of Utah School of Medicine, Huntsman Mental Health Institute, Salt Lake City, Utah

Matthew Macaluso, D.O.
Professor of Psychiatry, Bee McWane Reid Endowed Chair in Mood Disorders, and Vice Chair for Clinical Affairs, University of Alabama at Birmingham; Clinical Director, UAB Depression and Suicide Center, Birmingham, Alabama

Muniza Majoka, M.B.B.S.
Assistant Professor of Psychiatry, Yale School of Medicine, New Haven, Connecticut

Angela Mayorga, M.D.
Associate Professor, Departments of Psychiatry and Behavioral Sciences and General & Hospital Medicine; Director, Psychiatry Residency Program; and Co-Director, Internal Medicine/Psychiatry Residency Program, University of Kansas Medical Center, Kansas City, Kansas

Alexandra F. Muratore, Ph.D.
Assistant Professor, Department of Psychiatry, Columbia University Irving Medical Center; New York State Psychiatric Institute, New York, New York

J. Craig Nelson, M.D.
Professor Emeritus of Psychiatry, Leon J. Epstein Chair in Geriatric Psychiatry, Department of Psychiatry and Behavioral Sciences, UCSF Weill Institute for Neurosciences, University of California San Francisco

Andrew T. Olagunju, M.B.B.S., M.Sc., Ph.D., FMCPsych, FWACP
Assistant Professor, Department of Psychiatry and Behavioral Neurosciences, McMaster University/St. Joseph's Healthcare Hamilton, Hamilton, Canada; Research Fellow, Discipline of Psychiatry, University of Adelaide, Adelaide, Australia

Brandon S. Pruett, M.D., Ph.D.
Assistant Professor, Department of Psychiatry & Behavioral Neurobiology, Heersink School of Medicine, The University of Alabama at Birmingham

Mark H. Rapaport, M.D.
CEO, Huntsman Mental Health Institute, and Chair, Department of Psychiatry, University of Utah School of Medicine, Salt Lake City, Utah

M. Bates Redwine, M.D.
Professor of Psychiatry and Director of Ambulatory Services, Somatic Therapies, and Geriatric Division, Department of Psychiatry & Behavioral Neurobiology, The University of Alabama at Birmingham

Itamar Shapira, M.D., M.B.A.
Psychiatry Resident, Dell Medical School, The University of Texas at Austin

Richard C. Shelton, M.D.
Charles B. Ireland Professor, Department of Psychiatry & Behavioral Neurobiology, The University of Alabama at Birmingham

Claire Slavin-Stewart, M.Sc., M.D.
Child and Adolescent Psychiatry Fellow, Department of Psychiatry and Behavioral Neurosciences, McMaster University/St Joseph's Healthcare Hamilton, Hamilton, Ontario, Canada

B. Timothy Walsh, M.D.
Professor, Department of Psychiatry, Columbia University Irving Medical Center; New York State Psychiatric Institute, New York, New York

William M. Webb, M.D., Ph.D.
Resident Physician, Departments of Psychiatry and Behavioral Sciences and General & Hospital Medicine; University of Kansas Medical Center, Kansas City, Kansas

Samuel Wilkinson, M.D.
Associate Professor of Psychiatry and Associate Director, Yale Depression Research Program, Department of Psychiatry, Yale School of Medicine, New Haven, Connecticut

Laine Young-Walker, M.D.
Chair, Department of Psychiatry, University of Missouri–Columbia School of Medicine, Columbia, Missouri

Michael S. Ziffra, M.D.
Associate Professor, Psychiatry and Behavioral Sciences (General Psychiatry), Feinberg School of Medicine, Northwestern University, Chicago, Illinois

Disclosure of Interests

The following contributors have indicated a financial interest in or other affiliation with a commercial supporter, manufacturer of a commercial product, and/or provider of a commercial service, during the year preceding manuscript submission, as listed below:

Austin Campbell, Pharm.D., BCPP UpToDate paid coauthor, "Pharmacotherapy for schizophrenia: Long-acting injectable antipsychotic drugs"; Sunovion Pharmaceuticals Inc., speakers bureau; Intra-Cellular Therapies, grant-supported CE presentation: "Are we Ready to Embrace the Third-Generation Treatments for Schizophrenia?" (August 2021); Otsuka Pharmaceutical Co. Ltd., National Forum Panel (October 2020).

Joan A. Camprodon, M.D., M.P.H., Ph.D. Dr. Camprodon is an inventor named on patents and patent applications for neuromodulation targeting methods held by Massachusetts General Hospital. He is a member of the scientific advisory boards of Hyka Therapeutics and Flow Neuroscience and has been a paid consultant for Mifu Technologies, Neuroelectrics, and LivaNova.

Becky Kinkead, Ph.D. NIH Grant support (R33 AT012329-01, PI Rapaport; active 04/2023–03/2026), "Specialized pro-resolving lipid mediators and treatment-resistant depression." This study is evaluating whether omega-3 fatty acids added to ineffective antidepressant treatment increase compounds that resolve inflammation and whether the increase in these compounds is associated with improved antidepressant response.

Matthew Macaluso, D.O. Dr. Macaluso has conducted clinical trials research as principal investigator for the following pharmaceutical companies over the last 12 months: Acadia, Allergan, Alkermes, AssureRx/Myriad, Boehringer/Ingelheim, Eisai, Lundbeck, Liva Nova, Janssen, Novartis, Otsuka, SAGE Pharmaceuticals. All clinical trial and study contracts were with and payments made to the either the University of Alabama at Birmingham Medical Center or the Kansas University Medical Center Research Institute. From April 2019 to June of 2020, Dr Macaluso was a member of the speaker bureau for Janssen Pharmaceuticals (Spravato/esketamine). Dr Macaluso has also received royalties from Springer Nature for his work as co-editor of the textbook titled Antidepressants: From Biogenic Amines to New Mechanisms of Action. This book was published in May of 2019.

J. Craig Nelson, M.D. In the past 12 months, Dr. Nelson has received financial support from the following: Consultation from Biohaven Pharmaceuticals Inc, Cleio Biosciences Limited, Johnson & Johnson, Otsuka, Novartis; Royalties from UpToDate; and salary support from the National Institute of Mental Health.

Brandon S. Pruett, M.D., Ph.D. Dr. Pruett is funded by the National Institute of Mental Health (NIMH) of the National Institutes of Health (NIH) under Award Number K23MH127303.

Richard C. Shelton, M.D. Grant/Research Support: Abbvie, Alto Pharmaceuticals, Boehringer Ingelheim, Denovo Biopharma, Gate Neurosciences, InMune Bio, Intra-cellular Therapies, Johnson & Johnson Innovative Medicine, LivaNova PLC, Navitor Pharmaceuticals, Neumora, Neurocrine Biosciences, Novartis AG, Sumitomo Group, Supernus Pharmaceuticals; Consulting: Boehringer Ingelheim, Denovo Biopharma, Johnson & Johnson Innovative Medicine, NeuroRx, Novartis AG, Seelos Therapeutics, Inc.; Royalties: Springer-Nature Group, Wolters-Kluwer NV.

B. Timothy Walsh, M.D. Dr. Walsh reports receiving royalties and honoraria from Guilford Publications, Oxford University Press, UpToDate, and Wiley.

Samuel Wilkinson, M.D. Dr. Wilkinson has received contract research funding for the conduct of clinical trials (administered through Yale University) from Oui Therapeutics and Janssen. He has received consulting fees from LivaNova.

The following contributors stated that they had no competing interests during the year preceding manuscript submission:

Patricia Aguayo, M.D., M.P.H.; Shanon E. Astley, M.D., PMH-C; Sahand Babapoor-Farrokhran, M.D., Ph.D.; Gabrielle Bleich, M.D.; Bradley G. Burk, Pharm.D., BCPP; Erick Calvario-Sanchez, M.D.; Theadia L. Carey, M.D., M.S.; Lawrence J. Cohen, Pharm.D., BCPP, FASHP, FCCP, FCP, FNAP; Tammy Duong, M.D.; Matthew J. Ehrlich, M.D.; Cheryl Graber, M.D.; John Grissom, B.A.; L. Joy Houston, M.D.; Shailesh (Bobby) Jain, M.D.; Calley Johnston, M.D.; Linda Kang, M.D.; Laura Kenkel, M.D.; Muniza Majoka, M.B.B.S.; Angela Mayorga, M.D.; Alexandra F. Muratore, Ph.D.; Andrew T. Olagunju, M.B.B.S., M.Sc., Ph.D., FMCPsych, FWACP; Mark H. Rapaport, M.D.; M. Bates Redwine, M.D.; Itamar Shapira, M.D., M.B.A.; Claire Slavin-Stewart, M.Sc., M.D.; Kimberly A. Smith, Ph.D.; Abhishek Wadhwa, M.D.; Daniel Warren, M.D.; William M. Webb, M.D., Ph.D.; Laine Young-Walker, M.D.; Michael S. Ziffra, M.D.

Background and How to Use This Handbook

Matthew Macaluso, D.O.
Calley H. Johnston, M.D.

Background

This Handbook was created as a quick-reference tool for busy clinical practitioners, trainees, and others wanting high-yield, easy access to information on prescribing psychopharmacological agents. Below is information on 1) the vision for the Handbook, 2) limitations of the Handbook, and 3) how the Handbook was fact checked (peer reviewed), as well as a disclaimer on using the Handbook.

Vision

Our vision for this Handbook was to create an easy-access desk reference for frequent use by providers, staff, and learners in clinics, emergency departments, and hospital wards. Therefore, this Handbook contains—in one resource—information on indications, contraindications, dosing, drug interactions, clinical monitoring, and adverse effects of commonly prescribed psychopharmacological agents (and other somatic treatments such as ECT). It also contains "clinical pearls," which represent the authors' and editors' practical suggestions on prescribing these agents.

Peer Review

We have made great efforts to ensure that this Handbook contains up-to-date, factually correct, and evidence-based information. The Handbook's material was reviewed in detail by its editors as part of the editing process and was also reviewed by members of the Handbook's Advisory Board, who ascertained that the content was factually correct and based on the most reliable and current information at the time it was written. Despite these efforts to ensure the accuracy and currency of the Handbook's content, new papers and data are being released faster than ever before in medicine in general, and psychiatry in particular. In addition, sometimes data points may conflict or experts may have differing opinions on how to interpret data (or prescribe drugs). Therefore, the Handbook must be used judiciously and carefully and must not be relied on as fully comprehensive.

Limitations

In keeping with the spirit of a quick-reference resource, this Handbook is not an exhaustive, comprehensive, or encyclopedic manual, nor does it attempt to offer recommendations for individual patients or specific clinical scenarios. Rather, it is intended to be an accessible and practical tool for guidance on psychopharmacological prescribing. Readers seeking further information are referred to the manufacturer's package insert (prescribing information) for each drug, the medical literature, and the many textbooks and educational resources published on psychopharmacology.

Disclaimer

This Handbook is not a substitute for good clinical training, supervision, and judgment. To make wise clinical decisions, practitioners must possess experience and deep knowledge, and exercise sound clinical reasoning and judgment, when deciding what is best for patients. Finally, although this Handbook is a helpful tool for busy clinicians, they should have other tools "in the toolbox," because on its own and by its nature, a handbook is incomplete.

How to Use This Handbook

1. Each drug has a single entry in the Handbook providing basic information about its prescribing.
2. There are sections in the Handbook on prescribing in special situations, such as for older adults and for children and adolescents, as well as considerations for prescribing during pregnancy or lactation/breastfeeding.
3. The starting point to access the Handbook's information on specific drugs is to search for the drug in question within the larger chapter where the drug is classified. For example, if one was searching for information on fluoxetine, the starting point would be to find the entry on fluoxetine in the chapter on antidepressants, since fluoxetine was first FDA approved as an antidepressant. That entry will review the prescribing of fluoxetine across other indications as well.
4. Alternatively, and if easier for some readers, there is an index outlining each section where each drug is referenced by page number.
5. Some drug entries may appear in more than one chapter. For example, mirtazapine appears in both the antidepressants chapter and the hypnotics chapter. The antidepressants chapter covers the prescribing of the drug for depression, anxiety, and other common indications. Because there are special considerations for using mirtazapine off-label for insomnia, the authors and editors believed that an entry for mirtazapine in the hypnotics chapter was warranted.
6. The Handbook covers evidence-based off-label prescribing. Off-label prescribing is not illegal; however, it may be prudent for the prescriber to provide additional clinical documentation/justification in these instances. A drug may be prescribed for a non-approved indication if the prescriber has weighed the benefits against the risks, avail-

able evidence, and alternative options and has discussed these same considerations with the patient and/or their authorized representative (depending on the clinical scenario). Local practicing guidelines also need to be followed.

7. The Handbook is not an exhaustive guide and does not intend to be a substitute for good clinical decision making. By its nature, the Handbook is not comprehensive and may be incomplete.

Nomenclature in Psychopharmacology

The editors of this Handbook and authors of the Handbook's chapters recognize that drug nomenclature is a topic of discussion in the field of psychopharmacology. Traditional drug class names in psychopharmacology were often developed by industry or with marketing purposes in mind. The term "atypical antipsychotic" suggested that the "atypical" drug was new or different from its predecessors. To further understand the example of "typical" versus "atypical" or "first" versus "second generation" antipsychotic nomenclature, which is commonly used in clinical practice, Preskorn (2001) argued that there are four generations of antipsychotics based on their mechanisms of action.

To further confuse the issue, modern approaches to drug nomenclature, such as neuroscience-based nomenclature (NbN [ECNP 2024]), attempt to use nomenclature that moves away from a drug's target symptoms (e.g., antipsychotic or antidepressant) and toward a classification system that is based on drug mechanism of action (e.g., norepinephrine reuptake inhibitor or norepinephrine transporter [NET]). However, such modern nomenclature has not yet been widely adopted in clinical practice or medical education. Therefore, to avoid confusion or moving back and forth between different nomenclature systems, this Handbook uses the nomenclature system for each drug that is most common in clinical practice and medical education at the time of this writing.

References

Preskorn SH: Antipsychotic drug development in the pre-human-genome era: a full circle. J Psychiatr Pract. 2001 May;7(3):209–213, 2001 15990523

Preskorn SH: The evolution of antipsychotic drug therapy: reserpine, chlorpromazine, and haloperidol. J Psychiatr Pract 13(4):253–257, 2007 17667738

ECNP: Neuroscience-based Nomenclature (NbN) [website]. Utrecht, The Netherlands, European College of Neuropsychopharmacology. Available at: https://www.ecnp.eu/research-innovation/nomenclature. Accessed August 3, 2024.

List of Medications

PART I
Foundations

1

Basic Principles of Psychopharmacology

Itamar Shapira, M.D.
John Grissom, B.A.
Calley Johnston, M.D.
Matthew Macaluso, D.O.

Our aim in this chapter is to provide a concise summary of the most relevant general and psychopharmacological principles that will be encountered in clinical practice.

Pharmacokinetics

- Pharmacokinetics is often described as "what the body does to the drug." The four main pharmacokinetics parameters are absorption, distribution, metabolism, and excretion.

Absorption

- *Absorption* refers to the breakdown of drugs and their passage through specific barriers, primarily the stomach and small intestines. Most drugs exist as either weak acids or weak bases. Weak acids tend to be absorbed in the stomach, while weak bases are absorbed in the intestines due to their ionizing ability. Therefore, certain medications, such as weak acids, should be taken after eating. The presence of food slows gastric emptying and allows the drug to sit in the stomach longer to be absorbed.

- *Bioavailability* refers to the percentage of the drug that makes it into the systemic circulation. Several factors can affect bioavailability, such as the route of administration, drug formulation, rate of release, and chemical properties. Patient factors such as age, disease state, and pregnancy can also affect bioavailability. Through most routes of administration, drugs are subject to a *first-pass effect*. Drugs absorbed through the stomach or intestines travel to the liver initially through the hepatic portal system. They are metabolized by the liver, which will reduce the bioavailability of the drug, excluding prodrugs. Prodrugs require metabolism to be activated.

Distribution

- *Distribution* refers to the drug's travel into tissues and the interstitial fluid from the bloodstream. Distribution can be influenced by many factors, including capillary permeability, pH, and permeability of the cells in each tissue. Certain tissues (e.g., liver, kidney, brain) receive the drug more quickly than others (e.g., fat and other tissues with fewer blood vessels).
- Drugs reversibly bind to plasma proteins in the blood, such as albumin and alpha$_1$-acid glycoprotein. Only the unbound drug may cross the endothelium into target tissues. Disease states that affect plasma protein concentrations or two drugs administered simultaneously that both use the same plasma protein can affect total drug distribution.
- *Volume of distribution* (V_D) is an estimation of the volume occupied by the drug:

$$V_D = \frac{D}{C_p},$$

where D is the dose given and C_p is the plasma concentration of the drug. Large hydrophilic molecules tend to have a lower volume of distribution and are typically bound to a plasma protein. Small hydrophobic molecules tend to be unbound and to have a high V_D. Drugs with a high V_D usually distribute in adipose tissue.

Metabolism

- Drug *metabolism* can result in reduced biological effects of a drug, increased excretion, production of toxic metabolites, or metabolization of a prodrug to its active form. All tissues contain some ability to metabolize drugs, although drug metabolization primarily occurs in the liver and gastrointestinal epithelium.

Excretion

- *Excretion* is the elimination of the drug from the body. Excretion can occur through various routes such as renal, fecal, biliary, sweat, saliva, tears, and breast milk. Only a small portion of the drug is excreted into breast milk, although this should be considered when the drug is administered to a nursing mother.

Pharmacodynamics

Pharmacodynamics is typically defined as "what the drug does to the body."

Dissociation and Inhibition Constants (Kd/Ki)

- *Kd* refers to the equilibrium dissociation constant and denotes the ligand concentration at which receptor binding is at 50% capacity (Kd = [(L)(R)])/[LR], where L, R, and LR represent the free concentration of ligand, receptor, and ligand-receptor complex, respectively), independent of receptor concentration within the body. Having a ligand tightly bound to the receptor means that dissociation is unlikely ([LR] > [(L)(R)]), and thus the Kd value is small.
- Pharmacologically, the *Ki* is similar to the Kd but is specifically related to the *inhibitory* effect of a drug on a receptor (i.e., the concentration of the drug required to inhibit the activity of the receptor by 50%).
- As with the Kd, the Ki value is inversely proportional to the drug's inhibitory effect on the receptor; thus, the smaller the value, the greater the effect of the drug (i.e., only a small amount of the drug is required to lower the effect of receptor activity). In terms of antipsychotics, which inhibit the activity of endogenous ligands on various receptors (including dopaminergic receptors), the affinity is expressed as Ki. For example, assuming similar concentrations in the body, if an antipsychotic has a Ki of 0.7 nanomolar for the D_2 receptor, while the endogenous dopamine ligand has a Kd of 8 nanomolar for the same receptor, then the antipsychotic would bind more tightly to the receptor and block the activity of the endogenous dopamine, thus preventing its intrinsic activation of those dopaminergic receptors.

Drug Formulations

Oral Route

- Formulations taken orally—abbreviated as PO (from the Latin *per os*, meaning "by mouth")—are familiar to patients, are easily administered, and are often the most economical option.

Tablet

- Tablets are usually the most common and frequently least expensive formulations that patients will take. Amongst all formulations, tablets are usually the most readily splittable, often into halves, and sometimes into quarters. Tablets may have different coatings, such as enteric-coated tablets that target absorption of the medication in the intestine. Notably, orally disintegrating tablets (ODTs) are often indicated based on patient factors. ODTs may benefit patients with dysphagia, which is a symptomatic feature of some neurodegenerative disorders with associated psychiatric and behavioral disturbance. ODTs may also be useful in cases where patients are "cheeking" medications, a common occurrence on inpatient psychiatric units where involuntary medication compliance is required, or where adherence could become unclear.

Capsule

- Capsules are commonly prescribed because of their familiarity, ease of administration, and range of dosing as well as the frequent availability of both immediate-release and extended-release formulations. Because the capsule shields the medication it contains from the acidic stomach, it usually delays release to the intestine. Capsules generally can be opened by patients and the contents mixed in food, which may or may not be desirable, and may possibly affect pharmacokinetics. Sprinkle formulations are a specific subset of capsules—pellet-like contents are held in the capsule before the capsule is opened and the sprinkles deposited in and mixed with soft food. Sprinkle capsules are useful in dysphagia or pill aversion, and frequently are used to deliver stimulant medications to children—and can be the best way to deliver controlled-release formulations.

Liquid Suspension

- As with ODT formulations, liquid suspensions may provide a viable alternative for patients with dysphagia, impaired swallowing, pill aversion, or unclear adherence during medication administration. A liquid suspensions is sometimes cheaper than an ODT, and several formulations of liquid suspensions are commonly used in pediatric medicine.

Controlled Release

- Controlled-release formulations have diverse nomenclatures and mechanisms; for example, "extended release," "long acting," and "controlled release"—abbreviated as "ER" or "XR," "LA," and "CR," respectively). Given that the rate of absorption is partly related to the ability of a tablet, capsule, or liquid suspension to release medication during transit through the alimentary tract, different formulations have been developed that prolong this process and result in a more uniform distribution of the drug over time, with benefits on patient pill burden, shorter titration to effective dosing, minimization of adverse effects, and continuation of treatment effects overnight.

Sublingual Route

- While sublingual (often abbreviated "SL") medications do enter the oral cavity and could be swallowed, their intended site of absorption is the oral mucosa, whose venous drainage bypasses the portal circulation and enters straight into the superior vena cava. The sublingual route of administration is important for certain drugs that are susceptible to rapid first-pass metabolism in the liver. SL formulations often have a quicker onset of action than oral formulations, leading to clinician adoption in acute behavioral management and possibly avoiding more invasive intramuscular medication administration. Sublingual formulations may be available as films or tablets, such as some treatments for opioid use disorder.

Intramuscular Route

- Intramuscular administration is frequently associated with acute behavioral management in emergency department and inpatient settings. This is because of the rapidity of absorption through aqueous channels in the endothelium and the difficulty involved in self-administration.

Long-Acting Injectables

- In patients requiring long-term antipsychotic therapy, intramuscular administration of long-acting antipsychotics (both first generation and second generation) can provide medication release over a period ranging from weeks to months, depending on the agent. Long-acting injectables (LAIs) potentially offer improvement in medication adherence and may decrease the risk of inpatient admission. Initiation of LAIs may often require an "oral bridge" in some cases to cover the lag time until drug levels reach the therapeutic range.

Intravenous Route

- The intravenous route of administration is most frequently used in medical psychiatry, often in acute care settings (e.g., administration of IV haloperidol to a hospitalized patient who is experiencing delirium).

Transdermal Route

- Transdermal administration is advantageous for its ease of use, continuous and uniform rate of absorption over time, and avoidance of first-pass metabolism. There is inherent lag time to reach therapeutic levels, meaning that this route of administration is often inappropriate for acute needs. Consideration should also be given to intentional or unintentional drug discontinuation through patch removal.

Intranasal Route

- Intranasal medication formulations are an emerging area of development in psychopharmacology, with direct drug delivery to the CNS, bypassing the blood-brain barrier. An example is intranasal esketamine, which is FDA-approved for treatment-resistant major depressive disorder (MDD), as well as for depressive symptoms in adults with MDD with acute suicidal ideation or behavior.

Drug Precautions and Monitoring

Electrocardiogram and QTc Interval Monitoring

- Many psychiatric medications can cause prolongation of the corrected QT (QTc) interval. Such medications should be used carefully in the context of polypharmacy or personal or familial history of arrhythmia or cardiac risk factors.

Laboratory Monitoring for Adverse Effects

- Drug toxicity may produce detectable changes in diverse systems such as hematologic abnormalities, thyroid function, electrolyte disturbances, and metabolic disease. Monitoring may be indicated both prior to initiation and at regular intervals during maintenance therapy.

Therapeutic Drug-Level Monitoring

- Therapeutic drug monitoring (TDM) of medication blood levels is most commonly used with the antipsychotic clozapine, as well as the mood stabilizers valproate and lithium, both because such levels are important to guide further treatment and because these medications have a narrow therapeutic index. Levels may also be an indicator of patient adherence. TDM considerations are outlined in relation to specific drugs throughout this Handbook.

Screening for Drugs of Abuse

- Before prescribing a medication, providers might consider screening patients for objective evidence of substance use, an inexpensive and noninvasive test when performed on a urine sample, particularly if the patient will be receiving medications with abuse potential, such as stimulants or benzodiazepines. Careful history taking—including obtaining medical records, prescription drug monitoring program (PDMP) records, and collateral information—may be considered as well on a case-by-case basis.

Regulatory Considerations

- It is important to be aware of provider-specific prescribing privileges, often in the context of medication-assisted treatment for substance use disorders, or for clozapine, an antipsychotic regulated by the FDA's Risk Evaluation and Mitigation Strategy (REMS) program in the United States. Training or registration with regulatory bodies may be required to dispense restricted medications. Clinicians should be mindful of local and national prescribing regulations.

PART II
Medication Classes

2

Antidepressants

Calley Johnston, M.D.
Muniza Majoka, M.B.B.S.
Matthew Macaluso, D.O.
Samuel Wilkinson, M.D.

Antidepressants are among the most ubiquitous drugs prescribed today. Antidepressants are further divided into selective serotonin reuptake inhibitors (SSRIs), serotonin-norepinephrine reuptake inhibitors (SNRIs), tricyclic antidepressants (TCAs), monoamine oxidase inhibitors (MAOIs), and "atypical" antidepressants. Besides treating depression, this class of medications is used to treat a broad range of conditions, some on-label and many off-label. This includes anxiety disorders, eating disorders, chronic pelvic pain syndrome, ADHD, smoking cessation, and vasomotor symptoms associated with menopause. The "unintended" effects of antidepressants are sometimes used therapeutically, such as treating premature ejaculation ("side effect" becomes therapeutic effect).

This chapter aims to inform the reader of key facts related to common antidepressants. The chapter also provides a high-yield, yet nuanced, understanding of individual antidepressant drugs. By synthesizing each medication's mechanism of action, intended as well as unintended effects, and unique properties, clinicians can use their judgment and training to tailor pharmacological treatment plans to the unique needs of each patient.

Selective Serotonin Reuptake Inhibitors

- Of the antidepressant class, selective serotonin reuptake inhibitors (SSRIs) are commonly used. This is because SSRIs have a relatively lower risk of severe side effects. Because of this, SSRIs are often the first antidepressants selected in clinical practice. While all SSRIs involve the primary mechanism of blocking serotonin reuptake in the brain, each drug varies in the degree to which it acts on serotonin receptors and other receptors (e.g., norepinephrine, anticholinergic, histaminergic), side-effect profile, pharmacokinetics, and drug interactions. Their indications are far ranging, and go beyond major depressive disorder.

SSRI Class Warnings and Precautions

SSRI Class Warnings and Precautions

Boxed Warning: Suicidality and Antidepressant Drugs:* Potential increased risk of suicidal thoughts/behaviors in pediatric/young adult patients. Monitor closely for emergence of suicidal thoughts.
SSRI Class Effects: Gastrointestinal changes, sexual dysfunction, emotional blunting/apathy, weight gain/loss, bruxism, hyperhidrosis, increased sweating, hyponatremia/syndrome of inappropriate antidiuretic hormone secretion (SIADH), increased bleeding, serotonin syndrome, QTc prolongation, manic switch, bone fractures, acute angle-closure glaucoma.
Discontinuation Syndrome: May include nausea, sweating, headache, dysphoria, anxiety, irritability, insomnia, sensory disturbances.
**Note.* This warning on suicidality met with controversy. For a detailed discussion, the reader is referred to comprehensive sources in the literature (e.g., Fergusson et al. 2005).

References

Fergusson D, Doucette S, Glass KC, et al: Association between suicide attempts and selective serotonin reuptake inhibitors: systematic review of randomised controlled trials. BMJ 330(7488):396, 2005 15718539

Citalopram

I. **Brand Names**: Celexa
II. **Therapeutic Class**: Selective serotonin reuptake inhibitor (SSRI) antidepressant
III. **Mechanism-Based Class**: Serotonin reuptake inhibitor (SRI)
IV. **Mechanism(s) of Action**

A. CNS inhibition of the SERT (serotonin transporter), blocking reuptake and increasing synaptic serotonin (5-hydroxytryptamine [5-HT]) in several brain areas.

1. Ki=1.6 nM for SERT (Owens et al. 2001)

B. Weak inhibition at the histamine-1 receptor: Ki=283 nM (Owens et al. 2001)
C. Citalopram is a racemic mixture of *S*-citalopram and *R*-citalopram; escitalopram is the *S*-enantiomer alone.

V. **Indications**

A. FDA adult:

1. Major depressive disorder (MDD)
2. *Note*: Citalopram was released to the market with relatively little patent life remaining. As a result, it is often said that the manufacturer did relatively fewer studies, which is why citalopram has fewer FDA-approved indications than most other SSRIs, despite the fact that randomized controlled trials (RCTs) can be found in the literature of citalopram for indications other than MDD.

B. Evidence-based[1] off-label uses:

1. Generalized anxiety disorder
2. OCD
3. Panic disorder
4. PTSD
5. Premenstrual dysphoric disorder (PMDD)
6. Social anxiety disorder
7. Binge-eating disorder
8. Premature ejaculation
9. Vasomotor symptoms associated with menopause
10. Aggressive or agitated behavior associated with dementia

C. FDA pediatric: None

VI. **Major Contraindications and When to Use Caution**

A. Known allergy to citalopram or its components
B. Concomitant use of MAOI antidepressants or other MAO-inhibiting agents (e.g., linezolid, IV methylene blue): A 2-week washout is typically required.
C. Not recommended for patients with congenital long-QTc syndrome, bradycardia, hypokalemia, hypomagnesemia, recent myocardial infarction, or uncompensated congestive heart failure. Avoid use with other QTc-prolonging agents unless benefit outweighs risk.

---

[1]Evidence strength varies; readers are referred to the literature for more detailed information.

VII. Dosage Formulations

A. Brand tablet (10 mg, 20 mg [*scored*], 40 mg [*scored*])
B. Generic tablet (10 mg, 20 mg, 40 mg)
C. Generic capsule (30 mg)
D. Generic solution (10 mg/5 mL)

VIII. Dosage Ranges and Guidelines

A. Refer to Table 2–1 for dosage ranges (initial/maximum) and guidelines.
B. Start at 20 mg/day and increase by 10–20 mg/day every 1–2 weeks (FDA-approved maximum dosage is 40 mg/day). Benefits may be evident after 1–2 weeks, but it may take up to 6–8 weeks to reach the full effect at a given dosage.
C. Prior to the FDA warnings about potential QTc prolongation, citalopram dosages higher than 40 mg/day were commonly used.
D. Individuals who are sensitive to SSRIs could be started at dosages as low as 10 mg/day or even 5 mg/day, with the dosage increased slowly over time based on response and tolerability.
E. Maximum dosage of 20 mg/day for patients older than 60 years, for patients with hepatic impairment, and for individuals who are poor metabolizers of cytochrome P450 (CYP) 2C19 or who are taking CYP2C19 inhibitors.

Table 2–1. Citalopram indications and dosage ranges

Indications	Usual dosage range
MDD	20–40 mg/day
OCD, PTSD, binge-eating disorder, premature ejaculation (off-label)	20–40 mg/day
Generalized anxiety disorder, panic disorder, social anxiety disorder, vasomotor symptoms in menopause (off-label)	10–40 mg/day
PMDD (off-label)	10–40 mg/day (continuous dosing) 10–40 mg/day (luteal phase dosing)
Aggressive or agitated behavior associated with dementia (off-label)	10–30 mg/day (maximum of 20 mg/day if older than 60 years)

Note. For all off-label uses (generalized anxiety disorder, OCD, panic disorder, PTSD, PMDD, social anxiety disorder, binge-eating disorder, premature ejaculation, vasomotor symptoms associated with menopause, aggressive/agitated behavior associated with dementia), a general guideline for dosing is to start at 10–20 mg/day and gradually advance to 40 mg/day over time.

IX. Monitoring

A. Baseline and periodic serum potassium and magnesium for patients at increased risk of electrolyte disturbances
B. Periodic ECG monitoring in patients who have cardiac conditions (see "Major Contraindications") or who take other QTc-prolonging drugs.

X. Relevant Pharmacokinetics/Pharmacodynamics

A. **Metabolism**: Hepatic
B. **Time to peak plasma concentration**: ~4 hours (range: 1–6 hours)
C. **Half-life**: 24–48 hours (doubled in hepatic impairment and increased by 30%–50% in elderly individuals)
D. **Hepatic impairment**: Maximum dosage of 20 mg/day for hepatically impaired patients.
E. **Renal impairment**: If CrCl <20 mL/minute, start at 10 mg/day and gradually increase dosage, with close monitoring for adverse effects, including QTc prolongation. No dosage adjustment needed if CrCl ≥20 mL/minute.

XI. Clinically Relevant Drug Interactions

A. Metabolized by CYP2C19 (major), CYP3A4 (minor).

1. Use caution with CYP2C19 inhibitors, which can increase levels of citalopram and lead to greater risk of QTc prolongation (maximum dosage 20 mg/day in CYP2C19 inhibitors).

B. Mild CYP2D6 inhibitor
C. Could have pharmacodynamic interactions with other serotonergic drugs.

XII. Adverse Effects

A. **See "SSRI Class Warnings and Precautions" in introduction to SSRIs.**
B. **Most common**:

1. Gastrointestinal: Mainly nausea and dry mouth. Should improve; may need to take with food.
2. Somnolence: Related to higher antihistaminic effect
3. QTc prolongation: Dosage dependent, higher risk compared with escitalopram and other SSRIs. Average increase of 7.8 ms (10–20 mg/day) to 10.3 ms (30–40 mg/day) (Beach et al. 2018). Use caution with patients who are CYP2C19 poor metabolizers or who are taking CYP2C19 inhibitors, patients with other risk factors for QTc prolongation, and patients taking other medications that prolong the QTc. Risk factors include older age, structural heart disease, history of torsades de pointes, congenital long QT, electrolyte disturbances, and use of other QT-prolonging agents.
4. Sexual dysfunction: Decreased libido, anorgasmia, ejaculatory delay, erectile dysfunction. SSRI-induced sexual dysfunction may occur in up to 50% of patients taking these medications and is often dosage dependent.
5. Apathy, emotional numbness: Potentially related to 5-HT-mediated depletion of prefrontal dopamine (particularly via 5-HT_{2C}); may be dosage dependent, exact rates are unclear (Barnhart et al. 2004; De Deurwaerdère and Di Giovanni 2017).

C. **Other notable side effects**:

1. Diaphoresis
2. Rare: Priapism and decreased penile sensation

D. **Risks in pregnancy and lactation**: Citalopram was designated a Category C drug in the prior FDA classification and is present in breast milk. A thorough risk/benefit discussion with the patient is recommended on continuing versus stopping the medication, including consultation with an OB/GYN specialist and/or lactation expert. See Chapter 15 ("Women: Pregnancy, Postpartum, and Breastfeeding") for more information.

XIII. **Clinical Pearls/Prescribing Tips**

A. If possible, avoid use of citalopram in patients with risk factors for QTc prolongation (see "Major Contraindications").

B. Limit citalopram dosage to a maximum of 20 mg/day for patients older than 60 years, patients with hepatic impairment, and patients who are CYP2C19 poor metabolizers or who are also taking CYP2C19 inhibitors.

C. Citalopram may be less efficacious than escitalopram (Azorin et al. 2004; Owens et al. 2001).

D. Citalopram may be more cost-effective than escitalopram for some patients, although both medications are relatively inexpensive at present.

E. Citalopram is more sedating than many other SSRIs because of its relatively higher antihistamine effects.

Further Reading

Allergan USA: Celexa [package insert]. U.S. Food and Drug Administration website. Revised February 2022. Available at: https://www.accessdata.fda.gov/drugsatfda_docs/label/2022/020822s041lbl.pdf. Accessed June 21, 2024.

Roth BL, Driscoll J: PDSP Ki Database. Psychoactive Drug Screening Program (PDSP). University of North Carolina at Chapel Hill and the United States National Institute of Mental Health, 1999–present. Available at: https://pdsp.unc.edu/databases/pdsp.php. Accessed June 21, 2024.

References

Azorin JM, Llorca PM, Despiegel N, et al: Escitalopram is more effective than citalopram for the treatment of severe major depressive disorder [in French]. Encephale 30(2):158–166, 2004 15107719

Barnhart WJ, Makela EH, Latocha MJ: SSRI-induced apathy syndrome: a clinical review. J Psychiatr Pract 10(3):196–199, 2004 15330228

Beach SR, Celano CM, Sugrue AM, et al: QT prolongation, torsades de pointes, and psychotropic medications: a 5-year update. Psychosomatics 59(2):105–122, 2018 29275963

De Deurwaerdère P, Di Giovanni G: Serotonergic modulation of the activity of mesencephalic dopaminergic systems: therapeutic implications. Prog Neurobiol 151:175–236, 2017 27013075

Owens MJ, Knight DL, Nemeroff CB: Second-generation SSRIs: human monoamine transporter binding profile of escitalopram and R-fluoxetine. Biol Psychiatry 50(5):345–350, 2001 11543737

Escitalopram

I. **Brand Names**: Lexapro

II. **Therapeutic Class**: Selective serotonin reuptake inhibitor (SSRI) antidepressant

III. **Mechanism-Based Class**: Serotonin reuptake inhibitor (SRI)

IV. **Mechanism(s) of Action**

A. CNS inhibition of SERT (serotonin transporter), blocking reuptake and increasing synaptic serotonin (5-HT) in several brain areas.

1. Potent SERT blockade: Ki=0.8–1.1 nM (Owens et al. 2001)

B. Active *S*-isomer of the racemic mixture (citalopram)

V. **Indications**

A. FDA adult:

1. Major depressive disorder (MDD)
2. Generalized anxiety disorder (GAD)

B. Evidence-based[1] off-label uses:

1. OCD
2. Panic disorder
3. PTSD
4. Premenstrual dysphoric disorder (PMDD)
5. Binge-eating disorder
6. Body dysmorphic disorder
7. Bulimia nervosa
8. Premature ejaculation
9. Vasomotor symptoms associated with menopause

C. FDA pediatric: MDD (age 12–17 years)

VI. **Major Contraindications and When to Use Caution**

A. Known allergy to escitalopram or its components

B. Concomitant use of MAOI antidepressants or other MAO-inhibiting agents (e.g., linezolid, IV methylene blue)—A 2-week washout is typically required.

C. Concomitant use of pimozide

VII. **Dosage Formulations**

A. Brand tablet (5 mg, 10 mg [*scored*], 20 mg [*scored*])

B. Generic tablet (5 mg, 10 mg, 20 mg)

C. Generic solution (5 mg/5 mL)

VIII. **Dosage Ranges and Guidelines**

A. Refer to Table 2–2 for dosage ranges (initial/maximum) and guidelines.

B. Start at 10 mg/day and if needed, increase by 5–10 mg every 1–2 weeks to a maximum dosage of 20 mg/day.

---

[1]Evidence strength varies; readers are referred to the literature for more detailed information.

C. Individuals who are sensitive to SSRIs could be started at dosages as low as 5 mg/day or even 2.5 mg/day, with the dosage increased slowly over time based on response and tolerability.
D. Benefits may be evident after 1–2 weeks, but it may take up to 6–8 weeks to reach the full effect at a given dosage.
E. Start at a lower dosage (5 mg/day) for elderly patients. Some sources recommend a maximum dosage of 10 mg/day for this population (U.S. Department of Veterans Affairs/Department of Defense 2016).

Table 2–2. Escitalopram indications and dosage ranges

Indication	Usual dosage range
Major depressive disorder	Adult: 10–20 mg/day Adolescent: 10–20 mg/day
Generalized anxiety disorder	10–20 mg/day
OCD	10–40 mg/day*
Panic disorder	10–20 mg/day
PTSD	10–40 mg/day*
Premenstrual dysphoric disorder	5–20 mg/day (continuous) 5–20 mg/day (luteal phase)
Binge-eating disorder	10–30 mg/day*
Body dysmorphic disorder	10–60 mg/day*
Bulimia nervosa	10–30 mg/day*
Premature ejaculation	10–20 mg/day
Vasomotor symptoms associated with menopause	10–20 mg/day

*Dosages higher than 20 mg/day have been shown to be of benefit for the following conditions: OCD (Rabinowitz et al. 2008), PTSD (Qi et al. 2017), binge-eating disorder (Guerdjikova et al. 2008), body dysmorphic disorder (Phillips et al. 2016), and bulimia nervosa (Mitchell and Wonderlich 2014), but side effects may increase. Some sources recommend obtaining an electrocardiogram after every 10-mg increase in dosage past 30 mg/day, which is higher than the FDA maximum dosage (Phillips et al. 2016).

IX. **Monitoring**

A. Consider ECG monitoring in patients with risk factors for QTc prolongation, especially at higher dosages of escitalopram.

X. **Relevant Pharmacokinetics/Pharmacodynamics**

A. **Metabolism**: Hepatic
B. **Time to peak plasma concentration**: 5 hours for adults, 2.9 hours for adolescents
C. **Half-life**: 27–32 hours for adults, 19 hours for adolescents (doubled in hepatic impairment and increased by 50% in elderly individuals)
D. **Hepatic impairment**: Maximum dosage of 10 mg/day for most hepatically impaired patients
E. **Renal impairment**: No dosage adjustment necessary (not significantly dialyzed).

XI. **Clinically Relevant Drug Interactions**

A. No major interactions
B. Mild cytochrome P450 (CYP) 2D6 inhibitor
C. Metabolized by CYP2C19 (major), CYP3A4 (minor)
D. Escitalopram could have pharmacodynamic interactions with other serotonergic drugs.

XII. **Adverse Effects**

A. **See "SSRI Class Warnings and Precautions" in introduction to SSRIs.**
B. **Most common**:
  1. Gastrointestinal: Mainly nausea (15% with escitalopram vs. 7% with placebo) and diarrhea (8% with escitalopram vs. 5% with placebo). Symptoms may improve over time; may need to take dose with food (Allergan USA 2021).
  2. Insomnia/sedation: Insomnia (9% with escitalopram vs. 4% with placebo) or somnolence (6% with escitalopram vs. 2% with placebo) (Allergan USA 2021)
  3. Sexual dysfunction: Decreased libido, anorgasmia, ejaculatory delay, erectile dysfunction. SSRI-induced sexual dysfunction may occur in up to 50% of patients taking these medications and is often dosage dependent.
  4. Apathy, emotional numbness: Potentially related to 5-HT-mediated depletion of prefrontal dopamine (particularly via 5-HT_{2C}); may be dosage dependent; exact rates are unclear (Barnhart et al. 2004; De Deurwaerdère and Di Giovanni 2017).
  5. QTc prolongation (dosage dependent): Lower risk with escitalopram than with citalopram/TCAs (Beach et al. 2014; Hasnain et al. 2013); risk factors include older age, structural heart disease, history of torsades de pointes, congenital long QTc, electrolyte disturbances, and use of other QTc-prolonging agents.

C. **Other notable side effects**:
  1. Dry mouth, dizziness, sweating, headache
  2. Rare: Priapism and decreased penile sensation

D. **Risks in pregnancy and lactation**: Escitalopram was designated a Category C drug in the prior FDA classification and is present in breast milk. A thorough risk/benefit discussion with the patient is recommended on continuing versus stopping the medication, including consultation with an OB/GYN specialist and/or a lactation expert. See Chapter 15 ("Women: Pregnancy, Postpartum, and Breastfeeding") for more information.

XIII. **Clinical Pearls/Prescribing Tips**

A. Escitalopram is the therapeutically active *S*-enantiomer of citalopram and has been shown to be more efficacious than citalopram in various studies (Azorin et al. 2004). One study demonstrated that escitalopram's potency at the SERT receptor was 30 times greater than that of citalopram (Owens et al. 2001).
B. Escitalopram demonstrates a more selective SERT blockade compared with other SSRIs and has no other major receptor targets.
C. No major drug (pharmacokinetic) interactions occur with escitalopram.

Further Reading

Fava M: Weight gain and antidepressants. J Clin Psychiatry 61(Suppl 11):37–41, 2000 10926053

Roth BL, Driscoll J: PDSP Ki Database. Psychoactive Drug Screening Program (PDSP). University of North Carolina at Chapel Hill and the United States National Institute of Mental Health, 1999–present. Available at: https://pdsp.unc.edu/databases/pdsp.php. Accessed June 21, 2024.

References

Allergan USA: Lexapro (escitalopram) [package insert]. U.S. Food and Drug Administration website. Revised September 2021. Available at: https://www.accessdata.fda.gov/drugsatfda_docs/label/2021/021365s038,021323s053lbl.pdf. Accessed March 13, 2024.

Azorin JM, Llorca PM, Despiegel N, et al: Escitalopram is more effective than citalopram for the treatment of severe major depressive disorder [in French]. Encephale 30(2):158–166, 2004 15107719

Barnhart WJ, Makela EH, Latocha MJ: SSRI-induced apathy syndrome: a clinical review. J Psychiatr Pract 10(3):196–199, 2004 15330228

Beach SR, Kostis WJ, Celano CM, et al: Meta-analysis of selective serotonin reuptake inhibitor-associated QTc prolongation. J Clin Psychiatry 75(5):e441–e449, 2014 24922496

De Deurwaerdère P, Di Giovanni G: Serotonergic modulation of the activity of mesencephalic dopaminergic systems: therapeutic implications. Prog Neurobiol 151:175–236, 2017 27013075

Guerdjikova AI, McElroy SL, Kotwal R, et al: High-dose escitalopram in the treatment of binge-eating disorder with obesity: a placebo-controlled monotherapy trial. Hum Psychopharmacol 23(1):1–11, 2008 18058852

Hasnain M, Howland RH, Vieweg WV: Escitalopram and QTc prolongation. J Psychiatry Neurosci 38(4):E11, 2013 23791140

Mitchell JE, Wonderlich SA: Feeding and eating disorders, in The American Psychiatric Publishing Textbook of Psychiatry, 6th Edition. Edited by Hales RE, Yudofsky SC, Roberts LW. Washington, DC, American Psychiatric Publishing, 2014, pp 557–586

Owens MJ, Knight DL, Nemeroff CB: Second-generation SSRIs: human monoamine transporter binding profile of escitalopram and R-fluoxetine. Biol Psychiatry 50(5):345–350, 2001 11543737

Phillips KA, Keshaviah A, Dougherty DD, et al: Pharmacotherapy relapse prevention in body dysmorphic disorder: a double-blind, placebo-controlled trial. Am J Psychiatry 173(9):887–895, 2016 27056606

Qi W, Gevonden M, Shalev A: Efficacy and tolerability of high-dose escitalopram in posttraumatic stress disorder. J Clin Psychopharmacol 37(1):89–93, 2017 27977469

Rabinowitz I, Baruch Y, Barak Y: High-dose escitalopram for the treatment of obsessive-compulsive disorder. Int Clin Psychopharmacol 23(1):49–53, 2008 18090508

U.S. Department of Veterans Affairs/Department of Defense: VA/DoD Clinical Practice Guideline for the Management of Major Depressive Disorder. Updated April 2016. https://www.healthquality.va.gov/guidelines/MH/mdd/VADoDMDDCPGFINAL82916.pdf. Accessed May 2022.

Fluoxetine

I. **Brand Names**: Prozac, Prozac Weekly, Symbyax (combination product with olanzapine; also known as olanzapine-fluoxetine combination [OFC]), Sarafem

II. **Therapeutic Class**: Selective serotonin reuptake inhibitor (SSRI) antidepressant

III. **Mechanism-Based Class**: Serotonin reuptake inhibitor (SRI)

IV. **Mechanism(s) of Action**

A. CNS inhibition of SERT (serotonin transporter), blocking reuptake and increasing synaptic serotonin (5-HT) in several brain areas

1. Ki = 1.4 nM for SERT (Owens et al. 2001)
2. SERT is ~80% blocked at dosages of 10–20 mg/day (Sørensen et al. 2022), and higher dosages are effective in blocking 5-HT_{2C}, theoretically increasing dopamine and norepinephrine.

B. 5-HT_{2C} receptor inhibition: 5-HT_{2C} receptor blockade has been shown to increase dopamine and norepinephrine in the prefrontal cortex (Bymaster et al. 2002), demonstrating anxiolytic and antidepressant effects (Demireva et al. 2020). 5-HT_{2C} receptor blockade also has benefits in sleep and sexual function and may increase appetite (Millan 2005).

V. **Indications**

A. FDA adult:

1. Major depressive disorder (MDD)
2. OCD
3. Bulimia nervosa
4. Panic disorder
5. Bipolar I depression (Symbyax *with olanzapine*)
6. Treatment-resistant depression (Symbyax *with olanzapine*)

B. Evidence-based[1] off-label uses:

1. Generalized anxiety disorder
2. PTSD
3. Premenstrual dysphoric disorder
4. Social anxiety disorder
5. Premature ejaculation
6. Body dysmorphic disorder
7. Binge-eating disorder
8. Fibromyalgia

C. FDA pediatric:

1. MDD (age 8–18 years)
2. OCD (age 7–17 years)
3. Bipolar I depression (Symbyax *with olanzapine*) (age 10–17 years)

---

[1]Evidence strength varies; readers are referred to the literature for more detailed information.

VI. **Major Contraindications and When to Use Caution**

A. Known allergy to fluoxetine or its components
B. Concomitant use of MAOI antidepressants or other MAO-inhibiting agents (e.g., linezolid, IV methylene blue)—A 2-week washout is typically required.
C. Concomitant use of pimozide or thioridazine

VII. **Dosage Formulations**

A. Brand capsule (10 mg, 20 mg, 40 mg)
B. Generic capsule (10 mg, 20 mg, 40 mg)
C. Generic tablet (10 mg, 20 mg, 60 mg—*all scored*)
D. Generic delayed-release (DR) capsule (90 mg)
E. Generic solution (20 mg/5 mL)

VIII. **Dosage Ranges and Guidelines**

A. Refer to Table 2–3 for dosage ranges (initial/maximum) and guidelines.
B. Start at 10–20 mg/day and increase dosage every 1–2 weeks by 10–20 mg to a maximum dosage of 80 mg/day. Because of the long half-life, changes in dosage may not be fully reflected in plasma levels for several weeks.
C. Benefits may be evident after 1–2 weeks, but it may take up to 6–8 weeks to reach the full effect at a given dosage.

Table 2–3. Fluoxetine indications and dosage ranges

Indication	Usual dosage range
Bipolar I depression (in combination with olanzapine) (OFC; Symbyax[a])	Adult: 20 mg (+5 mg olanzapine) to 50 mg (+12 mg olanzapine) Child: 20 mg (+5 mg olanzapine) to 50 mg (+12 mg olanzapine)
Bulimia nervosa	20–60 mg/day[b]
Major depressive disorder	Adult: 20–80 mg/day Child (age ≤12 years): 10–20 mg/day, up to a maximum of 40 mg/day Adolescent (age >12 years): 10–20 mg/day, up to a maximum of 60–80 mg/day
OCD	Adult: 20–80 mg/day[c] Child: 10–60 mg/day
Panic disorder	10–60 mg/day
Treatment-resistant depression (OFC; Symbyax*)	20 mg (+5 mg olanzapine) to 50 mg (+20 mg olanzapine)
Binge-eating disorder (off-label)	20–80 mg/day
Body dysmorphic disorder (off-label)	20–80 mg/day
Fibromyalgia (off-label)	20–80 mg/day
Generalized anxiety disorder (off-label)	10–80 mg/day

Table 2–3. Fluoxetine indications and dosage ranges *(continued)*

Indication	Usual dosage range
Premature ejaculation (off-label)	10–40 mg/day
Premenstrual dysphoric disorder (off-label)	10–30 mg/day (continuous) 10–30 mg/day (luteal phase)
PTSD (off-label)	10–80 mg/day
Social anxiety disorder (off-label)	10–60 mg/day

[a]See Table 2–4 for approximate dosage correspondence between Symbyax and the combination of olanzapine and fluoxetine.
[b]Bulimia nervosa: Effective dosage is 60 mg/day per clinical trials, but higher dosages (e.g., 60–80 mg/day) may provide further benefit (Fluoxetine Bulimia Nervosa Collaborative Study Group 1992). Higher dosages may also be required for binge-eating disorder.
[c]OCD: Higher dosages, potentially up to 120 mg/day, have shown superior benefit compared with lower dosages (Bloch et al. 2010; Koran et al. 2007).

Table 2–4. Approximate dosage correspondence between Symbyax* and the combination of Prozac and olanzapine

	Use in combination (mg/day)	
For Symbyax (mg/day)	Olanzapine	Fluoxetine
3 mg olanzapine/25 mg fluoxetine	2.5	20
6 mg olanzapine/25 mg fluoxetine	5	20
12 mg olanzapine/25 mg fluoxetine	10 + 2.5	20
6 mg olanzapine/50 mg fluoxetine	5	40 + 10
12 mg olanzapine/50 mg fluoxetine	10 + 2.5	40 + 10

*Symbyax (olanzapine/fluoxetine hydrochloride) is a fixed-dosage combination of Prozac and olanzapine.
Source. Table 1 in Eli Lilly 2021.

IX. Monitoring

A. Not applicable

X. Relevant Pharmacokinetics/Pharmacodynamics

A. **Metabolism**: Hepatic
B. **Time to peak plasma concentration**: 6–8 hours
C. **Half-life**: 1–3 days for parent drug (4–6 if long-term use), 4–16 days for metabolite (norfluoxetine)
D. **Hepatic impairment**: Reduce dosage by 50% and use less frequent dosing intervals in patients with cirrhosis/chronic liver disease.
E. **Renal impairment**: No dosage adjustment necessary (not significantly dialyzed).

XI. Clinically Relevant Drug Interactions

A. Inhibitor of cytochrome P450 (CYP) 2D6, increasing blood levels of many commonly used medications (e.g., beta-blockers, TCAs, antidepressants, antipsychotics).

   1. Inhibition of CYP2D6 also affects conversion from prodrug to active drug for many medications, including tamoxifen and many opioids (codeine, hydrocodone, tramadol).

B. Mild CYP2C19 inhibitor

C. Metabolized by CYP1A2 (minor), CYP2B6 (minor), CYP2C19 (minor), CYP2C9 (minor), CYP2D6 (minor), CYP2E1 (minor), CYP3A4 (minor)

D. Fluoxetine could have pharmacodynamic interactions with other serotonergic drugs.

XII. Adverse Effects

A. **See "SSRI Class Warnings and Precautions" in introduction to SSRIs.**

B. **Most common**:

   1. Insomnia/anxiety/nervousness/irritability: Anxiety (6%–15% on drug vs. 2%–9% on placebo [Eli Lilly 2021]), potentially due to 5-HT_{2C} inhibition, increasing dopamine and norepinephrine. Daytime dosing is preferred.
   2. Gastrointestinal: Nausea (12%–29% on drug vs. 7%–13% on placebo), diarrhea, dyspepsia, increased gastric acid secretion (this should improve; dose may need to be taken with food [Eli Lilly 2021]).
   3. Sexual dysfunction: Decreased libido, anorgasmia, ejaculatory delay, erectile dysfunction. SSRI-induced sexual dysfunction may occur in up to 50% of patients taking these medications and is often dosage dependent.
   4. Apathy, emotional numbness: Potentially related to 5-HT-mediated depletion of prefrontal dopamine (particularly via 5-HT_{2C}); may be dosage dependent; exact rates are unclear (Barnhart et al. 2004; De Deurwaerdère and Di Giovanni 2017).

C. **Other notable side effects**:

   1. Anorexia/weight loss, asthenia, somnolence, dizziness, abnormal dreams
   2. Rare: Priapism and decreased penile sensation
   3. Relatively low risk of weight gain compared with other antidepressants (Uguz et al. 2015; White et al. 2013)

D. **Risks in pregnancy and lactation**:

   1. Fluoxetine was designated a Category C drug in the prior FDA classification and is present in breast milk. A thorough risk/benefit discussion with the patient is recommended on continuing versus stopping the medication, including consultation with an OB/GYN specialist and/or lactation expert. See Chapter 15 ("Women: Pregnancy, Postpartum, and Breastfeeding") for more information.
   2. Relative infant exposure in breastfeeding is higher for fluoxetine than for most other SSRIs (up to 12% [Chad et al. 2013]). Given fluoxetine's long half-life, levels may also be higher in utero (Chad et al. 2013).

XIII. **Clinical Pearls/Prescribing Tips**

A. Fluoxetine's dopaminergic/noradrenergic effects with 5-HT_{2C} inhibition make it unique among the SSRIs and could contribute to its antidepressant properties, but could also worsen anxiety/insomnia. Daytime dosing is recommended.

B. Fluoxetine is the only agent that has received FDA approval for use in treating bulimia nervosa. Dosages higher than those used for depression may be needed for the best response.

C. For OCD, fluoxetine dosages higher than 80 mg/day may have superior benefit.

D. Because of its long half-life, fluoxetine carries a lower risk of discontinuation syndrome compared with other SSRIs. Consider fluoxetine for patients who are likely to skip doses. A once-weekly formulation is also available (Prozac Weekly).

E. Another result of fluoxetine's long half-life is a longer washout period required (~5 weeks) prior to switching to an MAOI. Fluoxetine's long half-life should also be kept in mind when considering a switch to other antidepressants.

F. Be aware of CYP2D6 inhibition when combining with other medications.

Further Reading

Drugs and Lactation Database (LactMed) [Internet]: Fluoxetine. Bethesda, MD, National Library of Medicine (US), 2006–. Last Revision: August 15, 2023. Available at: https://www.ncbi.nlm.nih.gov/books/NBK501186/. Accessed June 21, 2024.

Fava M: Weight gain and antidepressants. J Clin Psychiatry 61(Suppl 11):37–41, 2000 10926053

Ni YG, Miledi R: Blockage of 5HT2C serotonin receptors by fluoxetine (Prozac). Proc Natl Acad Sci USA 94(5):2036–2040, 1997 9050900

Roth BL, Driscoll J: PDSP Ki Database. Psychoactive Drug Screening Program (PDSP). University of North Carolina at Chapel Hill and the United States National Institute of Mental Health, 1999–present. Available at: https://pdsp.unc.edu/databases/pdsp.php. Accessed June 21, 2024.

References

Barnhart WJ, Makela EH, Latocha MJ: SSRI-induced apathy syndrome: a clinical review. J Psychiatr Pract 10(3):196–199, 2004 15330228

Bloch MH, McGuire J, Landeros-Weisenberger A, et al: Meta-analysis of the dose-response relationship of SSRI in obsessive-compulsive disorder. Mol Psychiatry 15(8):850–855, 2010 19468281

Bymaster FP, Zhang W, Carter PA, et al: Fluoxetine, but not other selective serotonin uptake inhibitors, increases norepinephrine and dopamine extracellular levels in prefrontal cortex. Psychopharmacology (Berl) 160(4):353–361, 2002 11919662

Chad L, Pupco A, Bozzo P, et al: Update on antidepressant use during breastfeeding. Can Fam Physician 59(6):633–634, 2013 23766044

De Deurwaerdère P, Di Giovanni G: Serotonergic modulation of the activity of mesencephalic dopaminergic systems: therapeutic implications. Prog Neurobiol 151:175–236, 2017 27013075

Demireva EY, Suri D, Morelli E, et al: 5-HT2C receptor blockade reverses SSRI-associated basal ganglia dysfunction and potentiates therapeutic efficacy. Mol Psychiatry 25(12):3304–3321, 2020 30120415

Eli Lilly. Prozac (fluoxetine) [package insert]. U.S. Food and Drug Administration website. Revised October 2021. Available at: https://www.accessdata.fda.gov/drugsatfda_docs/label/2021/018936s111lbl.pdf. Accessed March 13, 2024.

Fluoxetine Bulimia Nervosa Collaborative Study Group: Fluoxetine in the treatment of bulimia nervosa: a multicenter, placebo-controlled, double-blind trial. Arch Gen Psychiatry 49(2):139–147, 1992 1550466

Koran LM, Hanna GL, Hollander E, et al; American Psychiatric Association: Practice guideline for the treatment of patients with obsessive-compulsive disorder. Am J Psychiatry 164(7)(Suppl):5–53, 2007 17849776

Millan MJ: Serotonin 5-HT2C receptors as a target for the treatment of depressive and anxious states: focus on novel therapeutic strategies. Therapie 60(5):441–460, 2005 16433010

Owens MJ, Knight DL, Nemeroff CB: Second-generation SSRIs: human monoamine transporter binding profile of escitalopram and R-fluoxetine. Biol Psychiatry 50(5):345–350, 2001 11543737

Sørensen A, Ruhé HG, Munkholm K: The relationship between dose and serotonin transporter occupancy of antidepressants—a systematic review. Mol Psychiatry 27(1):192–201, 2022 34548628

Uguz F, Sahingoz M, Gungor B, et al: Weight gain and associated factors in patients using newer antidepressant drugs. Gen Hosp Psychiatry 37(1):46–48, 2015 25467076

White W, Elmore L, Luthin DR, et al: Psychotropic-induced weight gain: a review of management strategies. Consultant 53(3):153–160, 2013

Fluvoxamine

I. **Brand Names**: Luvox, Luvox CR

II. **Therapeutic Class**: Selective serotonin reuptake inhibitor (SSRI) antidepressant

III. **Mechanism-Based Class**: Serotonin reuptake inhibitor (SRI)

IV. **Mechanism(s) of Action**

A. CNS inhibition of the SERT (serotonin transporter), blocking reuptake and increasing synaptic serotonin (5-HT) in several brain areas.

1. Ki=2.5 nM for SERT (Yahata et al. 2017)

B. Sigma-1 (σ_1) receptor agonism (Ki=36 nM): Potential anti-anxiety, antidepressant, antipsychotic, anti-obsessive, and procognitive effects (Hindmarch and Hashimoto 2010).

V. **Indications**

A. FDA adult:

1. OCD

B. Evidence-based[1] off-label uses:

1. Major depressive disorder (MDD)
2. Generalized anxiety disorder
3. Panic disorder

---

[1]Evidence strength varies; readers are referred to the literature for more detailed information.

4. Social anxiety disorder
5. PTSD
6. Bulimia nervosa

C. FDA pediatric: OCD (age 8–17 years)

VI. **Major Contraindications and When to Use Caution**

A. Known allergy to fluvoxamine or its components

B. Concomitant use of MAOI antidepressants or other MAO-inhibiting agents (e.g., linezolid, IV methylene blue)—A 2-week washout is typically required.

C. Concomitant use of pimozide, tizanidine, thioridazine, alosetron

VII. **Dosage Formulations**

A. Brand tablet (25 mg, 50 mg [*scored*], 100 mg [*scored*])

B. Brand extended-release (CR) capsule (100 mg, 150 mg)

C. Generic immediate-release (IR) tablet (25 mg, 50 mg [*scored*], 100 mg [*scored*])

D. Generic CR capsule (100 mg, 150 mg)

VIII. **Dosage Ranges and Guidelines**

A. Refer to Table 2–5 for dosage ranges (initial/maximum) and guidelines.

B. Adults: Start at 50 mg/day IR (100 mg/day CR) and increase by 50 mg every week to a maximum dosage of 300 mg/day. For IR forms, dosages higher than 100 mg/day should be divided.

C. Children/adolescents: Start at 25 mg/day IR at bedtime and increase by 25 mg every week to a maximum dosage of 200 mg/day (age 8–11 years) or 300 mg/day (age 12–17 years). Dosages higher than 50 mg/day should be divided.

D. May use IR tablet to determine a stable daily dosage, and then convert to once-daily CR formulation at the same total daily dosage.

E. Benefits may be evident after 1–2 weeks, but it may take up to 6–8 weeks to reach full effect at a given dosage.

Table 2–5. Fluvoxamine indications and dosage ranges

Indication	Usual dosage range
Obsessive-compulsive disorder	IR: 50–300 mg/day (start at 25 mg/day for children) CR: 100–300 mg/day
Major depressive disorder	IR: 50–300 mg/day
Generalized anxiety disorder	IR: 50–300 mg/day
Panic disorder	IR: 25–200 mg/day
Social anxiety disorder	IR: 50–300 mg/day CR: 100–300 mg/day
Posttraumatic stress disorder	IR: 75 mg BID
Bulimia nervosa	IR: 50–300 mg/day

IX. **Monitoring**

A. If used concomitantly with warfarin, monitor prothrombin time (PT)/international normalized ratio (INR).

X. **Relevant Pharmacokinetics/Pharmacodynamics**

A. **Metabolism**: Hepatic

B. **Time to peak plasma concentration**: 3–8 hours

C. **Half-life**: 14–16 hours (17–26 hours in elderly individuals)

D. **Hepatic impairment**: Use lower initial dosage and titrate slowly. Consider a maximum dosage of 150 mg/day for patients with moderate to severe impairment.

E. **Renal impairment**: No dosage adjustment necessary.

XI. **Clinically Relevant Drug Interactions**

A. Inhibitor of cytochrome P450 (CYP) 1A2

1. Increases levels of medications that utilize hepatic oxidation, including some benzodiazepines (i.e., alprazolam, diazepam), clozapine, olanzapine, duloxetine, methadone, mexiletine, ramelteon, and theophylline.
2. Warfarin may increase plasma concentrations by 98% and prolong PT/INR. Monitor PT if coadministered.

B. Weak inhibitor of CYP2C19, CYP2C9, CYP2D6, CYP3A4

1. May increase levels of carbamazepine, sumatriptan, tacrine, TCAs, tryptophan, diltiazem, beta-blockers.

C. Metabolized by CYP1A2 (minor) and CYP2D6 (minor).

1. Tobacco smoke (a CYP1A2 inducer) has been shown to reduce the serum concentration of fluvoxamine (Oliveira et al. 2017).

D. Fluvoxamine could have pharmacodynamic interactions with other serotonergic drugs.

XII. **Adverse Effects**

A. **See "SSRI Class Warnings and Precautions" in introduction to SSRIs.**

B. **Most common**:

1. Gastrointestinal: Notably nausea (34%–40% [ANI Pharmaceuticals 2021]), diarrhea, dry mouth, anorexia; symptoms should improve; may need to take dose with food.
2. Insomnia/drowsiness: Can lead to either insomnia or somnolence.
3. Sexual dysfunction: Decreased libido, anorgasmia, ejaculatory delay, erectile dysfunction. SSRI-induced sexual dysfunction may occur in up to 50% of patients taking these medications and is often dosage dependent.
4. Apathy, emotional numbness: Potentially related to 5-HT-mediated depletion of prefrontal dopamine (particularly via 5-HT_{2C}); may be dosage dependent; exact rates unclear (Barnhart et al. 2004; De Deurwaerdère and Di Giovanni 2017).

C. **Other notable side effects**:

1. Weakness, dizziness, sweating, headache, nervousness/agitation
2. Rare: Priapism and decreased penile sensation

D. **Risks in pregnancy and lactation**: Fluvoxamine was designated a Category C drug in the prior FDA classification and is present in breast milk. A thorough risk/benefit discussion with the patient is recommended on continuing versus stopping the medication, including consultation with an OB/GYN specialist and/or lactation expert. See Chapter 15 ("Women: Pregnancy, Postpartum, and Breastfeeding") for more information.

XIII. **Clinical Pearls/Prescribing Tips**

A. In addition to SERT blockade, fluvoxamine is a potent sigma-1 (σ_1) receptor agonist, potentially increasing antidepressant, anti-anxiety, procognitive, and even antipsychotic benefits. Furthermore, σ_1 receptor agonism may lead to a more rapid antidepressant/ant-anxiety effect compared with other SSRIs.

B. Nausea is the most common adverse effect, likely mediated by excessive serotonin agonism at the 5-HT_3 receptor. Tolerance should develop due to the downregulation of the 5-HT_3 receptor.

C. Fluvoxamine has numerous drug interactions. Before prescribing, use a formal interaction checker.

References

ANI Pharmaceuticals: Luvox [package insert]. U.S. Food and Drug Administration website. Revised July 2021. Available at: https://www.accessdata.fda.gov/drugsatfda_docs/label/2021/021519s018lbl.pdf. Accessed March 13, 2024.

Barnhart WJ, Makela EH, Latocha MJ: SSRI-induced apathy syndrome: a clinical review. J Psychiatr Pract 10(3):196–199, 2004 15330228

De Deurwaerdère P, Di Giovanni G: Serotonergic modulation of the activity of mesencephalic dopaminergic systems: therapeutic implications. Prog Neurobiol 151:175–236, 2017 27013075

Hindmarch I, Hashimoto K: Cognition and depression: the effects of fluvoxamine, a sigma-1 receptor agonist, reconsidered. Hum Psychopharmacol 25(3):193–200, 2010 20373470

Oliveira P, Ribeiro J, Donato H, et al: Smoking and antidepressants pharmacokinetics: a systematic review. Ann Gen Psychiatry 16:17, 2017 28286537

Yahata M, Chiba K, Watanabe T, et al: Possibility of predicting serotonin transporter occupancy from the in vitro inhibition constant for serotonin transporter, the clinically relevant plasma concentration of unbound drugs, and their profiles for substrates of transporters. J Pharm Sci 106(9):2345–2356, 2017 28501470

Paroxetine

I. **Brand Names**: Paxil, Paxil CR, Brisdelle (vasomotor), Pexeva

II. **Therapeutic Class**: Selective serotonin reuptake inhibitor (SSRI) antidepressant

III. **Mechanism-Based Class**: Serotonin-reuptake inhibitor (SRI)

IV. **Mechanism(s) of Action**—*Note*: Ki data obtained from PDSP Ki Database (Roth and Driscoll 1999–present).

A. CNS inhibition of the SERT (serotonin transporter), blocking reuptake and increasing synaptic serotonin (5-HT) in several brain areas

1. Very potent SERT inhibition: Ki=0.07–0.2 nM
2. A dosage of 20 mg/day given to rats occupied 88% of the SERT in the prefrontal cortex (Sanchez et al. 2014).

B. Weak CNS inhibition of the NET (norepinephrine transporter): Ki=40–85 nM

C. Inhibition of M_1 receptor (muscarinic acetylcholine [anticholinergic effects]): Ki=72 nM

D. Very weak CNS inhibition of the DAT (dopamine transporter): Ki=490 nM

V. **Indications**

A. FDA adult:

1. Major depressive disorder
2. OCD
3. Panic disorder
4. Social anxiety disorder
5. Generalized anxiety disorder
6. PTSD
7. Vasomotor symptoms of menopause—*Brisdelle*
8. Premenstrual dysphoric disorder (PMDD)—*Paxil controlled-release [CR] only*

B. Evidence-based[1] off-label uses:

1. Body dysmorphic disorder
2. Premature ejaculation

C. FDA pediatric: None

VI. **Major Contraindications and When to Use Caution**

A. Known allergy to paroxetine or its components

B. Concomitant use of MAOI antidepressants or other MAO-inhibiting agents (e.g., linezolid, IV methylene blue)—A 2-week washout is typically required.

C. Concomitant use of pimozide, thioridazine

VII. **Dosage Formulations**

A. Brand:

1. Paxil tablet (10 mg [*scored*], 20 mg [*scored*], 30 mg, 40 mg)

---

[1]Evidence strength varies; readers are referred to the literature for more detailed information.

2. Paxil CR tablet (12.5 mg, 25 mg, 37.5 mg)
    a. Do not cut CR tablet in half; cutting damages the controlled-release properties.
3. Brisdelle capsule (7.5 mg)
4. Pexeva tab (10 mg, 20 mg, 30 mg, 40 mg)
5. Oral suspension (10 mg/5 mL) (250 mL bottle)

B. Generic:
1. Capsule (7.5 mg)
2. Tablet (10 mg, 20 mg, 30 mg, 40 mg)
3. Paroxetine extended-release (ER) tab (*equivalent to Paxil CR*) (12.5 mg, 25 mg, 37.5 mg)
4. Oral suspension (10 mg/5 mL) (250 mL bottle)

VIII. **Dosage Ranges and Guidelines**

A. Refer to Table 2–6 for dosage ranges (initial/maximum) and guidelines.
B. Immediate-release (IR): Start at a dosage of 10–20 mg/day and increase in increments of 10 mg every 1–2 weeks. In sensitive individuals, a starting dosage as low as 5 mg/day may be necessary.
C. ER/CR: Start at a dosage of 12.5 mg/day and increase in increments of 12.5 mg every 1–2 weeks.
D. Benefits may be evident after 1–2 weeks, but it may take up to 6–8 weeks to reach full effect at a given dosage.
E. Do not break CR tablet in half. Cutting or splitting the CR formulation damages its controlled-release properties.
F. Consider using a lower starting dosage in elderly patients.
G. Dosing guidelines for pediatric use are not listed in the package insert. Caution and additional monitoring are recommended when paroxetine is used in pediatric patients.

Table 2–6. Paroxetine indications and dosage ranges

Indication	Usual dosage range
Major depressive disorder	IR: 20–50 mg/day CR/ER: 25.0–62.5 mg/day
Obsessive-compulsive disorder	IR: 20–60 mg/day
Panic disorder	IR: 10–60 mg/day CR/ER: 12.5–75.0 mg/day
Posttraumatic stress disorder	IR: 20–50 mg/day
Social anxiety disorder	IR: 10–60 mg/day CR/ER: 12.5–37.5 mg/day
Generalized anxiety disorder	IR: 10–50 mg/day

Table 2–6. Paroxetine indications and dosage ranges *(continued)*

Indication	Usual dosage range
Premenstrual dysphoric disorder (FDA approval for CR only)	Continuous dosing: IR: 10–40 mg/day CR/ER: 12.5–50.0 mg/day Luteal-phase dosing: IR: 10–30 mg/day CR/ER: 12.5–37.5 mg/day
Vasomotor symptoms of menopause (Brisdelle is FDA approved)	Brisdelle cap: 7.5 mg every night at bedtime Paroxetine tab: IR: 10–20 mg every night at bedtime ER 12.5–25.0 mg every night at bedtime
Body dysmorphic disorder (off-label)	20–60 mg/day (up to 100 mg/day)
Premature ejaculation (off-label)	10–40 mg/day

IX. Monitoring

A. Consider obtaining weight at baseline and monitoring periodically throughout treatment

X. Relevant Pharmacokinetics/Pharmacodynamics

A. **Metabolism**: Hepatic
B. **Time to peak plasma concentration**: 6–10 hours
C. **Half-life**:

1. Regular release: 21 hours; controlled release: 15–20 hours; Pexeva: 33.2 hours
2. The CR tablet contains a degradable polymeric matrix (GeoMatrix), which provides a more gradual release of active drug over a period of 4–5 hours, bypassing the stomach and leading to fewer gastrointestinal effects.

D. **Hepatic impairment**: Start at 10 mg/day; maximum dosage 40 mg/day
E. **Renal impairment**: Start at 10 mg/day; maximum dosage 40 mg/day

XI. Clinically Relevant Drug Interactions

A. Major inhibitor of cytochrome P450 (CYP) 2D6, increasing blood levels of many commonly used medications (e.g., beta-blockers, TCAs, other antidepressants, antipsychotics)

1. Inhibition of CYP2D6 also affects conversion from prodrug to active drug for many medications, including tamoxifen and many opioids (e.g., codeine, hydrocodone, tramadol).

B. Metabolized by CYP2D6 (major) and CYP3A4 (minor)
C. Paroxetine could have pharmacodynamic interactions with other serotonergic drugs.

XII. **Adverse Effects**

A. **See "SSRI Class Warnings and Precautions" in introduction to SSRIs.**

B. **Most common**:

1. Gastrointestinal: Nausea, constipation, diarrhea, decreased appetite
   a. Paroxetine CR may be the preferred choice for avoiding gastrointestinal side effects, particularly nausea (the CR formulation delivers active drug over a period of 4–5 hours, bypassing the stomach).
2. Sexual dysfunction: Shown to be more severe compared with other SSRIs (Jing and Straw-Wilson 2016). Includes decreased libido, anorgasmia, ejaculatory delay, erectile dysfunction. SSRI-induced sexual dysfunction may occur in up to 50% of patients taking these medications and is often dosage dependent.
3. Somnolence/sedation: More common with paroxetine than with other SSRIs; can dose at nighttime.
4. Anticholinergic effects: Constipation, dry mouth, urinary hesitancy, confusion
   a. Use caution in older adult patients, given the higher cognitive/delirium risk in this population.
5. Discontinuation syndrome: More pronounced with paroxetine than with other SSRIs because of paroxetine's short half-life (Tonks 2002). Taper slowly.
6. Apathy, emotional numbness: Potentially related to 5-HT-mediated depletion of prefrontal dopamine (particularly via 5-HT_{2C}). This effect may be dosage dependent, and exact rates are unclear (Barnhart et al. 2004; De Deurwaerdère and Di Giovanni 2017).
7. Weight gain may be more common with paroxetine than with other SSRIs (Fava 2000).

C. **Other notable side effects**:

1. Asthenia (weakness), dizziness, insomnia, sweating, tremor, paresthesias (pins/needles)
2. Rare: Priapism and decreased penile sensation

D. **Risks in pregnancy and lactation**: Category D per prior FDA classification and present in breast milk. Generally not recommended during pregnancy given the risks of pulmonary hypertension of the newborn and increased risk of cardiac defects. A thorough risk/benefit discussion with the patient is recommended on continuing versus stopping the medication, including consultation with an OB/GYN specialist and/or lactation expert. See Chapter 15 ("Women: Pregnancy, Postpartum, and Breastfeeding") for more information.

XIII. **Clinical Pearls/Prescribing Tips**

A. Paroxetine may be more calming/sedating compared with other SSRIs, and thus could be a more favorable choice for some patients with anxiety/insomnia.

B. Paroxetine's NET blockade (particularly at dosages above 30–40 mg/day) may confer additional antidepressant effects.

C. Notable side effects of paroxetine include sexual dysfunction (likely due to potent SERT binding), anticholinergic effects (avoid/use caution in older adults), and weight gain.
D. Use of paroxetine is not recommended in women of childbearing age, given its pregnancy risks (although paroxetine appears safer in breastfeeding because of its low relative infant dose). Consider consultation with an OB/GYN specialist and/or lactation expert.
E. Because of its controlled-release properties, the CR formulation may be beneficial for nausea.
F. Paroxetine should be tapered slowly because of its short half-life and high risk of discontinuation symptoms.
G. Be aware of CYP2D6 inhibition when combining paroxetine with other medications; check for drug interactions.

Further Reading

Chad L, Pupco A, Bozzo P, et al: Update on antidepressant use during breastfeeding. Can Fam Physician 59(6):633–634, 2013 23766044

Gilmor ML, Owens MJ, Nemeroff CB: Inhibition of norepinephrine uptake in patients with major depression treated with paroxetine. Am J Psychiatry 159(10):1702–1710, 2002 12359676

Paxil [package insert]. U.S. Food and Drug Administration website. Revised September 2021. Available at: https://www.accessdata.fda.gov/drugsatfda_docs/label/2021/020031s079,020710s047lbl.pdf#page=39. Accessed March 13, 2024.

References

Barnhart WJ, Makela EH, Latocha MJ: SSRI-induced apathy syndrome: a clinical review. J Psychiatr Pract 10(3):196–199, 2004 15330228

De Deurwaerdère P, Di Giovanni G: Serotonergic modulation of the activity of mesencephalic dopaminergic systems: therapeutic implications. Prog Neurobiol 151:175–236, 2017 27013075

Fava M: Weight gain and antidepressants. J Clin Psychiatry 61(Suppl 11):37–41, 2000 10926053

Jing E, Straw-Wilson K: Sexual dysfunction in selective serotonin reuptake inhibitors (SSRIs) and potential solutions: a narrative literature review. Ment Health Clin 6(4):191–196, 2016 29955469

Roth BL, Driscoll J: PDSP Ki Database. Psychoactive Drug Screening Program (PDSP). University of North Carolina at Chapel Hill and the United States National Institute of Mental Health, 1999–present. Available at: https://pdsp.unc.edu/databases/pdsp.php. Accessed June 21, 2024.

Sanchez C, Reines EH, Montgomery SA: A comparative review of escitalopram, paroxetine, and sertraline: are they all alike? Int Clin Psychopharmacol 29(4):185–196, 2014 24424469

Tonks A: Withdrawal from paroxetine can be severe, warns FDA. BMJ 324(7332):260, 2002 11823353

Sertraline

I. **Brand Names**: Zoloft, Lustral

II. **Therapeutic Class**: Selective serotonin reuptake inhibitor (SSRI) antidepressant

III. **Mechanism-Based Class**: Serotonin reuptake inhibitor (SRI)

IV. **Mechanism(s) of Action**—*Note*: Ki data obtained from PDSP Ki Database (Roth and Driscoll 1999–present).

A. CNS inhibition of the SERT (serotonin transporter), blocking reuptake and increasing synaptic serotonin (5-HT) in several brain areas.

1. At dosages of 200 mg/day, 95% blockade of the SERT (Ki=0.5–3.3 nM)

B. Weak CNS inhibition of the DAT (dopamine transporter)—Ki=22–300 nM. Exact clinical relevance is unclear, although it could partially explain sertraline's activating properties.

C. Very weak CNS inhibition of the NET (norepinephrine transporter)—Ki=400–900 nM. Exact clinical relevance is unclear.

V. **Indications**

A. FDA adult:

1. Major depressive disorder (MDD)
2. PTSD
3. Premenstrual dysphoric disorder (PMDD)
4. Panic disorder
5. OCD
6. Social anxiety disorder

B. Evidence-based[1] off-label uses:

1. Generalized anxiety disorder
2. Binge-eating disorder
3. Body dysmorphic disorder
4. Bulimia nervosa
5. Agitation/irritability in a number of disorders
6. Premature ejaculation

C. FDA pediatric: OCD (age 6–17 years)

VI. **Major Contraindications and When to Use Caution**

A. Known allergy to sertraline or its components

B. Concomitant use of MAOI antidepressants or other MAO-inhibiting agents (e.g., linezolid, IV methylene blue)—A 2-week washout is typically required.

C. Concomitant use of pimozide

D. The oral solution should not be combined with disulfiram (Pfizer 2016).

---

[1]Evidence strength varies; readers are referred to the literature for more detailed information.

VII. **Dosage Formulations**

A. Brand tablet (25 mg, 50 mg, 100 mg [*all scored*])
B. Brand concentrate (20 mg/mL) (60 mL bottle)
C. Generic capsule (150 mg, 200 mg)
D. Generic tablet (25 mg, 50 mg, 100 mg [*all scored*])
E. Generic concentrate (20 mg/mL)

VIII. **Dosage Ranges and Guidelines**

A. Refer to Table 2–7 for dosage ranges (initial/maximum) and guidelines.
B. Start at 25–50 mg/day and increase in increments of 25–50 mg every 1–2 weeks. Benefits may be evident after 1–2 weeks, but it may take up to 6–8 weeks to reach the full effect at a given dosage.
C. For patients who are sensitive to SSRIs, starting dosages as low as 12.5 mg/day could be considered.
D. Consider using lower starting dosages in elderly patients.

Table 2–7. Sertraline indications and dosage ranges

Indication	Usual dosage range
Major depressive disorder	50–200 mg/day
PTSD	25–200 mg/day
Premenstrual dysphoric disorder	50–150 mg/day (continuous) 50–100 mg/day (luteal phase)
Panic disorder	25–200 mg/day
OCD*	50–200 mg/day Pediatric (age 6–12 years): 25–200 mg/day
Social anxiety disorder	25–200 mg/day
Generalized anxiety disorder (off-label)	25–200 mg/day
Binge-eating disorder (off-label)	25–200 mg/day
Body dysmorphic disorder*, bulimia nervosa*, premature ejaculation (off-label)	50–200 mg/day

*Higher dosages (up to 400 mg/day) have been shown to be of benefit for bulimia nervosa, body dysmorphic disorder (Phillips 2017), and OCD (Bloch et al. 2010; Koran et al. 2007).

IX. **Monitoring**

A. Not applicable

X. **Relevant Pharmacokinetics/Pharmacodynamics**

A. **Metabolism**: Hepatic
B. **Time to peak plasma concentration**: 4.5–8.4 hours
C. **Half-life**: ~26 hours

D. **Hepatic impairment**: Reduce usual dosage by 50%; maximum dosage of 100 mg/day in patients with Child-Pugh class A disease. Do not use in patients with Child-Pugh class B or C disease.
E. **Renal impairment**: No dosage adjustment necessary (not dialyzable [Pfizer 2016]).

XI. **Clinically Relevant Drug Interactions**

A. No major drug interactions
B. Mild cytochrome P450 (CYP) 2D6 and CYP3A4 inhibitor at high dosages
C. Primarily metabolized by CYP2B6, but also metabolized by CYP1A2, CYP2C19, CYP2C9, CYP3A4, and CYP2D6.
D. Sertraline can have pharmacodynamic interactions with other serotonergic drugs.

XII. **Adverse Effects**

A. **See "SSRI Class Warnings and Precautions" in introduction to SSRIs.**
B. **Most common**:

1. Gastrointestinal: Nausea (26% on sertraline vs. 12% on placebo), diarrhea/loose stools (20% on sertraline vs. 10% on placebo), dry mouth (14% on sertraline vs. 9% on placebo), possible increased gastric acid secretion (Pfizer 2016). Symptoms should improve over time; medication may need to be taken with food.
2. Insomnia/activation or drowsiness/fatigue: Can potentially be both sedating or activating (somnolence [11% on sertraline vs. 6% on placebo], agitation [8% on sertraline vs. 5% on placebo], insomnia [20% on sertraline vs. 13% on placebo]). Adjust dosing time of day accordingly (Pfizer 2016).
3. Sexual dysfunction: Decreased libido, anorgasmia, ejaculatory delay, erectile dysfunction. SSRI-induced sexual dysfunction may occur in up to 50% of patients taking these medications and is often dosage dependent.
4. Apathy, emotional numbness: Potentially related to 5-HT-mediated depletion of prefrontal dopamine (particularly via 5-HT_{2C}); may be dosage dependent; exact rates are unclear (Barnhart et al. 2004; De Deurwaerdère and Di Giovanni 2017).

C. **Other notable side effects**:

1. Dizziness (12% on drug vs. 8% on placebo), hyperhidrosis (Pfizer 2016)
2. Rare: Priapism and decreased penile sensation
3. Relatively low risk of weight gain

D. **Risks in pregnancy and lactation**: Sertraline is one of the most extensively studied and safest antidepressants for use in pregnancy/breastfeeding (low placental exposure; low relative infant dose in breastfeeding). It was designated a Category C drug in the prior FDA classification and is present in breast milk. A thorough risk/benefit discussion with the patient is recommended on continuing versus stopping the medication, including consultation with an OB/GYN specialist and/or lactation expert. See Chapter 15 ("Women: Pregnancy, Postpartum, and Breastfeeding") for more information.

XIII. **Clinical Pearls/Prescribing Tips**

A. Sertraline's weak dopamine activity (especially at high dosages) may have additional benefits for depression and could contribute to activating effects. Given this potential for activating effects, sertraline may need to be started at lower dosages, especially in anxious patients. Consider daytime dosing if insomnia occurs.

B. Gastrointestinal effects are common but should subside with treatment (start low, go slow).

C. Among antidepressants, sertraline has one of the more favorable safety profiles for use in pregnancy/breastfeeding (see "Risks in pregnancy and lactation" under "Adverse Effects").

D. Sertraline has no significant drug interactions.

E. Sertraline dosages higher than 200 mg have been shown to have additional benefit in certain conditions (namely, OCD).

F. Well studied in post–myocardial infarction patients, with good effect (Glassman et al. 2002).

Further Reading

Chad L, Pupco A, Bozzo P, et al: Update on antidepressant use during breastfeeding. Can Fam Physician 59(6):633–634, 2013 23766044

Fava M: Weight gain and antidepressants. J Clin Psychiatry 61(Suppl 11):37–41, 2000 10926053

Kitaichi Y, Inoue T, Nakagawa S, et al: Sertraline increases extracellular levels not only of serotonin, but also of dopamine in the nucleus accumbens and striatum of rats. Eur J Pharmacol 647(1–3):90–96, 2010 20816814

Padala PR, Padala KP, Majagi AS, et al: Selective serotonin reuptake inhibitors-associated apathy syndrome: a cross sectional study. Medicine 99(33):e21497, 2020 32871995

References

Barnhart WJ, Makela EH, Latocha MJ: SSRI-induced apathy syndrome: a clinical review. J Psychiatr Pract 10(3):196–199, 2004 15330228

Bloch MH, McGuire J, Landeros-Weisenberger A, et al: Meta-analysis of the dose-response relationship of SSRI in obsessive-compulsive disorder. Mol Psychiatry 15(8):850–855, 2010 19468281

De Deurwaerdère P, Di Giovanni G: Serotonergic modulation of the activity of mesencephalic dopaminergic systems: therapeutic implications. Prog Neurobiol 151:175–236, 2017 27013075

Glassman AH, O'Connor CM, Califf RM, et al; Sertraline Antidepressant Heart Attack Randomized Trial (SADHART) Group: Sertraline treatment of major depression in patients with acute MI or unstable angina (correction appears in JAMA 288(14):1720, 2002). JAMA 288(6):701–709, 2002 12169073

Koran LM, Hanna GL, Hollander E, et al; APA: Practice guideline for the treatment of patients with obsessive-compulsive disorder. Am J Psychiatry 164(7)(Suppl):5–53, 2007 17849776

Pfizer. Zoloft (sertraline) [package insert]. U.S. Food and Drug Administration website. Revised December 2016. Available at: https://www.accessdata.fda.gov/drugsatfda_docs/label/2016/019839S74S86S87_20990S35S44S45lbl.pdf.

Phillips KA: Pharmacotherapy and other somatic treatments for body dysmorphic disorder, in Body Dysmorphic Disorder: Advances in Research and Clinical Practice. Edited by Phillips KA. New York, Oxford University Press, 2017, pp 333–356

Vilazodone

I. **Brand Names**: Viibryd
II. **Therapeutic Class**: Serotonin reuptake inhibitor and serotonin receptor modulator
III. **Mechanism-Based Class**: Multimodal serotonin agent
IV. **Mechanism(s) of Action**

A. Vilazodone's reuptake inhibition of the SERT (serotonin transporter) (Ki=0.1 nM) is 30 times more potent than that of fluoxetine (Page et al. 2002; Sahli et al. 2016).
B. 5-HT_{1A} partial agonism (IC_{50}=0.5 nM), much more selective for 5-HT_{1A} than buspirone (Singh and Schwartz 2012), potentially working in conjunction with SERT blockade to augment antidepressant and anxiolytic response and reduce response time to medication (Sahli et al. 2016). May also improve sexual function (Hull et al. 2004; Sukoff Rizzo et al. 2009).
C. Weak reuptake inhibition of the NET (norepinephrine transporter) (Ki=56 nM) and the DAT (dopamine transporter) (Ki=37 nM)

V. **Indications**

A. FDA adult:
  1. MDD
B. Evidence-based[1] off-label uses:
  1. Anxiety disorders
C. FDA pediatric: None

VI. **Major Contraindications and When to Use Caution**

A. Known allergy to vilazodone or its components
B. Concomitant use of MAOI antidepressants or other MAO-inhibiting agents (e.g., linezolid, IV methylene blue)—A 2-week washout is typically required.

VII. **Dosage Formulations**

A. Brand tablet (10 mg, 20 mg, 40 mg *not scored*)
B. Brand dose titration pack (10 mg and 20 mg, or 10 mg, 20 mg, 40 mg)

VIII. **Dosage Ranges and Guidelines**

A. For MDD, start at 10 mg/day (taken with food). After approximately 1 week, increase dosage in increments of 10 mg at weekly intervals to a maximum dosage of 40 mg/day as tolerated.
B. Food increases absorption by about 50%–60% compared with a fasting state. It is recommended that vilazodone be taken with food (at least 150 calories).

IX. **Monitoring**

A. No special monitoring is required, but clinical monitoring is recommended as it would be for any antidepressant and for managing depressed patients in general.

---

[1]Evidence strength varies; readers are referred to the literature for more detailed information.

X. **Relevant Pharmacokinetics/Pharmacodynamics**

A. **Metabolism**: Hepatic

B. **Time to peak plasma concentration**: 4–5 hours (food increases maximum concentration by about 50%–60%)

C. **Half-life**: 25 hours

D. **Use with food**: Vilazodone should be taken with food.

E. **Hepatic impairment**: No dosage adjustment necessary.

F. **Renal impairment**: No dosage adjustment necessary (Allergan 2021).

XI. **Clinically Relevant Drug Interactions**

A. Metabolized by cytochrome P450 (CYP) 3A4 (major), CYP2C19 (minor), CYP2D6 (minor).

1. Maximum dosage of 20 mg/day when used concomitantly with strong CYP3A4 inhibitors (e.g., some antifungals, antibiotics, antivirals, nefazodone) (Allergan 2021).
2. Consider doubling the dosage (up to 80 mg/day) when used concomitantly with strong CYP3A4 inducers (e.g., carbamazepine, St. John's wort) (Allergan 2021).
3. Vilazodone could have pharmacodynamic interactions with other drugs with similar mechanisms of action, including nonpsychiatric drugs that target similar receptors.

XII. **Adverse Effects**

A. **See "SSRI Class Warnings and Precautions" in introduction to SSRIs.**

B. **Most common**:

1. Gastrointestinal: Most notably diarrhea (29% on vilazodone vs. 10% on placebo for 40 mg) and nausea (24% on vilazodone vs. 7% on placebo for 40 mg) (Allergan 2021). The incidence of gastrointestinal effects may be higher with vilazodone than with other antidepressants (Hughes et al. 2017). Start low, go slow, and take with food.

C. **Other notable side effects**:

1. Sexual dysfunction risk appears to be low, potentially due to 5-HT_{1A} agonism (Hull et al. 2004; Sukoff Rizzo et al. 2009).
2. Insomnia (6% on vilazodone vs. 2% on placebo for 40 mg [Allergan 2021]), abnormal dreams (Hughes et al. 2017).
3. Weight gain appears to be minimal (Wang et al. 2013).
4. Vilazodone may have less emotional blunting effects compared with other antidepressants, but it may have a higher incidence of irritability and agitation (Hughes et al. 2017).

D. **Risks in pregnancy and lactation**: Vilazodone was designated a Category C drug in the prior FDA classification and is present in breast milk. A thorough risk/benefit discussion with the patient is recommended on continuing versus stopping the medication, including consultation with an OB/GYN specialist and/or lactation expert. See Chapter 15 ("Women: Pregnancy, Postpartum, and Breastfeeding") for more information.

XIII. **Clinical Pearls/Prescribing Tips**

A. Although head-to-head studies comparing vilazodone with other SSRIs are lacking, clinical trial data indicate that vilazodone is likely to have fewer sexual side effects, minimal weight gain, and a faster onset of action compared with other antidepressants (Wang et al. 2013). However, some clinical trials of vilazodone in depression showed questionable efficacy compared with placebo (Kirsch 2014) and recommended it as a second- or third-line option (Laughren et al. 2011; Stuivenga et al. 2019).

B. Vilazodone's combination of potent SERT blockade and potent 5-HT_{1A} partial agonism makes it analogous to combining an SSRI with buspirone, potentially adding to its anxiolytic and antidepressant effects.

C. Vilazodone should be taken with food. Start with a low dosage and titrate gradually to minimize gastrointestinal side effects.

References

Allergan: Viibryd (vilazodone) [package insert]. U.S. Food and Drug Administration website. Revised July 2021. Available at: https://www.accessdata.fda.gov/drugsatfda_docs/label/2021/022567s022lbl.pdf. Accessed March 13, 2024.

Hughes S, Lacasse J, Fuller RR, et al: Adverse effects and treatment satisfaction among online users of four antidepressants. Psychiatry Res 255:78–86, 2017 28531820

Hull EM, Muschamp JW, Sato S: Dopamine and serotonin: influences on male sexual behavior. Physiol Behav 83(2):291–307, 2004 15488546

Kirsch I: Antidepressants and the placebo effect. Z Psychol 222(3):128–134, 2014 25279271

Laughren TP, Gobburu J, Temple RJ, et al: Vilazodone: clinical basis for the US Food and Drug Administration's approval of a new antidepressant. J Clin Psychiatry 72(9):1166–1173, 2011 21951984

Page ME, Cryan JF, Sullivan A, et al: Behavioral and neurochemical effects of 5-{4-[4-(5-cyano-3-indolyl)-butyl)-butyl]-1-piperazinyl}-benzofuran-2-carboxamide (EMD 68843): a combined selective inhibitor of serotonin reuptake and 5-hydroxytryptamine(1A) receptor partial agonist. J Pharmacol Exp Ther 302(3):1220–1227, 2002 12183683

Sahli ZT, Banerjee P, Tarazi FI: The preclinical and clinical effects of vilazodone for the treatment of major depressive disorder. Expert Opin Drug Discov 11(5):515–523, 2016 26971593

Singh M, Schwartz TL: Clinical utility of vilazodone for the treatment of adults with major depressive disorder and theoretical implications for future clinical use. Neuropsychiatr Dis Treat 8:123–130, 2012 22536068

Stuivenga M, Giltay EJ, Cools O, et al: Evaluation of vilazodone for the treatment of depressive and anxiety disorders. Expert Opin Pharmacother 20(3):251–260, 2019 30475091

Sukoff Rizzo SJ, Pulicicchio C, Malberg JE, et al: 5-HT(1A) receptor antagonism reverses and prevents fluoxetine-induced sexual dysfunction in rats. Int J Neuropsychopharmacol 12(8):1045–1053, 2009 19435548

Wang SM, Han C, Lee SJ, et al: A review of current evidence for vilazodone in major depressive disorder. Int J Psychiatry Clin Pract 17(3):160–169, 2013 23578403

Serotonin-Norepinephrine Reuptake Inhibitors

- Serotonin-norepinephrine reuptake inhibitors (SNRIs) block both norepinephrine and serotonin reuptake. Each SNRI varies in terms of its affinity for blocking serotonin and/or norepinephrine reuptake inhibition, which can inform therapeutic use and predict adverse effects. In addition to treating many of the same disorders as selective serotonin reuptake inhibitors (SSRIs), the SNRIs are often used to treat neuropathic pain and have a favorable side-effect profile compared with tricyclic antidepressants (TCAs).

SNRI Class Warnings and Precautions

SNRI Class Warnings and Precautions

Boxed Warning: Suicidality and Antidepressant Drugs:* Potential increased risk of suicidal thoughts/behaviors in pediatric/young adult patients. Monitor closely for emergence of suicidal thoughts.
SNRI Class Effects: Gastrointestinal changes, sexual dysfunction, emotional blunting/apathy, weight gain/loss, bruxism, hyperhidrosis, increased sweating, hyponatremia/syndrome of inappropriate antidiuretic hormone secretion (SIADH), increased bleeding, serotonin syndrome, QTc prolongation, manic switch, bone fractures, acute angle-closure glaucoma, seizures, blood pressure increases, urinary retention/hesitation, skin reactions.
Discontinuation Syndrome: May include nausea, sweating, headache, dysphoria, anxiety, irritability, insomnia, sensory disturbances.
**Note.* This warning on suicidality met with controversy. For a detailed discussion, the reader is referred to comprehensive sources in the literature (e.g., Fergusson et al. 2005).

References

Fergusson D, Doucette S, Glass KC, et al: Association between suicide attempts and selective serotonin reuptake inhibitors: systematic review of randomised controlled trials. BMJ 330(7488):396, 2005 15718539

Desvenlafaxine

I. **Brand Names**: Pristiq

II. **Therapeutic Class**: Serotonin-norepinephrine reuptake inhibitor (SNRI) antidepressant

III. **Mechanism-Based Class**: Serotonin and norepinephrine reuptake inhibitor

IV. **Mechanism(s) of Action**

A. Desvenlafaxine is the major active metabolite of venlafaxine (*O*-desmethylvenlafaxine [ODV]), a product of metabolism via cytochrome P450 (CYP) 2D6.

B. CNS inhibition of the SERT (serotonin transporter), blocking reuptake and increasing synaptic serotonin (5-HT) in several brain areas.

1. Ki=~42 nM for the SERT (Roth and Driscoll 1999–present)
2. Desvenlafaxine is approximately 10 times more selective for the SERT than for the NET (norepinephrine transporter).

C. CNS inhibition of the NET, blocking reuptake and increasing synaptic norepinephrine in several brain areas

1. Ki=~558 nM for the NET (Roth and Driscoll 1999–present)
2. Inhibition of the NET in the prefrontal cortex has also been shown to boost dopamine levels, as the NET clears both norepinephrine and dopamine (Carboni et al. 1990; Kasper and Pail 2010; Saxon 2007).

V. **Indications**

A. FDA adult: Major depressive disorder

B. Evidence-based[1] off-label uses:

1. Vasomotor symptoms associated with menopause

C. FDA pediatric: None

VI. **Major Contraindications and When to Use Caution**

A. Known allergy to desvenlafaxine or its components

B. Concomitant use of MAOI antidepressants or other MAO-inhibiting agents (e.g., linezolid, IV methylene blue)—A 2-week washout is typically required.

VII. **Dosage Formulations**—*Note*: Do not crush or break ER/XR formulations.

A. Brand XR tablet (25 mg, 50 mg, 100 mg)

B. Generic ER tablet (25 mg, 50 mg, 100 mg)

VIII. **Dosage Ranges and Guidelines**

A. Refer to Table 2–8 for dosage ranges (initial/maximum) and guidelines.

B. Start at 25–50 mg/day and increase by 25–50 mg every 1–2 weeks to a maximum dosage of 50–100 mg/day.

C. Benefits may be evident after 1–2 weeks, but it may take up to 6–8 weeks to reach the full effect at a given dosage.

---

[1]Evidence strength varies; readers are referred to the literature for more detailed information.

Table 2–8. Desvenlafaxine indications and dosage ranges

Indication	Usual dosage range
Major depressive disorder	25–50 mg/day → 100 mg/day (usual maximum 50 mg/day)*
Vasomotor symptoms associated with menopause	25–50 mg/day → 100 mg/day (usual maximum 50 mg/day)*

*Dosages > 50 mg/day may not confer further benefit and may increase the risk of adverse effects (Berhan and Berhan 2014; Lieberman and Massey 2010; Reddy et al. 2010), although some studies show additional benefit with higher dosages up to 400 mg/day (Laoutidis and Kioulos 2015; Septien-Velez et al. 2007).

IX. **Monitoring**

A. Measure blood pressure and heart rate at baseline and monitor periodically throughout treatment, especially with high dosages.

B. Monitor cholesterol, low-density lipoprotein, and triglycerides periodically, given the potential for increases with desvenlafaxine.

X. **Relevant Pharmacokinetics/Pharmacodynamics**

A. **Metabolism**: Hepatic

B. **Time to peak plasma concentration**: ~7.5 hours

C. **Half-life**: 10–11 hours (prolonged with renal/hepatic failure)

D. **Hepatic impairment**: For patients with moderate to severe hepatic impairment (Child-Pugh score of 7–15), recommended dosage is 50 mg/day. Do not increase dosage beyond 100 mg/day for these patients.

E. **Renal impairment**: For patients with moderate renal impairment (CrCl = 30–50 mL/minute), use maximum dosage of 50 mg/day. For those with severe renal impairment or end-stage renal disease (CrCl ≤ 15 mL/minute), use maximum dosage of 25 mg/day or 50 mg every other day.

XI. **Clinically Relevant Drug Interactions**

A. Metabolized mainly via conjugation but also oxidation via CYP3A4 (minor).

B. No major drug interactions

XII. **Adverse Effects**

A. **See "SNRI Class Warnings and Precautions" in introduction to SNRIs.**

B. **Most common**:

1. Gastrointestinal: Notably nausea (35% on desvenlafaxine vs. 8% on placebo for 100 mg/day dosage), constipation, diarrhea, dry mouth, anorexia (Berhan and Berhan 2014; Lieberman and Massey 2010)
2. Sexual dysfunction: Some evidence for lower risk compared with other antidepressants (Montejo et al. 2019). However, it is difficult to predict which patients will experience which adverse effects with which drugs.
3. Discontinuation syndrome may be more common with desvenlafaxine than with other antidepressants, especially when at higher dosages prior to discontinuation (Fava et al. 2018). Taper slowly.

C. **Other notable side effects**:
   1. Headache, insomnia, somnolence, dizziness, mydriasis
   2. Sweating, heart rate increases, blood pressure increases (more likely at higher dosages)
   3. Potential increase in cholesterol and serum triglycerides

D. **Risks in pregnancy and lactation**: Desvenlafaxine was designated a Category C drug in the prior FDA classification and is present in breast milk. A thorough risk/benefit discussion with the patient is recommended on continuing versus stopping the medication, including consultation with an OB/GYN specialist and/or lactation expert. See Chapter 15 ("Women: Pregnancy, Postpartum, and Breastfeeding") for more information.

XIII. **Clinical Pearls/Prescribing Tips**

A. Serotonin and norepinephrine reuptake blockade is more balanced with desvenlafaxine compared with venlafaxine, although desvenlafaxine is still more serotonergic than noradrenergic.

B. In patients who are poor metabolizers of CYP2D6 or who are also taking CYP2D6 inhibitors, desvenlafaxine may be preferred because of its lack of reliance on CYP2D6 for metabolism (Colvard 2014).

C. Use caution with hepatic or renal impairment (see "Relevant Pharmacokinetics/Pharmacodynamics" above for recommended dosage adjustments).

D. Desvenlafaxine may have a lower risk of sexual side effects compared with venlafaxine but may be similar to venlafaxine when it comes to a significant risk of discontinuation syndrome when stopped abruptly.

E. In general, dosages higher than 50 mg/day do not appear to provide superior benefits compared with 50 mg/day. However, some patients may benefit from higher dosages.

Further Reading

Pfizer: Pristiq (desvenlafaxine) [package insert]. U.S. Food and Drug Administration website. Revised November 2021. Available at: https://www.accessdata.fda.gov/drugsatfda_docs/label/2021/021992s047lbl.pdf. Accessed March 13, 2024.

Serretti A, Chiesa A: Treatment-emergent sexual dysfunction related to antidepressants: a meta-analysis. J Clin Psychopharmacol 29(3):259–266, 2009 19440080

References

Berhan Y, Berhan A: Is desvenlafaxine effective and safe in the treatment of menopausal vasomotor symptoms? A meta-analysis and meta-regression of randomized double-blind controlled studies. Ethiop J Health Sci 24(3):209–218, 2014 25183927

Carboni E, Tanda GL, Frau R, et al: Blockade of the noradrenaline carrier increases extracellular dopamine concentrations in the prefrontal cortex: evidence that dopamine is taken up in vivo by noradrenergic terminals. J Neurochem 55(3):1067–1070, 1990 2117046

Colvard M: Key differences between venlafaxine XR and desvenlafaxine: an analysis of pharmacokinetic and clinical data. Ment Health Clin 4(1):35–39, 2014

Fava GA, Benasi G, Lucente M, et al: Withdrawal symptoms after serotonin-noradrenaline reuptake inhibitor discontinuation: systematic review. Psychother Psychosom 87(4):195–203, 2018 30016772

Kasper S, Pail G: Milnacipran: a unique antidepressant? Neuropsychiatr Dis Treat 6(Suppl 1):23–31, 2010 20856597

Laoutidis ZG, Kioulos KT: Desvenlafaxine for the acute treatment of depression: a systematic review and meta-analysis. Pharmacopsychiatry 48(6):187–199, 2015 26205685

Lieberman DZ, Massey SH: Desvenlafaxine in major depressive disorder: an evidence-based review of its place in therapy. Core Evid 4:67–82, 2010

Montejo AL, Becker J, Bueno G, et al: Frequency of sexual dysfunction in patients treated with desvenlafaxine: a prospective naturalistic study. J Clin Med 8(5):719, 2019

Reddy S, Kane C, Pitrosky B, et al: Clinical utility of desvenlafaxine 50 mg/d for treating MDD: a review of two randomized placebo-controlled trials for the practicing physician. Curr Med Res Opin 26(1):139–150, 2010 19919295

Roth BL, Driscoll J: PDSP Ki Database. Psychoactive Drug Screening Program (PDSP). University of North Carolina at Chapel Hill and the United States National Institute of Mental Health, 1999–present. Available at: https://pdsp.unc.edu/databases/pdsp.php. Accessed June 21, 2024.

Saxon AJ: Dopamine and depression. Arch Gen Psychiatry 64(9):1101, 2007 17768279

Septien-Velez L, Pitrosky B, Padmanabhan SK, et al: A randomized, double-blind, placebo-controlled trial of desvenlafaxine succinate in the treatment of major depressive disorder. Int Clin Psychopharmacol 22(6):338–347, 2007 17917552

Duloxetine

I. **Brand Names**: Cymbalta, Drizalma

II. **Therapeutic Class**: Serotonin-norepinephrine reuptake inhibitor (SNRI) antidepressant

III. **Mechanism-Based Class**: Serotonin and norepinephrine reuptake inhibitor

IV. **Mechanism(s) of Action**

A. CNS inhibition of the SERT (serotonin transporter), blocking reuptake and increasing synaptic serotonin (5-HT) in several brain areas

1. Duloxetine is approximately 10 times more selective for the SERT than for the NET (norepinephrine transporter).
2. SERT Ki=~0.8 nM; NET Ki=~7.5 nM (Bymaster et al. 2001)

B. CNS inhibition of the NET, blocking reuptake and increasing synaptic norepinephrine in several brain areas

1. NET occupancy is dosage dependent: 29.7% at 20 mg/day, 30.5% at 40 mg/day, 40% at 60 mg/day (Moriguchi et al. 2017), and 73% at 120 mg/day (Vincent et al. 2004), with higher NET blockade appearing to correlate with certain adverse effects (increased blood pressure, heart rate).
2. Inhibition of the NET in the prefrontal cortex has also been shown to boost dopamine levels, as the NET clears both norepinephrine and dopamine (Carboni et al. 1990; Kasper and Pail 2010; Saxon 2007).

V. **Indications**

A. FDA adult:

1. Major depressive disorder (MDD)
2. Generalized anxiety disorder (GAD)
3. Diabetic peripheral neuropathic pain
4. Fibromyalgia
5. Chronic musculoskeletal pain

B. Evidence-based[1] off-label uses:

1. Chemotherapy-induced peripheral neuropathy
2. Stress urinary incontinence (women and men)

C. FDA pediatric:

1. GAD (age ≥7 years)
2. Fibromyalgia (age ≥13 years)

VI. **Major Contraindications and When to Use Caution**

A. Known allergy to duloxetine or its components
B. Concomitant use of MAOI antidepressants or other MAO-inhibiting agents (e.g., linezolid, IV methylene blue)—A 2-week washout is typically required.

VII. **Dosage Formulations**

A. Brand delayed-release (DR) capsule (20 mg, 30 mg, 60 mg)
B. Brand (Drizalma) DR sprinkle capsule (20 mg, 30 mg, 40 mg, 60 mg)
C. Generic DR capsule (20 mg, 30 mg, 40 mg, 60 mg)

VIII. **Dosage Ranges and Guidelines**

A. Refer to Table 2–9 for dosage ranges (initial/maximum) and guidelines.
B. Start at 30–60 mg/day (depending on indication) and increase by 30 mg every 1–2 weeks to a maximum dosage of 60–120 mg/day.
C. Benefits may be evident after 1–2 weeks, but it may take up to 6–8 weeks to reach the full effect at a given dosage.

Table 2–9. Duloxetine indications and dosage ranges

Indication	Usual dosage range
Major depressive disorder	30–60 mg/day → 120 mg/day
Generalized anxiety disorder	Adults: 60–120 mg/day Children/elderly individuals: 30–60 mg/day
Fibromyalgia	Children and adults: 30–60 mg/day*
Chronic musculoskeletal pain	30–60 mg/day*
Diabetic peripheral neuropathic pain	60 mg/day*

[1]Evidence strength varies; readers are referred to the literature for more detailed information.

Table 2–9. Duloxetine indications and dosage ranges *(continued)*

Indication	Usual dosage range
Chemotherapy-induced peripheral neuropathy (off-label)	30–60 mg/day
Stress urinary incontinence (off-label)	20–40 mg BID

*A Cochrane Review indicated that pain syndromes responded best to dosages of 60–120 mg/day and that lower dosages were not as effective (Lunn et al. 2014). Pain benefit is likely mediated by the inhibition of sensory transmission in nociceptive fibers in the dorsal horn of the spinal cord by serotonin and norepinephrine (Micó et al. 2006). Additionally, duloxetine blocks voltage-gated sodium channels, which may also mediate this effect on pain (Wang et al. 2010).

IX. Monitoring

A. Measure blood pressure and heart rate at baseline and monitor periodically throughout treatment, especially with higher dosages.

B. Monitor liver function at baseline and periodically throughout treatment. Duloxetine is associated with small increases in alanine aminotransferase (ALT), aspartate transaminase (AST), creatine phosphokinase (CPK), and alkaline phosphatase and can in rare cases lead to hepatotoxicity. Avoid use of duloxetine in patients with substantial alcohol use or significant liver dysfunction (Lilly USA 2021).

X. Relevant Pharmacokinetics/Pharmacodynamics

A. **Metabolism**: Hepatic

B. **Time to peak plasma concentration**: 6 hours (2-hour lag until absorption begins; delayed absorption by ~2–4 hours if taken with food)

C. **Half-life**: 12 hours (range: 8–17 hours)

D. **Hepatic impairment**: Avoid use in hepatic impairment (chronic liver disease, cirrhosis).

E. **Renal impairment**: Avoid use in severe renal impairment (GFR <30 mL/minute).

XI. Clinically Relevant Drug Interactions

A. Metabolized by cytochrome P450 (CYP) 2D6 (major), CYP1A2 (major).

1. Decrease dosage if given with CYP2D6 or CYP1A2 inhibitors or in poor metabolizers of CYP2D6.

    a. Common CYP1A2 inhibitors: fluvoxamine, cimetidine, ciprofloxacin, enoxacin

    b. Common CYP2D6 inhibitors: fluoxetine, bupropion, paroxetine

2. Tobacco smoke is a CYP1A2 inducer, so dosages may need to be adjusted with changes in smoking status. Tobacco smoke has been shown to reduce the serum concentration of duloxetine (Oliveira et al. 2017).

B. Moderate inhibitor of CYP2D6

1. Use caution when combined with CYP2D6 substrates, most notably TCAs, beta-blockers, tamoxifen, and some opioids.

C. Duloxetine could have pharmacodynamic interactions with other drugs that have a similar mechanism of action and target the same receptors in the body.

XII. **Adverse Effects**

A. **See "SNRI Class Warnings and Precautions" in introduction to SNRIs.**

B. **Most common**:

1. Gastrointestinal: Notably nausea (23% on duloxetine vs. 8% on placebo), dry mouth, constipation, diarrhea (Lilly USA 2021)
   a. Nausea should largely resolve after week 2 and is significantly less severe in patients who start at the 30 mg/day dosage compared with those starting at the 60 mg/day dosage (Lee et al. 2012).
2. Sexual dysfunction: Decreased risk with duloxetine compared with venlafaxine and SSRIs, is potentially related to a more balanced serotonin and norepinephrine reuptake inhibition (Bitter et al. 2011; Clayton et al. 2007, 2014; Delgado et al. 2005; Dueñas et al. 2011; Nelson et al. 2006; Serretti and Chiesa 2009). However, it is difficult to predict which patients will develop which adverse effects with which medications.
3. Discontinuation syndrome may be relatively common (6%–55%) with duloxetine but appears to be less severe compared with venlafaxine and desvenlafaxine (Fava et al. 2018).

C. **Other notable side effects**:

1. Somnolence, hyperhidrosis, decreased appetite
2. Rare: Urinary retention/hesitation, blood pressure changes

D. **Risks in pregnancy and lactation**: Duloxetine was designated a Category C drug in the prior FDA classification and is present in breast milk. A thorough risk/benefit discussion with the patient is recommended on continuing versus stopping the medication, including consultation with an OB/GYN specialist and/or lactation expert. See Chapter 15 ("Women: Pregnancy, Postpartum, and Breastfeeding") for more information.

XIII. **Clinical Pearls/Prescribing Tips**

A. Duloxetine has notable efficacy in pain syndromes, including fibromyalgia, chronic musculoskeletal pain, and neuropathy, and may even reduce painful symptoms associated with MDD, including overall pain, back and shoulder pain, and time spent in pain while awake (Detke et al. 2002; Goldstein et al. 2002).

B. Use caution or avoid in patients with liver injury or heavy alcohol use. Monitor liver function tests periodically.

C. When prescribing duloxetine, consider the potential risk of drug interactions, including duloxetine's metabolism by CYP1A2 and CYP2D6 and its moderate inhibition of CYP2D6.

D. NET inhibition is dosage dependent, becoming more significant at dosages of 60 mg/day and higher. However, higher dosages also portend a higher risk of blood pressure and heart rate changes.

E. Duloxetine's relative balance of NET and SERT inhibition (1:10) likely mediates its lower risk of sexual side effects compared with SSRIs and venlafaxine.

Further Reading

Roth BL, Driscoll J: PDSP Ki Database. Psychoactive Drug Screening Program (PDSP). University of North Carolina at Chapel Hill and the United States National Institute of Mental Health, 1999–present. Available at: https://pdsp.unc.edu/databases/pdsp.php. Accessed June 21, 2024.

References

Bitter I, Filipovits D, Czobor P: Adverse reactions to duloxetine in depression. Expert Opin Drug Saf 10(6):839–850, 2011 21545241

Bymaster FP, Dreshfield-Ahmad LJ, Threlkeld PG, et al: Comparative affinity of duloxetine and venlafaxine for serotonin and norepinephrine transporters in vitro and in vivo, human serotonin receptor subtypes, and other neuronal receptors. Neuropsychopharmacology 25(6):871–880, 2001 11750180

Carboni E, Tanda GL, Frau R, et al: Blockade of the noradrenaline carrier increases extracellular dopamine concentrations in the prefrontal cortex: evidence that dopamine is taken up in vivo by noradrenergic terminals. J Neurochem 55(3):1067–1070, 1990 2117046

Clayton A, Kornstein S, Prakash A, et al: Changes in sexual functioning associated with duloxetine, escitalopram, and placebo in the treatment of patients with major depressive disorder. J Sex Med 4(4 Pt 1):917–929, 2007 17627739

Clayton AH, El Haddad S, Iluonakhamhe JP, et al: Sexual dysfunction associated with major depressive disorder and antidepressant treatment. Expert Opin Drug Saf 13(10):1361–1374, 2014 25148932

Delgado PL, Brannan SK, Mallinckrodt CH, et al: Sexual functioning assessed in 4 double-blind placebo- and paroxetine-controlled trials of duloxetine for major depressive disorder. J Clin Psychiatry 66(6):686–692, 2005 15960560

Detke MJ, Lu Y, Goldstein DJ, et al: Duloxetine, 60 mg once daily, for major depressive disorder: a randomized double-blind placebo-controlled trial. J Clin Psychiatry 63(4):308–315, 2002 12000204

Dueñas H, Brnabic AJ, Lee A, et al: Treatment-emergent sexual dysfunction with SSRIs and duloxetine: effectiveness and functional outcomes over a 6-month observational period. Int J Psychiatry Clin Pract 15(4):242–254, 2011 22121997

Fava GA, Benasi G, Lucente M, et al: Withdrawal symptoms after serotonin-noradrenaline reuptake inhibitor discontinuation: systematic review. Psychother Psychosom 87(4):195–203, 2018 30016772

Goldstein DJ, Mallinckrodt C, Lu Y, et al: Duloxetine in the treatment of major depressive disorder: a double-blind clinical trial. J Clin Psychiatry 63(3):225–231, 2002 11926722

Kasper S, Pail G: Milnacipran: a unique antidepressant? Neuropsychiatr Dis Treat 6(Suppl 1):23–31, 2010 20856597

Lee MS, Ahn YM, Chung S, et al: The effect of initial duloxetine dosing strategy on nausea in Korean patients with major depressive disorder. Psychiatry Investig 9(4):391–399, 2012 23251205

Lilly USA: Cymbalta (duloxetine) [package insert]. U.S. Food and Drug Administration website. Revised July 2021. Available at: https://www.accessdata.fda.gov/drugsatfda_docs/label/2021/021427s056lbl.pdf. Accessed March 13, 2024.

Lunn MP, Hughes RA, Wiffen PJ: Duloxetine for treating painful neuropathy, chronic pain or fibromyalgia. Cochrane Database Syst Rev (1):CD007115, 2014 24385423

Micó JA, Ardid D, Berrocoso E, et al: Antidepressants and pain. Trends Pharmacol Sci 27(7):348–354, 2006 16762426

Moriguchi S, Takano H, Kimura Y, et al: Occupancy of norepinephrine transporter by duloxetine in human brains measured by positron emission tomography with (S,S)-[18F]FMeNER-D2. Int J Neuropsychopharmacol 20(12):957–962, 2017 29016875

Nelson JC, Lu Pritchett Y, Martynov O, et al: The safety and tolerability of duloxetine compared with paroxetine and placebo: a pooled analysis of 4 clinical trials. Prim Care Companion J Clin Psychiatry 8(4):212–219, 2006 16964316

Oliveira P, Ribeiro J, Donato H, et al: Smoking and antidepressants pharmacokinetics: a systematic review. Ann Gen Psychiatry 16:17, 2017 28286537

Saxon AJ: Dopamine and depression. Arch Gen Psychiatry 64(9):1101, 2007 17768279

Serretti A, Chiesa A: Treatment-emergent sexual dysfunction related to antidepressants: a meta-analysis. J Clin Psychopharmacol 29(3):259–266, 2009 19440080

Vincent S, Bieck PR, Garland EM, et al: Clinical assessment of norepinephrine transporter blockade through biochemical and pharmacological profiles. Circulation 109(25):3202–3207, 2004 15184278

Wang SY, Calderon J, Kuo Wang G: Block of neuronal Na+ channels by antidepressant duloxetine in a state-dependent manner. Anesthesiology 113(3):655–665, 2010 20693878

Levomilnacipran

I. **Brand Names**: Fetzima

II. **Therapeutic Class**: Serotonin-norepinephrine reuptake inhibitor (SNRI) antidepressant

III. **Mechanism-Based Class**: Serotonin and norepinephrine reuptake inhibitor

IV. **Mechanism(s) of Action**

A. Levomilnacipran is the levorotatory enantiomer of milnacipran and is believed to be the more active form.

B. CNS inhibition of the SERT (serotonin transporter), blocking reuptake and increasing synaptic serotonin (5-hydroxytryptamine [5-HT]) in several brain areas.

1. Ki=~11 nM for the SERT (Auclair et al. 2013)

C. CNS inhibition of the NET (norepinephrine transporter), blocking reuptake and increasing synaptic norepinephrine in several brain areas.

1. Ki=~91 nM for the NET (Auclair et al. 2013)
2. Levomilnacipran is approximately 2 times more selective for the NET than for the SERT (Auclair et al. 2013), making it unique among the SNRIs. It demonstrates 17 and 27 times higher selectivity for norepinephrine reuptake inhibition compared with venlafaxine and duloxetine, respectively (Auclair et al. 2013).
3. Inhibition of the NET in the prefrontal cortex has also been shown to boost dopamine levels, as the NET clears both norepinephrine and dopamine (Carboni et al. 1990; Kasper and Pail 2010; Saxon 2007).

V. **Indications**

A. FDA adult: Major depressive disorder

B. Evidence-based[1] off-label uses:

1. Fibromyalgia (based on the efficacy of milnacipran)

C. FDA pediatric: None

---

[1]Evidence strength varies; readers are referred to the literature for more detailed information.

VI. **Major Contraindications and When to Use Caution**

A. Known allergy to levomilnacipran or its components

B. Concomitant use of MAOI antidepressants or other MAO-inhibiting agents (e.g., linezolid, IV methylene blue)—A 2-week washout is typically required.

VII. **Dosage Formulations**

A. Brand ER capsule (20 mg, 40 mg, 80 mg, 120 mg)

B. Brand ER dose titration pack (28 capsules of 20 mg and 40 mg)—*Note*: Do not crush or break ER/XR formulation.

VIII. **Dosage Ranges and Guidelines**

A. Start at 20 mg/day and increase to 40 mg/day after 2 days. Can increase by 40 mg/day thereafter every 2 or more days to a maximum dosage of 120 mg/day.

B. Benefits may be evident after 1–2 weeks, but it may take up to 6–8 weeks to reach full effect at a given dosage.

IX. **Monitoring**

A. Measure blood pressure and heart rate at baseline and monitor periodically throughout treatment, especially with high dosages.

B. Monitor liver function at baseline and periodically throughout treatment, given the low risk of increased aspartate transaminase (AST)/alanine aminotransferase (ALT).

X. **Relevant Pharmacokinetics/Pharmacodynamics**

A. **Metabolism**: Hepatic

B. **Time to peak plasma concentration**: ~6–8 hours

C. **Half-life**: 12 hours

D. **Hepatic impairment**: No dosage adjustment necessary.

E. **Renal impairment**: Adjust dosage for moderate or severe renal impairment (CrCl≤ 9 mL/minute). Use not recommended for patients with end-stage renal disease.

XI. **Clinically Relevant Drug Interactions**

A. Metabolized via cytochrome P450 (CYP) 3A4 (primary) as well as by CYP2D6, CYP2C19, CYP3C8, CYP2J2, and P-glycoprotein/ABCB1 (all minor)

B. Maximum dosage of 80 mg/day when combined with strong CYP3A4 inhibitors (e.g., ketoconazole, itraconazole, clarithromycin).

XII. **Adverse Effects**

A. **See "SNRI Class Warnings and Precautions" in introduction to SNRIs.**

B. **Most common**:

1. Gastrointestinal: Notably nausea (17% on levomilnacipran vs. 6% on placebo [Allergan 2021]), vomiting, constipation, anorexia
2. Sexual dysfunction: Likely lower than other SSRIs. Erectile dysfunction: 6% at 40 mg, 8% at 80 mg, 10% at 120 mg/day (vs. 2% on placebo) per clinical trial data (Allergan 2021).
3. Discontinuation syndrome may occur, although less commonly than with venlafaxine or desvenlafaxine (Fava et al. 2018). Taper slowly.

C. **Other notable side effects**:

1. Increased heart rate (6% on levomilnacipran vs. 1% on placebo [Allergan 2021]), with a mean increase of 9 beats per minute; tachycardia; palpitations; increased blood pressure (3% on levomilnacipran vs. 1% on placebo [Allergan 2021]), with a mean of 3.9/3.3 (Mago et al. 2013); urinary hesitation (4% on levomilnacipran vs. 0% on placebo [Allergan 2021]); hyperhidrosis (9% on levomilnacipran vs. 2% on placebo [Allergan 2021])
2. Rare risk of increased AST/ALT values (Mago et al. 2013)
3. Headache

D. **Risks in pregnancy and lactation**: Levomilnacipran was designated a Category C drug in the prior FDA classification and is present in breast milk. A thorough risk/benefit discussion with the patient is recommended on continuing versus stopping the medication, including consultation with an OB/GYN specialist and/or lactation expert. See Chapter 15 ("Women: Pregnancy, Postpartum, and Breastfeeding") for more information.

XIII. **Clinical Pearls/Prescribing Tips**

A. Among the SNRIs, only levomilnacipran is more selective for the NET than for the SERT. Potential benefits of norepinephrine reuptake inhibition include improvement in concentration, energy, and physical and mental slowing (Kasper et al. 2011).

B. Use caution with renal impairment and CYP3A4 inhibitors.

C. Sexual side effects have not been well studied for levomilnacipran, but may be less likely with levomilnacipran than with more serotonergic antidepressants.

Further Reading

Roth BL, Driscoll J: PDSP Ki Database. Psychoactive Drug Screening Program (PDSP). University of North Carolina at Chapel Hill and the United States National Institute of Mental Health, 1999–present. Available at: https://pdsp.unc.edu/databases/pdsp.php. Accessed June 21, 2024.

References

Allergan USA: Fetzima (levomilnacipran) [package insert]. U.S. Food and Drug Administration website. Revised September 2021. Available at: https://www.accessdata.fda.gov/drugsatfda_docs/label/2021/204168s007lbl.pdf. Accessed March 13, 2024.

Auclair AL, Martel JC, Assié MB, et al: Levomilnacipran (F2695), a norepinephrine-preferring SNRI: profile in vitro and in models of depression and anxiety. Neuropharmacology 70:338–347, 2013 23499664

Carboni E, Tanda GL, Frau R, et al: Blockade of the noradrenaline carrier increases extracellular dopamine concentrations in the prefrontal cortex: evidence that dopamine is taken up in vivo by noradrenergic terminals. J Neurochem 55(3):1067–1070, 1990 2117046

Fava GA, Benasi G, Lucente M, et al: Withdrawal symptoms after serotonin-noradrenaline reuptake inhibitor discontinuation: systematic review. Psychother Psychosom 87(4):195–203, 2018 30016772

Kasper S, Pail G: Milnacipran: a unique antidepressant? Neuropsychiatr Dis Treat 6(Suppl 1):23–31, 2010 20856597
Kasper S, Meshkat D, Kutzelnigg A: Improvement of the noradrenergic symptom cluster following treatment with milnacipran. Neuropsychiatr Dis Treat 7(Suppl 1):21–27, 2011 21750625
Mago R, Forero G, Greenberg WM, et al: Safety and tolerability of levomilnacipran ER in major depressive disorder: results from an open-label, 48-week extension study. Clin Drug Investig 33(10):761–771, 2013 23999912
Saxon AJ: Dopamine and depression. Arch Gen Psychiatry 64(9):1101, 2007 17768279

Milnacipran

I. **Brand Names**: Savella

II. **Therapeutic Class**: Serotonin-norepinephrine reuptake inhibitor (SNRI) antidepressant

III. **Mechanism-Based Class**: Serotonin and norepinephrine reuptake inhibitor

IV. **Mechanism(s) of Action**

A. Levomilnacipran is the levorotatory enantiomer of milnacipran and is believed to be the more active isomer form.

B. CNS inhibition of the SERT (serotonin transporter), blocking reuptake and increasing synaptic serotonin (5-hydroxytryptamine [5-HT]) in several brain areas.

1. Ki=~8.44 nM for the SERT
2. Milnacipran has 1.6 times higher selectivity for the SERT than for the NET (norepinephrine transporter), making it the most balanced of the SNRIs

C. CNS inhibition of the NET, blocking reuptake and increasing synaptic norepinephrine in several brain areas

1. Ki=~22 nM for the NET
2. Inhibition of the NET in the prefrontal cortex has also been shown to boost dopamine levels, as the NET clears both norepinephrine and dopamine (Carboni et al. 1990; Kasper and Pail 2010; Saxon 2007).

V. **Indications**

A. FDA adult:

1. Fibromyalgia

B. Evidence-based[1] off-label uses:

1. Major depressive disorder

C. FDA pediatric: None

[1]Evidence strength varies; readers are referred to the literature for more detailed information.

VI. **Major Contraindications and When to Use Caution**

A. Known allergy to milnacipran or its components
B. Concomitant use of MAOI antidepressants or other MAO-inhibiting agents (e.g., linezolid, IV methylene blue)—A 2-week washout is typically required.

VII. **Dosage Formulations**

A. Brand tablet (12.5 mg, 25 mg, 50 mg, 100 mg), *not scored*
B. Brand titration pack (55 tabs of each: 12.5 mg, 25 mg, 50 mg, 4 weeks)

VIII. **Dosage Ranges and Guidelines**

A. Refer to Table 2–10 for dosage ranges (initial/maximum) and guidelines.
B. Administer in two divided doses per day.
C. Start at 12.5 mg/day. After 2–3 days, increase to 12.5 mg BID. After 4–7 days, can increase to 25 mg BID as tolerated. After 7 days, can increase to 50 mg BID. Maximum dosage is 200 mg/day (100 mg BID).
D. Benefits may be evident after 1–2 weeks, but it may take up to 6–8 weeks to reach full effect at a given dosage.

Table 2–10. Milnacipran indications and dosage ranges

Indication	Usual dosage range
Fibromyalgia	12.5–200 mg/day (divided dosing)
Major depressive disorder (off-label)	25–50 mg BID → 100 mg BID

IX. **Monitoring**

A. Measure blood pressure and heart rate at baseline and monitor periodically throughout treatment, especially with high dosages.
B. Monitor liver function at baseline and periodically, given low risk of aspartate transaminase (AST)/alanine aminotransferase (ALT) increases. Avoid use in patients with substantial alcohol use or chronic liver disease.

X. **Relevant Pharmacokinetics/Pharmacodynamics**

A. **Metabolism**: Hepatic; no active metabolites
B. **Time to peak plasma concentration**: 2–4 hours
C. **Half-life**: 6–8 hours
D. **Hepatic impairment**: No dosage adjustment necessary.
E. **Renal impairment**: Use caution with moderate renal impairment. Reduce dosage by 50% for renal impairment (CrCl<29 mL/minute). Not recommended in end-stage renal disease.

XI. **Clinically Relevant Drug Interactions**

A. No significant drug interactions.

XII. **Adverse Effects**

A. **See "SNRI Class Warnings and Precautions" in introduction to SNRIs.**

B. **Most common:**

1. Gastrointestinal: Notably nausea (6% on milnacipran vs. 1% on placebo), low risk of vomiting, constipation, anorexia
2. Sexual dysfunction: Low risk; may actually improve sexual dysfunction in some patients (Baldwin et al. 2008; Kasper and Pail 2010).
3. Discontinuation syndrome risk is relatively low with milnacipran and appears less common than with venlafaxine and desvenlafaxine (Fava et al. 2018; Kasper and Pail 2010).
4. The risk of weight gain appears to be relatively low (Kasper and Pail 2010).

C. **Other notable side effects:**

1. Increased heart rate (1% on milnacipran vs. 0% on placebo), palpitations (3% on milnacipran vs. 1% on placebo); low risk of hyperhidrosis, headache, dizziness
2. Low risk of increased AST/ALT

D. **Risks in pregnancy and lactation**: Milnacipran was designated a Category C drug in the prior FDA classification and is present in breast milk. A thorough risk/benefit discussion with the patient is recommended on continuing versus stopping the medication, including consultation with an OB/GYN specialist and/or lactation expert. See Chapter 15 ("Women: Pregnancy, Postpartum, and Breastfeeding") for more information.

XIII. **Clinical Pearls/Prescribing Tips**

A. Milnacipran is one of three drugs approved for fibromyalgia treatment. Clinical trials have demonstrated efficacy of milnacipran for fibromyalgia. Patients experienced various levels of pain relief in the clinical trials of milnacipran in fibromyalgia, with an average of 30% reduction in pain. Studies have also shown improvements in fatigue, stiffness, and cognitive function (Cording et al. 2015; Ormseth et al. 2010).

B. Although not FDA approved for depression, in various clinical trials, milnacipran has shown efficacy comparable to that of fluoxetine, fluvoxamine, paroxetine, and TCAs, with better tolerability compared with TCAs (Guelfi et al. 1998; Kasper et al. 2011; Nakagawa et al. 2009; Sechter et al. 2004). In particular, increased norepinephrine reuptake inhibition may provide benefit for psychomotor retardation, concentration difficulties, and slowness in thought/speech (Kasper et al. 2011).

C. The need for twice-daily dosing may be difficult for some patients.

D. Milnacipran may actually improve sexual dysfunction and likely has a lower risk of weight gain and discontinuation symptoms compared with many other antidepressants.

E. Lack of active metabolites or dependence on the CYP system may be of benefit.

F. Use caution in moderate to severe renal impairment.

Further Reading

Allergan USA: Savella (milnacipran) [package insert]. U.S. Food and Drug Administration website. Revised September 2021. Available at: https://www.accessdata.fda.gov/drugsatfda_docs/label/2021/022256s025lbl.pdf. Accessed March 13, 2024.

Roth BL, Driscoll J: PDSP Ki Database. Psychoactive Drug Screening Program (PDSP). University of North Carolina at Chapel Hill and the United States National Institute of Mental Health, 1999–present. Available at: https://pdsp.unc.edu/databases/pdsp.php. Accessed June 21, 2024.

References

Baldwin D, Moreno RA, Briley M: Resolution of sexual dysfunction during acute treatment of major depression with milnacipran. Hum Psychopharmacol 23(6):527–532, 2008 18536065

Carboni E, Tanda GL, Frau R, et al: Blockade of the noradrenaline carrier increases extracellular dopamine concentrations in the prefrontal cortex: evidence that dopamine is taken up in vivo by noradrenergic terminals. J Neurochem 55(3):1067–1070, 1990 2117046

Cording M, Derry S, Phillips T, et al: Milnacipran for pain in fibromyalgia in adults. Cochrane Database Syst Rev (10):CD008244, 2015 26482422

Fava GA, Benasi G, Lucente M, et al: Withdrawal symptoms after serotonin-noradrenaline reuptake inhibitor discontinuation: systematic review. Psychother Psychosom 87(4):195–203, 2018 30016772

Guelfi JD, Ansseau M, Corruble E, et al: A double-blind comparison of the efficacy and safety of milnacipran and fluoxetine in depressed inpatients. Int Clin Psychopharmacol 13(3):121–128, 1998 9690979

Kasper S, Pail G: Milnacipran: a unique antidepressant? Neuropsychiatr Dis Treat 6(Suppl 1):23–31, 2010 20856597

Kasper S, Meshkat D, Kutzelnigg A: Improvement of the noradrenergic symptom cluster following treatment with milnacipran. Neuropsychiatr Dis Treat 7(Suppl 1):21–27, 2011 21750625

Nakagawa A, Watanabe N, Omori IM, et al: Milnacipran versus other antidepressive agents for depression. Cochrane Database Syst Rev (3):CD006529, 2009 19588396

Ormseth MJ, Eyler AE, Hammonds CL, et al: Milnacipran for the management of fibromyalgia syndrome. J Pain Res 3:15–24, 2010 21197306

Saxon AJ: Dopamine and depression. Arch Gen Psychiatry 64(9):1101, 2007 17768279

Sechter D, Vandel P, Weiller E, et al: A comparative study of milnacipran and paroxetine in outpatients with major depression. J Affect Disord 83(2–3):233–236, 2004 15555719

Venlafaxine

I. **Brand Names**: Effexor, Effexor XR

II. **Therapeutic Class**: Serotonin-norepinephrine reuptake inhibitor (SNRI) antidepressant

III. **Mechanism-Based Class**: Serotonin and norepinephrine reuptake inhibitor

IV. **Mechanism(s) of Action**

A. CNS inhibition of the SERT (serotonin transporter), blocking reuptake and increasing synaptic serotonin (5-hydroxytryptamine [5-HT]) in several brain areas.

1. Venlafaxine is approximately 30 times more selective for the SERT than for the NET (norepinephrine transporter).
2. Ki=~82 nM for the SERT; Ki=~2,480 nM for the NET (Bymaster et al. 2001)
    1. SERT occupancy is approximately 80% at a 75-mg/day dosage (Meyer et al. 2004), versus NET occupancy of only 20% at the 75-mg/day dosage (Arakawa et al. 2019).

B. CNS inhibition of the NET, blocking reuptake and increasing synaptic norepinephrine in several brain areas

1. NET occupancy is *dosage dependent*: Studies indicate significant NET activity only at a dosage of 150 mg/day (Arakawa et al. 2019) and at dosages of 225–375 mg/day (Debonnel et al. 2007). However, higher NET blockade appears to correlate with certain adverse effects (increased blood pressure, heart rate). Inhibition of the NET in the prefrontal cortex has also been shown to boost dopamine levels, as the NET clears both norepinephrine and dopamine (Carboni et al. 1990; Kasper and Pail 2010; Saxon 2007).

V. **Indications**

A. FDA adult:

1. Major depressive disorder
2. Generalized anxiety disorder
3. Social anxiety disorder
4. Panic disorder

B. Evidence-based[1] off-label uses:

1. OCD
2. PTSD
3. Premenstrual dysphoric disorder
4. Vasomotor symptoms associated with menopause

C. FDA pediatric: None

[1]Evidence strength varies; readers are referred to the literature for more detailed information.

VI. Major Contraindications and When to Use Caution

A. Known allergy to venlafaxine or its components
B. Concomitant use of MAOI antidepressants or other MAO-inhibiting agents (e.g., linezolid, IV methylene blue)—A 2-week washout is typically required.

VII. Dosage Formulations

A. Brand XR capsule (37.5 mg, 75 mg, 150 mg)—*Note*: Brand IR Effexor was discontinued by the manufacturer.
B. Generic ER capsule (37.5 mg, 75 mg, 150 mg)
C. Generic ER tablet (37.5 mg, 75 mg, 150 mg, 225 mg [*not scored*])
D. Generic IR tablet (25 mg, 37.5 mg, 50 mg, 75 mg, 100 mg—[*all scored*])

VIII. Dosage Ranges and Guidelines

A. Refer to Table 2–11 for dosage ranges (initial/maximum) and guidelines.
B. Start at 37.5–75 mg/day (depending on the indication) and increase by 37.5–75.0 mg every 1–2 weeks to a usual maximum dosage of 225 mg/day XR (or 375 mg/day IR). Some literature supports use of dosages up to 300 mg/day XR for additional effect, but this dosing is off-label.
C. Benefits may be evident after 1–2 weeks of treatment in some patients, but it may take up to 6–8 weeks to reach the full effect at a given dosage.
D. Although the package label recommends taking venlafaxine with food, some pharmacokinetic studies have not shown clinically relevant differences in blood levels between fed and fasted states.

Table 2–11. Venlafaxine indications and dosage ranges

Indication	Usual dosage range
Major depressive disorder	XR/ER: 37.5–75 mg/day → 225 mg/day IR: 37.5–75 mg/day → 375 mg/day[a]
Generalized anxiety disorder	XR/ER: 37.5–75 mg/day → 225 mg/day
Social anxiety disorder	XR/ER: 75–225 mg/day (usual maximum 75 mg/day)
Panic disorder	XR/ER: 37.5–225 mg/day
OCD (off-label)	XR/ER and IR: 75–350 mg/day[b]
PTSD (off-label)	XR/ER: 37.5 –300 mg/day[c]
Premenstrual dysphoric disorder (PMDD) (off-label)	XR/ER: 37.5–150 mg/day (continuous and luteal)[d]
Vasomotor symptoms associated with menopause (off-label)	XR/ER and IR: 37.5–75 mg/day[e]

[a]Per APA Practice Guideline for the Treatment of Patients With Major Depressive Disorder (American Psychiatric Association 2010).
[b]OCD: Clinical trials have demonstrated effects with dosages up to 350 mg/day (Albert et al. 2002; Denys et al. 2003; Koran et al. 2007).
[c]PTSD: Average dosages in clinical trials were ~170 mg/day (Davidson et al. 2006).
[d]PMDD: Maximum dosages averaged 130 mg/day (Freeman et al. 2001) or 150 mg/day (Hsiao and Liu 2003).
[e]Vasomotor symptoms: Studies indicate optimal dosing at 75 mg/day, with higher dosages leading to more side effects (Evans et al. 2005; Pachman et al. 2010).

IX. Monitoring

A. Measure blood pressure and heart rate at baseline and monitor periodically throughout treatment, especially with high dosages.

B. Monitor cholesterol, low-density lipoprotein, and triglycerides periodically, given the potential for increases with venlafaxine.

X. Relevant Pharmacokinetics/Pharmacodynamics

A. **Metabolism**: Hepatic

B. **Time to peak plasma concentration**:

1. Venlafaxine: 2 hours (IR), 3–8 hours (ER)
2. Metabolite (*O*-desmethylvenlafaxine [ODV]): 3 hours (IR), 8–14 hours (ER)

C. **Half-life**:

1. Venlafaxine: 3–7 hours (IR), ~7–13 hours (ER), prolonged with hepatic or renal impairment
2. Metabolite (ODV): 9–13 hours (IR), 9–15 hours (ER), prolonged with hepatic or renal impairment

D. **Hepatic impairment**: Reduce dosage by 25%–50% in patients with hepatic impairment and by 50% or more for severe hepatic impairment or hepatic cirrhosis.

E. **Renal impairment**: Reduce dosage by 25%–50% in patients with renal impairment and by 50% or more for severe renal impairment/dialysis.

XI. Clinically Relevant Drug Interactions

A. Metabolized by cytochrome P450 (CYP) 2D6 (major) and by CYP2C19 (minor), CYP2C9 (minor), and CYP3A4 (minor).

1. CYP2D6 is responsible for the conversion of venlafaxine to its metabolite (ODV/desvenlafaxine). Poor metabolizers of CYP2D6 show decreased metabolite (ODV) levels.

B. Weak inhibitor of CYP2D6

1. Use with caution when combined with CYP2D6 substrates, most notably TCAs, beta-blockers, tamoxifen, and some opioids.

C. Venlafaxine could have pharmacodynamic interactions with other drugs that have a similar mechanism of action and target the same receptors in the body.

XII. Adverse Effects

A. **See "SNRI Class Warnings and Precautions" in introduction to SNRIs.**

B. **Most common**:

1. Gastrointestinal: Notably nausea (30% on venlafaxine v. 11.8% on placebo [Pfizer 2021]), vomiting, dry mouth, constipation, anorexia (Debonnel et al. 2007; Harvey et al. 2000)
2. Sexual dysfunction: Increased risk with venlafaxine compared with other SNRIs and some SSRIs (Serretti and Chiesa 2009)—58%–73% for venlafaxine-treated patients (Montejo et al. 2001).

3. Discontinuation syndrome occurs frequently (up to 75%) and appears to be more common with venlafaxine than with most SSRIs and SNRIs (Fava et al. 2018; Montgomery et al. 2004), so taper slowly.

C. **Other notable side effects**:

1. Headache, insomnia, somnolence, dizziness
2. Sweating, heart rate increases, blood pressure increases (increased at higher dosages)
3. Increase in cholesterol and serum triglycerides (Pfizer 2021)

D. **Risks in pregnancy and lactation**: Venlafaxine was designated a Category C drug in the prior FDA classification and is present in breast milk. A thorough risk/benefit discussion with the patient is recommended on continuing versus stopping the medication, including consultation with an OB/GYN specialist and/or lactation expert. See Chapter 15 ("Women: Pregnancy, Postpartum, and Breastfeeding") for more information.

XIII. **Clinical Pearls/Prescribing Tips**

A. Venlafaxine is 30 times more selective for SERT receptors than for NET receptors. NET inhibition is dosage dependent, becoming more significant at dosages of 150 mg/day or greater. However, higher dosages also confer a higher risk of blood pressure and heart rate changes.

B. Venlafaxine confers a higher risk of discontinuation symptoms, sexual side effects, and nausea compared with other SSRIs and SNRIs.

C. CYP2D6 poor metabolizers will have decreased conversion of venlafaxine to its active metabolite ODV (or desvenlafaxine). For patients who are known to be poor metabolizers of CYP2D6 or who take other medications (e.g., CYP2D6 inhibitors) that functionally convert these patients into CYP2D6 poor metabolizers, consider prescribing desvenlafaxine to bypass CYP2D6 metabolism.

References

Albert U, Aguglia E, Maina G, et al: Venlafaxine versus clomipramine in the treatment of obsessive-compulsive disorder: a preliminary single-blind, 12-week, controlled study. J Clin Psychiatry 63(11):1004–1009, 2002 12444814

American Psychiatric Association: Practice Guideline for the Treatment of Patients With Major Depressive Disorder, 3rd Edition. Arlington, VA, American Psychiatric Association, November 2010. Available at: https://psychiatryonline.org/pb/assets/raw/sitewide/practice_guidelines/guidelines/mdd.pdf. Accessed March 13, 2024.

Arakawa R, Stenkrona P, Takano A, et al: Venlafaxine ER blocks the norepinephrine transporter in the brain of patients with major depressive disorder: a PET study using [18F]FMeNER-D2. Int J Neuropsychopharmacol 22(4):278–285, 2019 30649319

Bymaster FP, Dreshfield-Ahmad LJ, Threlkeld PG, et al: Comparative affinity of duloxetine and venlafaxine for serotonin and norepinephrine transporters in vitro and in vivo, human serotonin receptor subtypes, and other neuronal receptors. Neuropsychopharmacology 25(6):871–880, 2001 11750180

Carboni E, Tanda GL, Frau R, et al: Blockade of the noradrenaline carrier increases extracellular dopamine concentrations in the prefrontal cortex: evidence that dopamine is taken up in vivo by noradrenergic terminals. J Neurochem 55(3):1067–1070, 1990 2117046

Davidson J, Baldwin D, Stein DJ, et al: Treatment of posttraumatic stress disorder with venlafaxine extended release: a 6-month randomized controlled trial. Arch Gen Psychiatry 63(10):1158–1165, 2006 17015818

Debonnel G, Saint-André E, Hébert C, et al: Differential physiological effects of a low dose and high doses of venlafaxine in major depression. Int J Neuropsychopharmacol 10(1):51–61, 2007 16690006

Denys D, van der Wee N, van Megen HJ, et al: A double blind comparison of venlafaxine and paroxetine in obsessive-compulsive disorder. J Clin Psychopharmacol 23(6):568–575, 2003 14624187

Evans ML, Pritts E, Vittinghoff E, et al: Management of postmenopausal hot flushes with venlafaxine hydrochloride: a randomized, controlled trial. Obstet Gynecol 105(1):161–166, 2005 15625158

Fava GA, Benasi G, Lucente M, et al: Withdrawal symptoms after serotonin-noradrenaline reuptake inhibitor discontinuation: systematic review. Psychother Psychosom 87(4):195–203, 2018 30016772

Freeman EW, Rickels K, Yonkers KA, et al: Venlafaxine in the treatment of premenstrual dysphoric disorder. Obstet Gynecol 98(5 Pt 1):737–744, 2001 11704162

Harvey AT, Rudolph RL, Preskorn SH: Evidence of the dual mechanisms of action of venlafaxine. Arch Gen Psychiatry 57(5):503–509, 2000 10807491

Hsiao MC, Liu CY: Effective open-label treatment of premenstrual dysphoric disorder with venlafaxine. Psychiatry Clin Neurosci 57(3):317–321, 2003 12753573

Kasper S, Pail G: Milnacipran: a unique antidepressant? Neuropsychiatr Dis Treat 6(Suppl 1):23–31, 2010 20856597

Koran LM, Hanna GL, Hollander E, et al; American Psychiatric Association: Practice guideline for the treatment of patients with obsessive-compulsive disorder. Am J Psychiatry 164(7)(Suppl):5–53, 2007 17849776

Meyer JH, Wilson AA, Sagrati S, et al: Serotonin transporter occupancy of five selective serotonin reuptake inhibitors at different doses: an [11C]DASB positron emission tomography study. Am J Psychiatry 161(5):826–835, 2004 15121647

Montejo AL, Llorca G, Izquierdo JA, et al; Spanish Working Group for the Study of Psychotropic-Related Sexual Dysfunction: Incidence of sexual dysfunction associated with antidepressant agents: a prospective multicenter study of 1022 outpatients. J Clin Psychiatry 62(Suppl 3):10–21, 2001 11229449

Montgomery SA, Huusom AKT, Bothmer J: A randomised study comparing escitalopram with venlafaxine XR in primary care patients with major depressive disorder. Neuropsychobiology 50(1):57–64, 2004 15179022

Pachman DR, Jones JM, Loprinzi CL: Management of menopause-associated vasomotor symptoms: current treatment options, challenges and future directions. Int J Womens Health 2:123–135, 2010

Pfizer: Effexor XR [package insert]. U.S. Food and Drug Administration website. Revised November 2021. Available at: https://www.accessdata.fda.gov/drugsatfda_docs/label/2021/020699s113lbl.pdf. Accessed March 13, 2024.

Saxon AJ: Dopamine and depression. Arch Gen Psychiatry 64(9):1101, 2007 17768279

Serretti A, Chiesa A: Treatment-emergent sexual dysfunction related to antidepressants: a meta-analysis. J Clin Psychopharmacol 29(3):259–266, 2009 19440080

Monoamine Oxidase Inhibitors

General Considerations for Use of MAOIs

- Monoamine oxidase inhibitors (MAOIs) are underused (Balon et al. 1999), mostly because of fears about adverse effects and drug interactions, but they can be transformative for some patients with treatment-resistant depression. They exhibit a completely different mechanism of action from most traditional antidepressants (selective serotonin reuptake inhibitors [SSRIs], serotonin-norepinephrine reuptake inhibitors [SNRIs], tricyclic antidepressants [TCAs]) by inhibiting monoamine oxidase (MAO), the enzyme responsible for metabolizing endogenous monoamines (e.g., serotonin, norepinephrine, dopamine), thereby increasing the presynaptic stores of these transmitters available for release.
- MAOIs have been demonstrated to have particular efficacy in major depressive disorder with atypical features (Quitkin et al. 1988, 1990), which can include an excessive need for sleep, hyperphagia, lethargy/anergia, loss of motivation, sensitivity to interpersonal rejection, and mood reactivity (Łojko and Rybakowski 2017). MAOIs, and especially phenelzine, also have particular benefits for social anxiety disorder (Davidson 2003) and panic disorder (Sheehan 2002).

MAOI–Food and MAOI–Drug Interactions Leading to Hypertensive Crisis

- There are two potential interactions with MAOIs that can lead to a hypertensive crisis: dietary tyramine and sympathomimetic medications. These interactions and their symptoms are described in the following sections.

Dietary Tyramine

- Notably, monoamine oxidase is responsible for breaking down tyramine, which accumulates as a product of certain aged and fermented foods via tyrosine decarboxylation (Rapaport 2007). Tyramine is taken up via the norepinephrine transporter and displaces presynaptic epinephrine, norepinephrine, and dopamine (Brown et al. 1989), leading to a sudden increase in blood pressure, also known as the *tyramine trigger response*.
- Although patients should be advised on dietary guidelines and caution should be taken, it is notable that in the 1960s when MAOIs were widely prescribed, there were no dietary guidelines, and foods actually had much higher amounts of tyramine than they do now. Even then, only 14 patients out of 1.5 million had deaths related to a hypertensive crisis from tyramine (Gillman 2018).

- To prevent a hypertensive crisis, patients taking MAOI therapy must be advised to avoid excessive amounts of tyramine-rich foods (see Table 2–12 below).
- The cumulative effect of multiple foods in a meal must be considered. For example, a large serving of pizza with a craft beer may cause problems.
- Leftovers are safe if eaten within 48 hours. Longer storage in a refrigerator causes significant tyramine accumulation. Freezing is recommended if cooked food is stored for more than 2 days.
- Online recommendations regarding low-tyramine diets are extremely variable and often incorrect. Readers are referred to Gillman's (2018) excellent review of the medical literature on tyramine in foods.
- Many foods that are excluded by some low-tyramine diets actually have variable amounts of tyramine by brand. Patients can test very small amounts of a food and measure the effects on blood pressure.

Table 2–12. Dietary guidelines for MAOIs

Avoid	Likely safe
Cured meats (treated with salt/nitrite/nitrate) such as **dry (e.g., summer) sausages, mortadella, Cacciatore, Nostrano, chicken liver, paté, chorizo,** aged pepperoni, salami, most pickled/smoked fish (lox), anchovies, sardines caviar, hot dogs, bologna, corned beef, bacon, cured ham, game meat (e.g., deer)	Fresh meat, fresh fish and shellfish, eggs, lunch meats (other than salami), canned meats, kielbasa, sweet sausage. Most pepperoni made in the U.S. has low tyramine. Smoked salmon and uncured ham are usually safe.
Aged cheeses (aged Swiss, feta, aged Parmesan), **blue cheeses (Stilton, Gorgonzola)**, French Camembert, Italian goat cheese, some cheddar cheeses[a]	Cheeses made from pasteurized milk, such as American cheese, cottage cheese, ricotta, mozzarella (not Italian), Camembert (not French), farmer cheese, sour cream, cream cheese, Parmesan (not aged). Other cheeses considered safe are Romano, brie, Boursin, Havarti, Swiss (not aged), Cambozola, Muenster, Gruyere/Comté, Emmental, goat cheese (not Italian).
Certain alcoholic beverages, such as vermouth, craft/tap/home-brewed beers, high-tyramine red wines (Chianti, merlot, cabernet, Malbec)[b]	Coffee, tea, soda, milk, liquor. Wine and bottled/canned non-craft beer is generally safe except as noted. One serving of craft beer is likely safe.
Some yeast and bread products, such as concentrated yeast extracts **(Marmite, Vegemite), brewer's yeast**, sourdough bread	Most breads, pasta, grains, and sweets are low in tyramine.
Some condiments, such as certain **soy sauce products (e.g., Pearl River Bridge, Kimlan), fish/shrimp sauce or paste, teriyaki sauce, miso, concentrated yeast extract, kimchi, sauerkraut**	Mayonnaise, ketchup, mustard, Worcestershire sauce, salad dressing. Soybean oil is safe. Most soy sauce appears to be safe (e.g., Kikkoman, Ozeki, Wing's).

Table 2–12. Dietary guidelines for MAOIs *(continued)*

Avoid	Likely safe
Some fruits, vegetables: dried/overripe fruits such as raisins/prunes,[c] banana peel	Most fresh fruits and vegetables are safe except as noted. Unaged and unfermented black olives are safe.
Soy foods: soybeans and soybean products such as tofu, soy milk, soy sauce (see "Some condiments" above). Check labels for added soy.	
Other foods: Any pickled or fermented foods or overripe or spoiled foods; large amounts of peanuts (more than one-half cup); overripe avocados, figs, fava beans,[d] beef bouillon mix	Reasonable amounts of most U.S.-made pizzas are safe. Avoid products containing ingredients with high tyramine content (as noted above).

Note. Foods in **bold** have the highest tyramine content.

[a]Cheese typically requires aging for 3 months or more to accumulate sufficient tyramine to cause hypertensive reactions. Aged cheddar can cause a reaction, and tyramine accumulates in cheddar under refrigeration. Therefore, it is recommended that aged cheeses be avoided.

[b]The tyramine content of these wines is highly variable, but it is best that they be avoided. Also note that most published reports of very high tyramine content in red wines and craft beer are from older literature. Modern beer- and wine-making methods appear to have reduced tyramine content. Therefore, a single glass of craft beer or of one of the wines noted as problematic above is probably safe. However, it is a good idea for patients to test the effects by drinking 60 mL (2 oz.) of a wine and then measuring blood pressure every 15–20 minutes for 1 hour to see if it has increased. This test should be done with each new wine or beer that is introduced.

[c]Shulman et al. (1989) found that raisins, figs, and fava beans are safe.

[d]Many published MAOI diets recommend avoiding broad beans, including fava beans. However, experimental evidence does not support this prohibition. Also, the tyramine content of green olives and pickles can be variable.

Sympathomimetic Drugs and Stimulants

- MAOIs increase synaptic norepinephrine and dopamine. The pressor response with sympathomimetic decongestant drugs (e.g., pseudoephedrine, oral phenylephrine, phenylpropanolamine) results from an additive effect when these drugs are given with MAOIs. Direct-acting drugs are norepinephrine agonists (pseudoephedrine, phenylephrine) that directly stimulate α_1- and/or β_2-adrenergic receptors. Indirect-acting sympathomimetics (e.g., phenylpropanolamine) stimulate presynaptic release or block reuptake of norepinephrine, enhancing synaptic transmission. Some sympathomimetic decongestants (e.g., phenylephrine) are also metabolized by MAO, and inhibition leads to an increase in MAOI blood levels.
- Inhaled or insufflated sympathomimetics (e.g., albuterol) are usually safe because systemic exposure is low. However, it is recommended that patients measure blood pressure 30 minutes after administration for the first three exposures.

- MAOIs should be used with caution in combination with stimulants (amphetamines, methylphenidate). Patients should be on a stable dosage of an MAOI. An immediate-release stimulant medication should be selected, and should be started at the lowest dosage. Patients should measure blood pressure before dosing and then 30, 60, 90, and 120 minutes after administration. Patients should be instructed to seek acute care for blood pressure greater than 180/120. If blood pressure is elevated above 140/110 at 120 minutes, it should be monitored every 30 minutes until it declines. Blood pressure measurements should also be done after each dosage increase. After the dosage of the immediate-release stimulant is established, a switch to a long-acting preparation is possible.
- Table 2–13 summarizes the recommendations for avoiding MAOI–drug interactions.

Table 2–13. Sympathomimetic/stimulant use guidelines for MAOIs

Avoid	Likely safe
Decongestants such as pseudoephedrine (Sudafed), phenylpropanolamine, ephedrine, levomethamphetamine, propylhexedrine, naphazoline, oxymetazoline (Afrin), phenylephrine (Sudafed PE, DayQuil).	Saline nasal spray, plain guaifenesin (Mucinex), benzonatate (Tessalon Perles), antihistamines. Inhaled albuterol appears to be safe in most patients (see text).
Advise patients to check ingredients in common over-the-counter (OTC) drugs.	
Use with caution in combination with stimulants (e.g., amphetamines, methylphenidate). Do not use with atomoxetine or viloxazine.	

Signs of a Hypertensive Crisis

- Symptoms of hypertensive crisis include pounding occipital headache, palpitations, tachycardia, nausea, vomiting, sweating, photophobia, neck stiffness, and confusion. In rare instances, the elevated blood pressure can lead to cerebral hemorrhage and death.
- If patients experience the above symptoms or high blood pressure (>180/>120), either diastolic or systolic, advise them to check their resting blood pressure and recheck it every 5–10 minutes. If the blood pressure remains consistently elevated (three or more sequential blood pressure readings); or if any blood pressure is >200/>130); or if the heart rate is consistently greater than 130 beats per minute; or if patients experience symptoms of end-organ damage (e.g., chest pain, shortness of breath, symptoms of stroke), they should be instructed to present to the ER or call 911. It is ***not advisable*** for patients to take rapidly acting blood pressure–lowering medications such as nifedipine, because such medications carry the risk of hypotension and other adverse effects.
- Also keep in mind that blood pressure or pulse may naturally rise to very high levels during strenuous exercise (e.g., weight lifting), or when a person is very anxious, but these situational increases very rarely cause serious problems, such as a stroke.

MAOI–Drug Interactions Leading to Serotonin Syndrome

- All available MAOIs—including selegiline (Emsam) at higher dosages—are inhibitors of both MAO-A and MAO-B. Serotonin is metabolized primarily by MAO-A; MAOIs significantly increase serotonin levels throughout the body. Given the irreversible inhibition of MAO-A, concomitant use of MAOIs with other medications that increase synaptic serotonin can lead to serotonin syndrome (see Table 2–14 below).
- **Key symptoms of serotonin syndrome include muscular rigidity, hyperreflexia, clonus, bilateral Babinski sign, hyperthermia, mydriasis, and delirium/coma.** Several of these symptoms should be present for a definitive diagnosis of serotonin syndrome. Other symptoms include hypertension, diaphoresis, diarrhea, agitation, anxiety, excitement, tremor, akathisia, tachycardia, tachypnea, dry mucous membranes, flushed skin, vomiting, hyperactive bowel sounds, and arrhythmias. However, the latter symptoms are not considered pathognomonic because they can be the result of many other conditions. Serotonin syndrome can be fatal in 10% or less of affected persons.
- **Switching from another serotonergic antidepressant to an MAOI (and vice versa):**
  - Before a switch can be made from another serotonergic antidepressant to an MAOI, a drug washout of five half-lives or more is required, which can vary depending on half-life.
    - For example: Fluoxetine has a half life of 120 hours, and its primary metabolite, norfluoxetine, has a half-life of 7–9 days. A switch from fluoxetine to an MAOI would require a washout of 5 weeks. Sertraline has a half-life of about 26 hours (women=32 hours; men=22 hours), and its primary active metabolite has a half-life of 60–100 hours. Therefore, the minimum period after discontinuing sertraline would be 21 days. The variation in half-life depends on variability in cytochrome metabolism due to polymorphisms of metabolizing enzymes.
    - An approach to manage this situation is to switch to a medication with a shorter half-life for a period of 5–6 weeks prior to tapering. Most other antidepressants have half-lives of 20–35 hours, requiring a drug-free period of 5–7 days. However, venlafaxine and desvenlafaxine have shorter half-lives (5–11 hours), requiring shorter discontinuation periods.
  - The currently available MAOIs are irreversible, meaning that MAO has to be synthesized by the body to restore normal MAO levels. When switching from an MAOI to another medication that blocks the reuptake of serotonin or otherwise increases synaptic serotonin, a 2-week washout of the MAOI is required to allow for recovery of MAO enzyme levels.
- The principal mechanism mediating serotonin syndrome appears to be overactivation of 5-HT_{2A} (and possibly 5-HT_{1A}) receptors (Heise et al. 2017). Therefore, medications that block 5-HT_{2A} receptors, or that reduce 5-HT_{1A} activation relative to serotonin (e.g., buspirone), should not pose significant risks.

Table 2–14. Medications carrying risk for serotonin syndrome in combination with MAOIs

Avoid	Likely safe
Antidepressants: SSRIs, SNRIs, St. John's wort, vortioxetine, vilazodone, serotonergic TCAs	*Mixed evidence*: buspirone,[a,b] bupropion,[c] mirtazapine, trazodone
Pain: Tramadol, methadone, **meperidine (Demerol, pethidine)**, fentanyl,[d] pentazocine, cyclobenzaprine,[e] methadone (levomethadone)	Codeine, oxycodone, hydrocodone, buprenorphine, morphine
Antihistamines: Chlorpheniramine, brompheniramine	Diphenhydramine, doxylamine, hydroxyzine
Antibiotic: Linezolid	Other antibiotics appear safe
Drugs of abuse: Cocaine, methamphetamine, MDMA	
Others: Sumatriptan,[f,g,h] dextromethorphan (present in many OTC cold preparations), ziprasidone,[i] lumateperone	Carbamazepine, oxcarbazepine[j,k]

Note. MDMA=3,4-methylenedioxymethamphetamine; OTC=over-the-counter; SNRIs=serotonin-norepinephrine reuptake inhibitors; SSRIs=selective serotonin reuptake inhibitor; TCAs=tricyclic antidepressants.

[a]There were a few early case reports of elevated blood pressure with buspirone.
[b]Ciraulo and Shader 1990.
[c]Thomas et al. 2015.
[d]There is a single case report of a fentanyl–MAOI interaction (Rastogi et al. 2011).
[e]Keegan et al. 2006.
[f]Gardner and Lynd 1998.
[g]Gillman 2010.
[h]There are warnings about serotonin syndrome with sumatriptan and other triptans. However, there are no published case reports of definite serotonin syndrome (Gillman 2010). Sumatriptan is metabolized in part by MAO-A, and concurrent use doubles sumatriptan blood levels.
[i]Rim and Gitlin 2010.
[j]Dardis et al. 2012.
[k]Dursun et al. 1993.

Other Potential Adverse Effects of MAOIs

- **Boxed Warning: Suicidality and Antidepressant Drugs (see warning below)**: In common with all antidepressants, MAOIs carry an increased risk for suicidal thoughts/behaviors in pediatric and young adult patients. For detailed information, readers are referred to comprehensive sources in the literature (e.g., Fergusson et al. 2005).
- **Orthostatic hypotension**: Severe orthostasis leading to syncope may occur in 10%–20% of patients, with minor orthostatic hypotension being more common, although usually asymptomatic and minor (Rabkin et al. 1984). Patients will usually develop a tolerance to this in several weeks. Orthostasis may require dosage reduction or slower titration.
- **Weight gain**: More common with phenelzine and selegiline; less common with tranylcypromine

- **Sexual side effects**: More common with phenelzine and selegiline; less common with tranylcypromine
- **Anxiety**: More common with tranylcypromine and selegiline because of their stimulating effects
- **Insomnia**: Insomnia may occur with all MAOIs, but is more common with selegiline and tranylcypromine due to stimulating effects. Adjusting dosing to earlier in the day may be beneficial. Trazodone at dosages of 50–200 mg/day has been demonstrated to be safe and effective when administered with MAOIs (Nierenberg and Keck 1989).
- **Sedation**: May be more likely with phenelzine. Adjusting dosing to later in the day may be beneficial.
- **Vitamin B_6 deficiency**: May occur with phenelzine or isocarboxazid. Advise patients to monitor for paresthesias, edema, and muscle twitches.
- **Withdrawal effects**: Similar to SSRI withdrawal and may include return of severe depression, confusion, headache, diarrhea, nightmares, and, rarely, psychotic symptoms.
- **Transient liver injury**: Transient increases in serum aminotransferase levels may occur within 1–3 months of starting MAOIs and may represent possible hepatocellular damage, although the increases are usually small and asymptomatic, and usually do not necessitate a change in dosage. Monitor liver function tests routinely.

Boxed Warning: Suicidality and Antidepressant Drugs*

Increased risk of suicidal thoughts and behaviors in pediatric and young adult patients in the short term. Close monitoring of patients for emergence of suicidal thoughts and behaviors is required.

**Note.* This warning on suicidality met with controversy. For a detailed discussion, the reader is referred to comprehensive sources in the literature (e.g., Fergusson et al. 2005).

Further Reading

Moore JJ, Saadabadi A: Selegiline, in StatPearls. Treasure Island, FL, StatPearls Publishing, 2022

Mylan Specialty LP: Emsam (selegiline transdermal system) [package insert]. U.S. Food and Drug Administration website. Revised September 2014. Available at: https://www.accessdata.fda.gov/drugsatfda_docs/label/2014/021336s005s010,021708s000lbl.pdf. Accessed March 13, 2024.

Peck T, Wong A, Norman E: Anaesthetic implications of psychoactive drugs. Contin Educ Anaesth Crit Care Pain 10(6):177–181, 2010

Phenelzine, in LiverTox: Clinical and Research Information on Drug-Induced Liver Injury. Bethesda, MD, National Institute of Diabetes and Digestive and Kidney Diseases, 2012

Sidhu G, Marwaha R: Phenelzine, in StatPearls. Treasure Island, FL, StatPearls Publishing, 2022 32119395

Sub Laban T, Saadabadi A: Monoamine oxidase inhibitors (MAOI), in StatPearls. Treasure Island, FL, StatPearls Publishing, 2021 30969670

Zajecka JM, Fawcett J: Antidepressant combination and potentiation. Psychiatr Med 9(1):55–75, 1991 2017568

References

Balon R, Mufti R, Arfken CL: A survey of prescribing practices for monoamine oxidase inhibitors. Psychiatr Serv 50(7):945–947, 1999 10402617

Brown C, Taniguchi G, Yip K: The monoamine oxidase inhibitor–tyramine interaction. J Clin Pharmacol 29(6):529–532, 1989 2666453

Ciraulo DA, Shader RI: Question the experts. J Clin Psychopharmacol 10(4):306, 1990

Dardis C, Omoregie E, Ly V: Fatal serotonin syndrome precipitated by oxcarbazepine in a patient using an selective serotonin reuptake inhibitor. Neurologist 18(4):204–205, 2012 22735246

Davidson JR: Pharmacotherapy of social phobia. Acta Psychiatr Scand Suppl 417(417):65–71, 2003 12950437

Dursun SM, Mathew VM, Reveley MA. Toxic serotonin syndrome after fluoxetine plus carbamazepine. Lancet 342(8868):442–443, 1993

Fergusson D, Doucette S, Glass KC, et al: Association between suicide attempts and selective serotonin reuptake inhibitors: systematic review of randomised controlled trials. BMJ 330(7488):396, 2005 15718539

Gardner DM, Lynd LD: Sumatriptan contraindications and the serotonin syndrome. Ann Pharmacother 32(1):33–38, 1998 9475817

Gillman PK: Triptans, serotonin agonists, and serotonin syndrome (serotonin toxicity): a review. Headache 50(2):264–272, 2010 19925619

Gillman PK: A reassessment of the safety profile of monoamine oxidase inhibitors: elucidating tired old tyramine myths. J Neural Transm (Vienna) 125(11):1707–1717, 2018 30255284

Heise CW, Malashock H, Brooks DE: A review of vilazodone exposures with focus on serotonin syndrome effects. Clin Toxicol (Phila) 55(9):1004–1007, 2017 28594246

Keegan MT, Brown DR, Rabinstein AA: Serotonin syndrome from the interaction of cyclobenzaprine with other serotoninergic drugs. Anesth Analg 103(6):1466–1468, 2006 17122225

Łojko D, Rybakowski JK: Atypical depression: current perspectives. Neuropsychiatr Dis Treat 13:2447–2456, 2017 29033570

Nierenberg AA, Keck PE Jr: Management of monoamine oxidase inhibitor-associated insomnia with trazodone. J Clin Psychopharmacol 9(1):42–45, 1989 2708555

Quitkin FM, Stewart JW, McGrath PJ, et al: Phenelzine versus imipramine in the treatment of probable atypical depression: defining syndrome boundaries of selective MAOI responders. Am J Psychiatry 145(3):306–311, 1988 3278631

Quitkin FM, McGrath PJ, Stewart JW, et al: Atypical depression, panic attacks, and response to imipramine and phenelzine: a replication. Arch Gen Psychiatry 47(10):935–941, 1990 2222132

Rabkin J, Quitkin F, Harrison W, et al: Adverse reactions to monoamine oxidase inhibitors. Part I. A comparative study. J Clin Psychopharmacol 4(5):270–278, 1984 6386898

Rapaport MH: Dietary restrictions and drug interactions with monoamine oxidase inhibitors: the state of the art. J Clin Psychiatry 68(Suppl 8):42–46, 2007 17640157

Rastogi R, Swarm RA, Patel TA: Case scenario: opioid association with serotonin syndrome: implications to the practitioners. Anesthesiology 115(6):1291–1298, 2011 22037635

Rim CL, Gitlin MJ: Ziprasidone, monoamine oxidase inhibitors, and the serotonin syndrome. J Clin Psychopharmacol 30(4):470–471, 2010 20631570

Sheehan DV: The management of panic disorder. J Clin Psychiatry 63(Suppl 14):17–21, 2002 12562114

Shulman KI, Walker SE, MacKenzie S, et al: Dietary restriction, tyramine, and the use of monoamine oxidase inhibitors. J Clin Psychopharmacol 9(6):397–402, 1989 2592589

Thomas SJ, Shin M, McInnis MG, et al: Combination therapy with monoamine oxidase inhibitors and other antidepressants or stimulants: strategies for the management of treatment-resistant depression. Pharmacotherapy 35(4):433–449, 2015 25884531

Isocarboxazid

I. **Brand Names**: Marplan

II. **Therapeutic Class**: Monoamine oxidase inhibitor (MAOI) antidepressant

III. **Chemical Name**: 5-methyl-3-isoxazolecarboxylic acid 2-benzylhydrazide

IV. **Mechanism(s) of Action**

A. As a nonselective MAOI, isocarboxazid exerts its antidepressant effect by increasing the levels of norepinephrine, serotonin, and dopamine.

V. **Indications**

A. FDA adult: Depression (second-line treatment)

B. Evidence-based[1] off-label uses:

1. Bulimia nervosa

C. FDA pediatric: None

VI. **Major Contraindications and When to Use Caution**

A. Hypersensitivity to isocarboxazid

B. Pheochromocytoma

C. History of liver disease or abnormal liver function tests

D. Severe renal impairment

E. Confirmed or suspected cerebrovascular defect

F. History of hypertension

G. History of headache

H. Excessive use of caffeine

VII. **Dosage Formulations**

A. Brand tablet (Marplan): 10 mg (*scored*)

VIII. **Dosage Ranges and Guidelines**

A. Start with 10 mg BID. Dosage can be increased by 10 mg/day every 2–4 days up to a maximum of 40 mg/day after 1 week. Can be increased further in increments of 20 mg/week up to a maximum dosage of 60 mg/day (given in 2–4 doses per day).

IX. **Monitoring**

A. Sodium levels: Measure at baseline and 3–4 weeks after initiation to monitor for hyponatremia.

B. Blood pressure monitoring for hypertension.

C. Orthostatic blood pressure monitoring in elderly patients.

D. Liver function tests: Monitor over the first 3 months of use and periodically thereafter.

E. Weight changes: Check weight at 3, 6, and 12 months and yearly thereafter.

F. Risk of manic switch in bipolar patients: Needs to be appropriately monitored.

---

[1]Evidence strength varies; readers are referred to the literature for more detailed information.

X. Relevant Pharmacokinetics/Pharmacodynamics

A. **Metabolism**: Primarily hepatic. Approximately 40% is renally eliminated.

B. **Time to peak plasma concentration**: 3–5 hours

C. **Half-life**: 2.5 hours

D. **Hepatic impairment**: Avoid in patients with hepatic impairment or with history of abnormal liver function tests.

E. **Renal impairment**: Lower dosage in mild to moderate renal impairment and avoid in severe renal impairment.

F. **Elderly individuals**: Dosages lower than 60 mg/day are recommended.

XI. Clinically Relevant Drug Interactions

A. Isocarboxazid should not be used in combination with other MAOIs, tricyclic antidepressants, selective serotonin reuptake inhibitors, serotonin norepinephrine reuptake inhibitors, dextromethorphan, tramadol, methadone, meperidine, pentazocine, carbamazepine, or oxcarbazepine. It should be used with caution with disulfiram, as the combination may lead to toxicity.

B. See the subsections "MAOI–Food and MAOI–Drug Interactions Leading to Hypertensive Crisis" and "MAOI–Drug Interactions Leading to Serotonin Syndrome" in the introduction to MAOIs. Searchable online databases of drug interactions are available, as are specialized software and computer applications.

XII. Adverse Effects

A. **Increased risk of suicidality**:

1. See "Boxed Warning: Suicidality and Antidepressant Drugs" in the introduction to MAOIs. For detailed information, readers are referred to comprehensive sources in the literature (e.g., Fergusson et al. 2005).

B. **Hypertensive crisis**:

1. See "MAOI–Food and MAOI–Drug Interactions Leading to Hypertensive Crisis" in introduction to MAOIs.

C. **Serotonin syndrome**:

1. See "MAOI–Drug Interactions Leading to Serotonin Syndrome" in introduction to MAOIs.

D. **Other effects**:

1. Cardiovascular:
   a. Orthostatic hypotension
   b. New-onset hypertension
   c. Palpitations
2. Gastrointestinal:
   a. Constipation
   b. Nausea
   c. Xerostomia
3. Genitourinary:
   a. Sexual side effects

4. Neurological:
    a. Dizziness
    b. Headache
    c. Insomnia

E. **Risks in pregnancy and lactation**
    1. Isocarboxazid was designated a Category C drug in the prior FDA classification and should not be used in pregnant women unless the benefits outweigh the risk to the fetus.
    2. No clear evidence of presence in breast milk during lactation is seen. However, breastfeeding with ongoing use of isocarboxazid is not recommended.

XIII. **Clinical Pearls/Prescribing Tips**

A. Isocarboxazid is not recommended for use in patients younger than 16 years.
B. Use of isocarboxazid can suppress anginal pain and should be avoided in individuals with or at risk of angina and myocardial infarction.
C. Isocarboxazid should be used with caution at dosages higher than 40 mg/day.
D. Improvement in depressive symptoms may be noticed after 1–6 weeks of treatment with isocarboxazid.
E. Concomitant use of isocarboxazid and alcohol should be avoided.
F. Isocarboxazid can lower the seizure threshold and should be used with caution in patients with epilepsy.

Further Reading

Giller E Jr, Bialos D, Harkness L, et al: Assessing treatment response to the monoamine oxidase inhibitor isocarboxazid. J Clin Psychiatry 45(7 Pt 2):44–48, 1984 6376484

Isocarboxazid, in Drugs and Lactation Database (LactMed). Bethesda, MD, National Library of Medicine, 2018. Available at: https://www.ncbi.nlm.nih.gov/books/NBK501737/. Accessed March 13, 2024.

Isocarboxazid: PubChem Compound Summary for CID 3759. National Center for Biotechnology Information, 2022. Available at: https://pubchem.ncbi.nlm.nih.gov/compound/Isocarboxazid#section=ATC-Code. Accessed March 13, 2024.

Larsen JK, Rafaelsen OJ: Long-term treatment of depression with isocarboxazide. Acta Psychiatr Scand 62(5):456–463, 1980 7211430

Validus Pharmaceuticals: Marplan (isocarboxazid) [package insert]. Revised October 2020. Available at: https://marplan.com/marplan-prescribing-info-10-2020.pdf. Accessed March 13, 2024.

Zisook S: Side effects of isocarboxazid. J Clin Psychiatry 45(7 Pt 2):53–58, 1984 6376485

References

Fergusson D, Doucette S, Glass KC, et al: Association between suicide attempts and selective serotonin reuptake inhibitors: systematic review of randomised controlled trials. BMJ 330(7488):396, 2005 15718539

Phenelzine

I. **Brand Names**: Nardil

II. **Therapeutic Class**: Monoamine oxidase inhibitor (MAOI) antidepressant

III. **Chemical Name**: 2-phenylethylhydrazine

IV. **Mechanism(s) of Action**

A. As an irreversible nonselective MAOI, phenelzine exerts its antidepressant effect via increasing the levels of norepinephrine, serotonin, and dopamine.

B. GABA effects

C. Metabolite phenylethylidenehydrazine (PEH) leads to an elevation in brain GABA, with anxiolytic effects (Todd and Baker 1995).

V. **Indications**

A. FDA adult:

1. Major depressive disorder

B. Evidence-based[1] off-label uses:

1. Bulimia nervosa, social anxiety disorder

C. FDA pediatric: None

VI. **Major Contraindications and When to Use Caution**

A. Hypersensitivity to phenelzine

B. Pheochromocytoma

C. History of liver disease or abnormal liver function tests

D. Severe renal impairment

E. Congestive heart failure

VII. **Dosage Formulations**

A. Generic and brand tablet (15 mg)

VIII. **Dosage Ranges and Guidelines**

A. Start with 15 mg TID. The dosage can be increased to 60–90 mg/day in 3–4 divided doses. Can also dose nightly if better tolerated. Once-daily dosing is sufficient for the MAO-inhibitory effects of the drug.

IX. **Monitoring**

A. Blood pressure monitoring for hypertension

B. Orthostatic blood pressure monitoring in elderly patients

C. Weight should be monitored at approximately 3, 6, and 12 months.

D. Risk of manic switch in bipolar patients—needs to be appropriately monitored

X. **Relevant Pharmacokinetics/Pharmacodynamics**

A. **Metabolism**: Primarily by the monoamine oxidase enzyme. Metabolites are excreted renally.

[1]Evidence strength varies; readers are referred to the literature for more detailed information.

B. **Time to peak plasma concentration**: 45 minutes
C. **Half-life**: 11 hours
D. **Hepatic impairment**: Use lower dosage in mild to moderate hepatic impairment (Child-Pugh Score class A and B). Avoid use in severe hepatic impairment (Child-Pugh class C).
E. **Renal impairment**: No dosage adjustment required.
F. **Elderly individuals**: Can start with 15 mg/day and increase up to 30–60 mg/day in divided doses.

XI. **Clinically Relevant Drug Interactions**

A. No significant cytochrome P450 (CYP) interactions
B. Should not be used in combination with medications such as other MAOIs, tricyclic antidepressants, selective serotonin reuptake inhibitors, serotonin norepinephrine reuptake inhibitors, dextromethorphan, tramadol, meperidine, methadone, pentazocine, carbamazepine, oxcarbazepine.
C. See the subsections "MAOI–Food and MAOI–Drug Interactions Leading to Hypertensive Crisis" and "MAOI–Drug Interactions Leading to Serotonin Syndrome" in the introduction to MAOIs. Searchable online databases of drug interactions are available, as are specialized software and computer applications.

XII. **Adverse Effects**

A. **Increased risk of suicidality**:
   1. See "Boxed Warning: Suicidality and Antidepressant Drugs" in the introduction to MAOIs. For detailed information, readers are referred to comprehensive sources in the literature (e.g., Fergusson et al. 2005).

B. **Hypertensive crisis**:
   1. See "MAOI–Food and MAOI–Drug Interactions Leading to Hypertensive Crisis" in introduction to MAOIs.

C. **Serotonin syndrome**:
   1. See "MAOI–Drug Interactions Leading to Serotonin Syndrome" in introduction to MAOIs.

D. **Other effects**:
   1. Cardiovascular:
      a. Orthostatic hypotension—likely dosage dependent
      b. New-onset hypertension
      c. Edema
   2. Dermatological:
      a. Sweating
   3. Endocrine:
      a. Vitamin B_6 deficiency
      b. Weight gain

4. Gastrointestinal:
    a. Constipation
    b. Xerostomia
    c. Increased appetite
5. Genitourinary:
    a. Sexual side effects
6. Hematological:
    a. Leukopenia
    b. Methemoglobinemia
7. Hepatic:
    a. Hepatotoxicity
8. Neurological:
    a. Headache
    b. Insomnia
    c. Dizziness
    d. Sedation

E. **Risks in pregnancy and lactation**

1. The safety of use during pregnancy is not established. Phenelzine should not be used in pregnant women unless the benefits outweigh the risk to the fetus.
2. Evidence of presence in breast milk during lactation is not available. Patients should avoid breastfeeding during phenelzine treatment and up to 7 days after the last dose.

XIII. **Clinical Pearls/Prescribing Tips**

A. Sudden discontinuation can lead to symptoms of dizziness, nausea, headache, irritability, insomnia, anxiety, and even delirium. A gradual reduction in dosage is recommended.
B. Improvement in depressive symptoms may be noticed after 1–3 weeks of phenelzine treatment.
C. Consider use of phenelzine in depressed patients with comorbid anxiety, given its GABA-promoting effects.
D. Higher risks of sexual side effects and weight gain are seen with phenelzine compared with more activating MAOIs (selegiline, tranylcypromine).

Further Reading

Grant JE, Baldwin DS, Chamberlain SR. Time to reconsider monoamine oxidase inhibitors for obsessive compulsive disorder? A case series using phenelzine. J Clin Psychopharmacol 41(4):461–464, 2021

Mountjoy CQ, Roth M, Garside RF, Leitch IM: A clinical trial of phenelzine in anxiety depressive and phobic neuroses. Br J Psychiatry 131:486–492, 1977 338081

Parke-Davis: Nardil (phenelzine) [package insert]. Revised October 2008. Available at: https://cdn.pfizer.com/pfizercom/products/uspi_nardil.pdf. Accessed March 13, 2024.

Phenelzine, in Drugs and Lactation Database (LactMed). Bethesda, MD, National Library of Medicine, 2021. Available at: https://www.ncbi.nlm.nih.gov/books/NBK501172/. Accessed March 13, 2024.

Phenelzine, PubChem Compound Summary for CID 3675. National Center for Biotechnology Information, 2022

Sidhu G, Marwaha R: Phenelzine, in StatPearls. Treasure Island, FL, StatPearls Publishing, 2022

Robinson DS, Lerfald SC, Bennett B, et al: Continuation and maintenance treatment of major depression with the monoamine oxidase inhibitor phenelzine: a double-blind placebo-controlled discontinuation study. Psychopharmacol Bull 27(1):31–39, 1991

Walsh BT, Stewart JW, Roose SP, et al: Treatment of bulimia with phenelzine: a double-blind, placebo-controlled study. Arch Gen Psychiatry 41(11):1105–1109, 1984 6388524

References

Fergusson D, Doucette S, Glass KC, et al: Association between suicide attempts and selective serotonin reuptake inhibitors: systematic review of randomised controlled trials. BMJ 330(7488):396, 2005 15718539

Todd KG, Baker GB: GABA-elevating effects of the antidepressant/antipanic drug phenelzine in brain: effects of pretreatment with tranylcypromine, (-)-deprenyl and clorgyline. J Affect Disord 35(3):125–129, 1995 8749840

Selegiline

I. **Brand Names**: Eldepryl, Zelapar; Emsam (transdermal patch system)

II. **Therapeutic Class**: Monoamine oxidase inhibitor (MAOI) antidepressant

III. **Chemical Name**: (R)-(-)-N,2-dimethyl-N-2-propynylphenethylamine

IV. **Mechanism(s) of Action**

- A. Irreversible monoamine oxidase (MAO) inhibitor. At low dosages: blocks MAO-B, affecting dopamine levels. At higher levels, nonspecific monoamine oxidase inhibition (blocks MAO type A and B) leads to antidepressant effects via increased norepinephrine and serotonin.

V. **Indications**

- A. FDA adult:
  1. Oral formulations: Parkinson's disease with levodopa/carbidopa
  2. Transdermal formulation: Major depressive disorder
- B. Evidence-based off-label uses: None
- C. FDA pediatric: None

VI. **Major Contraindications and When to Use Caution**

- A. Hypersensitivity to selegiline

B. Children younger than 12 years

1. Use of selegiline transdermal patch is contraindicated in patients younger than 12 years because of an increased risk of hypertensive crisis.

C. Pheochromocytoma

VII. **Dosage Formulations**

A. Generic and brand capsule: 5 mg
B. ODT (Zelapar): 1.25 mg
C. Transdermal patch system (Emsam): 20 mg/20 cm^2—6 mg/24 hours, 9 mg/24 hours, 12 mg/24 hours

VIII. **Dosage Ranges and Guidelines**

A. Refer to Table 2–15 for dosage ranges (initial/maximum) and guidelines.
B. Major depressive disorder (transdermal patch): Start at 6 mg/day patch, and increase by 3 mg/day at 2-week intervals
C. Parkinson's disease (oral): Start at 5 mg/day or 5 mg BID. Increase to maximum dosage of 5 mg BID.

Table 2–15. Selegiline indications and dosage ranges

Indication	Usual dosage range
Major depressive disorder	Patch: 6–12 mg/day
Parkinson's disease	PO: 5 mg BID ODT: 1.25–1.5 mg/day

IX. **Monitoring**

A. Blood pressure monitoring for hypertension
B. Orthostatic blood pressure monitoring in elderly patients
C. Risk of manic switch in bipolar patients—needs to be appropriately monitored

X. **Relevant Pharmacokinetics/Pharmacodynamics**

A. **Metabolism**: Primarily hepatic; no renal involvement. Oral forms have a significant first-pass effect, although the transdermal form bypasses this. Cytochrome P450 (CYP) metabolism: CYP2B6, CYP2C9, CYP3A4/5.
B. **Major metabolites**: *N*-desmethyl selegiline and R(-)-methamphetamine
C. **Time to peak plasma concentration**: Oral form: <1 hour; transdermal form: 20 hours
D. **Half-life**: Oral form: 1.5–2 hours; transdermal form: 18–25 hours
E. **Time to steady-state drug levels (transdermal form)**: 5 days
F. **Hepatic impairment**: No dosage adjustment is needed for mild to moderate hepatic impairment (using the patch only; oral forms may require dosage adjustment).
G. **Renal impairment**: No dosage adjustment is needed for mild to moderate renal impairment (using the patch only; oral forms may require dosage adjustment).
H. **Elderly individuals**: Recommended dosage for elderly patients is 6 mg/day.

XI. **Clinically Relevant Drug Interactions**

A. Metabolized by CYP2B6, CYP2C9, and CYP3A4/5.
B. Competitive inhibitor of CYP2D6 and CYP3A4/5
C. See the subsections "MAOI–Food and MAOI–Drug Interactions Leading to Hypertensive Crisis" and "MAOI–Drug Interactions Leading to Serotonin Syndrome" in the introduction to MAOIs. Searchable online databases of drug interactions are available, as are specialized software and computer applications.
D. Selegiline should not be used in combination with medications such as other MAOIs, tricyclic antidepressants, selective serotonin reuptake inhibitors, serotonin norepinephrine reuptake inhibitors, dextromethorphan, tramadol, meperidine, methadone, pentazocine, carbamazepine, oxcarbazepine. Dietary modifications are required when using the transdermal patch at dosages greater than 6 mg/day.

XII. **Adverse Effects**

A. **Increased risk of suicidality**:
   1. See "Boxed Warning: Suicidality and Antidepressant Drugs" in the introduction to MAOIs. For detailed information, readers are referred to comprehensive sources in the literature (e.g., Fergusson et al. 2005).

B. **Hypertensive crisis**:
   1. Use of selegiline transdermal patch is contraindicated in patients younger than 12 years because of an increased risk of hypertensive crisis.
   2. See "MAOI–Food and MAOI–Drug Interactions Leading to Hypertensive Crisis" in introduction to MAOIs.

C. **Serotonin syndrome**:
   1. See "MAOI–Drug Interactions Leading to Serotonin Syndrome" in introduction to MAOIs.

D. **Other effects**:
   1. Cardiovascular:
      a. Orthostatic hypotension—likely dosage dependent
      b. New-onset hypertension
   2. Dermatological:
      a. Application site reactions with transdermal form.
      b. Use of selegiline transdermal patch is contraindicated in patients younger than 12 years because of an increased risk of hypertensive crisis.
   3. Gastrointestinal:
      a. Diarrhea
   4. Genitourinary:
      a. Sexual side effects
   5. Neurological:
      a. Headache
      b. Insomnia

E. **Risks in pregnancy and lactation**

1. Selegiline was previously designated a Pregnancy Category C drug and should not be used in pregnant women unless the benefits outweigh the risks to the fetus.
2. Rodent data show that selegiline is present in rodent milk. Patients should avoid breastfeeding during treatment and up to 7 days after the last dose.

XIII. **Clinical Pearls/Prescribing Tips**

A. The transdermal patch allows for ease of administration. It bypasses the first-pass metabolism and can easily be used in conditions where poor/limited gastrointestinal absorption is a concern.
B. Prolonged exposure to sun or sources of external heat should be avoided with the use of the transdermal patch, as such exposure may lead to an increase in selegiline absorption.
C. The patch should not be cut into smaller pieces or tampered with, as doing so may change drug levels.
D. Improvement in depressive symptoms may be noticed after 1–3 weeks of selegiline treatment.
E. Selegiline produces an amphetamine metabolite that may lead to positive drug screens. This metabolite also makes selegiline more activating, which can be beneficial for depression.

Further Reading

Amsterdam JD: A double-blind, placebo-controlled trial of the safety and efficacy of selegiline transdermal system without dietary restrictions in patients with major depressive disorder. J Clin Psychiatry 64(2):208–214, 2003 12633131

Amsterdam JD, Bodkin JA: Selegiline transdermal system in the prevention of relapse of major depressive disorder: a 52-week, double-blind, placebo-substitution, parallel-group clinical trial. J Clin Psychopharmacol 26(6):579–586, 2006 17110814

Bodkin JA, Amsterdam JD: Transdermal selegiline in major depression: a double-blind, placebo-controlled, parallel-group study in outpatients. Am J Psychiatry 159(11):1869–1875, 2002 12411221

Feiger AD, Rickels K, Rynn MA, et al: Selegiline transdermal system for the treatment of major depressive disorder: an 8-week, double-blind, placebo-controlled, flexible-dosage titration trial. J Clin Psychiatry 67(9):1354–1361, 2006 17017821

Mahmood I: Clinical pharmacokinetics and pharmacodynamics of selegiline: an update. Clin Pharmacokinet 33(2):91–102, 1997 9260033

Mizuno Y, Hattori N, Kondo T, et al: A randomized double-blind placebo-controlled Phase III trial of selegiline monotherapy for early Parkinson disease. Clin Neuropharmacol 40(5):201–207, 2017 28857772

Moore JJ: Selegiline, in StatPearls. Treasure Island, FL, StatPearls Publishing, 2022

Romberg RW, Needleman SB, Snyder JJ, et al: Methamphetamine and amphetamine derived from the metabolism of selegiline. J Forensic Sci 40(6):1100–1102, 1995 8522918

Rubinstein S, Malone MA, Roberts W, et al: Placebo-controlled study examining effects of selegiline in children with attention-deficit/hyperactivity disorder. J Child Adolesc Psychopharmacol 16(4):404–415, 2006 16958566

Selegiline, in Drugs and Lactation Database (LactMed). Bethesda, MD, National Library of Medicine, 2021. Available at: https://www.ncbi.nlm.nih.gov/books/NBK501755. Accessed March 13, 2024.

Somerset Pharmaceuticals: Eldepryl (selegiline) [package insert]. U.S. Food and Drug Administration website. January 2008. Available at: https://www.accessdata.fda.gov/drugsatfda_docs/label/2008/020647s006s007lbl.pdf. Accessed March 13, 2024.

Somerset Pharmaceuticals: Emsam (selegiline) [package insert]. U.S. Food and Drug Administration website. June 2007. Available at: https://www.accessdata.fda.gov/drugsatfda_docs/label/2007/021336s002lbl.pdf. Accessed March 13, 2024.

Valeant Pharmaceuticals North America: Zelapar ODT (selegiline) [package insert]. U.S. Food and Drug Administration website. February 2008. Available at: https://www.accessdata.fda.gov/drugsatfda_docs/label/2008/021479s003s004lbl.pdf. Accessed March 13, 2024.

References

Fergusson D, Doucette S, Glass KC, et al: Association between suicide attempts and selective serotonin reuptake inhibitors: systematic review of randomised controlled trials. BMJ 330(7488):396, 2005 15718539

Tranylcypromine

I. **Brand Names**: Parnate

II. **Therapeutic Class**: Monoamine oxidase inhibitor (MAOI) antidepressant

III. **Chemical Name**: (±)-trans-2-phenylcyclopropylamine sulfate

IV. **Mechanism(s) of Action**

A. As an irreversible nonselective MAOI, tranylcypromine exerts its antidepressant effect via increasing the levels of norepinephrine, serotonin, and dopamine.

V. **Indications**

A. FDA adult: Major depressive disorder (second-line treatment)

B. Evidence-based off-label uses: None

C. FDA pediatric: None

VI. **Major Contraindications and When to Use Caution**

A. Hypersensitivity to tranylcypromine

B. Pheochromocytoma

C. Confirmed or suspected cerebrovascular defect

D. History of liver disease

E. History of headache

VII. **Dosage Formulations**

A. Brand and generic tablet (10 mg)

VIII. **Dosage Ranges and Guidelines**

A. Initial dosage of 30 mg/day in divided doses. Dosage can be increased by 10 mg/day every 1 to 3 weeks up to a maximum dosage of 60 mg/day. Once daily dosing is sufficient for the MAO inhibitory effects of the drug.

IX. **Monitoring**

A. Blood pressure monitoring for hypertension.

B. Orthostatic blood pressure monitoring in elderly patients.

C. Liver function tests to be monitored over the first 3 months of use and then periodically.

D. Weight should be monitored at approximately 3, 6, and 12 months.

E. Risk of manic switch in bipolar patients; needs to be appropriately monitored.

X. **Relevant Pharmacokinetics/Pharmacodynamics**

A. **Metabolism**: Primarily hepatic

B. **Time to peak plasma concentration**: 0.67–3.5 hours

C. **Half-life**: 1.5–3.5 hours

D. **Elderly individuals**: Can start at a lower initial dosage and increase the dosage slowly.

XI. **Clinically Relevant Drug Interactions**

A. No significant cytochrome P450 (CYP) interactions

B. Tranylcypromine should not be used in combination with medications such as other MAOIs, tricyclic antidepressants, selective serotonin reuptake inhibitors, serotonin-norepinephrine reuptake inhibitors, dextromethorphan, tramadol, meperidine, methadone, pentazocine, carbamazepine, oxcarbazepine, dopamine, L-dopa, *S*-adenosyl-L-methionine (SAM-e), amphetamine, or methylphenidate.

C. See the subsections "MAOI–Food and MAOI–Drug Interactions Leading to Hypertensive Crisis" and "MAOI–Drug Interactions Leading to Serotonin Syndrome" in the introduction to MAOIs. Searchable online databases of drug interactions are available, as are specialized software and computer applications.

XII. **Adverse Effects**

A. **Increased risk of suicidality**:

1. See "Boxed Warning: Suicidality and Antidepressant Drugs" in the introduction to MAOIs. For detailed information, readers are referred to comprehensive sources in the literature (e.g., Fergusson et al. 2005).

B. **Hypertensive crisis**:

1. See "MAOI–Food and MAOI–Drug Interactions Leading to Hypertensive Crisis" in introduction to MAOIs.

C. **Serotonin syndrome**:

1. See "MAOI–Drug Interactions Leading to Serotonin Syndrome" in introduction to MAOIs.

D. **Other effects**:

1. Cardiovascular:
    a. Orthostatic hypotension (likely dosage dependent)
    b. New-onset hypertension
2. Endocrine:
    a. Syndrome of inappropriate antidiuretic hormone (SIADH)
3. Gastrointestinal:
    a. Nausea
    b. Diarrhea
4. Genitourinary:
    a. Sexual side effects
5. Hematological:
    a. Agranulocytosis
    b. Leukopenia
    c. Thrombocytopenia
6. Neurological:
    a. Headache
    b. Insomnia
    c. Akathisia
    d. Sedation

E. **Risks in pregnancy and lactation**:

1. Tranylcypromine's impact on fetal development during pregnancy is unclear. This medication should not be used in pregnant women unless the benefits outweigh the risks to the fetus.
2. Evidence of presence in breast milk during lactation is not available. Patients should avoid breastfeeding during treatment.

XIII. **Clinical Pearls/Prescribing Tips**

A. Sudden discontinuation can lead to symptoms of dizziness, nausea, headache, irritability, insomnia, anxiety, and even delirium. A gradual reduction in dosage is recommended.

B. Postural hypotension is a significant issue at dosages higher than 30 mg/day.

C. Some adverse effects of tranylcypromine can make driving and handling machinery potentially hazardous. Patients should be cautioned to avoid these activities until the effects of the medication are known

D. Improvement in depressive symptoms may be noticed after 1–6 weeks of tranylcypromine treatment.

E. The structure of tranylcypromine is more "amphetamine-like," although it does not produce true amphetamine metabolites like selegiline. It is one of the more activating MAOIs. One downside is that multiple daily dosing may be required.

Further Reading

Concordia Pharmaceuticals: Parnate (tranylcypromine) [package insert]. U.S. Food and Drug Administration website. Revised January 2018. Available at: https://www.accessdata.fda.gov/drugsatfda_docs/label/2018/012342s064lbl.pdf. Accessed March 13, 2024.

Parikh N, Yilanli M, Saadabadi A: Tranylcypromine, in StatPearls. Treasure Island, FL, StatPearls Publishing, 2022

Parnate. PubChem Compound Summary for CID 19493, National Center for Biotechnology Information, 2022. Available at: https://pubchem.ncbi.nlm.nih.gov/compound/Isocarboxazid#section=ATC-Code. Accessed March 13, 2024.

Tranylcypromine, in Drugs and Lactation Database (LactMed). Bethesda, MD, National Library of Medicine, 2021. Available at: https://www.ncbi.nlm.nih.gov/books/NBK501173/. Accessed March 13, 2024.

Versiani M, Mundim FD, Nardi AE, et al: Tranylcypromine in social phobia. J Clin Psychopharmacol 8(4):279–283, 1988 3209719

References

Fergusson D, Doucette S, Glass KC, et al: Association between suicide attempts and selective serotonin reuptake inhibitors: systematic review of randomised controlled trials. BMJ 330(7488):396, 2005 15718539

Tricyclic Antidepressants

General Considerations for Use of TCAs

- Previously used as first-line antidepressants, tricyclic antidepressants (TCAs) are generally considered to be second- or third-line antidepressants in modern practice because of their tolerability concerns and the potential for toxicity. However, specific properties of TCAs are harnessed in clinical practice today, including concomitant insomnia, neuropathic pain, irritable bowel syndrome, migraine, and treatment-resistant depression.
- TCAs are categorized as secondary amines or tertiary amines:
  - Tertiary amines include amitriptyline, imipramine, and clomipramine.
  - Secondary amines include nortriptyline (a metabolite of amitriptyline) and desipramine (a metabolite of imipramine).
  - Tertiary amines tend to be more potent inhibitors of the SERT (serotonin transporter) than of the NET (norepinephrine transporter), and the opposite is generally true for the secondary amines. Tertiary amines also tend to be more anticholinergic than secondary amines.
    1. Amitriptyline (SERT > NET) → Nortriptyline (NET > SERT)
    2. Imipramine (SERT > NET) → Desipramine (NET > SERT)

Overdose/Toxicity With TCAs

- TCAs generally have a narrow therapeutic index. Hence, toxicity from intentional or unintentional overdose is possible. Therapeutic drug monitoring can help ensure that medication levels remain within the normal range for patients.
- Overdose on TCAs can be life-threatening and potentially fatal. Some TCAs (e.g., desipramine, nortriptyline) are toxic at lower dosages than others (e.g., amitriptyline). Signs of toxicity can appear within 2 hours of ingestion.
- Symptoms of overdose include signs of anticholinergic toxicity (e.g., flushing, anhidrosis, dry mucous membranes, mydriasis, fever, urinary retention) as well as other signs (e.g., confusion, transient visual hallucinations, drowsiness, hypothermia, hypotension, tachycardia or other arrhythmias/ECG changes, convulsions, stupor, coma).
- Treatment for TCA overdose is symptomatic and supportive, with ongoing cardiac and respiratory monitoring. Early intubation for signs of CNS depression is indicated. Sodium bicarbonate may be used to maintain blood pH levels. Seizures may be controlled by using benzodiazepines. Use of physostigmine may reverse some of the cardiac and neurological effects.

TCA Warnings and Precautions

- **TCAs and Electroconvulsive Therapy**: TCAs are more commonly associated with prolonged QTc than are SSRIs. TCAs prolong the QTc interval by blocking sodium channels. TCAs are also associated with widening of the QRS complex on ECG.
- **TcAs and QTc Interval Prolongation**: TCAs are known to decrease the seizure threshold, and ECT should be used with caution in patients who are taking TCAs.

Boxed Warning: Suicidality and Antidepressant Drugs*
Increased risk of suicidal thoughts and behaviors in pediatric and young adult patients in the short term. Close monitoring of patients for emergence of suicidal thoughts and behaviors is required.
**Note.* This warning on suicidality met with controversy. For a detailed discussion, the reader is referred to comprehensive sources in the literature (e.g., Fergusson et al. 2005).

Further Reading

Moraczewski J, Aedma KK: Tricyclic antidepressants, in StatPearls. Treasure Island, FL, StatPearls Publishing, 2022

Khalid MM, Waseem M: Tricyclic antidepressant toxicity, in StatPearls. Treasure Island, FL, StatPearls Publishing; 2022

Nachimuthu S, Assar MD, Schussler JM: Drug-induced QT interval prolongation: mechanisms and clinical management. Ther Adv Drug Saf 3(5):241–253, 2012

References

Fergusson D, Doucette S, Glass KC, et al: Association between suicide attempts and selective serotonin reuptake inhibitors: systematic review of randomised controlled trials. BMJ 330(7488):396, 2005 15718539

Amitriptyline

I. **Brand Names**: Elavil

II. **Therapeutic Class**: Tricyclic antidepressant (TCA), tertiary amine

III. **Chemical Name**: *N,N*-dimethyl-3-(2-tricyclo[9.4.0.$0^{3,8}$]pentadeca-1(15),3,5,7,11,13-hexaenylidene)propan-1-amine

IV. **Mechanism(s) of Action**

A. In common with other TCAs, amitriptyline inhibits the membrane reuptake of norepinephrine and serotonin by adrenergic and serotonergic neurons at the presynaptic membranes, leading to increased levels of serotonin and norepinephrine in the synapse, which may potentiate or prolong neuronal activity and may be related to amitriptyline's antidepressant effects. The higher levels of norepinephrine and serotonin in the spinal cord are related to amitriptyline's effects on pain.

B. Amitriptyline is a tertiary amine and is metabolized to the secondary amine nortriptyline.

C. Amitriptyline exhibits more potent serotonin transporter (SERT) inhibition than norepinephrine transporter (NET) inhibition: SERT Ki=2.8–3.6 nM versus NET Ki=19–102 nM (Roth and Driscoll 1999–present). However, its metabolite, nortriptyline, is a more potent NET inhibitor.

D. Other notable receptor actions are histamine-1 (H_1) inhibition (Ki=0.5–11 nM), alpha-1 (α_1) inhibition (Ki=6.25–25 nM), cholinergic (muscarinic acetylcholine [mACh]) inhibition (M_2 Ki=11.8 nM), 5-HT_{2A} inhibition (Ki=18–23 nM), and 5-HT_{2C} inhibition (Ki=4–8 nM).

V. **Indications**

A. FDA adult: Major depressive disorder

B. Evidence-based[1] off-label uses:

1. Fibromyalgia
2. Migraine
3. Irritable bowel syndrome
4. Diabetic neuralgia
5. Postherpetic neuralgia
6. Tinnitus

C. FDA pediatric: None

VI. **Major Contraindications and When to Use Caution**

A. **Contraindications**:

1. Hypersensitivity to amitriptyline
2. Concomitant use with a monoamine oxidase inhibitor (MAOI)
3. Acute phase of recovery after myocardial infarction
4. Acute congestive heart failure
5. Children younger than 12 years

---

[1]Evidence strength varies; readers are referred to the literature for more detailed information.

B. **Use caution:**

1. History of seizures
2. Impaired liver function or history of liver impairment
3. Blood dyscrasias
4. Urinary retention
5. Narrow angle glaucoma
6. History of cardiovascular disease such as myocardial infarction or congestive heart failure
7. Concomitant electroconvulsive therapy (ECT)
8. Patients with hyperthyroidism or on medication for hypothyroidism

VII. **Dosage Formulations**

A. Generic tablet (10 mg, 25 mg, 75 mg, 100 mg, 150 mg)

VIII. **Dosage Ranges and Guidelines**

A. Depression: May start with 25 mg TID. Dosage can be increased to 150 mg/day. May be increased to a maximum of 300 mg/day. It may be possible to limit to once-a-day dosing at night for some patients.
B. Fibromyalgia (off-label): 25–50 mg/day at bedtime
C. Migraine prevention (off-label): 25 mg/day at bedtime
D. Diabetic neuropathy (off-label): 75–150 mg/day
E. Postherpetic neuralgia (off-label): 25–150 mg/day in divided doses
F. Tinnitus (off-label): 50 mg at bedtime for 1 week and then 100 mg at bedtime for 5 weeks
G. Irritable bowel syndrome (IBS) (off-label): 10–25 mg at bedtime; gradually increase to a dosage of 50–100 mg/day

IX. **Monitoring**

A. Therapeutic drug monitoring:

1. Timing of level: Draw trough level immediately prior to next dose (or at least 12–16 hours after the last dose) (Ziegler et al. 1977). If drawn too early, artificially elevated levels may be present.
2. Optimal response is correlated with combined serum levels of amitriptyline + nortriptyline of 80–200 ng/mL. Toxicity risk increases with levels of 300–500 ng/mL (Hiemke et al. 2018).
3. Plasma levels and therapeutic dosage levels are difficult to correlate. Plasma levels can be monitored to ensure nontoxic levels, given the heterogeneity of the cytochrome P450 (CYP) pathways involved in amitriptyline's metabolism.

B. Sodium levels: Measure at baseline and after 3–4 weeks.
C. Liver function tests: Monitor periodically.
D. Obtain an ECG at baseline, after dosage changes, and up to every 3 months for patients with specific cardiac risk factors.
E. Blood pressure: Measure at baseline, after dosage changes, and every 3–6 months once stabilized.
F. Weight changes: Check weight at 3, 6, and 12 months and yearly thereafter.
G. Risk of manic switch in bipolar patients: Needs to be appropriately monitored.

X. **Relevant Pharmacokinetics/Pharmacodynamics**

A. **Metabolism**: Rapidly absorbed after oral administration. Bioavailability is 30%–60% because of the high first-pass effect. Primarily metabolized in the liver, and metabolites are renally excreted. Nortriptyline is the major active metabolite. Primarily metabolized by CYP2D6, CYP3A4, and CYP2C19.

B. **Time to peak plasma concentration**: 2–12 hours

C. **Half-life**: 10–28 hours

D. **Hepatic impairment**: Reduced dosages should be used in patients with liver disease.

E. **Renal impairment**: No dosage adjustment required in mild to moderate renal impairment.

F. **Elderly individuals**: Amitriptyline use should be avoided in this population (per the Beers Criteria [American Geriatrics Society 2023]), as it may lead to sedation and orthostasis. If used, amitriptyline should be started at a lower dosage (e.g., 10 mg/day) and increased slowly based on tolerability. It may be used in divided doses (e.g., 10 mg during the day and 20 mg at night).

XI. **Clinically Relevant Drug Interactions**

A. Metabolized by CYP2D6 (major) and by CYP3A4, CYP2C19, CYP2C9, CYP2B6, and CYP1A2 (minor).

B. Caution should be used when prescribing amitriptyline to patients who are taking CYP2D6 inhibitors (e.g., quinidine, cimetidine, fluoxetine, bupropion) or who are known to be poor metabolizers of CYP2D6, as drug concentrations may be higher.

C. Caution should be used when prescribing amitriptyline in combination with other medications, such as the following:

1. Other serotonergic medications, including other TCAs, selective serotonin reuptake inhibitors, serotonin-norepinephrine reuptake inhibitors, monoamine oxidase inhibitors, dextromethorphan, tramadol, methadone, St. John's wort
2. Medications with anticholinergic effects (e.g., atropine, glycopyrrolate, benztropine, trihexyphenidyl, procyclidine, prochlorperazine, meclizine, scopolamine, hydroxyzine)
3. Medications that prolong QTc (e.g., cisapride, amiodarone, sotalol, quinidine, procainamide, fluoroquinolones, sumatriptan, ondansetron, haloperidol, risperidone, ziprasidone, olanzapine, quetiapine, methadone)

XII. **Adverse Effects**

A. Possible increased risk of suicidality:

1. See "Boxed Warning: Suicidality and Antidepressant Drugs" in the introduction to TCAs. For detailed information, readers are referred to comprehensive sources in the literature (e.g., Fergusson et al. 2005).

B. Serotonin syndrome

C. Neuroleptic malignant syndrome

D. Cardiovascular:

1. Arrhythmias
2. Prolonged QTc interval:
    a. Amitriptyline can cause QTc prolongation and other cardiac rhythm changes, especially at higher dosages.
3. Myocardial infarction

E. Gastrointestinal:

1. Nausea
2. Vomiting
3. Increased appetite
4. Amitriptyline may cause transient changes in liver function tests in up to 10% of patients, but these changes appear to be asymptomatic and transient in most cases. Dosage change or discontinuation is not required.

F. Neurological:

1. Dizziness
2. Headache
3. Somnolence
    a. Amitriptyline is well known for its sedative effects. The daily dosage should preferably be taken at night. If the medication is taken in the morning, patients should be advised to use caution with driving, operating machinery, or any activity requiring sustained attention.
4. Seizure
    a. Amitriptyline decreases the seizure threshold and leads to changes in EEG and sleep patterns.

G. Endocrine:

1. Weight gain.
2. Sexual dysfunction
3. Amitriptyline can cause increases in blood glucose levels.

H. Hematological:

1. Agranulocytosis

I. Hepatic:

1. Hepatotoxicity
2. Jaundice

J. Anticholinergic effects:

1. Urinary retention
2. Constipation
3. Paralytic ileus
4. Dry mouth
5. Hyperpyrexia
6. Mydriasis

7. Blurred vision
8. Narrow angle closure glaucoma

K. **Risks in pregnancy and lactation**

1. Amitriptyline was designated a Category C drug in the prior FDA classification and is present in breast milk. A thorough risk/benefit discussion with the patient is recommended on continuing versus stopping the medication, including consultation with an OB/GYN specialist and/or lactation expert. See Chapter 15 ("Women: Pregnancy, Postpartum, and Breastfeeding") for more information.
2. Amitriptyline passes into breast milk, and although it can be used with caution, there are reports of sedation in neonates. Therefore, it may be preferable to avoid breastfeeding during treatment.

XIII. **Clinical Pearls/Prescribing Tips**

A. Amitriptyline's potent antihistamine, anticholinergic, and anti-α_1 activity leads to a relatively high risk of sedation/weight gain, anticholinergic effects, and orthostatic hypotension, respectively.

B. Sedation, QTc prolongation, and a decrease in the seizure threshold are notable potential adverse effects of amitriptyline.

C. Amitriptyline should be discontinued before elective surgery because it may interact with agents used during anesthesia.

D. Improvement in depressive symptoms may be noticed after 2–4 weeks of amitriptyline treatment.

E. TCAs in general have been shown to be more efficacious than SNRIs—and significantly more efficacious than SSRIs—in treating neuropathic pain.

Further Reading

Amitriptyline, in LiverTox: Clinical and Research Information on Drug-Induced Liver Injury. Bethesda, MD, National Institute of Diabetes and Digestive and Kidney Diseases, 2016. Available at: https://www.ncbi.nlm.nih.gov/books/NBK548410/. Accessed March 13, 2024.

Amitryptiline, in PubChem Compound Summary for CID 2160. National Center for Biotechnology Information, 2022. Available at: https://pubchem.ncbi.nlm.nih.gov/compound/Amitriptyline. Accessed March 13, 2024.

Bayar N, Böke B, Turan E, et al: Efficacy of amitriptyline in the treatment of subjective tinnitus. J Otolaryngol 30(5):300–303, 2001 11771024

Gonçalves AL, Martini Ferreira A, Ribeiro RT, et al: Randomised clinical trial comparing melatonin 3 mg, amitriptyline 25 mg and placebo for migraine prevention. J Neurol Neurosurg Psychiatry 87(10):1127–1132, 2016 27165014

Kashani JH, Shekim WO, Reid JC: Amitriptyline in children with major depressive disorder: a double-blind crossover pilot study. J Am Acad Child Psychiatry 23(3):348–351, 1984 6736501

Leth-Møller KB, Hansen AH, Torstensson M, et al. Antidepressants and the risk of hyponatremia: a Danish register-based population study. BMJ Open 6(5):e011200, 2016

Price R, Smith D, Franklin G, et al: Oral and topical treatment of painful diabetic polyneuropathy: practice guideline update summary: report of the AAN Guideline Subcommittee. Neurology 98(1):31–43, 2022 34965987

Quality Care Products LLC: Amitriptyline package insert. U.S. Food and Drug Administration. Revised March 2023. Available at: https://www.accessdata.fda.gov/spl/data/661f467d-c49e-4d53-b736-e3ad591004d8/661f467d-c49e-4d53-b736-e3ad591004d8.xml. Accessed March 13, 2024.

Thour A, Marwaha R: Amitriptyline, in StatPearls. Treasure Island, FL, StatPearls Publishing, 2022

Uçeyler N, Häuser W, Sommer C: A systematic review on the effectiveness of treatment with antidepressants in fibromyalgia syndrome. Arthritis Rheum 59(9):1279–1298, 2008 18759260

Vieweg WV, Wood MA: Tricyclic antidepressants, QT interval prolongation, and torsade de pointes. Psychosomatics 45(5):371–377, 2004 15345781

References

American Geriatrics Society Beers Criteria Update Expert Panel: 2023 updated AGS Beers Criteria for potentially inappropriate medication use in older adults. J Am Geriatr Soc 71(7):2052–2081, 2023 37139824

Fergusson D, Doucette S, Glass KC, et al: Association between suicide attempts and selective serotonin reuptake inhibitors: systematic review of randomised controlled trials. BMJ 330(7488):396, 2005 15718539

Hiemke C, Bergemann N, Clement HW, et al: Consensus guidelines for therapeutic drug monitoring in neuropsychopharmacology: update 2017. Pharmacopsychiatry 51(1–2):9–62, 2018 28910830

Roth BL, Driscoll J: PDSP Ki Database. Psychoactive Drug Screening Program (PDSP). University of North Carolina at Chapel Hill and the United States National Institute of Mental Health, 1999–present. Available at: https://pdsp.unc.edu/databases/pdsp.php. Accessed June 21, 2024.

Ziegler VE, Clayton PJ, Biggs JT: A comparison study of amitriptyline and nortriptyline with plasma levels. Arch Gen Psychiatry 34(5):607–612, 1977 860894

Clomipramine

I. **Brand Names**: Anafranil
II. **Therapeutic Class**: Tricyclic antidepressant (TCA), tertiary amine
III. **Chemical Name**: 3-chloro-5-[3-(dimethylamino)propyl]-10,11-dihydro 5*H*-dibenz[*b*,*f*]azepine monohydrochloride
IV. **Mechanism(s) of Action**

A. Clomipramine inhibits the membrane reuptake of norepinephrine and serotonin by adrenergic and serotonergic neurons at the presynaptic membranes, leading to increased levels of serotonin and norepinephrine in the synapse.
B. Clomipramine is a tertiary amine.
C. Clomipramine exhibits more potent serotonin transporter (SERT) inhibition than norepinephrine transporter (NET) inhibition (SERT Ki=0.14–0.28 nM vs. NET Ki=38–53.7 nM), even more potent than that exhibited by most SSRIs (with the exception of paroxetine).
D. Other receptor effects include α_1-adrenergic receptor inhibition (Ki=3.2–38 nM), cholinergic (muscarinic acetylcholine [mACh]) receptor inhibition (mACh Ki=37 nM), and H_1 receptor inhibition (Ki=13–31 nM) (Roth and Driscoll 1999–present).

V. **Indications**

A. FDA adult: OCD
B. Evidence-based[1] off-label uses:
   1. Major depressive disorder
   2. Panic disorder
   3. Trichotillomania
   4. Premature ejaculation
C. FDA pediatric: None

VI. **Major Contraindications and When to Use Caution**

A. **Contraindications**:
   1. Hypersensitivity to clomipramine
   2. Concomitant use with a monoamine oxidase inhibitor (MAOI) or another TCA
   3. Acute phase of recovery after myocardial infarction
   4. Children younger than 10 years
B. **Use caution**:
   1. Older adults because of anticholinergic and sedating effects
   2. Concomitant alcohol use
   3. Acute angle-closure glaucoma
   4. History of seizures
   5. Patients with hyperthyroidism or on medication for hypothyroidism
   6. Patients who are poor metabolizers of cytochrome P450 (CYP) 2D6

[1]Evidence strength varies; readers are referred to the literature for more detailed information.

VII. **Dosage Formulations**

A. Generic and brand capsule (25 mg, 50 mg, 75 mg)

VIII. **Dosage Ranges and Guidelines**

A. OCD (adult): Start with 25 mg/day and increase by 25 mg every 1–3 days up to 100 mg/day. Maximum dosage: 250 mg/day.

B. OCD (pediatric): Start with 25 mg/day and increase to 3 mg/kg or 100 mg/day (whichever is less) during the initial 2 weeks of treatment. Maximum dosage is 200 mg/day or 3 mg/kg/day (whichever is less).

C. Depression: Up to 200 mg/day in divided doses.

D. Panic disorder: 60–150 mg/day

E. Trichotillomania: 50–250 mg/day

F. Premature ejaculation: Up to 50 mg/day

IX. **Monitoring**

A. Therapeutic drug monitoring:

1. Plasma levels should be monitored after desired target dosage is reached.
2. Timing: Draw trough just before the next dose.
3. Clomipramine's therapeutic range is 230–450 ng/mL (clomipramine+*N*-desmethyl-clomipramine) (Hiemke et al. 2018)
4. Concern for toxicity at levels >450 ng/mL
5. Plasma levels may vary among individuals, given the heterogeneity of the CYP2D6 pathways involved in clomipramine's metabolism.

B. Sodium levels: Measure at baseline and after 3–4 weeks of treatment.

C. Liver function tests: Monitor periodically.

D. Obtain an ECG at baseline, after dosage changes, and up to every 3 months for those with cardiac risk factors.

E. Blood pressure: Measure at baseline, after dosage changes, and every 3–6 months once the dosage is stabilized.

F. Weight changes: Check weight at 3, 6, and 12 months and yearly thereafter.

G. Risk of manic switch in bipolar patients: Needs to be appropriately monitored.

X. **Relevant Pharmacokinetics/Pharmacodynamics**

A. **Metabolism**: Rapidly absorbed after oral administration, with bioavailability of 20%–70%. Primarily metabolized in the liver, with metabolites excreted in urine and feces. Desmethylclomipramine is the major active metabolite. CYP metabolism: CYP2D6, CYP2C19, CYP3A4, and CYP1A2.

B. **Time to peak plasma concentration**: 2–6 hours

C. **Half-life**: 19–37 hours; desmethylclomipramine: 69 hours

D. **Hepatic impairment**: Reduced dosages should be used in patients with liver disease.

E. **Renal impairment**: Reduced dosages may be needed in patients with moderate to severe renal impairment.

F. **Elderly individuals**: Clomipramine use should be avoided in this population (per the Beers Criteria [American Geriatrics Society 2023]), as it may lead to sedation and orthostasis. If used, clomipramine should be started at a lower dosage and increased slowly based on tolerability.

XI. Clinically Relevant Drug Interactions

A. Metabolized by CYP1A2 and CYP2D6 (major) and CYP3A4 and CYP2C19 (minor).

1. Caution should be used when prescribing clomipramine to patients who are taking CYP2D6 inhibitors (e.g., quinidine, cimetidine, fluoxetine, bupropion) or who are known to be poor metabolizers of CYP2D6, as drug concentrations may be higher.
2. Caution patients regarding concomitant use of CYP1A2 inhibitors (e.g., fluvoxamine, fluoroquinolones).
3. Tobacco smoke (a CYP1A2 inducer) may reduce clomipramine concentrations.

B. Caution should be used when prescribing clomipramine in combination with other medications, such as the following:

1. Other serotonergic medications, including other TCAs, selective serotonin reuptake inhibitors, serotonin-norepinephrine reuptake inhibitors, monoamine oxidase inhibitors, dextromethorphan, tramadol, methadone, St. John's wort
2. Medications with anticholinergic effects (e.g., atropine, glycopyrrolate, benztropine, trihexyphenidyl, procyclidine, prochlorperazine, meclizine, scopolamine, hydroxyzine)
3. Medications that prolong QTc (e.g., cisapride, amiodarone, sotalol, quinidine, procainamide, fluoroquinolones, sumatriptan, ondansetron, haloperidol, risperidone, ziprasidone, olanzapine, quetiapine, methadone)

XII. Adverse Effects

A. Possible increased risk of suicidality:

1. See "Boxed Warning: Suicidality and Antidepressant Drugs" in the introduction to TCAs. For detailed information, readers are referred to comprehensive sources in the literature (e.g., Fergusson et al. 2005).

B. Serotonin syndrome

C. Cardiovascular:

1. Tachycardia
2. Arrhythmias
3. Prolonged QTc interval and QRS widening
   a. Clomipramine can cause QTc prolongation and other cardiac rhythm changes, especially at higher dosages.
4. Myocardial infarction

D. Gastrointestinal:

1. Nausea
2. Vomiting
3. Diarrhea

E. Neurological:

1. Dizziness
2. Headache

3. Tremor
4. Seizure

F. Endocrine:

1. Weight gain
2. Hyperglycemia

G. Hematological:

1. Agranulocytosis
2. Leukopenia
3. Thrombocytopenia

H. Hepatic:

1. Altered liver function

a. Among all TCAs, clomipramine is the most likely to cause liver injury. Alternative medications should be used in patients with preexisting liver injury.

I. Anticholinergic effects:

1. Urinary retention
2. Constipation
3. Paralytic ileus
4. Dry mouth
5. Hyperthermia
6. Blurred vision
7. Narrow angle closure glaucoma

J. **Risks in pregnancy and lactation**:

1. Clomipramine was designated a Category C drug in the prior FDA classification and is present to a minimal extent in breast milk. A thorough risk/benefit discussion with the patient is recommended on continuing versus stopping the medication, including consultation with an OB/GYN specialist and/or lactation expert. See Chapter 15 ("Women: Pregnancy, Postpartum, and Breastfeeding") for more information.

XIII. Clinical Pearls/Prescribing Tips

A. Starting clomipramine at a low dosage, using slow titration, using divided dosing, and taking the medication with food can minimize gastrointestinal side effects.

B. QTc prolongation is a notable potential adverse effect with clomipramine. Use caution with other serotonergic medications given clomipramine's potent SERT blockade.

C. Clomipramine should be discontinued before elective surgery because it may interact with agents used during anesthesia.

D. Among all TCAs, clomipramine is the most likely to cause liver injury, and alternatives should be used in patients with preexisting liver injury.

E. Improvement in depressive symptoms may be noticed after 2–4 weeks of clomipramine treatment; however, it often takes at least 6–10 weeks before any improvement in OCD symptoms is noticed.

Further Reading

Caillard V, Rouillon F, Viel JF, et al; French University Antidepressant Group: Comparative effects of low and high dosages of clomipramine and placebo in panic disorder: a double-blind controlled study. Acta Psychiatr Scand 99(1):51–58, 1999 10066007

Clomipramine, in Drugs and Lactation Database (LactMed). Bethesda, MD, National Library of Medicine, 2022. Available at: https://www.ncbi.nlm.nih.gov/books/NBK501175/. Accessed March 13, 2024.

Clomipramine, in PubChem Compound Summary for CID 2801. National Center for Biotechnology Information, 2022. Available at: https://pubchem.ncbi.nlm.nih.gov/compound/Clomipramine. Accessed June 13, 2022.

Danish University Antidepressant Group: Citalopram: clinical effect profile in comparison with clomipramine: a controlled multicenter study. Psychopharmacology (Berl) 90(1):131–138, 1986 2876451

Insel TR, Murphy DL, Cohen RM, et al: Obsessive-compulsive disorder: a double-blind trial of clomipramine and clorgyline. Arch Gen Psychiatry 40(6):605–612, 1983 6342562

Patheon Inc: Anafranil (clomipramine) [package insert]. U.S. Food and Drug Administration website. Revised October 2012. Available at: https://www.accessdata.fda.gov/drugsatfda_docs/label/2012/019906s037lbl.pdf. Accessed March 13, 2024.

Swedo SE, Leonard HL, Rapoport JL, et al: A double-blind comparison of clomipramine and desipramine in the treatment of trichotillomania (hair pulling). N Engl J Med 321(8):497–501, 1989 2761586

Wilson M, Tripp J: Clomipramine, in StatPearls. Treasure Island, FL, StatPearls Publishing, 2022

Wu PC, Hung CS, Kang YN, et al: Tolerability and optimal therapeutic dosage of clomipramine for premature ejaculation: a systematic review and meta-analysis. Sex Med 9(1):100283, 2021 33291044

References

American Geriatrics Society Beers Criteria Update Expert Panel: 2023 updated AGS Beers Criteria for potentially inappropriate medication use in older adults. J Am Geriatr Soc 71(7):2052–2081, 2023 37139824

Fergusson D, Doucette S, Glass KC, et al: Association between suicide attempts and selective serotonin reuptake inhibitors: systematic review of randomised controlled trials. BMJ 330(7488):396, 2005 15718539

Hiemke C, Bergemann N, Clement HW, et al: Consensus guidelines for therapeutic drug monitoring in neuropsychopharmacology: update 2017. Pharmacopsychiatry 51(1–2):9–62, 2018 28910830

Roth BL, Driscoll J: PDSP Ki Database. Psychoactive Drug Screening Program (PDSP). University of North Carolina at Chapel Hill and the United States National Institute of Mental Health, 1999–present. Available at: https://pdsp.unc.edu/databases/pdsp.php. Accessed June 21, 2024.

Desipramine

I. **Brand Names**: Norpramin

II. **Therapeutic Class**: Tricyclic antidepressant (TCA), secondary amine

III. **Chemical Name**: 5*H*-dibenz[*bf*]azepine-5-propanamine,10,11-dihydro-*N*-methyl-monohydrochloride

IV. **Mechanism(s) of Action**

A. Desipramine inhibits the membrane reuptake of norepinephrine and serotonin by adrenergic and serotonergic neurons at the presynaptic membranes, leading to increased levels of both in the synapse. As a secondary amine, desipramine has a greater affinity for norepinephrine. Additionally, it blocks adrenergic receptors.

B. Desipramine is a product of the metabolism of imipramine.

C. Desipramine has much more potent NET inhibition compared with SERT inhibition (NET Ki=0.63–3.5 nM vs. SERT Ki=17.6–163 nM) (Roth and Driscoll 1999–present).

D. Effects on other receptors are relatively mild: α_1 receptor inhibition (Ki=23–130 nM), H_1 receptor inhibition (Ki=60–110 nM), and muscarinic acetylcholine (mACh) receptor inhibition (mACh Ki=66–198 nM).

V. **Indications**

A. FDA adult:

1. Depression

B. Evidence-based[1] off-label uses:

1. ADHD (pediatric)
2. Diabetic neuropathy
3. Postherpetic neuralgia

C. FDA pediatric: None

VI. **Major Contraindications and When to Use Caution**

A. **Contraindications**:

1. Hypersensitivity to desipramine
2. Concomitant use with a monoamine oxidase inhibitor (MAOI) or another TCA
   a. See comment under "Clinical Pearls" regarding desipramine combination treatment.
3. Acute phase of recovery after myocardial infarction

B. **Use caution**:

1. Older adults because of anticholinergic and sedating effects
2. Heart conduction defects or arrhythmias
3. Congestive heart failure
4. Concomitant alcohol use

---

[1]Evidence strength varies; readers are referred to the literature for more detailed information.

5. Acute angle-closure glaucoma
6. History of seizures
7. Patients with hyperthyroidism or on medication for hypothyroidism
8. Patients who are poor metabolizers of cytochrome P450 (CYP) 2D6

VII. **Dosage Formulations**

A. Generic tablet (10 mg, 25 mg, 50 mg, 75 mg, 100 mg, 150 mg)
B. Brand tablet (10 mg, 25 mg)

VIII. **Dosage Ranges and Guidelines**

A. Depression: Start with 50–100 mg/day. Can be increased to a maximum dosage of 200–300 mg/day.
B. ADHD (pediatric): 25 mg/day to start, up to a maximum dosage of 5 mg/kg/day.

IX. **Monitoring**

A. Therapeutic drug monitoring:
   1. Plasma levels should be monitored as desired dosages are achieved.
   2. Timing: Draw trough just prior to next dose.
   3. The reference range for the drug is 50–300 ng/mL (desipramine) (Hiemke et al. 2018). Below a plasma level of 115 ng/mL, there is limited clinical response.
   4. At levels higher than 300 ng/mL, there is often a higher side-effect burden.
   5. Plasma levels may vary among individuals, given the heterogeneity of the CYP2D6 pathways involved in desipramine's metabolism.
B. Sodium levels: Measure at baseline and after 3–4 weeks of treatment.
C. Liver function tests: Monitor periodically.
D. Obtain ECG at baseline, after dosage changes, and up to every 3 months thereafter.
E. Blood pressure: Measure at baseline, after dosage changes, and every 3–6 months once the dosage is stabilized.
F. Weight changes: Check weight at 3, 6, and 12 months and yearly thereafter.
G. Risk of manic switch in bipolar patients: Needs to be appropriately monitored.

X. **Relevant Pharmacokinetics/Pharmacodynamics**

A. **Metabolism**: Rapidly absorbed after oral administration and undergoes significant first-pass effect. Primarily metabolized in the liver (70% of metabolites are excreted in urine). CYP metabolism: CYP2D6 with some contribution of CYP1A2.
B. **Time to peak plasma concentration**: 4–6 hours
C. **Half-life**: 22 hours
D. **Hepatic impairment**: Use with caution in patients with liver impairment; may use reduced dosages.
E. **Renal impairment**: Use with caution in patients with renal impairment; may use reduced dosages.
F. **Elderly individuals**: Desipramine use should be avoided in this population (per the Beers Criteria [American Geriatrics Society 2023]), as it may lead to sedation and orthostasis. If used, desipramine should be started at 25 mg/day and increased slowly, based on tolerability, up to a maximum dosage of 150 mg/day.

XI. Clinically Relevant Drug Interactions

A. Metabolized by CYP2D6 (major) and CYP1A2 (minor).

1. Caution should be used when prescribing desipramine to patients who are taking CYP2D6 inhibitors (e.g., quinidine, cimetidine, fluoxetine, bupropion) or who are known to be poor metabolizers of CYP2D6, as drug concentrations may be higher.

B. Caution should be used when prescribing desipramine in combination with other medications, such as the following:

1. Other serotonergic medications, including other TCAs, selective serotonin reuptake inhibitors, serotonin norepinephrine reuptake inhibitors, monoamine oxidase inhibitors, dextromethorphan, tramadol, methadone, St. John's wort
2. Medications with anticholinergic effects (e.g., atropine, glycopyrrolate, benztropine, trihexyphenidyl, procyclidine, prochlorperazine, meclizine, scopolamine, hydroxyzine)
3. Medications that prolong QTc (e.g., cisapride, amiodarone, sotalol, quinidine, procainamide, fluoroquinolones, sumatriptan, ondansetron, haloperidol, risperidone, ziprasidone, olanzapine, quetiapine, methadone)

XII. Adverse Effects

A. Possible increased risk of suicidality:

1. See "Boxed Warning: Suicidality and Antidepressant Drugs" in the introduction to TCAs. For detailed information, readers are referred to comprehensive sources in the literature (e.g., Fergusson et al. 2005).

B. Serotonin syndrome

C. Cardiovascular:

1. Tachycardia
2. Arrhythmias
3. Prolonged QTc interval and QRS widening
   a. Desipramine can cause prolongation of QTc, QRS, and PR intervals as well as other cardiac rhythm changes, and ECG monitoring is recommended.
4. Myocardial infarction
5. Orthostatic hypotension

D. Gastrointestinal:

1. Nausea
2. Vomiting
3. Diarrhea

E. Neurological:

1. Dizziness
2. Paresthesia
3. Tremor
4. Seizure

F. Endocrine:
   1. Weight gain
   2. Hyperglycemia
G. Hematological:
   1. Agranulocytosis
   2. Eosinophilia
H. Hepatic:
   1. Altered liver function
I. Anticholinergic effects:
   1. Urinary retention
   2. Constipation
   3. Paralytic ileus
   4. Dry mouth
   5. Hyperthermia
   6. Mydriasis
   7. Blurred vision
   8. Narrow angle closure glaucoma
J. **Risks in pregnancy and lactation**
   1. Desipramine's effects on fetal development are unclear, and it should not be used in pregnant women unless the benefits outweigh the risk to the fetus. Consultation with an OB/GYN specialist is advised.
   2. A minimal amount of the medication passes into breast milk. Therefore, it may be used with caution in patients as they breastfeed, especially with infants older than 2 months. Consultation with a lactation expert is advised.

XIII. **Clinical Pearls/Prescribing Tips**

A. Desipramine is the least likely of the TCAs to have significant side effects and generally causes the least sedation. Monitor QTc.
B. Desipramine's potent NET blockade and low risk of sedation likely account for its efficacy in ADHD, although it is not a first-line choice for this indication.
C. If desipramine is used in adolescents, lower dosages are recommended.
D. Desipramine should be discontinued before elective surgery because it may interact with agents used during anesthesia.
E. In some patients, improvement in depressive symptoms may be noticed after 2–3 weeks of desipramine treatment.
F. Certain TCAs—particularly those with less notable SERT blockade, such as nortriptyline and desipramine (secondary amines)—may be safer in combination with SSRIs, other TCAs, and MAOIs than previously thought. Patients would still need to be monitored closely for adverse effects, including serotonin syndrome, hypertension, headache, insomnia, and constipation (Amsterdam and Kim 2019; Gillman 2007; Goldberg and Thornton 1978).
G. TCAs in general have been shown to be more efficacious than SNRIs—and significantly more efficacious than SSRIs—in treating neuropathic pain.

Further Reading

Biederman J, Baldessarini RJ, Wright V, et al: A double-blind placebo controlled study of desipramine in the treatment of ADD, I: efficacy. J Am Acad Child Adolesc Psychiatry 28(5):777–784, 1989 2676967

Desipramine package insert. U.S. Food and Drug Administration, 2020. Available at: https://www.accessdata.fda.gov/spl/data/a7e6d256-7227-3334-e053-2995a90aa96d/a7e6d256-7227-3334-e053-2995a90aa96d.xml. Accessed March 13, 2024.

Desipramine, in Drugs and Lactation Database (LactMed). Bethesda, MD, National Library of Medicine, 2022. Available at: https://www.ncbi.nlm.nih.gov/books/NBK501179/. Accessed March 13, 2024.

Desipramine, in PubChem Compound Summary for CID 2995. National Center for Biotechnology Information, 2022. Available at: https://pubchem.ncbi.nlm.nih.gov/compound/Desipramine. Accessed June 2022.

Maan JS, Rosani A, Saadabadi A: Desipramine, in StatPearls. Treasure Island, FL, StatPearls Publishing, 2022

Sanofi-Aventis US: Norpramin (desipramine) [package insert]. U.S. Food and Drug Administration website. 2012. Available at: https://www.accessdata.fda.gov/drugsatfda_docs/label/2012/014399s066s067lbl.pdf. Accessed March 13, 2024.

Stewart JW, Quitkin F, Liebowitz MR, et al: Efficacy of desipramine in mildly depressed patients: a double-blind, placebo-controlled trial. Psychopharmacol Bull 17(1):136–138, 1981 7015394

References

American Geriatrics Society Beers Criteria Update Expert Panel: 2023 updated AGS Beers Criteria for potentially inappropriate medication use in older adults. J Am Geriatr Soc 71(7):2052–2081, 2023 37139824

Amsterdam JD, Kim TT: Relative effectiveness of monoamine oxidase inhibitor and tricyclic antidepressant combination therapy for treatment-resistant depression. J Clin Psychopharmacol 39(6):649–652, 2019 31688401

Fergusson D, Doucette S, Glass KC, et al: Association between suicide attempts and selective serotonin reuptake inhibitors: systematic review of randomised controlled trials. BMJ 330(7488):396, 2005 15718539

Gillman PK: Tricyclic antidepressant pharmacology and therapeutic drug interactions updated. Br J Pharmacol 151(6):737–748, 2007 17471183

Goldberg RS, Thornton WE: Combined tricyclic-MAOI therapy for refractory depression: a review, with guidelines for appropriate usage. J Clin Pharmacol 18(2–3):143–147, 1978 342553

Hiemke C, Bergemann N, Clement HW, et al: Consensus guidelines for therapeutic drug monitoring in neuropsychopharmacology: update 2017. Pharmacopsychiatry 51(1–2):9–62, 2018 28910830

Roth BL, Driscoll J: PDSP Ki Database. Psychoactive Drug Screening Program (PDSP). University of North Carolina at Chapel Hill and the United States National Institute of Mental Health, 1999–present. Available at: https://pdsp.unc.edu/databases/pdsp.php. Accessed June 21, 2024.

Doxepin

I. **Brand Names**: Sinequan, Silenor, Zonalon
II. **Therapeutic Class**: Tricyclic antidepressant (TCA), tertiary amine
III. **Chemical Name**: 1-propanamine, 3-dibenzo[*b*,*e*]oxepin-11(6*H*)-ylidene-*N*,*N*-dimethylpropan-1-amine
IV. **Mechanism(s) of Action**

A. Doxepin inhibits the membrane reuptake of norepinephrine and serotonin by adrenergic and serotonergic neurons at the presynaptic membranes, leading to increased levels of both in the synapse. It also blocks adrenergic, muscarinic, and histaminergic receptors.
B. Doxepin's antihistamine effects (H_1 Ki=0.09–1.23 nM) greatly outperform its SERT (serotonin transporter) and NET (norepinephrine transporter) inhibition effects (NET Ki=30–58 nM; SERT Ki=68–95 nM). As a result, relatively high doxepin dosages are required to obtain antidepressant/anti-anxiety effects.
C. Notable receptor effects include moderate α_1 inhibition (Ki=24 nM), 5-HT_{2A} inhibition (Ki=11–27 nM), 5-HT_{2C} inhibition (Ki=8.8–200 nM), and cholinergic (muscarinic acetylcholine [mACh]) inhibition (Ki=23–80 nM) (Roth and Driscoll 1999–present).

1. The additive effects of H_1 inhibition and 5-HT_{2C} inhibition may increase the risk of weight gain.

V. **Indications**

A. FDA adult:

1. Sinequan:

a. Depression
b. Anxiety
c. Depression and anxiety associated with alcoholism
d. Psychotic depression

2. Silenor:

a. Insomnia

3. Zonalon:

a. Pruritus

B. Evidence-based[1] off-label uses:

1. Neuropathic pain
2. Urticaria

C. FDA pediatric: None

[1]Evidence strength varies; readers are referred to the literature for more detailed information.

VI. Major Contraindications and When to Use Caution

A. **Contraindications:**

1. Hypersensitivity to doxepin
2. Concomitant use with a monoamine oxidase inhibitor (MAOI) or another TCA
3. Acute phase of recovery after myocardial infarction (MI)
4. Children younger than 12 years
5. Acute angle-closure glaucoma
6. Urinary retention

B. **Use caution:**

1. Older adults because of anticholinergic and sedating effects
2. Heart conduction defects or arrhythmias
3. Congestive heart failure
4. Concomitant alcohol use
5. History of seizures
6. Patients with hyperthyroidism or on medication for hypothyroidism
7. Patients who are poor metabolizers of cytochrome P450 (CYP) 2D6

VII. Dosage Formulations

A. Generic capsule (10 mg, 25 mg, 50 mg, 75 mg, 100 mg, 150 mg)
B. Generic oral concentrate (10 mg/mL) (118 mL bottle, 120 mL bottle)
C. Generic and brand (Silenor) tablet (3 mg, 6 mg)
D. A topical cream for neuropathic pain and pruritus is also available.

VIII. Dosage Ranges and Guidelines

A. Depression/anxiety/alcoholism: Start with 75 mg/day. Can be increased to a 150–300 mg/day maximum dosage. Can be administered on a once-daily or twice-daily dosing schedule.
B. Insomnia: Take a 6-mg dose 30 minutes before bedtime. For elderly adults: 3 mg at bedtime.
C. Pruritus: Apply a thin film (5%) four times daily for short-term therapy (up to 8 days).
D. Neuropathic pain: Topical dosing: 3.3%–5% daily topical application.
E. Urticaria: 10–30 mg/day has been effective in treating idiopathic cold urticaria; 25 mg TID has been shown to be effective in treating chronic idiopathic urticaria.

IX. Monitoring

A. Therapeutic drug monitoring:

1. Timing: Draw trough just prior to next dose.
2. The reference range for the drug is 50–150 ng/mL (doxepin + *N*-desmethyl-doxepin) (Hiemke et al. 2018)
3. At plasma levels 300 ng/mL, there is often a higher side-effect burden.
4. Plasma levels may vary among individuals, given the heterogeneity of the CYP2D6 pathways involved in doxepin's metabolism.

B. Sodium levels: Measure at baseline and after 3–4 weeks.
C. Liver function tests: Monitor periodically.

D. Obtain ECG at baseline, after dosage changes, and up to every 3 months thereafter.
E. Blood pressure: Measure at baseline, after dosage changes, and every 3–6 months once the dosage is stabilized.
F. Weight changes: Check weight at 3, 6, and 12 months and yearly thereafter.
G. Risk of manic switch in bipolar patients: Needs to be appropriately monitored.

X. **Relevant Pharmacokinetics/Pharmacodynamics**

A. **Metabolism**: Rapidly absorbed after oral administration and undergoes a significant first-pass effect. Primarily metabolized in the liver (metabolites are excreted in the urine). Nordoxepin is the major metabolite. CYP metabolism: CYP2D6 and CYP2C19 with some contribution of CYP1A2 and CYP2C9.
B. **Time to peak plasma concentration**: 2–3.5 hours
C. **Half-life**: 15 hours. Nordoxepin: 31 hours
D. **Use with food**: Doxepin should not be taken within 3 hours after a meal.
E. **Hepatic impairment**: Use with caution in those with liver impairment; consider reduced dosages.
F. **Renal impairment**: Use with caution in those with renal impairment; consider reduced dosages.
G. **Elderly individuals**: Doxepin use should be avoided in this population (per the Beers Criteria [American Geriatrics Society 2023]), as it may lead to sedation and orthostasis. If used for depression, doxepin should be started at a low dosage and increased slowly based on tolerability. For insomnia, elderly patients can be given 3 mg/day at bedtime.

XI. **Clinically Relevant Drug Interactions**

A. Metabolized by CYP2D6 (major) and by CYP3A4, CYP2C19, and CYP1A2 (minor).
   1. Caution should be used when prescribing doxepin to patients who are taking CYP2D6 inhibitors (e.g., quinidine, cimetidine, fluoxetine, bupropion) or who are known to be poor metabolizers of CYP2D6, as drug concentrations may be higher.

B. Caution should be used when prescribing doxepin in combination with other medications, such as the following:
   1. Other serotonergic medications, including other TCAs, selective serotonin reuptake inhibitors, serotonin norepinephrine reuptake inhibitors, monoamine oxidase inhibitors, dextromethorphan, tramadol, methadone, St. John's wort
   2. Medications with anticholinergic effects (e.g., atropine, glycopyrrolate, benztropine, trihexyphenidyl, procyclidine, prochlorperazine, meclizine, scopolamine, hydroxyzine)
   3. Medications that prolong QTc (e.g., cisapride, amiodarone, sotalol, quinidine, procainamide, fluoroquinolones, sumatriptan, ondansetron, haloperidol, risperidone, ziprasidone, olanzapine, quetiapine, methadone)

C. Coadministration of doxepin with a high-fat meal delays the peak concentration by approximately 3 hours, so patients should not take doxepin within 3 hours after eating.

XII. Adverse Effects

A. Possible increased risk of suicidality:

1. See "Boxed Warning: Suicidality and Antidepressant Drugs" in the introduction to TCAs. For detailed information, readers are referred to comprehensive sources in the literature (e.g., Fergusson et al. 2005).

B. Serotonin syndrome

C. Cardiovascular:

1. Tachycardia
2. Hypertension
3. Arrhythmias
4. Prolonged QTc interval and QRS widening
    a. Doxepin can cause QTc prolongation as well as other cardiac rhythm changes, and ECG monitoring is recommended.
5. Orthostatic hypotension

D. Gastrointestinal:

1. Nausea
2. Vomiting
3. Diarrhea

E. Neurological:

1. Drowsiness
2. Dizziness
3. Paresthesia
4. Tremor
5. Seizure

F. Endocrine:

1. Weight gain
2. Sexual dysfunction

G. Hematological:

1. Agranulocytosis
2. Eosinophilia

H. Hepatic:

1. Altered liver function

I. Anticholinergic effects:

1. Urinary retention
2. Constipation
3. Paralytic ileus
4. Dry mouth
5. Hyperthermia
6. Mydriasis
7. Blurred vision
8. Narrow angle closure glaucoma

J. **Risks in pregnancy and lactation**

1. Doxepin was designated a Category C drug in the prior FDA classification and is present to a significant extent in breast milk. A thorough risk/benefit discussion with the patient is recommended on continuing versus stopping the medication, including consultation with an OB/GYN specialist and/or lactation expert. See Chapter 15 ("Women: Pregnancy, Postpartum, and Breastfeeding") for more information.
2. While breastfeeding is generally not recommended with oral use of doxepin, there are no contraindications to topical use at a site away from the breast while breastfeeding.

XIII. **Clinical Pearls/Prescribing Tips**

A. Doxepin is notably antihistaminergic, which accounts for its efficacy in insomnia. Antidepressant effects require higher dosages. Be aware of the risk of weight gain with H_1 and 5-HT_{2C} inhibition. QTc prolongation is also a notable potential adverse effect.

B. Doxepin should be discontinued before elective surgery because it may interact with agents used during anesthesia.

C. Coadministration with a high-fat meal delays the peak concentration by approximately 3 hours, so patients should not take doxepin within 3 hours after eating.

D. Improvement in depressive symptoms may be noticed after 2–3 weeks of doxepin treatment. When used for insomnia, the effect should be apparent within 7–10 days of use.

Further Reading

Almasi A, Meza CE: Doxepin, in StatPearls. Treasure Island, FL, StatPearls Publishing, 2022

Currax Pharmaceuticals LLC: Silenor (doxepin) [package insert]. U.S. Food and Drug Administration website. Revised October 2020. Available at: https://www.accessdata.fda.gov/drugsatfda_docs/label/2020/022036s006lbl.pdf. Accessed March 13, 2024.

Doxepin, in Drugs and Lactation Database (LactMed). Bethesda, MD, National Library of Medicine, 2022. Available at: https://www.ncbi.nlm.nih.gov/books/NBK501181/. Accessed March 13, 2024.

Doxepin, in PubChem Compound Summary for CID 3158. National Center for Biotechnology Information, 2022. Available at: https://pubchem.ncbi.nlm.nih.gov/compound/Doxepin. Accessed June 2022.

Mylan Pharmaceuticals: Zonalon (doxepin HCl) cream, 5%. Morgantown, WV, Mylan Pharmaceuticals, 2017. Available at: https://dailymed.nlm.nih.gov/dailymed/fda/fdaDrugXsl.cfm?setid=5f302247-525e-4acc-852b-00eb1d79af4b&type=display. Accessed March 13, 2024.

Roerig: Sinequan (doxepin HCl) capsules, oral concentrate [package insert]. U.S. Food and Drug Administration website. May 2007. Available at: https://www.accessdata.fda.gov/drugsatfda_docs/label/2007/016798s054,017516s023lbl.pdf. Accessed March 13, 2024.

References

American Geriatrics Society Beers Criteria Update Expert Panel: 2023 updated AGS Beers Criteria for potentially inappropriate medication use in older adults. J Am Geriatr Soc 71(7):2052–2081, 2023 37139824

Fergusson D, Doucette S, Glass KC, et al: Association between suicide attempts and selective serotonin reuptake inhibitors: systematic review of randomised controlled trials. BMJ 330(7488):396, 2005 15718539

Hiemke C, Bergemann N, Clement HW, et al: Consensus guidelines for therapeutic drug monitoring in neuropsychopharmacology: update 2017. Pharmacopsychiatry 51(1–2):9–62, 2018 28910830

Roth BL, Driscoll J: PDSP Ki Database. Psychoactive Drug Screening Program (PDSP). University of North Carolina at Chapel Hill and the United States National Institute of Mental Health, 1999–present. Available at: https://pdsp.unc.edu/databases/pdsp.php. Accessed June 21, 2024.

Imipramine

I. **Brand Names**: Tofranil

II. **Therapeutic Class**: Tricyclic antidepressant (TCA), tertiary amine

III. **Chemical Name**: 5-3-(dimethylamino) propyl-10, 11-dihydro-5*H* dibenz ['b, f]-azepine monohydrochloride

IV. **Mechanism(s) of Action**

A. Imipramine inhibits the membrane reuptake of norepinephrine and serotonin by adrenergic and serotonergic neurons at the presynaptic membranes, leading to increased levels of both in the synapse. As a tertiary amine, imipramine has a greater affinity for serotonin. It also has anticholinergic properties through blockade of muscarinic receptors. Additionally, imipramine blocks dopamine (D_2), α_1- and α_2-adrenergic, and H_1 receptors.

B. Imipramine is a tertiary amine and is metabolized to the secondary amine desipramine.

C. Imipramine's serotonin transporter (SERT) inhibition is much more potent than its norepinephrine transporter (NET) inhibition (SERT Ki=1.3–1.4 nM vs. NET Ki=20–37 nM) (Roth and Driscoll 1999–present).

D. Other notable receptor targets include moderate α_1 inhibition (Ki=32 nM), H_1 inhibition (Ki=7.6–37 nM), and cholinergic (muscarinic acetylcholine [mACh]) inhibition (Ki=46 nM).

V. **Indications**

A. FDA adult:

1. Depression

B. Evidence-based[1] off-label uses:

1. Panic disorder
2. Chronic neuropathic pain

C. FDA pediatric:

1. Nocturnal enuresis

VI. **Major Contraindications and When to Use Caution**

A. **Contraindications**:

1. Hypersensitivity to imipramine
2. Concomitant use with a monoamine oxidase inhibitor (MAOI) or another TCA
3. Acute phase of recovery after myocardial infarction
4. Children younger than 6 years

B. **Use caution**:

1. Elderly adults because of anticholinergic and sedating effects
2. Heart conduction defects or arrhythmias
3. Congestive heart failure
4. Concomitant alcohol use
5. Acute angle-closure glaucoma
6. History of seizures
7. Patients with hyperthyroidism or on medication for hypothyroidism
8. Patients who are poor metabolizers of cytochrome P450 (CYP) 2D6

VII. **Dosage Formulations**

A. Generic capsule (75 mg, 100 mg, 125 mg, 150 mg)
B. Generic tablet (10 mg, 25 mg, 50 mg)

VIII. **Dosage Ranges and Guidelines**

A. Depression: Start with 75–100 mg/day in divided doses. Can be increased to a maximum dosage of 200–300 mg/day after a few weeks.
B. Nocturnal enuresis (pediatric): 25–50 mg at bedtime for children ages 6–12 years; patients older than 12 years can be given up to 75 mg at bedtime.
C. Panic disorder: Up to 100–200 mg/day in divided doses
D. Chronic neuropathic pain: 50–150 mg/day

IX. **Monitoring**

A. Therapeutic drug monitoring:

1. Plasma levels should be monitored as desired dosages are achieved.
2. Timing: Draw trough just prior to next dose.
3. The reference range for the drug is 175–300 ng/mL (imipramine + desipramine) (Hiemke et al. 2018). At 300 ng/mL, imipramine is effective for severe depression.

---

[1]Evidence strength varies; readers are referred to the literature for more detailed information.

4. At plasma levels >300 ng/mL, there is often a higher side-effect burden.
5. Plasma levels may vary among individuals, given the heterogeneity of the CYP2D6 pathways involved in imipramine's metabolism.

B. Sodium levels: Measure at baseline and after 3–4 weeks of treatment.
C. Liver function tests: Monitor periodically.
D. Obtain ECG at baseline, after dosage changes, and as often as every 3 months for patients with specific cardiac risk factors.
E. Blood pressure: Measure at baseline, after dosage changes, and every 3–6 months once the dosage is stabilized.
F. Weight changes: Check weight at 3, 6, and 12 months and yearly thereafter.
G. Closely monitor blood sugar and hemoglobin A1c (HbA1c) in patients with diabetes mellitus.
H. Risk of manic switch in bipolar patients: Needs to be appropriately monitored.

X. **Relevant Pharmacokinetics/Pharmacodynamics**

A. **Metabolism**: Rapidly absorbed after oral administration, with bioavailability of 22%–77%. Primarily metabolized in the liver (metabolites excreted in the urine). Desipramine is the major active metabolite. CYP metabolism: CYP2D6, CYP2C19, CYP3A4, CYP1A2.
B. **Time to peak plasma concentration**: 2–6 hours
C. **Half-life**: 12 hours; desipramine: 22 hours
D. **Hepatic impairment**: Use with caution in patients with liver impairment; may need reduced dosages.
E. **Renal impairment**: Use with caution in patients with renal impairment; may need reduced dosages.
F. **Elderly individuals**: Imipramine use should be avoided in this population (per the Beers Criteria [American Geriatrics Society 2023]), as it may lead to sedation and orthostasis. If used, imipramine should be started at a lower dosage and increased slowly based on tolerability.

XI. **Clinically Relevant Drug Interactions**

A. Metabolized by CYP2D6 (major), and by CYP1A2, CYP2B6, CYP2C19, and CYP3A4 (minor).

1. Caution should be used when prescribing imipramine to patients who are taking CYP2D6 inhibitors (e.g., quinidine, cimetidine, fluoxetine, bupropion) or who are known to be poor metabolizers of CYP2D6, as drug concentrations may be higher.

B. Caution should be used when prescribing imipramine in combination with other medications, such as the following:

1. Other serotonergic medications, including other TCAs, selective serotonin reuptake inhibitors, serotonin-norepinephrine reuptake inhibitors, monoamine oxidase inhibitors, dextromethorphan, tramadol, methadone, St. John's wort
2. Medications with anticholinergic effects (e.g., atropine, glycopyrrolate, benztropine, trihexyphenidyl, procyclidine, prochlorperazine, meclizine, scopolamine, hydroxyzine)

3. Medications that prolong QTc (e.g., cisapride, amiodarone, sotalol, quinidine, procainamide, fluoroquinolones, sumatriptan, ondansetron, haloperidol, risperidone, ziprasidone, olanzapine, quetiapine, methadone)

XII. **Adverse Effects**

A. Possible increased risk of suicidality:

1. See "Boxed Warning: Suicidality and Antidepressant Drugs" in the introduction to TCAs. For detailed information, readers are referred to comprehensive sources in the literature (e.g., Fergusson et al. 2005).

B. Serotonin syndrome

C. Cardiovascular:

1. Tachycardia
2. Arrhythmias
3. Prolonged QTc interval and QRS interval

D. Imipramine causes QTc prolongation and other cardiac rhythm changes, and ECG monitoring is recommended. Monitoring should be more frequent in patients with known cardiac disease.

1. Myocardial infarction
2. Orthostatic hypotension

E. Gastrointestinal:

1. Nausea
2. Vomiting
3. Diarrhea

F. Neurological:

1. Dizziness
2. Paresthesia
3. Tremor
4. Seizure

G. Dermatological

1. Photosensitivity

   a. Imipramine may cause photosensitization; excessive sun exposure should be avoided.

H. Endocrine:

1. Weight gain.
2. Hyperglycemia

   a. Imipramine could cause fluctuations in blood sugar levels, and this should be monitored closely in patients with diabetes.

I. Hematological:

1. Agranulocytosis
2. Eosinophilia

J. Hepatic:
   1. Altered liver function
   2. Jaundice

K. Anticholinergic effects:
   1. Urinary retention
   2. Constipation
   3. Paralytic ileus
   4. Dry mouth
   5. Hyperthermia
   6. Mydriasis
   7. Blurred vision
   8. Narrow angle closure glaucoma

L. **Risks in pregnancy and lactation**
   A. Imipramine's effects on fetal development are unclear, and it should not be used in pregnant women unless the benefits outweigh the risk to the fetus. Consultation with an OB/GYN specialist is recommended.
   B. A minimal amount of imipramine passes into breast milk. Therefore, it may be used with caution in patients as they breastfeed, especially with infants older than 2 months. Consultation with a lactation expert is recommended.

XIII. **Clinical Pearls/Prescribing Tips**
   A. Notable adverse effects include photosensitization, QTc prolongation, and fluctuations in blood sugar levels.
   B. Imipramine should be discontinued before elective surgery because it may interact with agents used during anesthesia.
   C. In some patients, improvement in depressive symptoms may be noticed after 4–5 weeks of imipramine treatment.
   D. TCAs in general have been shown to be more efficacious than SNRIs—and significantly more efficacious than SSRIs—in treating neuropathic pain.

Further Reading

Excellium Pharmaceutical: Imipramine hydrochloride tablet, film coated [package insert]. U.S. Food and Drug Administration. Revised October 2012. Available at: https://www.accessdata.fda.gov/drugsatfda_docs/label/2012/040903lbl.pdf. Accessed March 13, 2024.

Fayez R, Gupta V: Imipramine, in StatPearls. Treasure Island, FL, StatPearls Publishing, 2022

Fritz GK, Rockney RM, Yeung AS: Plasma levels and efficacy of imipramine treatment for enuresis. J Am Acad Child Adolesc Psychiatry 33(1):60–64, 1994 8138522

Hearn L, Derry S, Phillips T, et al: Imipramine for neuropathic pain in adults. Cochrane Database Syst Rev (5):CD010769, 2014 24838845

Imipramine, in Drugs and Lactation Database (LactMed). Bethesda, MD, National Library of Medicine (US), 2022. Available at: https://www.ncbi.nlm.nih.gov/books/NBK501180/. Accessed March 13, 2024.

Imipramine, in PubChem Compound Summary for CID 3696. National Center for Biotechnology Information, 2022. Available at: https://pubchem.ncbi.nlm.nih.gov/compound/Imipramine. Accessed June 2022.

Kocsis JH, Frances AJ, Voss C, et al: Imipramine treatment for chronic depression. Arch Gen Psychiatry 45(3):253–257, 1988 3277579

Mallinckrodt Inc: Tofranil-PM (imipramine pamoate) capsules [package insert]. U.S. Food and Drug Administration, 2014. Available at: https://www.accessdata.fda.gov/drugsatfda_docs/label/2014/017090s078lbl.pdf. Accessed March 13, 2024.

Mavissakalian MR, Perel JM: Imipramine dose-response relationship in panic disorder with agoraphobia: preliminary findings. Arch Gen Psychiatry 46(2):127–131, 1989 2643933

Rochester MP, Kane AM, Linnebur SA, et al: Evaluating the risk of QTc prolongation associated with antidepressant use in older adults: a review of the evidence. Ther Adv Drug Saf 9(6):297–308, 2018 29854391

References

American Geriatrics Society Beers Criteria Update Expert Panel: 2023 updated AGS Beers Criteria for potentially inappropriate medication use in older adults. J Am Geriatr Soc 71(7):2052–2081, 2023 37139824

Fergusson D, Doucette S, Glass KC, et al: Association between suicide attempts and selective serotonin reuptake inhibitors: systematic review of randomised controlled trials. BMJ 330(7488):396, 2005 15718539

Hiemke C, Bergemann N, Clement HW, et al: Consensus guidelines for therapeutic drug monitoring in neuropsychopharmacology: update 2017. Pharmacopsychiatry 51(1–2):9–62, 2018 28910830

Roth BL, Driscoll J: PDSP Ki Database. Psychoactive Drug Screening Program (PDSP). University of North Carolina at Chapel Hill and the United States National Institute of Mental Health, 1999–present. Available at: https://pdsp.unc.edu/databases/pdsp.php. Accessed June 21, 2024.

Nortriptyline

I. **Brand Names**: Pamelor, Aventyl

II. **Therapeutic Class**: Tricyclic antidepressant (TCA), secondary amine

III. **Chemical Name**: 3-(10,11-dihydro-5*H*-dibenzo[*a,d*]cyclohepten-5-ylidene)-*N*-methyl-1-propanamine

IV. **Mechanism(s) of Action**

A. Nortriptyline inhibits the membrane reuptake of norepinephrine and serotonin by adrenergic and serotonergic neurons at the presynaptic membranes, leading to increased levels of serotonin and norepinephrine in the synapse. Additionally, nortriptyline inhibits histamine, 3-hydroxytyramine, and acetylcholine. Nortriptyline also causes desensitization of adenylyl cyclase, downregulation of β-adrenergic receptors, and downregulation of serotonin receptors.

B. Nortriptyline is a secondary amine, a product of the metabolism of amitriptyline.

C. Nortriptyline's NET (norepinephrine transporter) inhibition is approximately 10-fold higher than its SERT (serotonin transporter) inhibition (Takano et al. 2014): SERT Ki=15–18 nM vs. NET Ki=1.8–4.4 nM (Roth and Driscoll 1999–present).

D. Nortriptyline's H_1 antagonism (Ki=3.0–15 nM), α_1 antagonism (Ki=55 nM), and cholinergic (muscarinic acetylcholine [mACh]) activity (mACh: Ki=37 nM; M_1: Ki=3 nM; M_2: Ki=110 nM) are less potent than those of nortriptyline's parent molecule, amitriptyline. Nortriptyline also exhibits 5-HT_{2C} inhibition (Ki=5.0–41 nM).

V. **Indications**

A. FDA adult: Major depressive disorder

B. Evidence-based[1] off-label uses:

1. ADHD
2. Low back pain
3. Pain associated with diabetic neuropathy
4. Smoking cessation
5. Neurogenic bladder
6. Migraine prophylaxis

C. FDA pediatric: None

VI. **Major Contraindications and When to Use Caution**

A. **Contraindications**

1. Hypersensitivity to nortriptyline
2. Concomitant use with a monoamine oxidase inhibitor (MAOI)
   a. See comment under "Clinical Pearls" regarding nortriptyline combination treatment.
3. Acute phase of recovery after myocardial infarction
4. Children younger than 12 years

[1]Evidence strength varies; readers are referred to the literature for more detailed information.

B. **Use caution**:

1. Elderly adults because of anticholinergic and sedating effects
2. Brugada syndrome
3. Concomitant alcohol use
4. Acute angle-closure glaucoma
5. History of seizures
6. Patients with hyperthyroidism or on medication for hypothyroidism
7. Patients who are poor metabolizers of cytochrome P450 (CYP) 2D6

VII. Dosage Formulations

A. Brand and generic capsule (10 mg, 25 mg, 50 mg, 75 mg)

B. Generic oral solution (10 mg/5 mL) (473 mL bottle)

VIII. Dosage Ranges and Guidelines

A. Depression: 25 mg taken 3–4 times daily. Alternatively, nortriptyline can be taken once a day, generally at night. Start with a lower dosage and increase with appropriate monitoring of plasma levels.

B. ADHD: 10 mg/day at bedtime (up to 25 mg BID)

C. Lower back pain: Up to 100 mg/day

D. Diabetic neuropathy: 25–150 mg/day as a single dose or in divided doses

E. Smoking cessation: Up to 75–100 mg/day for 6–14 weeks

F. Migraine prophylaxis: 10–150 mg/day

IX. Monitoring

A. Therapeutic drug monitoring:

1. For dosages higher than 100 mg/day, plasma levels should be monitored.
2. The therapeutic range of the drug is 50–150 ng/mL, with a curvilinear dose-response relationship, meaning that nortriptyline levels higher than 150 ng/mL are associated with a poorer clinical response (Montgomery et al. 1978; Ziegler et al. 1976).
3. Plasma-level monitoring is recommended to ensure that blood levels are within the therapeutic range. Plasma levels may vary among patients, given the heterogeneity of the CYP2D6 pathways involved in nortriptyline's metabolism.

B. Sodium levels: Measure at baseline and after 3–4 weeks.

C. Liver function tests: Monitor periodically.

D. Obtain ECG at baseline, after dosage changes, and up to every 3 months for patients with specific cardiac risk factors.

E. Blood pressure: Measure at baseline, after dosage changes, and every 3–6 months once the dosage is stabilized.

F. Weight changes: Check weight at 3, 6, and 12 months and yearly thereafter.

G. Risk of manic switch in bipolar patients: Needs to be appropriately monitored.

X. Relevant Pharmacokinetics/Pharmacodynamics

A. **Metabolism**: Rapidly absorbed after oral administration. Bioavailability is 45%–85% due to the high first-pass effect. Primarily metabolized in the liver, with metabolites renally excreted. 10-hydroxynortriptyline is the major active metabolite. CYP metabolism: Primarily CYP2D6.

B. **Time to peak plasma concentration**: 7–8.5 hours
C. **Half-life**: 36 hours
D. **Hepatic impairment**: Use reduced dosages in patients with liver disease.
E. **Renal impairment**: Reduced dosages may be needed in patients with moderate to severe renal impairment.
F. **Elderly individuals**: Nortriptyline use should be avoided in elderly adults (per the Beers Criteria [American Geriatrics Society 2023]), as it may lead to sedation and orthostasis. If used, nortriptyline should be started at a lower dosage and increased slowly based on tolerability.

XI. Clinically Relevant Drug Interactions

A. Metabolized by CYP2D6 (major) and by CYP3A4, CYP2C19, and CYP1A2 (all minor).
   1. Caution should be used when prescribing nortriptyline to patients who are taking CYP2D6 inhibitors (e.g., quinidine, cimetidine, fluoxetine, bupropion) or who are known to be poor metabolizers of CYP2D6, as drug concentrations may be higher.

B. Caution should be used when prescribing nortriptyline in combination with other medications, such as the following:
   1. Other serotonergic medications, including other TCAs, selective serotonin reuptake inhibitors, serotonin-norepinephrine reuptake inhibitors, MAOIs, dextromethorphan, tramadol, methadone, St. John's wort
   2. Medications with anticholinergic effects (e.g., atropine, glycopyrrolate, benztropine, trihexyphenidyl, procyclidine, prochlorperazine, meclizine, scopolamine, hydroxyzine)
   3. Medications that prolong QTc (e.g., cisapride, amiodarone, sotalol, quinidine, procainamide, fluoroquinolones, sumatriptan, ondansetron, haloperidol, risperidone, ziprasidone, olanzapine, quetiapine, methadone)

XII. Adverse Effects

A. Possible increased risk of suicidality:
   1. See "Boxed Warning: Suicidality and Antidepressant Drugs" in the introduction to TCAs. For detailed information, readers are referred to comprehensive sources in the literature (e.g., Fergusson et al. 2005).

B. Serotonin syndrome
C. Cardiovascular:
   1. Arrhythmias
   2. Prolonged QTc interval and QRS widening
      a. Nortriptyline can cause QTc prolongation and other cardiac rhythm changes, especially at higher dosages.
   3. Myocardial infarction

D. Gastrointestinal:

1. Nausea
2. Vomiting
3. Anorexia

E. Neurological:

1. Numbness
2. Tingling
3. Somnolence
4. Seizure
    a. Nortriptyline decreases the seizure threshold and leads to changes in EEG and sleep patterns.

F. Endocrine:

1. Weight gain
2. Sexual dysfunction

G. Hematological:

1. Agranulocytosis
2. Eosinophilia
3. Thrombocytopenia

H. Hepatic:

1. Altered liver function
2. Jaundice

I. Anticholinergic effects:

1. Urinary retention
2. Constipation
3. Paralytic ileus
4. Dry mouth
5. Hyperpyrexia
6. Mydriasis
7. Blurred vision
8. Narrow angle closure glaucoma

J. **Risks in pregnancy and lactation**

1. Nortriptyline's effects on fetal development are unclear. It should not be used in pregnant women unless the benefits outweigh the risk to the fetus.
2. A minimal amount of the medication passes into breast milk. Therefore, it may be acceptable for patients to breastfeed during treatment. Consultation with an OB/GYN is recommended.

XIII. **Clinical Pearls/Prescribing Tips**

A. Nortriptyline may be sedating for some individuals; for these patients, the entire daily dose can be taken at bedtime. However, nortriptyline is less sedating than amitriptyline. Overall, nortriptyline's side-effect profile is more favorable than that of tertiary amines such as amitriptyline, clomipramine, and imipramine.

B. QTc prolongation and decreases in the seizure threshold are notable potential adverse effects of nortriptyline.
C. Nortriptyline should be discontinued before elective surgery because it may interact with agents used during anesthesia.
D. In some patients, improvement in depressive symptoms may be noticed after 2–4 weeks of nortriptyline treatment.
E. Certain TCAs—particularly those with less notable SERT blockade, such as nortriptyline and desipramine (secondary amines)—may be safer in combination with SSRIs, other TCAs, and MAOIs than previously thought, although patient should still be monitored closely for adverse effects, including serotonin syndrome, hypertension, headache, insomnia, and constipation (Amsterdam and Kim 2019; Gillman 2007; Goldberg and Thornton 1978).
F. TCAs in general have been shown to be more efficacious than SNRIs—and significantly more efficacious than SSRIs—in treating neuropathic pain.

Further Reading

Atkinson HJ, Slater MA, Williams RA, et al: A placebo-controlled randomized clinical trial of nortriptyline for chronic low back pain. Pain 76(3):287–296, 1998 9718247

Cadila Healthcare Ltd: Nortriptyline capsules [package insert]. U.S. Food and Drug Administration website. Revised August 2019. Available at: https://www.accessdata.fda.gov/spl/data/2e1c5e82-2293-4241-87ff-df3a7398f7fc/2e1c5e82-2293-4241-87ff-df3a7398f7fc.xml. Accessed March 13, 2024.

Dodd S, Malhi GS, Tiller J, et al: A consensus statement for safety monitoring guidelines of treatments for major depressive disorder. Aust NZ J Psychiatry 45(9):712–725, 2011 21888608

Finnerup NB, Attal N, Haroutounian S, et al: Pharmacotherapy for neuropathic pain in adults: a systematic review and meta-analysis. Lancet Neurol 14(2):162–173, 2015 25575710

Hughes JR, Stead LF, Hartmann-Boyce J, et al: Antidepressants for smoking cessation. Cochrane Database Syst Rev (1):CD000031, 2014 24402784

Mallinckrodt Inc: Pamelor (nortriptyline HCl) capsules, oral solution [package insert]. U.S. Food and Drug Administration website. Revised October 2012. Available at: https://www.accessdata.fda.gov/drugsatfda_docs/label/2012/018012s029,018013s061lbl.pdf. Accessed March 13, 2024.

Merwar G, Gibbons JR, Hosseini SA, et al: Nortriptyline, in StatPearls. Treasure Island, FL, StatPearls Publishing, 2022

Nortriptyline, in Drugs and Lactation Database (LactMed). Bethesda, MD, National Library of Medicine, 2022. Available at: https://www.ncbi.nlm.nih.gov/books/NBK501176/. Accessed March 13, 2024.

Nortriptyline, in PubChem Compound Summary for CID 4543. National Center for Biotechnology Information, 2022. Available at: https://pubchem.ncbi.nlm.nih.gov/compound/Nortriptyline. Accessed March 13, 2024.

Saul RC: Nortriptyline in attention deficit disorder (letter). Clin Neuropharmacol 8(4):382–383, 1985 4075308

References

American Geriatrics Society Beers Criteria Update Expert Panel: 2023 updated AGS Beers Criteria for potentially inappropriate medication use in older adults. J Am Geriatr Soc 71(7):2052–2081, 2023 37139824

Amsterdam JD, Kim TT: Relative effectiveness of monoamine oxidase inhibitor and tricyclic antidepressant combination therapy for treatment-resistant depression. J Clin Psychopharmacol 39(6):649–652, 2019 31688401

Fergusson D, Doucette S, Glass KC, et al: Association between suicide attempts and selective serotonin reuptake inhibitors: systematic review of randomised controlled trials. BMJ 330(7488):396, 2005 15718539

Gillman PK: Tricyclic antidepressant pharmacology and therapeutic drug interactions updated. Br J Pharmacol 151(6):737–748, 2007 17471183

Goldberg RS, Thornton WE: Combined tricyclic-MAOI therapy for refractory depression: a review, with guidelines for appropriate usage. J Clin Pharmacol 18(2–3):143–147, 1978 342553

Montgomery S, Braithwaite R, Dawling S, et al: High plasma nortriptyline levels in the treatment of depression. I. Clin Pharmacol Ther 23(3):309–314, 1978 627137

Roth BL, Driscoll J: PDSP Ki Database. Psychoactive Drug Screening Program (PDSP). University of North Carolina at Chapel Hill and the United States National Institute of Mental Health, 1999–present. Available at: https://pdsp.unc.edu/databases/pdsp.php. Accessed June 21, 2024.

Takano H, Arakawa R, Nogami T, et al: Norepinephrine transporter occupancy by nortriptyline in patients with depression: a positron emission tomography study with (S,S)-[18F]FMeNER-D2. Int J Neuropsychopharmacol 17(4):553–560, 2014 24345533

Ziegler VE, Clayton PJ, Taylor JR, et al: Nortriptyline plasma levels and therapeutic response. Clin Pharmacol Ther 20(4):458–463, 1976 788992

Protriptyline

I. **Brand Names**: Vivactil

II. **Therapeutic Class**: Tricyclic antidepressant (TCA), secondary amine

III. **Chemical Name**: *N*-methyl-5*H* dibenzo[*a,d*]-cycloheptene-5-propanamine hydrochloride

IV. **Mechanism(s) of Action**

A. Protriptyline inhibits the membrane reuptake of norepinephrine and serotonin by adrenergic and serotonergic neurons at the presynaptic membranes, leading to increased levels of both in the synapse. Additionally, it blocks adrenergic and muscarinic receptors.

B. Protriptyline has more potent NET inhibition than SERT inhibition (NET Ki = 1.41 nM vs. SERT Ki = 19.6 nM) (Roth and Driscoll 1999–present).

C. Other notable receptor actions include H_1 inhibition (Ki = 7.2–25 nM) and moderate to low α_1 inhibition (Ki = 130 nM) and cholinergic (muscarinic acetylcholine [mACh]) inhibition (Ki = 25 nM).

V. **Indications**

A. FDA adult: Depression

B. Evidence-based[1] off-label uses:

1. Narcolepsy (cataplexy)

C. FDA pediatric: None

VI. **Major Contraindications and When to Use Caution**

A. **Contraindications**:

1. Hypersensitivity to protriptyline
2. Concomitant use of a monoamine oxidase inhibitor (MAOI) or another TCA
3. Acute phase of recovery after myocardial infarction
4. Concomitant use of cisapride, as it can lead to significant QTc prolongation

B. **Use caution**:

1. Older adults because of anticholinergic and sedating effects
2. Heart conduction defects or arrhythmias
3. Congestive heart failure
4. Concomitant alcohol use
5. Acute angle-closure glaucoma
6. History of seizures
7. Urinary retention
8. Patients with hyperthyroidism or on medication for hypothyroidism
9. Risk of arrhythmias
10. Patients who are poor metabolizers of cytochrome P450 (CYP) 2D6

[1]Evidence strength varies; readers are referred to the literature for more detailed information.

VII. **Dosage Formulations**

A. Generic and brand tablet (5 mg, 10 mg)

VIII. **Dosage Ranges and Guidelines**

A. Depression: 15–40 mg/day taken as a single dose or multiple divided doses. Maximum dosage is 60 mg/day.
B. Narcolepsy: 30 mg/day at bedtime

IX. **Monitoring**

A. Therapeutic drug monitoring:
   1. Timing: Draw trough just prior to next dose.
   2. Optimal ranges are not fully clarified, but some data suggest that optimal antidepressant effect is associated with 70–260 ng/mL (Orsulak and Schildkraut 1979).
   3. Plasma levels may vary among individuals, given the heterogeneity of the CYP2D6 pathways involved in protriptyline's metabolism.
B. Sodium levels: Measure at baseline and after 3–4 weeks.
C. Liver function tests: Monitor periodically.
D. Obtain ECG at baseline, after dosage changes, and up to every 3 months thereafter.
E. Blood pressure: Measure at baseline, after dosage changes, and every 3–6 months once the dosage is stabilized
F. Weight changes: Check weight at 3, 6, and 12 months and yearly thereafter.
G. Risk of manic switch in bipolar patients: Needs to be appropriately monitored.

X. **Relevant Pharmacokinetics/Pharmacodynamics**

A. **Metabolism**: Rapidly absorbed after oral administration and undergoes significant first-pass effect. Primarily metabolized in the liver; ultimately excreted in the urine. CYP metabolism: CYP2D6.
B. **Time to peak plasma concentration**: 8–12 hours
C. **Half-life**: 74 hours
D. **Hepatic impairment**: Use with caution in individuals with liver impairment; may require reduced dosages.
E. **Renal impairment**: Use with caution in individuals with renal impairment; may require reduced dosages.
F. **Elderly individuals**: Protriptyline use should be avoided in this population (per the Beers Criteria [American Geriatrics Society 2023]), as it may lead to sedation and orthostasis. If used, protriptyline should be started at 5 mg TID and increased slowly. Dosages higher than 20 mg/day require close cardiac monitoring.

XI. **Clinically Relevant Drug Interactions**

A. Metabolized by CYP2D6 (minor).
   1. Caution should be used with CYP2D6 inhibitors (e.g., quinidine, cimetidine, fluoxetine, bupropion) or in known CYP2D6 poor metabolizers, as drug concentrations may be higher.

B. Caution should be used when prescribing protriptyline in combination with other medications, such as the following:

  1. Other serotonergic medications, including other TCAs, selective serotonin reuptake inhibitors, serotonin-norepinephrine reuptake inhibitors, MAOIs, dextromethorphan, tramadol, methadone, St. John's wort
  2. Medications with anticholinergic effects (e.g., atropine, glycopyrrolate, benztropine, trihexyphenidyl, procyclidine, prochlorperazine, meclizine, scopolamine, hydroxyzine)
  3. Medications that prolong QTc (e.g., cisapride, amiodarone, sotalol, quinidine, procainamide, fluoroquinolones, sumatriptan, ondansetron, haloperidol, risperidone, ziprasidone, olanzapine, quetiapine, methadone)

XII. Adverse Effects

A. Possible increased risk of suicidality:

  1. See "Boxed Warning: Suicidality and Antidepressant Drugs" in the introduction to TCAs. For detailed information, readers are referred to comprehensive sources in the literature (e.g., Fergusson et al. 2005).

B. Serotonin syndrome

C. Cardiovascular:

  1. Tachycardia
  2. Arrhythmias
  3. Prolonged QTc interval and QRS widening
     a. Protriptyline can cause QTc prolongation as well as other cardiac rhythm changes, and close monitoring is recommended.
  4. Myocardial infarction
  5. Orthostatic hypotension

D. Gastrointestinal:

  1. Nausea
  2. Vomiting
  3. Diarrhea

E. Neurological:

  1. Dizziness
  2. Paresthesia
  3. Tremor
  4. Seizure

F. Endocrine:

  1. Weight gain.
  2. Hyperglycemia

G. Hematological:

  1. Agranulocytosis
  2. Eosinophilia

H. Hepatic:

1. Altered liver function

I. Anticholinergic effects:

1. Urinary retention
2. Constipation
3. Paralytic ileus
4. Dry mouth
5. Hyperthermia
6. Mydriasis
7. Blurred vision
8. Narrow angle closure glaucoma

J. **Risks in pregnancy and lactation**

1. Protriptyline's effects on fetal development are unclear; therefore, it should not be used in pregnant women unless the benefits outweigh the risks to the fetus.
2. Presence of protriptyline in breast milk is unclear. Therefore, it may be preferable to avoid use in patients who are breastfeeding. Consultation with an OB/GYN specialist is recommended.

XIII. **Clinical Pearls/Prescribing Tips**

A. Protriptyline is less likely than other TCAs to have anticholinergic effects and generally causes less sedation. Monitor QTc.

B. Protriptyline should be discontinued before elective surgery because it may interact with agents used during anesthesia.

C. Improvement in depressive symptoms may be noticed after 3–4 weeks of protriptyline treatment.

Further Reading

Henry GK, Hart RP, Kwentus JA, et al: Effects of protriptyline on vigilance and information processing in narcolepsy. Psychopharmacology (Berl) 95(1):109–112, 1988 3133688

Epic Pharma LLC: Protriptyline hydrochloride tablets [package insert]. U.S. Food and Drug Administration website. Revised May 2020. Available at: https://www.accessdata.fda.gov/spl/data/8d390c9f-eabf-4ee1-8f21-d752d6aa5d1b/8d390c9f-eabf-4ee1-8f21-d752d6aa5d1b.xml. Accessed June 21, 2024.

Protriptyline, in PubChem Compound Summary for CID 4976. National Center for Biotechnology Information, 2022. Available at: https://pubchem.ncbi.nlm.nih.gov/compound/Protriptyline. Accessed June 2022.

Saef MA, Yilanli M, Saadabadi A: Protriptyline, in StatPearls. Treasure Island, FL, StatPearls Publishing, 2022

Teva Pharmaceuticals USA: Vivactil (protriptyline hydrochloride) tablets [package insert]. U.S. Food and Drug Administration website. Revised May 2014. Available at: https://www.accessdata.fda.gov/drugsatfda_docs/label/2014/073645s028,073644s023lbl.pdf. Accessed March 13, 2024.

References

American Geriatrics Society Beers Criteria Update Expert Panel: 2023 updated AGS Beers Criteria for potentially inappropriate medication use in older adults. J Am Geriatr Soc 71(7):2052–2081, 2023 37139824

Fergusson D, Doucette S, Glass KC, et al: Association between suicide attempts and selective serotonin reuptake inhibitors: systematic review of randomised controlled trials. BMJ 330(7488):396, 2005 15718539

Orsulak PJ, Schildkraut JJ: Guidelines for therapeutic monitoring of tricyclic antidepressant plasma levels. Ther Drug Monit 1(2):199–208, 1979 555572

Roth BL, Driscoll J: PDSP Ki Database. Psychoactive Drug Screening Program (PDSP). University of North Carolina at Chapel Hill and the United States National Institute of Mental Health, 1999–present. Available at: https://pdsp.unc.edu/databases/pdsp.php. Accessed June 21, 2024.

Other Antidepressants

Bupropion

I. **Brand Names**: Aplenzin, Budeprion SR, Buproban, Forfivo XL, Wellbutrin, Wellbutrin XL, Wellbutrin SR, Zyban

II. **Therapeutic Class**: Antidepressant, smoking cessation aid

III. **Mechanism-Based Class**: Norepinephrine and dopamine reuptake inhibitor and releaser

IV. **Mechanism(s) of Action**

A. The active metabolites of bupropion—S,S-hydroxybupropion (the primary metabolite), threohydrobupropion, and erythrohydrobupropion—reach higher plasma levels than the parent molecule (Costa et al. 2019).

B. CNS inhibition of the DAT (dopamine transporter), reducing reuptake of dopamine in the CNS

1. DAT inhibition for bupropion: Ki = 0.66 nM; DAT inhibition for S,S-hydroxybupropion: Ki = 0.63 nM (Lukas et al. 2010)
2. At 150 mg/day, bupropion occupies nearly zero DAT receptor sites, but at 300 mg/day, bupropion occupies approximately 20% of the sites, compared with >50% occupancy for methylphenidate at therapeutic dosages (Carroll et al. 2014; Verbeeck et al. 2017).

C. CNS inhibition of the NET (norepinephrine transporter), reducing reuptake of norepinephrine in the CNS

1. NET inhibition for bupropion: Ki = 1.85 nM; NET inhibition for S,S-hydroxybupropion: Ki = 0.24 nM (Lukas et al. 2010)
2. S,S-hydroxybupropion is an active metabolite and has more affinity for the NET than does the parent molecule.

D. Antagonism of nicotinic acetylcholine receptors ($\alpha_3\beta_4$, $\alpha_4\beta_2$, $\alpha_1\beta_1\gamma\delta$)

1. This antagonism occurs with both the parent molecule and (to varying degrees) the metabolites.
2. Antagonism of nicotinic receptors is likely helpful for smoking cessation, but may also treat depression by decreasing overactivation of cholinergic activity, thought to be a factor in the development of depression (Shytle et al. 2002).

V. **Indications**

A. FDA adult:

1. Major depressive disorder
2. Prevention of seasonal affective disorder (XL only)
3. Smoking cessation (the Zyban brand was discontinued)

B. Evidence-based[1] off-label uses:
   1. ADHD
   2. Bipolar depression
   3. SSRI-induced sexual dysfunction

C. FDA pediatric: None

VI. **Major Contraindications and When to Use Caution**

A. Known allergy to bupropion or its components
B. Concomitant use of MAOI antidepressants or other MAO-inhibiting agents (e.g., linezolid, IV methylene blue)—A 2-week washout is typically required.
C. Seizure disorder or other risk factors for seizure: Withdrawal from alcohol, benzodiazepines, barbiturates, antiepileptic drugs, head injury, metabolic disorders, other medications that lower seizure threshold, illicit drug use/abuse
D. Current or prior diagnosis of bulimia or anorexia nervosa, which is also a risk factor for electrolyte abnormalities and seizures
E. Bupropion may decrease alcohol tolerance.

VII. **Dosage Formulations**—*Note*: For SR/XL/ER forms, do not break, cut, or crush.

A. Generic IR tablet (75 mg, 100 mg), *not scored*
B. Brand SR tablet (100 mg, 150 mg, 300 mg)
C. Generic SR tablet (100 mg, 150 mg, 300 mg)
D. Brand ER/XL tablet (150 mg, 300 mg, 450 mg)
E. Generic ER tablet (150 mg, 300 mg)

VIII. **Dosage Ranges and Guidelines**

A. Refer to Table 2–16 for dosage ranges (initial/maximum) and guidelines.
B. Bupropion IR (dosed three times daily): Start at 100 mg BID. After 1 week, increase to 100 mg TID. Can further increase to a maximum of 450 mg/day in 3–4 divided doses.
C. Bupropion SR (12 hours, BID): Start at 150 mg/day. After 1 week, increase to 150 mg BID. Can further increase to a maximum of 200 mg BID (400 mg/day total).
D. Bupropion ER/XL (24 hours, once daily): Start at 150 mg/day. After 1 week, increase to 300 mg/day. Can further increase to a maximum of 450 mg/day.

Table 2–16. Bupropion indications and dosage ranges

Indication	Usual dosage range
Major depressive disorder	IR: 100 mg BID → 150 mg TID (or 450 mg/day split into 3–4 doses) SR: 100 mg/day → 200 mg BID (400 mg total, split dose) ER/XL: 150–450 mg/day
Prevention of seasonal affective disorder	ER/XL: 150–300 mg/day (start in the fall prior to onset of symptoms and continue through winter)

[1]Evidence strength varies; readers are referred to the literature for more detailed information.

Table 2–16. Bupropion indications and dosage ranges *(continued)*

Indication	Usual dosage range
ADHD[a] (off-label)	IR: 100 mg/day → 200 mg BID ER/XL: 150–450 mg/day
Bipolar depression[b] (off-label)	SR: 100 mg/day → 225 mg BID (450 mg/day maximum)
SSRI-induced sexual dysfunction, as augmentation[c] (off-label)	SR: 150 mg/day → 150 mg BID
Smoking cessation[d] (off-label)	SR: 150 mg/day → 150 mg BID (start 1 week prior to quit date; continue for at least 12 weeks)

Note. Conversion between formulations: Keep the same total daily dosage but adjust frequency. IR 3–4 times daily, SR 2 times daily, and ER/XL 1 time daily.

[a]Bupropion is an effective second-line agent for ADHD symptoms (Bond et al. 2012; Verbeeck et al. 2017; Wilens et al. 2001, 2005) and has demonstrated efficacy similar to that of methylphenidate in children/adolescents (Jafarinia et al. 2012).

[b]Numerous trials have indicated bupropion's effectiveness in bipolar depression (Grossman et al. 1999; McIntyre et al. 2002), with a potentially lower risk of manic switch compared with many other antidepressants (Leverich et al. 2006; Sachs et al. 1994), although this is somewhat controversial (Fogelson et al. 1992; Li et al. 2016). Risk of manic switch could be dosage-related (Goren and Levin 2000).

[c]Bupropion may be an effective augmenting agent for patients with antidepressant-related sexual dysfunction (Montejo et al. 2019), as it has been shown to increase self-reported feelings of sexual desire and frequency of sexual activity (Clayton et al. 2004), as well as desire, arousal, lubrication, orgasm, and satisfaction for women (Safarinejad 2011).

[d]Bupropion has been shown to aid in long-term smoking cessation, either alongside or independent of nicotine replacement therapy, although it was less effective than varenicline (Hughes et al. 2014; Wu et al. 2006). Studies indicate that bupropion can alleviate some nicotine withdrawal symptoms, including irritability, concentration difficulties, increased appetite, and depressed mood, as well as smoking cravings (Mooney and Sofuoglu 2006).

IX. Monitoring

A. Monitor blood pressure periodically, especially if used in combination with nicotine replacement therapy (NRT).

X. Relevant Pharmacokinetics/Pharmacodynamics

A. **Metabolism**: Hepatic to R,R- and S,S-hydroxybupropion; non–cytochrome P450 (CYP) metabolism (liver and intestine) to erythrohydrobupropion and threohydrobupropion

B. **Time to peak plasma concentration**:

1. IR bupropion: 1–2 hours; IR hydroxybupropion: 3 hours
2. SR bupropion: up to 3 hours; SR hydroxybupropion: 6–7 hours
    a. *Note*: The SR and XL formulations have a slightly lower maximum concentration of drug and fewer daily plasma peaks, potentially leading to better tolerability (Fava et al. 2005).
3. XL/ER bupropion: 5 hours; XL/ER hydroxybupropion: 6–7 hours
    a. *Note*: The XL tablet has a moisture-barrier coating and a controlled-release coating surrounding the tablet, extending the release of the drug. Crushing/chewing or cutting destroys this matrix (Fava et al. 2005).

C. **Half-life**:
   1. Bupropion: 8–10 hours
   2. Metabolites: ~24 hours
D. **Hepatic impairment**: Consider lowering the dosage or dose frequency in patients with hepatic impairment. In patients with moderate to severe impairment, limit dosage to 150 mg every other day.
E. **Renal impairment**: Consider lowering the dosage or dose frequency in patients with renal impairment, given decreased elimination and accumulation of metabolites in renal impairment (Bausch Health US 2022; GlaxoSmithKline 2020).

XI. **Clinically Relevant Drug Interactions**

A. Metabolized via CYP2B6 to R,R- and S,S-hydroxybupropion.
   1. May need to increase bupropion dosage when coadministered with CYP2B6 inducers, such as ritonavir, lopinavir, efavirenz, carbamazepine, phenobarbital, or phenytoin (Bausch Health US 2022; GlaxoSmithKline 2020.
   2. May need to decrease bupropion dosage when coadministered with CYP2B6 inhibitors, such as clopidogrel or ticlopidine (Bausch Health US 2022; GlaxoSmithKline 2020.
B. Inhibitor of CYP2D6
   1. May need to decrease dosages of drugs metabolized by CYP2D6, including many antidepressants, antipsychotics, beta-blockers, and antiarrhythmics.
      a. Use caution with drugs that lower the seizure threshold.
      b. Use caution with dopaminergic drugs (e.g., levodopa, amantadine), given the potential for additive dopaminergic effects, such as restlessness, agitation, tremor, dizziness, ataxia, vertigo, and gait disturbance.

XII. **Adverse Effects**

A. **Boxed warning: suicidality and antidepressant drugs**:
   1. In common with all antidepressants, bupropion may carry an increased risk for suicidal thoughts/behaviors in pediatric and young adult patients. Patients should be monitored closely for emergence of suicidal thoughts. For detailed information, readers are referred to comprehensive sources in the literature (e.g., Fergusson et al. 2005).
B. **Most common**:
   1. Insomnia (16% for SR 400 mg/day vs. 5%–6% placebo [GlaxoSmithKline 2020]): Take XL in the morning and avoid taking IR/SR formulations too close to bedtime.
   2. Gastrointestinal: Dry mouth (24% for SR 400 mg/day vs. 7% placebo), abdominal pain, nausea, constipation, anorexia (all <20%) (GlaxoSmithKline 2020)
   3. Other: Headache, dizziness, sweating, tinnitus, tremor, hypertension, agitation

C. **Other notable side effects**:

1. Anxiety: Although commonly believed to increase anxiety in some cases, bupropion may actually treat anxiety (Bystritsky et al. 2008; Rush et al. 2001). Data from registration trials showed a similar incidence of anxiety compared with placebo (6%–7% vs. 5% placebo [[GlaxoSmithKline 2020]). Starting low and slowly titrating can be helpful for anxious patients.
2. Seizures: Low risk; higher risk with IR formulation and dosages higher than 300 mg/day (Hughes et al. 2014). For SR formulation, an overall seizure incidence of 0.07% was reported at dosages up to 400 mg/day (Stahl et al. 2004). Use caution or avoid bupropion in patients with risk factors for seizures (see "Major Contraindications").

D. **Rare**:

1. Activation of hypomania/mania, psychosis, or other neuropsychiatric events, angle-closure glaucoma, hypersensitivity reactions (e.g., anaphylactoid/anaphylactic reactions, erythema multiforme, Stevens-Johnson syndrome, serum sickness), neuropsychiatric adverse effects, and suicide risk in smoking cessation treatment (Bausch Health US 2022; GlaxoSmithKline 2020).

E. **Risks in pregnancy and lactation**: Bupropion was designated a Category C drug in the prior FDA classification and is present in breast milk. A thorough risk/benefit discussion with the patient is recommended on continuing versus stopping the medication, including consultation with an OB/GYN specialist and/or lactation expert. See Chapter 15 ("Women: Pregnancy, Postpartum, and Breastfeeding") for more information.

XIII. **Clinical Pearls/Prescribing Tips**

A. Bupropion is unique in that it has three distinct bioequivalent formulations (IR, SR, ER/XL), mainly differing in their time to peak absorption (as a result of their different drug delivery systems).
B. Bupropion may be especially beneficial in patients with depression in which lack of motivation and low energy are core features, given its potential to improve these symptoms.
C. Efficacy has been established for bupropion in aiding long-term smoking cessation, as a second-line treatment for ADHD (in patients for whom stimulants are not a good choice), and as an augmentation agent in patients with antidepressant-induced sexual dysfunction.
D. Bupropion historically was believed to be relatively safe in treating bipolar depression, with a lower risk of manic switch compared with other antidepressants, although this finding is controversial.
E. Bupropion's lack of serotonergic activity results in a lack of associated serotonergic side effects, such as weight gain, sexual dysfunction, and sedation (Stahl et al. 2004).
F. False-positive urine drug screens for amphetamine have occurred with bupropion (Casey et al. 2011; Reidy et al. 2011; Weintraub and Linder 2000).

Further Reading

Papakostas GI, Fava M: A meta-analysis of clinical trials comparing the serotonin (5-HT)-2 receptor antagonists trazodone and nefazodone with selective serotonin reuptake inhibitors for the treatment of major depressive disorder. Eur Psychiatry 22(7):444–447, 2007 17418537

Roth BL, Driscoll J: PDSP Ki Database. Psychoactive Drug Screening Program (PDSP). University of North Carolina at Chapel Hill and the United States National Institute of Mental Health, 1999–present. Available at: https://pdsp.unc.edu/databases/pdsp.php. Accessed June 21, 2024.

References

Bausch Health US: Wellbutrin XL (bupropion hydrochloride) extended-release tablets [package insert]. U.S. Food and Drug Administration website. Revised March 2022. Available at: https://www.accessdata.fda.gov/drugsatfda_docs/label/2022/021515s044lbl.pdf. Accessed March 13, 2024.

Bond DJ, Hadjipavlou G, Lam RW, et al; Canadian Network for Mood and Anxiety Treatments (CANMAT) Task Force: The Canadian Network for Mood and Anxiety Treatments (CANMAT) task force recommendations for the management of patients with mood disorders and comorbid attention-deficit/hyperactivity disorder. Ann Clin Psychiatry 24(1):23–37, 2012 22303520

Bystritsky A, Kerwin L, Feusner JD, et al: A pilot controlled trial of bupropion XL versus escitalopram in generalized anxiety disorder. Psychopharmacol Bull 41(1):46–51, 2008 18362870

Carroll FI, Blough BE, Mascarella SW, et al: Bupropion and bupropion analogs as treatments for CNS disorders. Adv Pharmacol 69:177–216, 2014 24484978

Casey ER, Scott MG, Tang S, et al: Frequency of false positive amphetamine screens due to bupropion using the Syva EMIT II immunoassay. J Med Toxicol 7(2):105–108, 2011 21191682

Clayton AH, Warnock JK, Kornstein SG, et al: A placebo-controlled trial of bupropion SR as an antidote for selective serotonin reuptake inhibitor-induced sexual dysfunction. J Clin Psychiatry 65(1):62–67, 2004 14744170

Costa R, Oliveira NG, Dinis-Oliveira RJ: Pharmacokinetic and pharmacodynamic of bupropion: integrative overview of relevant clinical and forensic aspects. Drug Metab Rev 51(3):293–313, 2019 31124380

Fergusson D, Doucette S, Glass KC, et al: Association between suicide attempts and selective serotonin reuptake inhibitors: systematic review of randomised controlled trials. BMJ 330(7488):396, 2005 15718539

Fava M, Rush AJ, Thase ME, et al: 15 years of clinical experience with bupropion HCl: from bupropion to bupropion SR to bupropion XL. Prim Care Companion J Clin Psychiatry 7(3):106–113, 2005 16027765

Fogelson DL, Bystritsky A, Pasnau R: Bupropion in the treatment of bipolar disorders: the same old story? J Clin Psychiatry 53(12):443–446, 1992 1487473

GlaxoSmithKline: Wellbutrin SR (bupropion hydrochloride sustained-release tablets) [package insert]. U.S. Food and Drug Administration website. Revised October 2020. Available at: https://www.accessdata.fda.gov/drugsatfda_docs/label/2020/020358s064lbl.pdf. Accessed March 13, 2024.

Goren JL, Levin GM: Mania with bupropion: a dose-related phenomenon? Ann Pharmacother 34(5):619–621, 2000 10852090

Grossman F, Potter WZ, Brown EA, et al: A double-blind study comparing idazoxan and bupropion in bipolar depressed patients. J Affect Disord 56(2-3):237–243, 1999 10701483

Hughes JR, Stead LF, Hartmann-Boyce J, et al: Antidepressants for smoking cessation. Cochrane Database Syst Rev (1):CD000031, 2014 24402784

Jafarinia M, Mohammadi MR, Modabbernia A, et al: Bupropion versus methylphenidate in the treatment of children with attention-deficit/hyperactivity disorder: randomized double-blind study. Hum Psychopharmacol 27(4):411–418, 2012 22806822

Leverich GS, Altshuler LL, Frye MA, et al: Risk of switch in mood polarity to hypomania or mania in patients with bipolar depression during acute and continuation trials of venlafaxine, sertraline, and bupropion as adjuncts to mood stabilizers. Am J Psychiatry 163(2):232–239, 2006 16449476

Li DJ, Tseng PT, Chen YW, et al: Significant treatment effect of bupropion in patients with bipolar disorder but similar phase-shifting rate as other antidepressants: a meta-analysis following the PRISMA guidelines. Medicine (Baltimore) 95(13):e3165, 2016 27043678

Lukas RJ, Muresan AZ, Damaj MI, et al: Synthesis and characterization of in vitro and in vivo profiles of hydroxybupropion analogues: aids to smoking cessation. J Med Chem 53(12):4731–4748, 2010 20509659

McIntyre RS, Mancini DA, McCann S, et al: Topiramate versus bupropion SR when added to mood stabilizer therapy for the depressive phase of bipolar disorder: a preliminary single-blind study. Bipolar Disord 4(3):207–213, 2002 12180276

Montejo AL, Prieto N, de Alarcón R, et al: Management strategies for antidepressant-related sexual dysfunction: a clinical approach. J Clin Med 8(10):1640, 2019 31591339

Mooney ME, Sofuoglu M: Bupropion for the treatment of nicotine withdrawal and craving. Expert Rev Neurother 6(7):965–981, 2006 16831112

Reidy L, Walls HC, Steele BW: Crossreactivity of bupropion metabolite with enzyme-linked immunosorbent assays designed to detect amphetamine in urine. Ther Drug Monit 33(3):366–368, 2011 21436763

Rush AJ, Trivedi MH, Carmody TJ, et al: Response in relation to baseline anxiety levels in major depressive disorder treated with bupropion sustained release or sertraline. Neuropsychopharmacology 25(1):131–138, 2001 11377926

Sachs GS, Lafer B, Stoll AL, et al: A double-blind trial of bupropion versus desipramine for bipolar depression. J Clin Psychiatry 55(9):391–393, 1994 7929019

Safarinejad MR: Reversal of SSRI-induced female sexual dysfunction by adjunctive bupropion in menstruating women: a double-blind, placebo-controlled and randomized study. J Psychopharmacol 25(3):370–378, 2011 20080928

Shytle RD, Silver AA, Lukas RJ, et al: Nicotinic acetylcholine receptors as targets for antidepressants. Mol Psychiatry 7(6):525–535, 2002 12140772

Stahl SM, Pradko JF, Haight BR, et al: A review of the neuropharmacology of bupropion, a dual norepinephrine and dopamine reuptake inhibitor. Prim Care Companion J Clin Psychiatry 6(4):159–166, 2004 15361919

Verbeeck W, Bekkering GE, Van den Noortgate W, et al: Bupropion for attention deficit hyperactivity disorder (ADHD) in adults. Cochrane Database Syst Rev (10):CD009504, 2017 28965364

Weintraub D, Linder MW: Amphetamine positive toxicology screen secondary to bupropion. Depress Anxiety 12(1):53–54, 2000 10999247

Wilens TE, Spencer TJ, Biederman J, et al: A controlled clinical trial of bupropion for attention deficit hyperactivity disorder in adults. Am J Psychiatry 158(2):282–288, 2001 11156812

Wilens TE, Haight BR, Horrigan JP, et al: Bupropion XL in adults with attention-deficit/hyperactivity disorder: a randomized, placebo-controlled study. Biol Psychiatry 57(7):793–801, 2005 15820237

Wu P, Wilson K, Dimoulas P, et al: Effectiveness of smoking cessation therapies: a systematic review and meta-analysis. BMC Public Health 6:300, 2006 17156479

Mirtazapine

I. **Brand Names**: Remeron

II. **Therapeutic Class**: Noradrenergic and specific serotonergic antidepressant (NaSSA)

III. **Mechanism-Based Class**: Norepinephrine and serotonin receptor antagonist

IV. **Mechanism(s) of Action**—*Note*: Ki data obtained from PDSP Ki Database (Roth and Driscoll 1999–present).

A. Dosage-dependent effects: At low dosages, mirtazapine is more selective for H_1, $5\text{-}HT_{2A}$, and $5\text{-}HT_{2C}$ receptor antagonism, causing sedating effects. However, at dosages higher than 15 mg/day, noradrenergic activation (via α_2-adrenergic receptor inhibition) overrides the sedating antihistamine activity, increasing activation (Barkin et al. 1999).

B. α_2-adrenergic receptor inhibition (Ki for α_{2A}=10 nM, α_{2B}=88 nM, α_{2C}=18 nM)

1. Blockade at autoreceptors on *adrenergic* neurons leads to disinhibition of norepinephrine release (Croom et al. 2009).
2. Blockade at heteroreceptors on *serotonergic* neurons leads to disinhibition of 5-HT release (Croom et al. 2009).

   a. Specifically, mirtazapine's α_2-adrenergic receptor antagonist activity and $5\text{-}HT_{1A}$ receptor agonist activity have been shown to increase dopamine levels in the medial prefrontal cortex, potentially contributing to its antidepressant effects (Berendsen and Broekkamp 1997; Nakayama et al. 2004).

C. H_1 antagonism (Ki=0.14–1.6 nM): Potent inhibitor, likely accounting for sedation, weight gain

D. $5\text{-}HT_{2A}$ antagonism (Ki=6.3–69 nM): Sedating, anxiolytic effects (Barkin et al. 1999; Millan 2005)

E. $5\text{-}HT_{2C}$ antagonism (Ki=8.9–39 nM): $5\text{-}HT_{2C}$ receptor blockade has been shown to increase dopamine and norepinephrine in the prefrontal cortex and likely potentiates the antidepressant/anxiolytic effects of SSRIs and SNRIs (Barkin et al. 1999; Demireva et al. 2020). $5\text{-}HT_{2C}$ receptor antagonism has benefits in sleep and sexual function and may increase appetite (Millan 2005); it may also be implicated in weight gain.

F. $5\text{-}HT_3$ antagonism (Ki=8.1): $5\text{-}HT_3$ receptor blockade inhibits the vomiting signal in the chemoreceptor trigger zone of the brain (Kast and Foley 2007) and may also be anxiolytic (Barkin et al. 1999).

V. **Indications**

A. FDA adult: Major depressive disorder (MDD)

B. Evidence-based[1] off-label uses:

1. Panic disorder
2. Headache, chronic tension-type, prophylaxis
3. Anxiety

---

[1]Evidence strength varies; readers are referred to the literature for more detailed information.

4. Nausea, vomiting
5. Insomnia

C. FDA pediatric: None

VI. **Major Contraindications and When to Use Caution**

A. Known allergy to mirtazapine or its components
B. Concomitant use of MAOI antidepressants or other MAO-inhibiting agents (e.g., linezolid, IV methylene blue)—A 2-week washout is typically required.

VII. **Dosage Formulations**

A. Brand tablet (15 mg, 30 mg—*both scored*)
B. Brand disintegrating tablet (15 mg, 30 mg, 45 mg)
C. Generic tablet (7.5 mg, 15 mg [*scored*], 30 mg [*scored*], 45 mg)
D. Generic disintegrating tablet (15 mg, 30 mg, 45 mg)

VIII. **Dosage Ranges and Guidelines**

A. Refer to Table 2–17 for dosage ranges (initial/maximum) and guidelines.
B. For MDD, start at 15 mg once daily; after 1 week, increase by 15 mg/day to a maximum dosage of 60 mg/day. Typically taken at bedtime.
C. For individuals sensitive to medication or to clinically harness mirtazapine's more sedating effects, could start at 7.5 mg/day taken at bedtime.

Table 2–17. Mirtazapine indications and dosage ranges

Indication	Usual dosage range
Major depressive disorder[a]	15–45 mg/day (dosages up to 60 mg/day have been used)
Panic disorder (off label)[b]	15–45 mg/day
Headache, chronic tension-type, prophylaxis (off-label)[c]	15–30 mg QHS (every night at bedtime)
Other off-label uses[d,e]	7.5–60 mg QHS

[a]MDD: Mirtazapine has shown efficacy similar to that of other antidepressants, although it may have an earlier onset of therapeutic benefit (Anttila and Leinonen 2001; Bech 2001; Benkert et al. 2000; Guelfi et al. 2001; Quitkin et al. 1979; Watanabe et al. 2008). It has also been shown to work synergistically with other antidepressants (Marek et al. 2003).
[b]Panic disorder: Mirtazapine has shown benefit (Boshuisen et al. 2001) and performed better than fluoxetine in one study (Ribeiro et al. 2001).
[c]Headache: Bendtsen and Jensen (2004) recommended mirtazapine 30 mg/day as an option for the prophylactic management of tension-type headaches due to a finding that it reduced headache index by 34% more than placebo in nondepressed patients with chronic tension-type headaches, even those who had not responded to amitriptyline).
[d]Insomnia: Mirtazapine has been shown to improve sleep efficiency, total sleep time, and sleep quality, with an efficacy similar to that of TCAs (Dolder et al. 2012; Winokur et al. 2000), making it a potentially good option for depressed patients with insomnia. Dosages are sometimes lower for insomnia, especially when augmenting the effects of other antidepressants; however, titration to higher dosages is sometimes necessary when treating depression (7.5–15 mg QHS).
[e]Nausea: Mirtazapine has shown positive therapeutic effects in treating nausea in cancer patients with depression and insomnia (Cao et al. 2020; Kim et al. 2008), post-ECT headaches/nausea (Li et al. 2011), postoperative nausea (Chang et al. 2010; Chen et al. 2008), and nausea after gastric bypass (Teixeira et al. 2005).

IX. Monitoring

A. Consider periodic monitoring of CBC, liver function tests, and lipids, given mirtazapine's rare potential to cause agranulocytosis, increased liver transaminases, and cholesterol and triglyceride increases, respectively.

B. Monitor weight at baseline and periodically given the potential for weight gain.

X. Relevant Pharmacokinetics/Pharmacodynamics

A. **Metabolism**: Hepatic

B. **Time to peak plasma concentration**: 2 hours

C. **Half-life**: 20–40 hours (increased in women and patients with renal/hepatic impairment)

D. **Hepatic impairment**: Use caution in hepatic impairment, given decreased clearance; consider reducing the dosage by at least 50% (Mauri et al. 2014; Mullish et al. 2014).

E. **Renal impairment**: Use caution in kidney impairment, as clearance is reduced; consider a decreased dosage. Not significantly dialyzed (Merck Sharp & Dohme 2021).

XI. Clinically Relevant Drug Interactions

A. Metabolized by cytochrome P450 (CYP) 3A4 (major) and by CYP1A2, CYP2C19, and CYP2D6 (all minor).

1. Adjust dosage with CYP3A4 inhibitors (e.g., some antifungals, antibiotics, antivirals, nefazodone) and CYP3A4 inducers (e.g., carbamazepine, St. John's wort).
2. Tobacco smoke (a CYP1A2 inducer) has been shown to reduce the serum concentration of mirtazapine (Oliveira et al. 2017).

B. Mirtazapine may counteract the antihypertensive action of clonidine, given these two agents' opposite actions on α_2 receptors (Abo-Zena et al. 2000).

C. Mirtazapine could have pharmacodynamic interactions with other drugs with similar mechanisms of action, including nonpsychiatric drugs that target similar receptors.

XII. Adverse Effects

A. **Boxed warning: suicidality and antidepressant drugs**:

1. In common with all antidepressants, mirtazapine may carry an increased risk for suicidal thoughts/behaviors in pediatric and young adult patients. Patients should be monitored closely for emergence of suicidal thoughts. For detailed information, readers are referred to comprehensive sources in the literature (e.g., Fergusson et al. 2005).

B. **Most common**:

1. Drowsiness, sedation, somnolence: Primarily due to H_1 antagonism. Up to 54% of patients in clinical trials reported drowsiness/sedation/somnolence with mirtazapine, which led to discontinuation in 10% of patients (Merck Sharp & Dohme 2021); higher dosages may actually cause less sedation (see mechanism of action). The sedating effects may also diminish in intensity/severity with time.

2. Increased appetite and weight gain: Likely due to 5-HT_{2C} and H_1 antagonism. Increased appetite may occur (17% of patients on mirtazapine vs. 2% on placebo). Weight gain rates vary but are significant (Serretti and Mandelli 2010; Uguz et al. 2015; White et al. 2013), although likely less than rates with TCAs and SSRIs/SNRIs (Drieling et al. 2007). Weight gain may be more common early in the course of treatment with mirtazapine (Goodnick et al. 1998).
3. Low risk of sexual side effects: Incidence actually *less than* with placebo—0.6% on mirtazapine vs. 1.7% on placebo (Anttila and Leinonen 2001; Sitsen and Zivkov 1995), and mirtazapine may actually improve sexual function (Farah 1998; Gelenberg et al. 1998), perhaps due to 5-HT_{2C} and 5-HT_{2A} blockade (Barkin et al. 1999).
4. Relatively low risk of serotonin syndrome due to lower 5-HT_{1A} agonism (Barkin et al. 1999).
5. Other: Dry mouth (35.3% on mirtazapine vs. 15.9% on placebo), dizziness (7% on mirtazapine vs. 3% on placebo), discontinuation symptoms (including mania/hypomania), constipation.

C. **Other notable side effects**:

1. Elevated cholesterol and triglycerides: Increases in cholesterol (15% on mirtazapine vs. 7% on placebo) and triglycerides (6% on mirtazapine vs. 3% on placebo) occurred in clinical trials (Merck Sharp & Dohme 2021), but it was unclear if this was related to weight gain (Nicholas et al. 2003).
2. Transaminase elevations: alanine aminotransferase (ALT) ≥3 times the upper limit of normal (2% on mirtazapine vs. 0.3% on placebo); may spontaneously improve (Merck Sharp & Dohme 2021).
3. Hematological abnormalities: Neutropenia, leukopenia, agranulocytosis, and immune thrombocytopenia have occurred, although these are very rare (Ahmed 2002; Civalier et al. 2009; Dholakia et al. 2010; Liu and Sahud 2003; Merck Sharp & Dohme 2021).
4. Drug-induced movement disorders: Akathisia is potentially related to α_2 receptor blockade, occurring more often at higher dosages (whereas lower dosages may treat akathisia). Dystonia/dyskinesia is potentially related to 5-HT_2 blockade, leading to a dopamine/norepinephrine imbalance, often occurring at lower dosages. Restless legs syndrome may be due to α_2-related 5-HT_1 activation and 5-HT_2/5-HT_3 blockade (Gulsun and Doruk 2008; Hutchins et al. 2019; Makiguchi et al. 2015; Raveendranathan and Swaminath 2015; Rissardo and Caprara 2020).
5. Rare: Angle-closure glaucoma, QTc prolongation, skin reactions (e.g., drug rash with eosinophilia and systemic symptoms [DRESS], Stevens-Johnson syndrome [SJS], bullous dermatitis, erythema multiforme, toxic epidermal necrolysis), activation of mania/hypomania, seizures, hyponatremia, orthostatic hypotension.

D. **Risks in pregnancy and lactation**: Mirtazapine was designated a Category C drug in the prior FDA classification and is present in breast milk. A thorough risk/benefit discussion with the patient is recommended on continuing versus stopping the medication, including consultation with an OB/GYN specialist and/or lactation expert. See Chapter 15 ("Women: Pregnancy, Postpartum, and Breastfeeding") for more information.

XIII. **Clinical Pearls/Prescribing Tips**

A. Mirtazapine is similar in efficacy to other antidepressants but may work faster. It may also work synergistically with other antidepressants.

B. Mirtazapine is unique in that it has dosage-dependent effects (see "Mechanism[s] of Action"): lower dosages tend to be more sedating, and higher dosages tend to be more activating. The drug is usually taken at bedtime.

C. In addition to depression, mirtazapine may be beneficial in anxiety, insomnia, decreased appetite, and nausea.

D. Increased hunger and weight gain are relatively common. Caution should be used with potential weight gain. Sometimes weight gain is an intended effect when using mirtazapine, but this can be problematic for other patients.

E. Mirtazapine has a very low risk of sexual side effects and may improve sexual function.

F. Interestingly, low-dosage mirtazapine (15 mg/day) may treat akathisia (Poyurovsky et al. 2003), but high-dosage mirtazapine (30 mg/day) may actually cause akathisia.

References

Abo-Zena RA, Bobek MB, Dweik RA: Hypertensive urgency induced by an interaction of mirtazapine and clonidine. Pharmacotherapy 20(4):476–478, 2000 10772378

Ahmed A: Neutropenia associated with mirtazapine use: is a drop in the neutrophil count in a symptomatic older adults a cause for concern? J Am Geriatr Soc 50(8):1461–1463, 2002 12165012

Anttila SA, Leinonen EV: A review of the pharmacological and clinical profile of mirtazapine. CNS Drug Rev 7(3):249–264, 2001 11607047

Barkin RL, Chor PN, Braun BG, et al: A trilogy case review highlighting the clinical and pharmacologic applications of mirtazapine in reducing polypharmacy for anxiety, agitation, insomnia, depression, and sexual dysfunction. Prim Care Companion J Clin Psychiatry 1(5):142–145, 1999 15014675

Bech P: Meta-analysis of placebo-controlled trials with mirtazapine using the core items of the Hamilton Depression Scale as evidence of a pure antidepressive effect in the short-term treatment of major depression. Int J Neuropsychopharmacol 4(4):337–345, 2001 11806859

Bendtsen L, Jensen R: Mirtazapine is effective in the prophylactic treatment of chronic tension-type headache. Neurology 62(10):1706–1711, 2004 15159466

Benkert O, Szegedi A, Kohnen R: Mirtazapine compared with paroxetine in major depression. J Clin Psychiatry 61(9):656–663, 2000 11030486

Berendsen HH, Broekkamp CL: Indirect in vivo 5-HT1A-agonistic effects of the new antidepressant mirtazapine. Psychopharmacology (Berl) 133(3):275–282, 1997 9361334

Boshuisen ML, Slaap BR, Vester-Blokland ED, et al: The effect of mirtazapine in panic disorder: an open label pilot study with a single-blind placebo run-in period. Int Clin Psychopharmacol 16(6):363–368, 2001 11712626

Cao J, Ouyang Q, Wang S, et al: Mirtazapine, a dopamine receptor inhibitor, as a secondary prophylactic for delayed nausea and vomiting following highly emetogenic chemotherapy: an open label, randomized, multicenter phase III trial. Invest New Drugs 38(2):507–514, 2020 32036491

Chang FL, Ho ST, Sheen MJ: Efficacy of mirtazapine in preventing intrathecal morphine-induced nausea and vomiting after orthopaedic surgery. Anaesthesia 65(12):1206–1211, 2010 21182602
Chen CC, Lin CS, Ko YP, et al: Premedication with mirtazapine reduces preoperative anxiety and postoperative nausea and vomiting. Anesth Analg 106(1):109–113, 2008 18165563
Civalier KA, Krahn LE, Agrwal N: Repeated episodes of neutropenia triggered by mirtazapine. Psychosomatics 50(3):299–300, 2009 19567774
Croom KF, Perry CM, Plosker GL: Mirtazapine: a review of its use in major depression and other psychiatric disorders. CNS Drugs 23(5):427–452, 2009 19453203
Demireva EY, Suri D, Morelli E, et al: 5-HT2C receptor blockade reverses SSRI-associated basal ganglia dysfunction and potentiates therapeutic efficacy. Mol Psychiatry 25(12):3304–3321, 2020 30120415
Dholakia R, Schleifer SJ, Ahmad YJ, et al: Delayed-onset mirtazapine-related leukopenia and rechallenge. J Clin Psychopharmacol 30(6):758, 2010 21057250
Dolder CR, Nelson MH, Iler CA: The effects of mirtazapine on sleep in patients with major depressive disorder. Ann Clin Psychiatry 24(3):215–224, 2012 22860241
Drieling T, Biedermann NC, Schärer LO, et al: Psychotropic drug-induced change of weight: a review [in German]. Fortschr Neurol Psychiatr 75(2):65–80, 2007 16586261
Farah A: Lack of sexual adverse effects with mirtazapine [letter]. Am J Health System Pharm 55(20):2195–2196, 1998
Fergusson D, Doucette S, Glass KC, et al: Association between suicide attempts and selective serotonin reuptake inhibitors: systematic review of randomised controlled trials. BMJ 330(7488):396, 2005 15718539
Gelenberg AJ, Laukes C, McGahuey C, et al: Mirtazapine substitution in SSRI-induced sexual dysfunction. Biol Psychiatry 15(43)(Suppl):104S, 1998
Goodnick PJ, Kremer C, Wingard P: Weight change during mirtazapine therapy. Prim Psychiatry 3:103–108, 1998
Guelfi JD, Ansseau M, Timmerman L, et al; Mirtazapine-Venlafaxine Study Group: Mirtazapine versus venlafaxine in hospitalized severely depressed patients with melancholic features. J Clin Psychopharmacol 21(4):425–431, 2001 11476127
Gulsun M, Doruk A: Mirtazapine-induced akathisia. J Clin Psychopharmacol 28(4):467, 2008 18626283
Hutchins D, Hall J, Sharma A: Mirtazapine-induced transient dyskinesia. Prim Care Companion CNS Disord 21(2):18102377, 2019
Kast RE, Foley KF: Cancer chemotherapy and cachexia: mirtazapine and olanzapine are 5-HT3 antagonists with good antinausea effects. Eur J Cancer Care (Engl) 16(4):351–354, 2007 17587360
Kim SW, Shin IS, Kim JM, et al: Effectiveness of mirtazapine for nausea and insomnia in cancer patients with depression. Psychiatry Clin Neurosci 62(1):75–83, 2008 18289144
Li TC, Shiah IS, Sun CJ, et al: Mirtazapine relieves post-electroconvulsive therapy headaches and nausea: a case series and review of the literature. J ECT 27(2):165–167, 2011 21602639
Liu X, Sahud MA: Glycoprotein IIb/IIIa complex is the target in mirtazapine-induced immune thrombocytopenia. Blood Cells Mol Dis 30(3):241–245, 2003 12737939
Makiguchi A, Nishida M, Shioda K, et al: Mirtazapine-induced restless legs syndrome treated with pramipexole. J Neuropsychiatry Clin Neurosci 27(1):e76, 2015 25716506
Marek GJ, Carpenter LL, McDougle CJ, et al: Synergistic action of 5-HT2A antagonists and selective serotonin reuptake inhibitors in neuropsychiatric disorders. Neuropsychopharmacology 28(2):402–412, 2003 12589395
Mauri MC, Fiorentini A, Paletta S, et al: Pharmacokinetics of antidepressants in patients with hepatic impairment. Clin Pharmacokinet 53(12):1069–1081, 2014 25248846

Merck Sharp & Dohme. Remeron package insert. Merck Sharp & Dohme, 2021. Available at: https://www.accessdata.fda.gov/drugsatfda_docs/label/2021/020415s038,021208s028lbl.pdf. Accessed March 13, 2024.

Millan MJ: Serotonin 5-HT2C receptors as a target for the treatment of depressive and anxious states: focus on novel therapeutic strategies. Therapie 60(5):441–460, 2005 16433010

Mullish BH, Kabir MS, Thursz MR, et al: Review article: depression and the use of antidepressants in patients with chronic liver disease or liver transplantation. Aliment Pharmacol Ther 40(8):880–892, 2014 25175904

Nakayama K, Sakurai T, Katsu H: Mirtazapine increases dopamine release in prefrontal cortex by 5-HT1A receptor activation. Brain Res Bull 63(3):237–241, 2004 15145142

Nicholas LM, Ford AL, Esposito SM, et al: The effects of mirtazapine on plasma lipid profiles in healthy subjects. J Clin Psychiatry 64(8):883–889, 2003 12927002

Oliveira P, Ribeiro J, Donato H, et al: Smoking and antidepressants pharmacokinetics: a systematic review. Ann Gen Psychiatry 16:17, 2017 28286537

Poyurovsky M, Epshtein S, Fuchs C, et al: Efficacy of low-dose mirtazapine in neuroleptic-induced akathisia: a double-blind randomized placebo-controlled pilot study. J Clin Psychopharmacol 23(3):305–308, 2003 12826992

Quitkin F, Rifkin A, Klein DF: Monoamine oxidase inhibitors: a review of antidepressant effectiveness. Arch Gen Psychiatry 36(7):749–760, 1979 454092

Raveendranathan D, Swaminath GR: Mirtazapine induced akathisia: understanding a complex mechanism. Indian J Psychol Med 37(4):474–475, 2015 26702190

Ribeiro L, Busnello JV, Kauer-Sant'Anna M, et al: Mirtazapine versus fluoxetine in the treatment of panic disorder. Braz J Med Biol Res 34(10):1303–1307, 2001 11593305

Rissardo JP, Caprara ALF: Mirtazapine-associated movement disorders: a literature review. Tzu Chi Med J 32(4):318–330, 2020

Roth BL, Driscoll J: PDSP Ki Database. Psychoactive Drug Screening Program (PDSP). University of North Carolina at Chapel Hill and the United States National Institute of Mental Health, 1999–present. Available at: https://pdsp.unc.edu/databases/pdsp.php. Accessed June 21, 2024.

Serretti A, Mandelli L: Antidepressants and body weight: a comprehensive review and meta-analysis. J Clin Psychiatry 71(10):1259–1272, 2010 21062615

Sitsen JMA, Zivkov M: Mirtazapine: clinical profile. CNS Drugs 4(Suppl 1):39–48, 1995

Teixeira FV, Novaretti TM, Pilon B, et al: Mirtazapine (Remeron) as treatment for non-mechanical vomiting after gastric bypass. Obes Surg 15(5):707–709, 2005 15946465

Uguz F, Sahingoz M, Gungor B, et al: Weight gain and associated factors in patients using newer antidepressant drugs. Gen Hosp Psychiatry 37(1):46–48, 2015 25467076

Watanabe N, Omori IM, Nakagawa A, et al; Multiple Meta-Analyses of New Generation Antidepressants (MANGA) Study Group: Mirtazapine versus other antidepressants in the acute-phase treatment of adults with major depression: systematic review and meta-analysis. J Clin Psychiatry 69(9):1404–1415, 2008 19193341

White W, Elmore L, Luthin DR, et al: Psychotropic-induced weight gain: a review of management strategies. Consultant 53(3):153–160, 2013

Winokur A, Sateia MJ, Hayes JB, et al: Acute effects of mirtazapine on sleep continuity and sleep architecture in depressed patients: a pilot study. Biol Psychiatry 48(1):75–78, 2000 10913511

Nefazodone

I. **Brand Names**: Serzone (discontinued)

II. **Therapeutic Class**: Serotonin antagonist and reuptake inhibitor (SARI) antidepressant

III. **Mechanism-Based Class**: Serotonin antagonist and reuptake inhibitor

IV. **Mechanism(s) of Action**

A. 5-HT_{2A} receptor antagonist (Ki=26 nM): Sedating antidepressant and antipsychotic effects; may complement the effects of serotonin transporter inhibition in depression (Marek et al. 2003; Meltzer et al. 2003).

B. 5-HT_{1A} receptor partial agonist (Ki=80 nM): Potential anti-anxiety, antidepressant, and anti-impulsive effects (Schreiber and De Vry 1993; ?lifirski et al. 2021)

C. 5-HT_{2C} receptor antagonist (Ki=72 nM): 5-HT_{2C} receptor blockade has been shown to increase dopamine and norepinephrine in the prefrontal cortex and likely potentiates the antidepressant/anxiolytic effects of SSRIs (Bubar et al. 2011; Demireva et al. 2020; Opal et al. 2014). 5-HT_{2C} receptor antagonism also has benefits in sleep and sexual function (Millan 2005).

D. Weak inhibitor of the NET (Ki>300 nM), the SERT (Ki>200 nM), and the DAT (Ki>300 nM).

E. α_1 receptor agonist (Ki=5.5–48 nM) and α_2 receptor agonist (Ki>80 nM) (Cusack et al. 1994; Owens et al. 1997; Roth and Kroeze 2006; Tatsumi et al. 1997)

V. **Indications**

A. FDA adult: Major depressive disorder

B. Evidence-based[1] off-label uses: None

C. FDA pediatric: None

VI. **Major Contraindications and When to Use Caution**

A. Known allergy to nefazodone or its components.

B. Avoid with coadministration of terfenadine, astemizole, cisapride, pimozide, carbamazepine (label)

C. Do not use in patients who were previously withdrawn from nefazodone due to evidence of liver injury.

D. Concomitant use with alprazolam or triazolam can lead to significantly increased levels of these benzodiazepines (Teva Pharmaceuticals 2014).

VII. **Dosage Formulations**

A. Generic tablet (50 mg, 100 mg [*scored*], 150 mg [*scored*], 200 mg, 250 mg)

VIII. **Dosage Ranges and Guidelines**

A. Start at 100 mg BID (may start lower at 50–100 mg/day) and increase every 1–2 weeks by 100–200 mg/day to a maximum of 300 mg BID (600 mg total).

---

[1]Evidence strength varies; readers are referred to the literature for more detailed information.

IX. **Monitoring**

A. Monitor for signs and symptoms of liver failure and obtain baseline and periodic liver transaminases given potential risk of hepatotoxicity (see adverse effects).
B. Monitor blood pressure at baseline and periodically given the risk of orthostatic hypotension with treatment.

X. **Relevant Pharmacokinetics/Pharmacodynamics**

A. **Metabolism**: Hepatic to metabolites (triazoledione, hydroxynefazodone [active], *m*-chlorophenylpiperazine [active, mCPP])
B. **Time to peak plasma concentration**: 1 hour (prolonged with food)
C. **Half-life**:
   1. Nefazodone: 2–4 hours
   2. Active metabolites: 1.4–8 hours (persist longer than the parent molecule)
D. **Hepatic impairment**: Use with caution in patients with liver disease or elevated baseline serum transaminases. Do not reintroduce in patients with prior liver injury due to nefazodone.
E. **Renal impairment**: No dosage adjustment necessary (Teva Pharmaceuticals 2014).

XI. **Clinically Relevant Drug Interactions**

A. Inhibitor of cytochrome P450 (CYP) 3A4
   1. Substantial increases in alprazolam and triazolam (triazolobenzodiazepines) have been noted with nefazodone. Use a 50% lower dosage of alprazolam and a 75% lower dosage of triazolam (may need to avoid) (Teva Pharmaceuticals 2014).
   2. Decrease dosages of concomitant CYP3A4 substrates including many antidepressants, antipsychotics, calcium channel blockers, hormones, pain medications, immunological medications
B. Metabolized by CYP2D6 (minor) and CYP3A4 (minor).
C. Nefazodone could have pharmacodynamic interactions with other drugs with similar mechanisms of action, including nonpsychiatric drugs that target similar receptors.

XII. **Adverse Effects**

A. **Boxed warning: suicidality and antidepressant drugs**:
   1. In common with all antidepressants, nefazodone may carry an increased risk for suicidal thoughts/behaviors in pediatric and young adult patients. Patients should be monitored closely for emergence of suicidal thoughts. For detailed information, readers are referred to comprehensive sources in the literature (e.g., Fergusson et al. 2005).

B. **Boxed warning: hepatotoxicity**:

1. Risk of life-threatening hepatic failure associated with nefazodone is 1 case per 250,000–300,000 patient-years[1] of nefazodone treatment (U.S.).
   a. No evidence that underlying liver disease increases the likelihood, but it may complicate monitoring. Avoid use of nefazodone in patients with active liver disease, elevated baseline serum transaminases, or significant risk factors for liver disease.
   b. Stop use if there is evidence of hepatocellular injury (aspartate transaminase [AST] or alanine aminotransferase [ALT] three times the upper limit of normal) or signs of liver failure (look out for jaundice, anorexia, gastrointestinal complaints, malaise).
   c. Do not reintroduce nefazodone if stopped because of liver dysfunction.

C. **Most common**:

1. Gastrointestinal: dry mouth (35% on nefazodone vs. 13% on placebo, nausea (22% on nefazodone vs. 12% on placebo), constipation (14% on nefazodone vs. 8% on placebo) (Teva Pharmaceuticals 2014)
2. Sedation (25% on nefazodone vs. 14% on placebo) (Teva Pharmaceuticals 2014)
3. Other: Headache (36% on nefazodone vs. 33% on placebo), asthenia/weakness (11% on nefazodone vs. 5% on placebo), postural hypotension (4% on nefazodone vs. 1% on placebo), dizziness (17% on nefazodone vs. 5% on placebo), lightheadedness (10% on nefazodone vs. 3% on placebo), confusion (8% on nefazodone vs. 1% on placebo), abnormal vision (10% on nefazodone vs. 2% on placebo) (Teva Pharmaceuticals 2014)

D. **Other notable side effects**:

1. Rare: Priapism, seizures, activation of mania/hypomania

E. **Risks in pregnancy and lactation**: Nefazodone was designated a Category C drug in the prior FDA classification and is present in breast milk. A thorough risk/benefit discussion with the patient is recommended on continuing versus stopping the medication, including consultation with an OB/GYN specialist and/or a lactation expert. See Chapter 15 ("Women: Pregnancy, Postpartum, and Breastfeeding") for more information.

XIII. **Clinical Pearls/Prescribing Tips**

A. Nefazodone is rarely used due to the risk of hepatotoxicity (black box warning) as well as its significant drug interactions and has been withdrawn from the market in Europe, Australia, New Zealand, and Canada.

B. Nefazodone is related to trazodone, and they have similar side effects, including priapism, orthostatic hypotension, and sedation, although trazodone does not have a black box warning for hepatotoxicity.

---

[1]Total patient-years is a summation of each patient's duration of exposure expressed in years. For example, 1 patient-year is equal to 2 patients each treated for 6 months, 3 patients each treated for 4 months, etc.

C. Trazodone could be considered clinically for patients with treatment-resistant depression or in patients with known prior response to nefazodone, but only after careful consideration and weighing of the risks versus benefits.

Further Reading

Roth BL, Driscoll J: PDSP Ki Database. Psychoactive Drug Screening Program (PDSP). University of North Carolina at Chapel Hill and the United States National Institute of Mental Health, 1999–present. Available at: https://pdsp.unc.edu/databases/pdsp.php. Accessed June 21, 2024.

References

Bubar MJ, Stutz SJ, Cunningham KA: 5-HT(2C) receptors localize to dopamine and GABA neurons in the rat mesoaccumbens pathway. PLoS One 6(6):e20508, 2011 21687728

Cusack B, Nelson A, Richelson E: Binding of antidepressants to human brain receptors: focus on newer generation compounds. Psychopharmacology (Berl) 114(4):559–565, 1994 7855217

Demireva EY, Suri D, Morelli E, et al: 5-HT2C receptor blockade reverses SSRI-associated basal ganglia dysfunction and potentiates therapeutic efficacy. Mol Psychiatry 25(12):3304–3321, 2020 30120415

Fergusson D, Doucette S, Glass KC, et al: Association between suicide attempts and selective serotonin reuptake inhibitors: systematic review of randomised controlled trials. BMJ 330(7488):396, 2005 15718539

Marek GJ, Carpenter LL, McDougle CJ, et al: Synergistic action of 5-HT2A antagonists and selective serotonin reuptake inhibitors in neuropsychiatric disorders. Neuropsychopharmacology 28(2):402–412, 2003 12589395

Meltzer HY, Li Z, Kaneda Y, et al: Serotonin receptors: their key role in drugs to treat schizophrenia. Prog Neuropsychopharmacol Biol Psychiatry 27(7):1159–1172, 2003 14642974

Millan MJ: Serotonin 5-HT2C receptors as a target for the treatment of depressive and anxious states: focus on novel therapeutic strategies. Therapie 60(5):441–460, 2005 16433010

Opal MD, Klenotich SC, Morais M, et al: Serotonin 2C receptor antagonists induce fast-onset antidepressant effects. Mol Psychiatry 19(10):1106–1114, 2014 24166413

Owens MJ, Morgan WN, Plott SJ, et al: Neurotransmitter receptor and transporter binding profile of antidepressants and their metabolites. J Pharmacol Exp Ther 283(3):1305–1322, 1997 9400006

Roth BL, Kroeze WK: Screening the receptorome yields validated molecular targets for drug discovery. Curr Pharm Des 12(14):1785–1795, 2006 16712488

Schreiber R, De Vry J: 5-HT1A receptor ligands in animal models of anxiety, impulsivity and depression: multiple mechanisms of action? Prog Neuropsychopharmacol Biol Psychiatry 17(1):87–104, 1993 8416603

Ślifirski G, Król M, Turło J: 5-HT Receptors and the development of new antidepressants. Int J Mol Sci 22(16):9015, 2021

Tatsumi M, Groshan K, Blakely RD, et al: Pharmacological profile of antidepressants and related compounds at human monoamine transporters. Eur J Pharmacol 340(2–3):249–258, 1997 9537821

Teva Pharmaceuticals: Nefazodone hydrochloride package insert. 2014. Available at: https://www.accessdata.fda.gov/drugsatfda_docs/label/2014/076037s011lbl.pdf. Accessed March 13, 2024.

Trazodone

I. **Brand Names**: Desyrel (discontinued), Oleptro (extended release [ER], discontinued)
II. **Therapeutic Class**: Serotonin antagonist and reuptake inhibitor (SARI) antidepressant
III. **Mechanism-Based Class**: Serotonin antagonist and reuptake inhibitor (SARI)
IV. **Mechanism(s) of Action**

A. Both trazodone and its active metabolite *m*-chlorophenylpiperazine (mCPP) variably affect multiple receptors.
B. Blockade of 5-HT_{2A}, H_1, and α_1-adrenergic receptors at lower dosages (25–100 mg/day) likely causes the hypnotic effects of trazodone, and the combination of 5-HT_{2A} and SERT blockade at higher dosages (150–600 mg/day) likely treats depression (Jaffer et al. 2017; Stahl 2009).
   1. 5-HT_{2A} antagonism (Ki=20–45 nM for trazodone, 32–398 nM for mCPP)—may complement the effects of serotonin transporter inhibition in depression (Marek et al. 2003; Meltzer et al. 2003).
   2. H_1 antagonism (Ki=220–1,100 nM for trazodone, 326 nM for mCPP)
   3. α_1 receptor antagonism (Ki=12–42 nM for trazodone) and α_2 receptor antagonism (Ki=106–490 nM for trazodone) explain trazodone's potential to cause orthostatic hypotension.
   4. SERT antagonism
      a. The metabolite mCPP is a more potent blocker of SERT than trazodone (mCPP Ki=202–432 nM vs. trazodone Ki=160–10,000 nM).
      b. Trazodone's SERT occupancy is 86% at 100 mg/day and 90% at 150 mg/day (Settimo and Taylor 2018; Stahl 2009).

C. 5-HT_{2B} receptor antagonism (Ki=74–189 nM for trazodone, 3.2–63 nM for mCPP)
D. 5-HT_{2C} receptor antagonism (Ki=224–402 nM for trazodone, 3.4–251 for mCPP): 5-HT_{2C} receptor blockade has been shown to increase dopamine and norepinephrine in the prefrontal cortex and likely potentiates the antidepressant/anxiolytic effects of SSRIs when used in combination (Demireva et al. 2020). 5-HT_{2C} receptor antagonism also has benefits in sleep and sexual function (Millan 2005).
E. 5-HT_{1A} receptor partial agonism (Ki=96–118 nM for trazodone, 44–400 nM for mCPP): Potential anti-anxiety, antidepressant, and anti-impulsive effects (Odagaki et al. 2005; Schreiber and De Vry 1993; Ślifirski et al. 2021; Stahl 2009)

V. **Indications**

A. FDA adult:
   1. Major depressive disorder (MDD)

B. Evidence-based[1] off-label uses:
   1. Insomnia
   2. Aggressive or agitated behavior associated with dementia

C. FDA pediatric: None

---

[1]Evidence strength varies; readers are referred to the literature for more detailed information.

VI. **Major Contraindications and When to Use Caution**

A. Known allergy to trazodone or its components
B. Concomitant use of MAOI antidepressants or other MAO-inhibiting agents (e.g., linezolid, IV methylene blue)—A 2-week washout is typically required.

VII. **Dosage Formulations**

A. Generic tablet (50 mg, 100 mg, 150 mg, 300 mg—*all scored*)
B. Brand formulations not available
C. ER form discontinued

VIII. **Dosage Ranges and Guidelines**

A. Refer to Table 2–18 for dosage ranges (initial/maximum) and guidelines.
B. For MDD, start at 50 mg BID and increase by 50 mg every week to a maximum of 600 mg/day.

Table 2–18. Trazodone indications and dosage ranges

Indication	Usual dosage range
Major depressive disorder[a]	150–400 mg/day (manufacturer's labeling) 50 mg BID → 600 mg/day (alternative dosing)
Insomnia (off-label)[b]	50–300 mg QHS (Note: Although dosages for insomnia are typically lower than antidepressant dosages, dosages of up to 600 mg/day have been used for insomnia.)
Agitated behavior associated with dementia (off-label)[c]	25–50 mg QHS → 300 mg/day (as a single dose or 2–3 divided doses)

[a]Clinical trials show that trazodone's efficacy for MDD is similar to that of other antidepressants, particularly in patients with comorbid anxiety (Cunningham et al. 1994; Feighner and Boyer 1988; Papakostas and Fava 2007; Rickels and Case 1982; Schatzberg 1987), but may be limited by side effects (Cunningham et al. 1994), as higher dosages are likely required for antidepressant effects (Cuomo et al. 2019; Settimo and Taylor 2018).

[b]There are limited clinical trials on trazodone as a sleep agent, but discontinuation due to side effects such as sedation, dizziness, psychomotor impairment, tolerance, and potential arrhythmias is of concern, especially in the treatment of older adults (James and Mendelson 2004; Mendelson 2005). A meta-analysis performed in 2017 showed evidence of trazodone's benefit in both primary and secondary insomnia (Jaffer et al. 2017). Specifically, in primary insomnia, it improved sleep latency (although the effect waned after 2 weeks). Low-dosage trazodone was helpful for sleep maintenance in another study.
In secondary insomnia, trazodone demonstrated improved sleep quality in depressed patients with insomnia, although drowsiness was reported as a side effect (Jaffer et al. 2017). Efficacy in antidepressant-induced insomnia and insomnia in patients with Alzheimer's disease has also been demonstrated (Camargos et al. 2014; Jaffer et al. 2017). One study showed low-dosage trazodone was helpful for insomnia and nightmares in cancer patients (Tanimukai et al. 2013).

[c]There is some evidence of trazodone's efficacy in agitation associated with frontotemporal dementia (Lebert et al. 2004) as well as efficacy similar to that of haloperidol in patients with dementia (major neurocognitive disorder) (Sultzer et al. 1997).

IX. **Monitoring**

A. Monitor blood pressure at baseline and periodically given the risk of orthostatic hypotension.

X. **Relevant Pharmacokinetics/Pharmacodynamics**

A. **Metabolism**: Hepatic to active metabolite *m*-chlorophenylpiperazine (mCPP)
B. **Time to peak plasma concentration**: 30–100 minutes; delayed up to 2.5 hours with food
C. **Half-life**: 5–9 hours
D. **Hepatic impairment**: No dosage adjustment necessary.
E. **Renal impairment**: No dosage adjustment necessary. Not significantly dialyzed (Teva Pharmaceuticals 2014).

XI. **Clinically Relevant Drug Interactions**

A. Metabolized by cytochrome P450 (CYP) 3A4 (major) and CYP2D6 (minor).

1. Adjust dosage with CYP3A4 inhibitors (e.g., some antifungals, antibiotics, antivirals, nefazodone) and CYP3A4 inducers (e.g., carbamazepine, St. John's wort).

B. Trazodone could have pharmacodynamic interactions with other drugs with similar mechanisms of action, including nonpsychiatric drugs that target similar receptors.

XII. **Adverse Effects**

A. **Boxed warning (antidepressant class effect)**:

1. In common with all antidepressants, trazodone may carry an increased risk for suicidal thoughts/behaviors in pediatric and young adult patients. Patients should be monitored closely for emergence of suicidal thoughts. For detailed information, readers are referred to comprehensive sources in the literature (e.g., Fergusson et al. 2005).

B. **Most common**:

1. Somnolence/sedation, drowsiness, fatigue (rates of 24%–41%) (Pragma Pharmaceuticals 2018)
2. Orthostatic hypotension, dizziness, and syncope: Likely dosage related. Rates vary, but one study estimated that trazodone was associated with a 58% prevalence of orthostatic hypotension in older adult veterans (Poon and Braun 2005). Use caution in elderly individuals or patients with cardiac diseases (Nambudiri et al. 1989; Rivasi et al. 2020).
3. Gastrointestinal: Nausea (rates of 10%–13%), diarrhea, dry mouth (15%–34%), constipation (Pragma Pharmaceuticals 2018)
4. Other: Blurred vision (14% on trazodone vs. 4% on placebo), headache, vivid dreams, edema, nasal congestion, weight loss (Pragma Pharmaceuticals 2018; Teva Pharmaceuticals 2014)

C. **Other notable side effects**:

1. Priapism: This effect appears to be related to medications with alpha-adrenergic-blocking properties, such as trazodone, antipsychotics, and prazosin (Patel et al. 1996; Thompson et al. 1990). Priapism occurs in 1/1,000–1/10,000 patients (Jaffer et al. 2017). Use particular caution in men with other risk factors for priapism, although all male patients should be warned about priapism as a potential adverse effect.

2. Low risk of sexual side effects (and may actually improve libido [Fink et al. 2003])
   a. Trazodone's antagonism at 5-HT_{2A} and 5-HT_{2C} receptors likely leads to decreased risk of anxiety and sexual dysfunction (Millan 2005; Stahl 2009).
3. Low risk of weight gain
   a. Trazodone's moderate affinity for 5-HT_{2C} and H_1 receptors may limit the risk of weight gain. May actually cause weight loss.
4. Rare: QTc prolongation, abnormal bleeding, hyponatremia, acute angle glaucoma, serotonin syndrome, NMS, cardiac issues, switch into mania/hypomania, discontinuation symptoms (Pragma Pharmaceuticals 2018; Teva Pharmaceuticals 2014)

D. **Risks in pregnancy and lactation**: Trazodone was designated a Category C drug in the prior FDA classification and is present in breast milk. A thorough risk/benefit discussion with the patient is recommended on continuing versus stopping the medication, including consultation with an OB/GYN specialist and/or lactation expert. See Chapter 15 ("Women: Pregnancy, Postpartum, and Breastfeeding") for more information.

XIII. **Clinical Pearls/Prescribing Tips**

A. Trazodone may be a good choice for patients with comorbid insomnia or insomnia as a result of depression. However, trazodone's use as a monotherapy for depression is limited by its sedative effects and the need for higher dosages to produce antidepressant effects.

B. In comparison with most other antidepressants, trazodone has a relatively lower risk of weight gain or adverse sexual side effects due to its receptor profile. Priapism is a very rare side effect, but male patients should be advised of this possibility.

C. Trazodone is a relatively potent α_1 receptor antagonist, leading to a risk of orthostatic hypotension (often dosage related). Use caution, especially in older adults. However, trazodone at low dosages may have efficacy in agitation associated with major neurocognitive disorders.

References

Camargos EF, Louzada LL, Quintas JL, et al: Trazodone improves sleep parameters in Alzheimer disease patients: a randomized, double-blind, and placebo-controlled study. Am J Geriatr Psychiatry 22(12):1565–1574, 2014 24495406

Cunningham LA, Borison RL, Carman JS, et al: A comparison of venlafaxine, trazodone, and placebo in major depression. J Clin Psychopharmacol 14(2):99–106, 1994 8195464

Cuomo A, Ballerini A, Bruni AC, et al: Clinical guidance for the use of trazodone in major depressive disorder and concomitant conditions: pharmacology and clinical practice. Riv Psichiatr 54(4):137–149, 2019 31379379

Demireva EY, Suri D, Morelli E, et al: 5-HT2C receptor blockade reverses SSRI-associated basal ganglia dysfunction and potentiates therapeutic efficacy. Mol Psychiatry 25(12):3304–3321, 2020 30120415

Feighner JP, Boyer WF: Overview of USA controlled trials of trazodone in clinical depression. Psychopharmacology (Berl) 95(Suppl):S50–S53, 1988 3133715

Fergusson D, Doucette S, Glass KC, et al: Association between suicide attempts and selective serotonin reuptake inhibitors: systematic review of randomised controlled trials. BMJ 330(7488):396, 2005 15718539

Fink HA, MacDonald R, Rutks IR, et al: Trazodone for erectile dysfunction: a systematic review and meta-analysis. BJU Int 92(4):441–446, 2003 12930437

Jaffer KY, Chang T, Vanle B, et al. Trazodone for insomnia: a systematic review. Innov Clin Neurosci 14(7–8):24–34, 2017

James SP, Mendelson WB: The use of trazodone as a hypnotic: a critical review. J Clin Psychiatry 65(6):752–755, 2004 15291651

Lebert F, Stekke W, Hasenbroekx C, et al: Frontotemporal dementia: a randomised, controlled trial with trazodone. Dement Geriatr Cogn Disord 17(4):355–359, 2004 15178953

Marek GJ, Carpenter LL, McDougle CJ, et al: Synergistic action of 5-HT2A antagonists and selective serotonin reuptake inhibitors in neuropsychiatric disorders. Neuropsychopharmacology 28(2):402–412, 2003 12589395

Meltzer HY, Li Z, Kaneda Y, et al: Serotonin receptors: their key role in drugs to treat schizophrenia. Prog Neuropsychopharmacol Biol Psychiatry 27(7):1159–1172, 2003 14642974

Mendelson WB: A review of the evidence for the efficacy and safety of trazodone in insomnia. J Clin Psychiatry 66(4):469–476, 2005 15816789

Millan MJ: Serotonin 5-HT2C receptors as a target for the treatment of depressive and anxious states: focus on novel therapeutic strategies. Therapie 60(5):441–460, 2005 16433010

Nambudiri DE, Mirchandani IC, Young RC: Two more cases of trazodone-related syncope in the elderly. J Geriatr Psychiatry Neurol 2(4):225, 1989 2635019

Odagaki Y, Toyoshima R, Yamauchi T: Trazodone and its active metabolite m-chlorophenylpiperazine as partial agonists at 5-HT1A receptors assessed by [35S]GTPgammaS binding. J Psychopharmacol 19(3):235–241, 2005 15888508

Papakostas GI, Fava M: A meta-analysis of clinical trials comparing the serotonin (5HT)-2 receptor antagonists trazodone and nefazodone with selective serotonin reuptake inhibitors for the treatment of major depressive disorder. Eur Psychiatry 22(7):444–447, 2007 17418537

Patel AG, Mukherji K, Lee A: Priapism associated with psychotropic drugs. Br J Hosp Med 55(6):315–319, 1996 8696624

Poon IO, Braun U: High prevalence of orthostatic hypotension and its correlation with potentially causative medications among elderly veterans. J Clin Pharm Ther 30(2):173–178, 2005 15811171

Pragma Pharmaceuticals: Desyrel (trazodone hydrochloride) tablets [package insert]. U.S. Food and Drug Administration website. Revised October 2018. Available at: https://www.accessdata.fda.gov/drugsatfda_docs/label/2018/018207s033lbl.pdf. Accessed March 13, 2024.

Rickels K, Case WG: Trazodone in depressed outpatients. Am J Psychiatry 139(6):803–806, 1982 7044154

Rivasi G, Rafanelli M, Mossello E, et al: Drug-related orthostatic hypotension: beyond anti-hypertensive medications. Drugs Aging 37(10):725–738, 2020 32894454

Schatzberg AF: Trazodone: a 5-year review of antidepressant efficacy. Psychopathology 20(Suppl 1):48–56, 1987 3321130

Schreiber R, De Vry J: 5-HT1A receptor ligands in animal models of anxiety, impulsivity and depression: multiple mechanisms of action? Prog Neuropsychopharmacol Biol Psychiatry 17(1):87–104, 1993 8416603

Settimo L, Taylor D: Evaluating the dose-dependent mechanism of action of trazodone by estimation of occupancies for different brain neurotransmitter targets. J Psychopharmacol 32(1):96–104, 2018 29332554

Ślifirski G, Król M, Turło J: 5-HT receptors and the development of new antidepressants. Int J Mol Sci 22(16):9015, 2021

Stahl SM: Mechanism of action of trazodone: a multifunctional drug. CNS Spectr 14(10):536–546, 2009 20095366

Sultzer DL, Gray KF, Gunay I, et al: A double-blind comparison of trazodone and haloperidol for treatment of agitation in patients with dementia. Am J Geriatr Psychiatry 5(1):60–69, 1997 9169246

Tanimukai H, Murai T, Okazaki N, et al: An observational study of insomnia and nightmare treated with trazodone in patients with advanced cancer. Am J Hosp Palliat Care 30(4):359–362, 2013 22777411

Teva Pharmaceuticals: Trazodone hydrochloride package insert. 2014. Available at: https://www.accessdata.fda.gov/drugsatfda_docs/label/2015/071196s062lbl.pdf. Accessed March 13, 2024.

Thompson JW Jr, Ware MR, Blashfield RK: Psychotropic medication and priapism: a comprehensive review. J Clin Psychiatry 51(10):430–433, 1990 2211542

Vortioxetine

I. **Brand Names**: Trintellix, Brintellix (discontinued)

II. **Therapeutic Class**: Serotonin reuptake inhibitor (SRI) and serotonin receptor modulator

III. **Mechanism-Based Class**: Serotonin multimodal agent

IV. **Mechanism(s) of Action**

A. CNS inhibition of SERT (serotonin transporter), blocking reuptake and increasing synaptic serotonin (5-hydroxytryptamine [5-HT]) in several brain areas.

1. Ki = 1.6 nM for SERT
2. Vortioxetine's SERT occupancy in the raphe nuclei was ~50% at 5 mg/day, 65% at 10 mg/day, and >80% at 20 mg/day, and it may require lower levels of SERT occupancy to exert antidepressant activity compared with SSRI/SNRIs, given its additional 5-HT receptor effects (Sanchez et al. 2015).

B. 5-HT_3 receptor antagonism (Ki = 3.7 nM): Potential anti-anxiety and anti-nausea effects. Because 5-HT_3 receptors regulate many interneurons in the brain, blockade can also lead to increased levels of serotonin, dopamine, norepinephrine, acetylcholine, and histamine (D'Agostino et al. 2015).

C. 5-HT_7 antagonism (Ki = 19 nM) releases additional serotonin via a downstream mechanism, increases dopamine, and is thought to have procognitive effects (Sanchez et al. 2015).

D. 5-HT_{1A} receptor agonism (Ki = 15 nM) and 5-HT_{1B} partial agonism likely lead to further serotonin release. 5-HT_{1A} agonism may potentially improve sexual function (Sanchez et al. 2015).

V. **Indications**

A. FDA adult: Major depressive disorder

B. Off-label: None, but often considered by clinicians for anxiety disorders, especially those not responsive to usual FDA-approved treatments.

C. FDA pediatric: None

VI. Major Contraindications and When to Use Caution

A. Known allergy to vortioxetine or its components
B. Concomitant use of MAOI antidepressants or other MAO-inhibiting agents (e.g., linezolid, IV methylene blue)—A 2-week washout is typically required.

VII. Dosage Formulations

A. Brand tablet (5 mg, 10 mg, 20 mg)
B. No generic form available at this time.

VIII. Dosage Ranges and Guidelines

A. Start at 10 mg/day and increase by 5–10 mg every 1–2 weeks to a maximum dosage of 20 mg/day. Benefits may be evident after 1–2 weeks, but it may take up to 6 weeks to reach the full effect at a given dosage.

IX. Monitoring

A. Not applicable

X. Relevant Pharmacokinetics/Pharmacodynamics

A. **Metabolism**: Hepatic
B. **Time to peak plasma concentration**: 7–11 hours
C. **Half-life**: ~66 hours
D. **Hepatic impairment**: No dosage adjustment necessary.
E. **Renal impairment**: No dosage adjustment necessary (Takeda Pharmaceuticals America 2021).

XI. Clinically Relevant Drug Interactions

A. Metabolized by cytochrome P450 (CYP) 2D6 (major) and also by CYP3A4/5, CYP2C19, CYP2C9, CYP2A6, CYP2C8, and CYP2B6.
   1. The maximum recommended dosage is 10 mg/day for genetically poor metabolizers of CYP2D6 or patients taking strong CYP2D6 inhibitors (functional CYP2D6 poor metabolizers).

B. Vortioxetine could have pharmacodynamic interactions with other drugs with similar mechanisms of action, including nonpsychiatric drugs that target similar receptors.

XII. Adverse Effects

A. **Boxed warning: suicidality and antidepressant drugs**:
   1. In common with all antidepressants, vortioxetine may carry an increased risk for suicidal thoughts/behaviors in pediatric and young adult patients. Patients should be monitored closely for emergence of suicidal thoughts. For detailed information, readers are referred to comprehensive sources in the literature (e.g., Fergusson et al. 2005).

B. **SSRI class effects**:
   1. Vortioxetine's side-effect profile is similar to that of the SSRIs, although it appears to have a lower level of discontinuation symptoms (Sanchez et al. 2015).

C. **Most common**:

1. Gastrointestinal: Notably nausea (21%–32%), constipation, diarrhea, dry mouth. Nausea should improve within 2 weeks and is less prevalent with vortioxetine than with venlafaxine or duloxetine (Baldwin et al. 2016).
2. Sexual dysfunction: Vortioxetine appears to carry lower risk for sexual effects compared with other antidepressants (<2% for vortioxetine vs. 12.4% for venlafaxine and 4.5% for duloxetine) (Baldwin et al. 2016; D'Agostino et al. 2015). Effects (often dosage dependent) may include decreased libido, anorgasmia, ejaculatory delay, erectile dysfunction, and (in rare cases) priapism or decreased penile sensation.
3. Compared with most other antidepressants, vortioxetine may have a lower risk of emotional blunting but a higher risk of agitation and irritability (Hughes et al. 2017).

D. **Other notable side effects**:

1. Less common: Dizziness, insomnia, headache, nasopharyngitis, upper respiratory tract infection, weight gain (although studies indicate that weight gain is minimal [i.e., <1 kg])

E. **Risks in pregnancy and lactation**: Vortioxetine was designated a Category C drug in the prior FDA classification and is present in breast milk. A thorough risk/benefit discussion with the patient is recommended on continuing versus stopping the medication, including consultation with an OB/GYN specialist and/or lactation expert. See Chapter 15 ("Women: Pregnancy, Postpartum, and Breastfeeding") for more information.

XIII. **Clinical Pearls/Prescribing Tips**

A. Vortioxetine may be a more favorable medication choice for certain patients, given its lower risk of sexual side effects and weight gain (D'Agostino et al. 2015), although its gastrointestinal side effects may still be significant (Hughes et al. 2017).

B. Various studies indicate that vortioxetine produces greater improvement in cognitive performance compared with other antidepressants, seemingly independent of the alleviation of depressive symptoms (Bennabi et al. 2019; Harrison et al. 2016). This effect may be attributable to vortioxetine's enhancement of cholinergic, histaminergic, and glutamatergic neurotransmission via 5-HT_{1A}, 5-HT_{1B}, 5-HT_3, and 5-HT_7 receptor action (Sanchez et al. 2015).

1. In a network meta-analysis that used the DSST (Digit Symbol Substitution Test, a measure of processing speed) to compare the effects of various antidepressant classes, vortioxetine was found to be statistically significantly more efficacious than escitalopram, nortriptyline, SSRIs, and TCAs in improving DSST scores (Baune et al. 2018).

References

Baldwin DS, Chrones L, Florea I, et al: The safety and tolerability of vortioxetine: analysis of data from randomized placebo-controlled trials and open-label extension studies. J Psychopharmacol 30(3):242–252, 2016 26864543

Baune BT, Brignone M, Larsen KG: A network meta-analysis comparing effects of various antidepressant classes on the digit symbol substitution test (DSST) as a measure of cognitive dysfunction in patients with major depressive disorder. Int J Neuropsychopharmacol 21(2):97–107, 2018 29053849

Bennabi D, Haffen E, Van Waes V: Vortioxetine for cognitive enhancement in major depression: from animal models to clinical research. Front Psychiatry 10:771, 2019

D'Agostino A, English CD, Rey JA: Vortioxetine (brintellix): a new serotonergic antidepressant. PT 40(1):36–40, 2015 25628505

Fergusson D, Doucette S, Glass KC, et al: Association between suicide attempts and selective serotonin reuptake inhibitors: systematic review of randomised controlled trials. BMJ 330(7488):396, 2005 15718539

Harrison JE, Lophaven S, Olsen CK: Which cognitive domains are improved by treatment with vortioxetine? Int J Neuropsychopharmacol 19(10):pyw054, 2016

Hughes S, Lacasse J, Fuller RR, et al: Adverse effects and treatment satisfaction among online users of four antidepressants. Psychiatry Res 255:78–86, 2017 28531820

Sanchez C, Asin KE, Artigas F: Vortioxetine, a novel antidepressant with multimodal activity: review of preclinical and clinical data. Pharmacol Ther 145:43–57, 2015 25016186

Takeda Pharmaceuticals America: Trintellix (vortioxetine) package insert. 2021. Available at: https://www.accessdata.fda.gov/drugsatfda_docs/label/2021/204447s024lbl.pdf. Accessed March 13, 2024.

Newer Antidepressants

Brexanolone and Zuranolone

- In 2019 and 2023, respectively, the neuroactive steroid $GABA_A$ receptor positive allosteric modulator agents brexanolone (Zulresso, intravenous injection; patients 15 years and older) and zuranolone (Zurzuvae, capsule for oral use; adults) were approved by the FDA for the treatment of postpartum depression. Chapter 15 ("Women: Pregnancy, Postpartum, and Breastfeeding") in this Handbook contains a broad overview of brexanolone and zuranolone.

Esketamine

- In 2019, the noncompetitive *N*-methyl D-aspartate (NMDA) receptor antagonist esketamine (Spravato, nasal spray; adults) received FDA approval for use in treatment-resistant major depressive disorder (MDD) as well as for treatment of depressive symptoms with acute suicidal ideation/behavior. Chapter 14 ("Interventional Psychiatry") in this Handbook provides further information on esketamine (as well as intravenous ketamine, which has been in use for many years for treating depression).

Gepirone

- The recently approved antidepressant agent gepirone was first developed in the 1980s but was rejected by the FDA for approval in 2002, 2004, 2012, and 2015, when clinical trial data examining depression and/or anxiety were reviewed. However, in 2016, the FDA reversed its decision on the gepirone extended-release (ER) clinical trial data, and the manufacturer was told that it could resubmit a New Drug Application. In September 2023, gepirone ER (marketed under the brand name Exxua) received FDA approval for use in the treatment of MDD in adults. Many have argued that gepirone was a victim of common difficulties in psychiatric drug development, including the impact of study design on trial outcomes and the conundrum of how to interpret negative trials and the designs of those trials in the context of subsequent positive trials.
- Gepirone is a partial agonist of $5\text{-}HT_{1A}$, which is the same mechanism of action attributed to buspirone, which is FDA approved for the treatment of generalized anxiety disorder and is commonly used off-label for treatment-resistant major depression. Buspirone is reviewed at length in Chapter 3 ("Anxiolytics: Benzodiazepines and Nonbenzodiazepines") of this Handbook. Although the two drugs are similar (both have

an active metabolite that is an antagonist at α_2-adrenergic receptors), gepirone differs from buspirone in several key ways:

- Gepirone is more potent than buspirone in activating 5-HT_{1A} receptors.
- Unlike buspirone, gepirone also acts as an antagonist at 5-HT_{2A} receptors. 5-HT_{2A} receptor antagonists have antipsychotic and antidepressant properties. 5-HT_{2A} receptors may have effects related to cognition and learning, and are an active area of study.
- Gepirone has a lower affinity for D_2 receptors than buspirone, although this D_2 effect is likely not of clinical significance for either drug.

3

Anxiolytics

Benzodiazepines and Nonbenzodiazepines

Cheryl Graber, M.D.
Gabrielle Bleich, M.D.

Chapter Highlights

- Both benzodiazepine and nonbenzodiazepine medications are effective in treating anxiety disorders.
- Both benzodiazepine and nonbenzodiazepine medications have FDA-approved and evidence-based off-label uses in treating anxiety.
- The choice of medication is based on patient-specific factors.
- A history of substance use disorder often warrants selection of a nonbenzodiazepine anxiolytic.
- When used to treat anxiety disorders, anxiolytic medications are most often prescribed to augment selective serotonin reuptake inhibitor (SSRI) and/or serotonin-norepinephrine reuptake inhibitor (SNRI) antidepressants (which are covered elsewhere in this Handbook [see Chapter 2, "Antidepressants"]).

Overview of Benzodiazepine Class Characteristics

As a class, benzodiazepines

- Are effective in treating anxiety, insomnia, seizures, and catatonia and can be used for sedation and multiple other purposes.
- Are dangerous in overdose and withdrawal.
- Can be habit-forming.
- Cause tolerance to develop over time.
- Are short-term treatments.

- Should be used at the lowest effective dosage.
- Can cause memory loss.
- Can be reversed by flumazenil in overdose.
- Can cause dosage-dependent CNS and respiratory depression.
- Can cause seizures if stopped abruptly; must be tapered slowly when discontinued.
- Should be avoided or used with caution in older adults; meet American Geriatrics Society (2023) Beers Criteria regarding concern for increased risk of falls, fractures, sedation, dependence, confusion, respiratory depression in chronic obstructive pulmonary disease (COPD), and incontinence.
- Should be avoided in pregnancy and breastfeeding.
- Can worsen confusion in delirium.
- Can cause complex sleep behaviors (e.g., driving, preparing food, making phone calls, having sex without retaining a memory of behaviors).
- Are U.S. Drug Enforcement Agency (DEA) Schedule IV controlled substances.
- Are metabolized by the liver, often through cytochrome P450 (CYP) enzymes.
- Should not be combined with opioids or other CNS depressants.

Benzodiazepine Class Effects

- **Side effects and adverse effects of benzodiazepines:** Altered sensorium, drowsiness, sedation, fatigue, ataxia, slurred speech, weakness, dizziness, syncope, diplopia, confusion, forgetfulness, amnesia, impaired concentration, disinhibition, dependency, abuse, increased suicidality, hallucinations (rare), edema, rash, dry mouth, asthenia, extrapyramidal symptoms, dystonia, hypotension, nausea, constipation, appetite changes, incontinence, urinary retention, menstrual irregularities, changes in libido.
- **Paradoxical effects of benzodiazepines:** Nervousness, hyperexcitability, irritability.

Benzodiazepine Class Warnings and Precautions

Benzodiazepine Class Boxed Warnings

Risks From Concomitant Use With Opioids

- Concomitant use with opioids may result in profound sedation, respiratory depression, coma, and death.
- Reserve concomitant use for patients with inadequate alternative treatment options after carefully weighing risks, benefits, and alternatives. Proceed with caution and ensure adequate informed consent.
- Limit concomitant benzodiazepine and opioid use to the minimum required dosage and duration of treatment.
- Monitor patients closely for signs and symptoms of respiratory depression and sedation.
- The reader is also referred to the FDA warnings on this topic.

Risks From Abuse, Misuse, and Addiction

- Benzodiazepines expose users to the risk of abuse, misuse, diversion, and the development of a substance use disorder (addiction). Patients need to be screened for a history of substance use disorder.
- Benzodiazepines are classified as DEA Schedule IV controlled substances.

Benzodiazepine Class Boxed Warnings *(continued)*

Risks From Abuse, Misuse, and Addiction ***(continued)***

- Use can lead to overdose or death.
- Use often involves concomitant use with other medications, alcohol, and/or illicit substances, which is associated with increased frequency of serious adverse outcomes. Patients need to be counseled about lifestyle changes, such as avoiding alcohol. Concomitant use of CNS depressants should be avoided whenever possible.
- Assess risk for abuse, misuse, and addiction before prescribing and throughout treatment.

Risks From Dependence and Withdrawal Reactions

- Benzodiazepine use may lead to clinically significant physical or psychological dependence.
- Risk of dependence and withdrawal increases with longer treatment duration and higher daily dosages.
- Gradually taper to discontinue after long-term use, as abrupt discontinuation or rapid dosage reduction may cause acute withdrawal reactions, including an increased risk of seizures, which may be potentially life-threatening.

Benzodiazepine Approximate Equivalencies

Table 3–1. Benzodiazepine equivalency chart (approximate)

Drug	Equivalent dose (oral)[a]	Half-life (hours) (includes active metabolites)	Time to peak (hours unless otherwise specified)
Alprazolam	0.5 mg	12–15 (short acting)	<1
Chlordiazepoxide	10–25 mg	24–200 (long acting)	1–4
Clonazepam	0.25–0.5 mg	20–50 (long acting)	1–4
Diazepam	5 mg	30–100 (long acting)	1–2
Estazolam	0.33–1.0 mg	10–24 (medium acting)	0.5–6.0
Flurazepam	15 mg	40–100 (long acting)	0.5–1.0
Lorazepam	1 mg	12–15 (medium acting)	1–2
Midazolam	1.25–1.7 mg (1 mg IV lorazepam to 2 mg IV midazolam)]	2–3 (very short acting)	PO: 10–20 minutes IM: 30–60 minutes IV: 3–5 minutes
Oxazepam	15 mg	5–15 (short acting)	1–4
Quazepam	10–20 mg	25–41 (long acting)	1.5–2.0
Temazepam	15 mg	10–20 (medium acting)	1.5–3.0
Triazolam	0.1–0.25 mg	1.5–5.5 (short acting)	1–2

[a]Approximate oral dose equivalent to 5 mg diazepam.
Source. Borrelli et al. 2022; Brett and Murnion 2015; Griffin et al. 2013.

Benzodiazepine Safety in Pregnancy

Table 3–2. Benzodiazepines in pregnancy

• Carefully weigh risks versus benefits. Consider consultation with an OB/GYN specialist.
• Most benzodiazepines were classified as Pregnancy Category D in the prior FDA classification system.
• Avoid use in the first trimester and peripartum whenever possible.
• Use is associated with possible increased risk of teratogenicity, based on conflicting human data.
• Risk of early miscarriage and preterm birth is low, according to human data.
• Use is associated with increased risk of floppy infant syndrome and neonatal withdrawal syndrome near term, based on human data.
• If use is necessary, consider use of shorter-acting before longer-acting benzodiazepines and ensure that the benefits of use outweigh the risks.

Source. Lee et al. 2022.

Further Reading

Stahl SM: Prescriber's Guide: Stahl's Essential Psychopharmacology, 7th Edition. Cambridge, UK, Cambridge University Press, 2020

References

American Geriatrics Society Beers Criteria® Update Expert Panel: 2023 updated AGS Beers Criteria for potentially inappropriate medication use in older adults. J Am Geriatr Soc 71(7):2052–2081, 2013 37139824

Borrelli EP, Bratberg J, Hallowell BD, et al: Application of a diazepam milligram equivalency algorithm to assess benzodiazepine dose intensity in Rhode Island in 2018. J Manag Care Spec Pharm 28(1):58–68, 2022 34949119

Brett J, Murnion B: Management of benzodiazepine misuse and dependence. Aust Prescr 38(5):152–155, 2015 26648651

Griffin CE III, Kaye AM, Bueno FR, et al: Benzodiazepine pharmacology and central nervous system-mediated effects. Ochsner J 13(2):214–223, 2013 23789008

Lee H, Koh JW, Kim YA, et al: Pregnancy and neonatal outcomes after exposure to alprazolam in pregnancy. Front Pharmacol 13:854562, 2022 35548333

FDA-Indicated Anxiolytic Benzodiazepines

Alprazolam

I. **Brand Names**: Xanax, Xanax XR

II. **Therapeutic Class**: Benzodiazepine (short acting), anxiolytic

III. **Mechanism-Based Class**: GABA positive allosteric modulator (GABA PAM)

IV. **Mechanism(s) of Action**

A. Enhances GABA inhibitory binding to stereo-specific benzodiazepine receptors on postsynaptic GABA neurons, leading to hyperpolarization.

B. Enhances the inhibitory effects of GABA.

C. Inhibits neuronal activity (presumably in the amygdala, regulating fear centers to provide anxiolytic effects).

V. **Indications**

A. FDA adult:

1. Generalized anxiety disorder (IR)
2. Panic disorder (IR and XR)

B. Evidence-based[1] off-label uses:

1. Other anxiety disorders
2. Anxiety associated with depression
3. Premenstrual dysphoric disorder
4. Insomnia
5. Acute mania (adjunctive)
6. Acute psychosis (adjunctive)
7. Irritable bowel syndrome/other somatic anxiety symptoms
8. Catatonia

C. FDA pediatric: None

VI. **Major Contraindications and When to Use Caution**

A. **Contraindications**:

1. Known hypersensitivity to class or medication
2. Acute narrow-angle glaucoma

---

[1]Evidence strength varies; readers are referred to the literature for more detailed information.

B. **Use caution**:

1. Substance use history, obstructive sleep apnea, elderly individuals or those with high fall risk, debilitated patients, concurrent use of other CNS depressant medications, concurrent use of opioids, severe respiratory disease, severe liver disease, renal impairment, seizure history, depression, porphyria, delirium, dementia
2. A change in smoking habits—Alprazolam concentrations can be decreased by as much as 50% in smokers in comparison with nonsmokers.

C. **Avoid abrupt withdrawal**: Gradually taper to discontinue after long-term use, as abrupt discontinuation or rapid dosage reduction may cause acute withdrawal reactions, including increased risk of seizures, which may be life-threatening.

VII. Dosage Formulations

A. Brand: IR tablet (0.25 mg, 0.5 mg, 1 mg, 2 mg); ER tablet (0.5 mg, 1 mg, 2 mg, 3 mg)

B. Generic: IR tablet (0.25 mg [*scored*], 0.5 mg [*scored*], 1 mg [*scored*], 2 mg [*multi-scored*]); ER tablet (0.5 mg, 1 mg, 2 mg, 3 mg); ODT tablet (0.25 mg, 0.5 mg, 1 mg, 2 mg); oral concentrate (1 mg/mL)

1. Patients with decreased gastric pH or salivary flow (caused either by a disease or by a drug) may experience slowed or reduced absorption of the ODT formulation.
2. Patients with phenylketonuria should be informed that the ODT formulation contains phenylalanine.

VIII. Dosage Ranges and Guidelines

A. Dosage varies greatly based on indication and tolerance (see Table 3–3 for usual dosage ranges).

B. Use a reduced dosage for elderly individuals and those with fall risk, hepatic or respiratory disease, or concurrent opioid use.

1. Start at 0.25 mg BID–TID in elderly adults and 0.5–1 mg/day for the ER formulation.

C. **Titration**: Start at dosage listed in Table 3–3. Increase by up to 1 mg/day every 3–4 days.

1. Typical dosage is less than 4 mg/day, but some severely ill patients may require up to 10 mg/day.
2. Maximum dosage range for anxiety is 4–10 mg/day.

D. **Tapering**: Taper dosage by no more than 0.5 mg every 3 days to discontinue.

1. Some individuals may require a slower taper.

Table 3–3. Alprazolam indications and dosage ranges

Indications	Usual dosage range
Anxiety disorder (IR)	Start: 0.25–0.5 mg TID, increase every 3–4 days as needed Typical IR dosage range: 1–4 mg/day (in 3–4 divided doses) Maximum: 4 mg/day
Panic disorder (IR)	Start: 0.5 mg TID, increase 1 mg/day or less every 3–4 days as needed Typical IR dosage range: 5–6 mg/day (in 3–4 divided doses) Maximum: 10 mg/day (severe cases)
Panic disorder (XR)	Start: 0.5–1 mg/day, increase by up to 1 mg/day every 3–4 days as needed Typical XR dosage range: 3–6 mg/day (1–2 times daily) Maximum: 10 mg/day (severe cases)

IX. **Monitoring**

A. Monitor baseline and periodic vital signs, complete blood count, creatinine, liver function tests, urinalysis, and physical and psychiatric evaluations.

1. Potential risk of hepatic dysfunction (aspartate transaminase [AST]/alanine aminotransferase [ALT] elevation), renal dysfunction, blood dyscrasias, jaundice
2. Leukopenia and elevated lactate dehydrogenase have been found in patients with long-term use of benzodiazepines.

B. Abuse/dependence/tolerance/withdrawal:

1. Alprazolam is a Schedule IV controlled substance. Routinely assess for use of other narcotics (boxed warning with opioids).
2. Consider periodic urine drug screens to monitor for other narcotic/substance use.
3. Monitor for abuse, dependence, and tolerance.
4. Monitor for withdrawal effects; abrupt withdrawal can precipitate seizures and may be fatal.

C. Monitor for behavioral changes, alertness, and mental status (e.g., depression, suicidality).

X. **Relevant Pharmacokinetics/Pharmacodynamics**

A. **Metabolism**: Hepatic cytochrome P450 (CYP) 3A4; no active metabolite
B. **Time to peak plasma concentration**: <1 hour
C. **Half-life**: 12–15 hours (short acting)
D. **Effect of food**: Food does not affect absorption.
E. **Hepatic impairment**: Start at lower dosage of 0.25 mg PO BID–TID, with gradual titration.
F. **Renal impairment**: No dosage adjustment needed.

XI. Clinically Relevant Drug Interactions

A. Metabolized by CYP3A4

1. CYP3A4 inhibitors may decrease clearance and increase serum concentrations and effects. CYP3A4 inhibitors include nefazodone, fluvoxamine, fluoxetine, ketoconazole, itraconazole, isoniazid, and the HIV protease inhibitors ritonavir, indinavir, nelfinavir, saquinavir, and lopinavir, as well as grapefruit juice.
2. CYP3A4 inducers (e.g., carbamazepine, oxcarbazepine) may increase clearance and decrease serum concentrations and effects.

   a. Tobacco smoke may decrease serum concentrations.

B. Avoid concomitant use with opioids and other narcotics.

C. Avoid concomitant use with other CNS depressants. If used, dosage adjustments may be necessary.

D. Other sleep aids, including zolpidem and eszopiclone, should not be used with benzodiazepines.

E. Coadministration of benzodiazepines with antihypertensives or other medications that can lower blood pressure may result in additive hypotensive effects.

XII. Adverse Effects

A. **Boxed warnings**: See "Benzodiazepine Class Boxed Warnings" in the "Benzodiazepine Class Warnings and Precautions" section at the beginning of this chapter.

B. **Most common**:

1. Drowsiness, sedation, fatigue, ataxia, slurred speech, weakness, dizziness, syncope, diplopia, confusion, forgetfulness, euphoric mood, anterograde amnesia, impaired concentration, disinhibition, psychomotor impairment
2. Nervousness, hyperexcitability, irritability

C. **Benzodiazepine class effects**:

1. Nausea and constipation, appetite changes, incontinence, urinary retention, menstrual irregularities, changes in libido, dry mouth, asthenia, hallucinations (rare), extrapyramidal symptoms, dystonia, sialorrhea, hypotension

D. **Serious reactions**:

1. Stevens-Johnson syndrome, angioedema, hypersensitivity reaction, anaphylactoid reaction: Monitor for skin changes, particularly during initiation and reintroduction, and titrate slowly.
2. If abruptly discontinued, respiratory depression and CNS depression, dependency, abuse, depression with suicidality, and/or wit*hdrawal with possible seizures can result. Use the lowest effective dosage for the shortest possible time; taper slowly to discontinue use.
3. Hepatic dysfunction with ALT/AST elevation, renal dysfunction, blood dyscrasias, jaundice: Monitor laboratory values at baseline and periodically.

E. **Risks in pregnancy and lactation**: Most benzodiazepines were designated Category D drugs in the prior FDA classification. See Table 3–2 ("Benzodiazepines in pregnancy") in the introduction to this chapter; see also Chapter 15 ("Women: Pregnancy, Postpartum, and Breastfeeding"). For current information on benzodiazepine use in lactation, readers are referred to the Drugs and Lactation Database (LactMed; www.ncbi.nlm.nih.gov/books/NBK501922/).

XIII. **Clinical Pearls/Prescribing Tips**

A. Alprazolam may be less sedating compared with most other benzodiazepines.

B. Alprazolam is highly psychoactive. Patients may obtain immediate relief with the first dose, but the effect builds with continued use. Alprazolam may have a higher abuse potential compared with other benzodiazepines; its rapid onset of action increases its "likability" and produces a euphoric effect, and these characteristics may lead to habit formation and dependency, especially in patients with past or present substance use disorders. Development of tolerance is common.

C. Because of its short half-life, IR alprazolam may be more difficult to taper than the ER formulation. Consider a crossover to the ER form or an alternative benzodiazepine for tapering if needed.

1. IR formulation: Short duration of action and pronounced on/off effect may increase the addiction potential of the IR formulation.
2. ER formulation: Longer duration of action and less prominent on/off effect makes the ER formulation easier to taper.

D. Alprazolam is recommended for short-term use only (as needed or just for a few weeks). Beware of the "clock-watching" phenomenon, especially with PRN dosing in anxious patients.

E. Hypomania/mania with alprazolam has occurred in some patients.

F. Benzodiazepine class use guidelines:

1. Use the lowest effective dosage for the shortest possible period of time. Regularly assess the need for continued treatment. Benzodiazepines are not recommended for long-term treatment of anxiety disorders; consider switching to an SSRI or SNRI for long-term maintenance. Consider augmenting with gabapentin or pregabalin for anxiety disorders to reduce benzodiazepine requirements.
2. When helping patients through the process of gradually tapering and discontinuing benzodiazepines, clinicians must be able to distinguish among reemergence of chronic anxiety disorder symptoms, rebound anxiety symptoms, and acute withdrawal symptoms.
3. **Caution**: Benzodiazepines can be fatal in overdose and withdrawal. Taper slowly. Protracted withdrawal effects can occur. Do not combine with other CNS depressants (e.g., other benzodiazepines, opioids). The benzodiazepine receptor antagonist flumazenil can be used in acute overdose but can precipitate seizures.

Further Reading

Ait-Daoud N, Hamby AS, Sharma S, et al: A review of alprazolam use, misuse, and withdrawal. J Addict Med 12(1):4–10, 2018 28777203

Xanax (alprazolam) [package insert]. U.S. Food and Drug Administration website. Revised August 2011. Available at: https://www.accessdata.fda.gov/drugsatfda_docs/label/2011/018276s045lbl.pdf. Accessed May 29, 2022.

Chlordiazepoxide

I. **Brand Names**: Librium (brand discontinued in U.S.)

II. **Therapeutic Class**: Benzodiazepine (long acting), anxiolytic

III. **Mechanism-Based Class**: GABA positive allosteric modulator (GABA PAM)

IV. **Mechanism(s) of Action**

A. Enhances GABA inhibitory binding to stereo-specific benzodiazepine receptors on postsynaptic GABA neurons, leading to hyperpolarization.

B. Enhances inhibitory effects of GABA.

C. Inhibits neuronal activity (presumably in the amygdala, regulating fear centers to provide anxiolytic effects)

V. **Indications**

A. FDA adult:

1. Anxiety disorders
2. Short-term relief of anxiety symptoms
3. Withdrawal symptoms of acute alcoholism
4. Preoperative anxiety

B. Evidence-based[1] off-label uses:

1. Catatonia

C. FDA pediatric: None

VI. **Major Contraindications and When to Use Caution**

A. **Contraindications**:

1. Known hypersensitivity to medication or class
2. Myasthenia gravis
3. Angle-closure glaucoma

B. **Use caution**: Substance use history, obstructive sleep apnea, elderly individuals or those with high fall risk, debilitated patients, concurrent use of other CNS depressant medications, concurrent use of opioids, severe respiratory disease, severe liver disease, renal impairment, seizure history, depression, porphyria, delirium, dementia.

C. **Avoid abrupt withdrawal**: Gradually taper to discontinue after long-term use, as abrupt discontinuation or rapid dosage reduction may cause acute withdrawal reactions, including increased risk of seizures, which may be life-threatening.

VII. **Dosage Formulations**

A. Generic capsules (5 mg, 10 mg, 25 mg)

B. Chlordiazepoxide is also available in an injectable form intended for short-term use (see package labeling and prescribing information)

---

[1]Evidence strength varies; readers are referred to the literature for more detailed information.

VIII. **Dosage Ranges and Guidelines**

A. Dosage varies according to indication and tolerance (see Table 3–4 for usual dosage ranges).

B. Use a reduced dosage for elderly individuals and those with fall risk, hepatic or respiratory disease, or concurrent opioid use.

1. In elderly adults, the usual starting dosage is 5 mg/day to 5 mg BID, with slow upward titration.

C. **Titration**: Start at dosage listed in Table 3–4. Titration varies depending on indication, but increases can be made in increments of 5–50 mg as needed and tolerated. In general, the maximum dosage for anxiety is about 100 mg/day.

D. For alcohol withdrawal, dosing may be symptom-triggered or scheduled. If scheduled, decrease the daily dosage by 25%–50% each day by reducing the dosage and/or frequency (American Society of Addiction Medicine 2020).

E. **Tapering**: Taper by 10 mg every 3 days to reduce the risk of withdrawal effects. Inpatient tapers may progress more rapidly because closer monitoring is possible in this setting. Consider use of a slower taper (e.g., reduction by 5 mg or less per week) in difficult-to-taper patients. Some individuals may require an even slower taper (e.g., reduction by 1% every 3 days over a period of up to several months), especially those who need behavioral desensitization because of psychological dependence.

Table 3–4. Chlordiazepoxide indications and dosage ranges

Indications	Usual dosage range
Mild to moderate anxiety	5–10 mg TID–QID Maximum dosage: 100 mg/day
Severe anxiety	20–25 mg TID–QID Maximum dosage: 100 mg/day
Alcohol withdrawal (acute)	25–100 mg (every 4–6 hours) PRN or scheduled Maximum dosage: 300–400 mg/day
Preoperative anxiety	5–10 mg PO TID–QID Maximum dosage: 100 mg/day
Geriatric patients	5 mg BID–QID
Pediatric patients	5 mg BID–QID

IX. **Monitoring**

A. Monitor baseline and periodic vital signs, complete blood count, creatinine, liver function tests, urinalysis, and physical and psychiatric evaluations.

1. Potential risk of hepatic dysfunction (aspartate transaminase [AST]/alanine aminotransferase [ALT] elevation), renal dysfunction, blood dyscrasias, jaundice
2. Leukopenia and elevated lactate dehydrogenase have been found in patients with long-term use of benzodiazepines.

B. **Abuse/dependence/tolerance/withdrawal**:

1. Chlordiazepoxide is a Schedule IV controlled substance. Routinely assess patients for use of other narcotics (boxed warning with opioids).
2. Consider periodic urine drug screens to monitor for other narcotic/substance use.
3. Monitor for abuse, dependence, and tolerance.
4. Monitor for withdrawal symptoms; abrupt withdrawal can precipitate seizures and may be fatal.

C. Monitor for behavioral changes, alertness, and mental status (e.g., depression, suicidality).

X. Relevant Pharmacokinetics/Pharmacodynamics

A. **Metabolism**: Hepatic cytochrome P450 (CYP) 3A4 partial substrate; active metabolites present

B. **Time to peak plasma concentration**: 0.5–2 hours

C. **Half-life**: 24–48 hours (long acting)

1. Elimination half-life: 5–30 hours
2. Half-life of active metabolites: 3–200 hours
3. Active metabolites can accumulate.

D. **Hepatic impairment**: Caution is advised, given chlordiazepoxide's hepatic metabolism and risk of metabolite accumulation.

E. **Renal impairment**: If CrCl is <10 mL/minute, decrease dosage by 50%. Accumulation of active metabolites can occur, so use with caution.

XI. Clinically Relevant Drug Interactions

A. Metabolized by CYP3A4

1. CYP3A4 inhibitors may decrease clearance and increase serum concentrations and effects. CYP3A4 inhibitors include nefazodone, fluvoxamine, fluoxetine, ketoconazole, itraconazole, isoniazid, and the HIV protease inhibitors ritonavir, indinavir, nelfinavir, saquinavir, and lopinavir, as well as grapefruit juice.
2. CYP3A4 inducers (e.g., carbamazepine, oxcarbazepine) and smoking may increase clearance, resulting in decreased concentration and effect.

B. Avoid concomitant use with opioids and other narcotics.

C. Avoid concomitant use with other CNS depressants. If used, dosage adjustments may be necessary.

D. Other sleep aids, including zolpidem and eszopiclone, should not be used with benzodiazepines.

E. Coadministration of benzodiazepines with antihypertensives or other medications that can lower blood pressure may result in additive hypotensive effects.

XII. Adverse Effects

A. **Boxed warnings**: See "Benzodiazepine Class Boxed Warnings" in the "Benzodiazepine Class Warnings and Precautions" section at the beginning of this chapter.

B. **Most common**:

1. Drowsiness, sedation, fatigue, ataxia, slurred speech, weakness, dizziness, syncope, diplopia, confusion, forgetfulness, euphoric mood, anterograde amnesia, impaired concentration, disinhibition, psychomotor impairment: Side effects are dosage dependent. Use the lowest effective dosage and titrate slowly to effect.
2. Nervousness, hyperexcitability, irritability: Monitor for potential paradoxical response.

C. **Benzodiazepine class effects**:

1. Nausea and constipation, appetite changes, incontinence, urinary retention, menstrual irregularities, changes in libido, dry mouth, asthenia, hallucinations (rare), extrapyramidal symptoms, dystonia, sialorrhea, hypotension

D. **Serious reactions**:

1. Stevens-Johnson syndrome, angioedema, hypersensitivity reaction, anaphylactoid reaction: Monitor for skin changes, particularly during initiation and reintroduction, and titrate slowly.
2. Respiratory depression and CNS depression, dependency, abuse, depression with suicidality, withdrawal with possible seizures if abrupt discontinuation: Use lowest effective dosage for shortest possible time; taper slowly to discontinue use.
3. Hepatic dysfunction with ALT/AST elevation, renal dysfunction, blood dyscrasias, jaundice: Monitor laboratory values at baseline and periodically.

E. **Risks in pregnancy and lactation**: Most benzodiazepines were designated Category D drugs in the prior FDA classification. See Table 3–2 ("Benzodiazepines in pregnancy") in the introduction to this chapter; see also Chapter 15 ("Women: Pregnancy, Postpartum, and Breastfeeding"). For current information on benzodiazepine use in lactation, readers are referred to the Drugs and Lactation Database (LactMed; www.ncbi.nlm.nih.gov/books/NBK501922/).

XIII. **Clinical Pearls/Prescribing Tips**

A. Chlordiazepoxide is sedating. Advise patients to take the largest dose at night to avoid daytime sedation.
B. Chlordiazepoxide's longer half-life can lead to daytime sedation and impaired motor and cognitive functioning, which can increase over time due to active metabolite accumulation. Use caution and decrease the dosage if accumulation is suspected. Avoid use in elderly patients, as long-term accumulation of active metabolites can lead to insidious onset of falls or confusion.
C. Because of the long half-life of its active metabolites, chlordiazepoxide is often a preferred medication in treating alcohol withdrawal and for tapering patients off other shorter-acting benzodiazepines (except in patients with liver disease).
D. Chlordiazepoxide is not recommended for long-term daily use. Risk of dependence increases with dosage and duration of treatment. Long-term adaptation of benzodiazepine receptors may explain tolerance, dependence, and withdrawal.

E. If breakthrough anxiety occurs, consider either 1) increasing the dosage or 2) lowering the dosage but increasing the dosing frequency (for the same total daily dosage [TDD]).
F. Some severely ill patients may require dosages higher than the generally recommended maximum dosages.
G. Because of the long half-life of its metabolites, chlordiazepoxide may "taper itself"; however, withdrawal can still occur (see "Tapering" under "Dosage Ranges and Guidelines").
H. Benzodiazepine class use guidelines:
    1. Use the lowest effective dosage for the shortest possible period of time. Regularly assess the need for continued treatment. Use is not recommended for long-term treatment of anxiety disorders; consider switching to an SSRI or SNRI for long-term maintenance. Consider augmenting with gabapentin or pregabalin for anxiety disorders to reduce benzodiazepine requirements.
    2. When helping patients through the process of gradually tapering and discontinuing benzodiazepines, clinicians must be able to distinguish among reemergence of chronic anxiety disorder symptoms, rebound anxiety symptoms, and acute withdrawal symptoms.
    3. **Caution**: Benzodiazepines can be fatal in overdose and withdrawal. Taper slowly. Protracted withdrawal effects can occur. Do not combine with other CNS depressants (e.g., other benzodiazepines, opioids). The benzodiazepine receptor antagonist flumazenil can be used in acute overdose but can precipitate seizures.

Further Reading

Greenblatt DJ, Shader RI, MacLeod SM, et al: Clinical pharmacokinetics of chlordiazepoxide. Clin Pharmacokinet 3(5):381–394, 1978359214

Librium (chlordiazepoxide) [package insert]. U.S Food and Drug Administration website. Revised July 2005. Available at: https://www.accessdata.fda.gov/drugsatfda_docs/label/2016/012249s049lbl.pdf. Accessed May 28, 2022.

Reference

American Society of Addiction Medicine: The ASAM clinical practice guideline on alcohol withdrawal management. J Addict Med 14(3S)(Suppl 1):1–72, 2020 32511109

Clonazepam

I. **Brand Names**: Klonopin, Klonopin Wafer (brand discontinued in U.S.)

II. **Therapeutic Class**: Benzodiazepine (long acting), anxiolytic, hypnotic, muscle relaxant, anticonvulsant

III. **Mechanism-Based Class**: GABA positive allosteric modulator (GABA PAM)

IV. **Mechanism(s) of Action**:

A. Enhances GABA inhibition binding to stereo-specific benzodiazepine receptors on postsynaptic GABA neurons leading to hyperpolarization

B. Positive allosteric modulator of $GABA_A$ receptor, benzodiazepine site, causing increased permeability of neuronal membrane to chloride ions, results in hyperpolarization and depressed activity

V. **Indications**

A. FDA adult:

1. Panic disorder
2. Seizure disorder (akinetic, myoclonic, absence, Lennox-Gastaut)

B. Evidence-based[1] off-label uses:

1. Agitation
2. Anxiety
3. Catatonia
4. Adjunct to antipsychotics for treatment of acute mania or psychosis
5. Rapid eye movement (REM) sleep behavior disorder
6. Restless legs syndrome
7. Sleep terrors
8. Sleepwalking
9. Confusional arousals
10. Tourette syndrome
11. Insomnia
12. Myoclonus
13. Tardive dyskinesia
14. Acute vertigo

C. FDA pediatric: None

VI. **Major Contraindications and When to Use Caution**

A. **Contraindications**:

1. Known hypersensitivity to medication or class
2. Myasthenia gravis
3. Angle-closure glaucoma

---

[1]Evidence strength varies; readers are referred to the literature for more detailed information.

B. **Use caution**: Substance use history, obstructive sleep apnea, elderly individuals or those with high fall risk, debilitated patients, concurrent use of other CNS depressant medications, concurrent use of opioids, severe respiratory disease, severe liver disease, renal impairment, seizure history, depression, porphyria, delirium, dementia.

C. **Avoid abrupt withdrawal**: Gradually taper to discontinue after long-term use, as abrupt discontinuation or rapid dosage reduction may cause acute withdrawal reactions, including increased risk of seizures, which may be life-threatening.

VII. **Dosage Formulations**

A. Generic: tablet (0.5 mg, 1 mg, 2 mg); ODT (0.125 mg, 0.25 mg, 0.5 mg, 1 mg, 2 mg)
B. Brand tablet (0.5 mg, 1 mg, 2 mg)

VIII. **Dosage Ranges and Guidelines**

A. Dosage varies based on indication and tolerance (see Table 3–5 for usual dosage ranges).
B. Use a reduced dosage for elderly individuals and those with fall risk, hepatic or respiratory disease, or concurrent opioid use.
C. **Titration**: Start at dosages listed in Table 3–5. Escalate dosage by 0.25–0.5 mg every 3 days; use the lowest effective dosage. In general, the maximum dosage for anxiety is around 4–8 mg/day.
D. **Tapering**: Taper dosage by 0.25–0.5 mg every 3 days.
   1. Some individuals may require a slower taper/discontinuation.

Table 3–5. Clonazepam indications and dosage ranges

Indications	Usual dosage range
Seizures	0.5–1.5 mg up to 20 mg/day (taken as a single dose or in 2 divided doses)
Panic disorder Other anxiety disorders (off-label)	0.25–4 mg/day (either divided or at bedtime) Scheduled or as needed
Severe agitation (off-label)	0.5–8 mg/day (2–4 divided doses) Scheduled or as needed

IX. **Monitoring**

A. Monitor baseline and periodic vital signs, complete blood count, creatinine, liver function tests, urinalysis, and physical and psychiatric evaluations.
   1. Potential risk of hepatic dysfunction (aspartate transaminase [AST]/alanine aminotransferase [ALT] elevation), renal dysfunction, blood dyscrasias, jaundice
   2. Leukopenia and elevated lactate dehydrogenase have been found in patients with long-term use of benzodiazepines.

B. Abuse/dependence/tolerance/withdrawal:

1. Clonazepam is a Schedule IV controlled substance. Routinely assess for use of other narcotics (boxed warning with opioids).
2. Consider periodic urine drug screens to monitor for other narcotic use.
3. Monitor for abuse, dependence, and tolerance.
4. Monitor for withdrawal symptoms; abrupt withdrawal can precipitate seizures and may be fatal.

C. Monitor for behavioral changes, alertness, and mental status (e.g., depression, suicidality).

D. Monitor for skin changes (Stevens-Johnson syndrome [SJS], toxic epidermal necrolysis [TEN]).

X. **Relevant Pharmacokinetics/Pharmacodynamics**

A. **Metabolism**: Hepatic cytochrome P450 (CYP) 3A4
B. **Time to peak plasma concentration**: 1–4 hours
C. **Half-life**: 22–33 hours in children, 20–50 hours in adults (long acting)
D. **Hepatic impairment**: No adjustment needed. Accumulation of active metabolites can occur, so use with caution.
E. **Renal impairment**: Clonazepam use is contraindicated in patients with significant impairment.

XI. **Clinically Relevant Drug Interactions**

A. Metabolized by CYP3A4

1. CYP3A4 inhibitors may decrease clearance and increase serum concentrations and effects. CYP3A4 inhibitors include nefazodone, fluvoxamine, fluoxetine, ketoconazole, itraconazole, isoniazid, and the HIV protease inhibitors ritonavir, indinavir, nelfinavir, saquinavir, and lopinavir, as well as grapefruit juice.
2. CYP3A4 inducers (e.g., carbamazepine, oxcarbazepine) and smoking may increase clearance, resulting in decreased concentration and effect.

B. Avoid concomitant use with opioids and other narcotics.

C. Avoid concomitant use with other CNS depressants. If used, dosage adjustments may be necessary.

D. Other sleep aids, including zolpidem and eszopiclone, should not be used with benzodiazepines.

E. Coadministration of benzodiazepines with antihypertensives or other medications that can lower blood pressure may result in additive hypotensive effects.

XII. **Adverse Effects**

A. **Boxed warnings**: See "Benzodiazepine Class Boxed Warnings" in the "Benzodiazepine Class Warnings and Precautions" section at the beginning of this chapter.

B. **Most common**:

1. Drowsiness, sedation, fatigue, ataxia, slurred speech, weakness, dizziness, syncope, diplopia, confusion, forgetfulness, euphoric mood, anterograde amnesia, impaired concentration, disinhibition, psychomotor impairment; side effects are dosage dependent. Use the lowest effective dosage and titrate slowly to effect.

2. Nervousness, hyperexcitability, irritability: Monitor for potential paradoxical response.

C. **Benzodiazepine class effects**:

1. Nausea and constipation, appetite changes, incontinence, urinary retention, menstrual irregularities, changes in libido, dry mouth, asthenia, hallucinations (rare), extrapyramidal symptoms, dystonia, sialorrhea, hypotension

D. **Serious reactions**:

1. Stevens-Johnson syndrome, angioedema, hypersensitivity reaction, anaphylactoid reaction: Monitor for skin changes, particularly during initiation and reintroduction, and titrate slowly.
2. Respiratory depression and CNS depression, dependency, abuse, depression with suicidality, withdrawal with possible seizures if abrupt discontinuation: Use lowest effective dosage for the shortest possible time; taper slowly to discontinue.
3. Hepatic dysfunction with ALT/AST elevation, renal dysfunction, blood dyscrasias, jaundice: Monitor laboratory values at baseline and periodically.

E. **Risks in pregnancy and lactation**: Most benzodiazepines were designated Category D drugs in the prior FDA classification. See Table 3–2 ("Benzodiazepines in pregnancy") in the introduction to this chapter; see also Chapter 15 ("Women: Pregnancy, Postpartum, and Breastfeeding"). For current information on benzodiazepine use in lactation, readers are referred to the Drugs and Lactation Database (LactMed; www.ncbi.nlm.nih.gov/books/NBK501922/).

XIII. Clinical Pearls/Prescribing Tips

A. In comparison with other benzodiazepines, clonazepam is more potent but has a weaker binding affinity for $GABA_A$.

B. Clonazepam has low lipid solubility and therefore a slower absorption and onset of action, which may lower the potential for tolerance or misuse ("likability") and theoretically confers lower risk of habit formation compared with other benzodiazepines.

C. Clonazepam's longer half-life may make it easier to taper/discontinue.

D. Clonazepam may also be less likely than most other benzodiazepines to cause anterograde amnesia.

E. Clonazepam has shown some efficacy in reducing tardive dyskinesia symptoms (Thaker et al. 1990).

F. Benzodiazepine class use guidelines:

1. Use the lowest effective dosage for the shortest possible period of time. Regularly assess the need for continued treatment. Benzodiazepines are not recommended for long-term treatment of anxiety disorders; consider switching to an SSRI or SNRI for long-term maintenance. Consider augmenting with gabapentin or pregabalin for anxiety disorders to reduce benzodiazepine requirements.
2. When helping patients through the process of gradually tapering and discontinuing benzodiazepines, clinicians must be able to distinguish among reemergence of chronic anxiety disorder symptoms, rebound anxiety symptoms, and acute withdrawal symptoms.

3. **Caution**: Benzodiazepines can be fatal in overdose and withdrawal. Taper slowly. Protracted withdrawal can occur. Do not combine with other CNS depressants (e.g., other benzodiazepines, opioids). The benzodiazepine receptor antagonist flumazenil can be used in acute overdose but can precipitate seizures.

Further Reading

Chouinard G: Issues in the clinical use of benzodiazepines: potency, withdrawal, and rebound. J Clin Psychiatry 65(Suppl 5):7–12, 200415078112

Griffin CE III, Kaye AM, Bueno FR, et al: Benzodiazepine pharmacology and central nervous system-mediated effects. Ochsner J 13(2):214–223, 2013 23789008

Klonopin package insert. U.S Food and Drug Administration, 2023. Available at: https://www.accessdata.fda.gov/spl/data/d0072d65-bc19-4229-a957-a4608506f713/d0072d65-bc19-4229-a957-a4608506f713.xml. Accessed March 13, 2024.

Salpekar JA, Basu T, Thangaraj S, Maguire J: The intersections of stress, anxiety and epilepsy. Int Rev Neurobiol 152:195–219, 2020 32450996

References

Thaker GK, Nguyen JA, Strauss ME, et al: Clonazepam treatment of tardive dyskinesia: a practical GABAmimetic strategy. Am J Psychiatry 147(4):445–451, 1990 1969244

Diazepam

I. **Brand Names**: Valium, Diastat, Valtoco

II. **Therapeutic Class**: Benzodiazepine (long acting), anxiolytic, hypnotic, sedative, muscle relaxant, anticonvulsant

III. **Mechanism-Based Class**—GABA positive allosteric modulator (GABA PAM)

IV. **Mechanism(s) of Action**

A. Enhances GABA inhibition binding to stereo-specific benzodiazepine receptors on postsynaptic GABA neurons leading to hyperpolarization

B. Positive allosteric modulator of $GABA_A$ receptor at the benzodiazepine site, causing increased permeability of the neuronal membrane to chloride ions, results in hyperpolarization and depressed activity

V. **Indications**

A. FDA adult:

1. Anxiety disorders
2. Acute alcohol withdrawal
3. Spasticity
4. Spasms
5. Rigidity
6. Tremor
7. Athetosis

8. Seizure disorder (adjunctive)
9. Status epilepticus
10. Situational/procedural anxiety
11. Sedation, preoperative/pre-procedural

B. Evidence-based[1] off-label uses:

1. Insomnia
2. Catatonia
3. Sympathomimetic intoxication
4. Neuroleptic malignant syndrome
5. Opioid withdrawal (adjunctive)
6. Serotonin syndrome (adjunctive)
7. Acute vertigo

C. FDA pediatric: None

VI. **Major Contraindications and When to Use Caution**

A. **Contraindications**:

1. Known hypersensitivity to medication or class
2. Myasthenia gravis
3. Angle-closure glaucoma

B. **Use caution**: Substance use history, obstructive sleep apnea, elderly individuals or those with high fall risk, debilitated patients, concurrent use of other CNS depressant medications, concurrent use of opioids, severe respiratory disease, severe liver disease, renal impairment, seizure history, depression, porphyria, delirium, dementia.

C. **Avoid abrupt withdrawal**: Gradually taper to discontinue after long-term use, as abrupt discontinuation or rapid dosage reduction may cause acute withdrawal reactions, including increased risk of seizures, which may be life-threatening.

VII. **Dosage Formulations**

A. Brand: tablet (2 mg, 5 mg, 10 mg), intranasal (dose titration kits: 5 mg, 10 mg, 15 mg, 20 mg), rectal (gel: 2.5 mg, 10 mg, 20 mg/applicator)

B. Generic: tablet (2 mg, 5 mg, 10 mg), concentrate (5 mg/5 mL, 5 mg/mL), injectable (5 mg/mL), auto-injector (10 mg), rectal (gel: 2.5 mg, 10 mg, 20 mg/applicator)

VIII. **Dosage Ranges and Guidelines**

A. Dosage varies based on indication and tolerance (see Table 3–6 for usual dosage ranges).

B. Use a reduced dosage for elderly individuals and those with fall risk, hepatic or respiratory disease, or concurrent opioid use.

C. **Titration**: Start at dosages listed in Table 3–6. For anxiety, increase gradually in increments of 5–10 mg based on response and tolerability. In general, the maximum dosage is 40 mg/day.

---

[1]Evidence strength varies; readers are referred to the literature for more detailed information.

D. **Tapering**: Taper dosage by 25%–50% every 1–2 weeks based on response, tolerability, and patient factors. Reduce the dosage more slowly as the taper progresses. May require up to 6 months for full taper/discontinuation.

Table 3–6. Diazepam indications and dosage ranges

Indications	Usual dosage ranges
Anxiety	PO: 2–5 mg/day or BID → 40 mg/day (2–4 divided doses) IM/IV: 2–10 mg every 3–4 hours PRN
Procedural anxiety (sedation)	PO: 2–10 mg 30–60 minutes prior to procedure, may repeat at 50% of initial dose after 30–60 minutes IV: 2–10 mg 5–15 minutes prior to procedure, may repeat at 50% of initial dose after 5–30 minutes
Alcohol withdrawal	**Fixed dosage**: IV: 2–10 mg 5–15 minutes prior to procedure, may repeat at 50% of initial dose after 5–30 minutes **Symptom triggered**: PO/IV: 5–20 mg as needed based on institution-specific protocol
Muscle spasm	PO: 2–10 mg PO BID–QID → 40–60 mg/day (3–4 divided doses)
Seizure (acute, non-status)	IV: 5–10 mg every 3–5 minutes PRN IV, rectal gel, intranasal formulations available (see package insert for dosing). IM diazepam not recommended for seizures because of its erratic absorption and slow time to peak concentration.
Status epilepticus	IV: 5–10 mg every 3–5 minutes PRN A rectal gel is also available.
Acute agitation (e.g., intoxication) (off-label)	IV: 2–10 mg every 3–10 minutes PRN
Parasomnias (off-label)	PO: 5–10 mg QHS
Serotonin syndrome (off-label)	IV: 5–10 mg every 10–60 minutes PRN until symptoms resolve

IX. **Monitoring**

A. Monitor baseline and periodic vital signs, complete blood count, creatinine, liver function tests, urinalysis, and physical and psychiatric evaluations.

1. Potential risk of hepatic dysfunction (aspartate transaminase [AST]/alanine aminotransferase [ALT] elevation), renal dysfunction, blood dyscrasias, jaundice
2. Leukopenia and elevated lactate dehydrogenase have been found in patients with long-term use of benzodiazepines.

...ependence/tolerance/withdrawal:

1. ...iazepam is a Schedule IV controlled substance. Routinely assess for use of other narcotics (boxed warning with opioids).
2. Consider periodic urine drug screens to monitor for other narcotic use.
3. Monitor for abuse, dependence, and tolerance.
4. Monitor for withdrawal symptoms; abrupt withdrawal can precipitate seizures and may be fatal.

C. Monitor for behavioral changes, alertness, and mental status (e.g., depression, suicidality).

D. Monitor for skin changes (Stevens-Johnson syndrome [SJS], toxic epidermal necrolysis [TEN]).

E. Monitor for signs of propylene glycol toxicity, including serum lactate and osmolar gap, in individuals receiving high-dosage or long-duration IV medication.

X. Relevant Pharmacokinetics/Pharmacodynamics

A. **Metabolism**: Hepatic extensively; cytochrome P450 (CYP) 3A4 and CYP2C19

1. Major and minor metabolites: *N*-desmethyldiazepam, temazepam, and oxazepam are all active metabolites, eliminated via hepatic glucuronidation.

B. **Time to peak plasma concentration**: 1–4 hours

C. **Half-life**:

1. Parent drug: 30–60 hours (long acting)
2. Active metabolites: 30–100 hours

D. **Hepatic impairment**: Caution is advised for mild/moderate impairment; use is contraindicated for severe impairment.

E. **Renal impairment**: Accumulation of active metabolites is possible, so use with caution; however, no dosage adjustment is required. CNS adverse effects increase with hypoalbuminemia, which is common in end-stage renal disease (ESRD). Diazepam is not significantly dialyzable.

XI. Clinically Relevant Drug Interactions

A. Metabolized by CYP3A4 and CYP219

1. CYP3A4 inhibitors may decrease clearance and increase serum concentrations and effects. CYP3A4 inhibitors include nefazodone, fluvoxamine, fluoxetine, ketoconazole, itraconazole, isoniazid, and the HIV protease inhibitors ritonavir, indinavir, nelfinavir, saquinavir, and lopinavir, as well as grapefruit juice.
2. CYP3A4 inducers (e.g., carbamazepine, oxcarbazepine) and smoking may increase clearance, resulting in decreased concentration and effect.

B. Avoid concomitant use with opioids and other narcotics.

C. Avoid concomitant use with other CNS depressants. If used, dosage adjustments may be necessary.

D. Other sleep aids, including zolpidem and eszopiclone, should not be used with benzodiazepines.

E. Coadministration of benzodiazepines with antihypertensives or other medications that can lower blood pressure may result in additive hypotensive effects.

XII. Adverse Effects

A. **Boxed warnings**: See "Benzodiazepine Class Boxed Warnings" in the "Benzodiazepine Class Warnings and Precautions" section at the beginning of this chapter.

B. **Most common**:

1. Drowsiness, sedation, fatigue, ataxia, slurred speech, weakness, dizziness, syncope, diplopia, confusion, forgetfulness, euphoric mood, anterograde amnesia, impaired concentration, disinhibition, psychomotor impairment: Side effects are dosage dependent. Use the lowest effective dosage and titrate slowly to effect.
2. Nervousness, hyperexcitability, irritability: Monitor for potential paradoxical response.

C. **Benzodiazepine class effects**:

1. Nausea and constipation, appetite changes, incontinence, urinary retention, menstrual irregularities, changes in libido, dry mouth, asthenia, hallucinations (rare), extrapyramidal symptoms, dystonia, sialorrhea, hypotension

D. **Serious reactions**:

1. Stevens-Johnson syndrome, angioedema, hypersensitivity reaction, anaphylactoid reaction: Monitor for skin changes, particularly during initiation and reintroduction, and titrate slowly.
2. Respiratory depression and CNS depression, dependency, abuse, depression with suicidality, withdrawal with possible seizures if abruptly discontinued: Use the lowest effective dosage for the shortest possible time; taper slowly to discontinue use.
3. Hepatic dysfunction with ALT/AST elevation, renal dysfunction, blood dyscrasias, jaundice: Monitor laboratory values at baseline and periodically.
4. Cardiovascular collapse, venous thrombosis, phlebitis: Use caution with IV/IM administration.

E. **Risks in pregnancy and lactation**: Most benzodiazepines were designated Category D drugs in the prior FDA classification. See Table 3–2 ("Benzodiazepines in pregnancy") in the introduction to this chapter; see also Chapter 15 ("Women: Pregnancy, Postpartum, and Breastfeeding"). For current information on benzodiazepine use in lactation, readers are referred to the Drugs and Lactation Database (LactMed; www.ncbi.nlm.nih.gov/books/NBK501922/).

XIII. Clinical Pearls/Prescribing Tips

A. Diazepam has a rapid onset of action and multiple formulations. It is commonly used for treating muscle spasms, sleep disorders, and alcohol withdrawal.

B. All benzodiazepines should be prescribed with caution, given their CNS depressant effects and addiction potential.

C. Benzodiazepines are generally used as short-term therapy until other medications such as SSRIs can take effect. They may also be used long term at low dosages in selected patients with refractory conditions, or as an adjunct to SSRI/SNRI or mood-stabilizing medication.

D. The longer half-life of diazepam's active metabolites can lead to excessive sedation and impaired motor and cognitive functioning, which can increase over time. Use caution and taper the dosage if accumulation is suspected.
E. Avoid use in elderly individuals; long-term accumulation of active metabolites can lead to insidious onset of falls or confusion.
F. Long-term daily use of benzodiazepines is not recommended.
G. Benzodiazepine class use guidelines:
   1. Use the lowest effective dosage for the shortest possible period of time. Regularly assess the need for continued treatment. Benzodiazepines are not recommended for long-term treatment of anxiety disorders; consider switching to an SSRI or SNRI for long-term maintenance. Consider augmenting with gabapentin or pregabalin for anxiety disorders to reduce benzodiazepine requirements.
   2. When helping patients through the process of gradually tapering and discontinuing benzodiazepines, clinicians must be able to distinguish among reemergence of chronic anxiety disorder symptoms, rebound anxiety symptoms, and acute withdrawal symptoms.
   3. **Caution**: Benzodiazepines can be fatal in overdose and withdrawal. Taper slowly. Protracted withdrawal can occur. Do not combine with other CNS depressants (e.g., other benzodiazepines, opioids). The benzodiazepine receptor antagonist flumazenil can be used in acute overdose but can precipitate seizures.

Further Reading

Dhaliwal JS, Rosani A: Diazepam, in StatPearls. Treasure Island, FL, StatPearls Publishing, 2022

Salpekar JA, Basu T, Thangaraj S, Maguire J: The intersections of stress, anxiety and epilepsy. Int Rev Neurobiol 152:195–219, 2020 32450996

Valium package insert. U.S Food and Drug Administration, 2023. Available at: https://www.accessdata.fda.gov/spl/data/f7e32540-6fc4-a744-e053-6294a90ab11a/f7e32540-6fc4-a744-e053-6294a90ab11a.xml. Accessed March 13, 2024.

Lorazepam

I. **Brand Names**: Ativan, Loreev XR

II. **Therapeutic Class**: Benzodiazepine (intermediate acting), anxiolytic, hypnotic, sedative, antiemetic, anticonvulsant

III. **Mechanism-Based Class**: GABA positive allosteric modulator (GABA PAM)

IV. **Mechanism(s) of Action**

A. Enhances GABA inhibition binding to stereo-specific benzodiazepine receptors on postsynaptic GABA neurons leading to hyperpolarization

V. **Indications**

A. FDA adult:

1. Short-term anxiolytic effects
2. Anxiety-related symptoms in patients with depression
3. Status epilepticus
4. Pre-anesthesia/procedural anxiety

B. Evidence-based[1] off-label uses:

1. Muscle spasm
2. Insomnia
3. Panic disorder
4. Acute mania (adjunctive)
5. Headache
6. Alcohol withdrawal, delirium tremens
7. Psychosis (adjunctive)
8. Catatonia
9. Akathisia

C. FDA pediatric: None

VI. **Major Contraindications and When to Use Caution**

A. **Contraindications**:

1. Known hypersensitivity to medication or class
2. Acute narrow-angle glaucoma/angle-closure glaucoma

B. **Use caution**:

1. Patients with underlying depression, which may increase the risk of suicidality.
2. Substance use history, obstructive sleep apnea, elderly individuals or those with high fall risk, debilitated patients, concurrent use of other CNS depressant medications, concurrent use of opioids, severe respiratory disease, severe liver disease, renal impairment, seizure history, depression, porphyria, delirium, dementia.

C. **Avoid abrupt withdrawal**: Gradually taper to discontinue after long-term use, as abrupt discontinuation or rapid dosage reduction may cause acute withdrawal reactions, including increased risk of seizures, which may be life-threatening.

---

[1]Evidence strength varies; readers are referred to the literature for more detailed information.

VII. **Dosage Formulations**

A. Brand: tablet (0.5 mg, 1 mg, 2 mg); ER capsule (1 mg, 1.5 mg, 2 mg, 3 mg); injection (2 mg/mL, 4 mg/mL)

B. Generic: tablet (0.5 mg, 1 mg, 2 mg); concentrate (2 mg/mL); injection (2 mg/mL, 4 mg/mL)

VIII. **Dosage Ranges and Guidelines**

A. Dosage varies based on indication and tolerance (see Table 3–7 for usual dosage ranges).

B. Use a reduced dosage for elderly individuals and those with fall risk, hepatic or respiratory disease, or concurrent opioid use.

1. For elderly adults, start at 1–2 mg/day (may divide BID–TID).

C. **Titration**: Start at dosages listed in Table 3–7. For anxiety, increase gradually by 1 mg/day based on response and tolerability. In general, the maximum dosage is 6 mg/day.

D. **Tapering**: Taper dosage by 25%–50% every 1–2 weeks based on response, tolerability, and patient factors. Reduce the dosage more slowly as the taper progresses. May require up to 6 months for full taper/discontinuation.

1. Taper by 0.5 mg every 3 days to reduce chances of withdrawal. Inpatient tapers may progress more rapidly because closer monitoring is possible in this setting.

Table 3–7. Lorazepam indications and dosage ranges

Indications	Usual dosage ranges
Anxiety	PO/IM/IV: 1–6 mg/day divided BID–TID ER form: Can switch once stabilized on IR form; give daily in the morning at the equivalent IR daily dosage.
Procedural anxiety	IV: 1–4 mg once every 5–20 minutes prior to procedure; may repeat dose at 50% after 5 or more minutes
Status epilepticus	IV: 4 mg; repeat once after 10–15 minutes
Insomnia (off-label)	PO: 2–4 mg nightly PRN
Alcohol withdrawal (off-label)	PO/IM/IV: 1–4 mg PRN or scheduled; it is often helpful to refer to established institutional protocols
Delirium tremens (off-label)	IV: 1–4 mg every 5–15 minutes PRN; refer to institutional protocols
NMS (off-label)	IM/IV: 1–4 mg every 4–6 hours until symptoms resolve; higher dosages are used for muscle rigidity
Nausea, chemo-related (off-label)	0.5–1 mg every 4–6 hours as needed, or 2.5 mg PO administered twice—the night before, and just after chemo
Catatonia (off-label)	PO/IM/IV: 1–2 mg TID; dosages up to 30 mg/day have been reported
Akathisia (off-label)	0.5–3 mg BID

Note. NMS=neuroleptic malignant syndrome.

IX. Monitoring

A. Monitor baseline and periodic vital signs, complete blood count, creatinine, liver function tests, urinalysis, and physical and psychiatric evaluations.

1. Potential risk of hepatic dysfunction (aspartate transaminase [AST]/alanine aminotransferase [ALT] elevation), renal dysfunction, blood dyscrasias, jaundice
2. Leukopenia and elevated lactate dehydrogenase have been found in patients with long-term use of benzodiazepines.

B. Abuse/dependence/tolerance/withdrawal:

1. Lorazepam is a Schedule IV controlled substance. Routinely assess for use of other narcotics (boxed warning with opioids).
2. Consider periodic urine drug screens to monitor for other narcotic use.
3. Monitor for abuse, dependence, and tolerance.
4. Monitor for withdrawal symptoms; abrupt withdrawal can precipitate seizures and may be fatal.

C. Monitor for behavioral changes, alertness, and mental status (e.g., depression, suicidality).

D. Monitor for skin changes (Stevens-Johnson syndrome [SJS], toxic epidermal necrolysis [TEN]).

X. Relevant Pharmacokinetics/Pharmacodynamics

A. **Metabolism**: Hepatic glucuronidation; no active metabolites

B. **Time to peak plasma concentration**: 2 hours

C. **Half-life**: 12–15 hours (intermediate acting)

D. **Elimination**: 10–20 hours

E. **Effect of food**: Food does not affect absorption.

F. **Hepatic impairment**: Caution advised; decrease dosage to 1–2 mg/day in 2–3 divided doses

G. **Renal impairment**: Avoid use of IM/IV formulation in patients with renal failure; decrease dosage to 1–2 mg/day taken in 2–3 doses.

XI. Clinically Relevant Drug Interactions

A. Lorazepam has no known CYP interactions; remember the mnemonic "OTL": oxazepam, temazepam, and lorazepam are all metabolized "outside the liver."

B. Both lorazepam and valproic acid are substrates of the uridine 5′-diphospho-glucuronosyltransferase (UGT) B27 enzyme, so valproic acid may increase concentrations and reduce the clearance of lorazepam, likely via this interaction of hepatic glucuronidation (Chung et al. 2008).

C. Concomitant use with clozapine can cause excessive sedation, salivation, hypotension, ataxia, delirium, and respiratory arrest.

D. Oral contraceptives may increase clearance and decrease concentrations of lorazepam.

E. Concomitant use with theophylline or amitriptyline may reduce the antiepileptic and sedative effects of lorazepam.

F. Avoid concomitant use with opioids and/or other narcotics.

G. Avoid concomitant use with other CNS depressants. If used, dosage adjustments may be necessary.
H. Other sleep aids, including zolpidem and eszopiclone, should not be used with benzodiazepines.
I. Coadministration of benzodiazepines with antihypertensives or other medications that can lower blood pressure may result in additive hypotensive effects.

XII. **Adverse Effects**

A. **Boxed warnings**: See "Benzodiazepine Class Boxed Warnings" in the "Benzodiazepine Class Warnings and Precautions" section at the beginning of this chapter.

B. **Most common**:

1. Drowsiness, sedation, fatigue, ataxia, slurred speech, weakness, dizziness, syncope, diplopia, confusion, forgetfulness, euphoric mood, anterograde amnesia, impaired concentration, disinhibition, psychomotor impairment: Side effects are dosage dependent. Use the lowest effective dosage and titrate slowly to effect.
2. Nervousness, hyperexcitability, irritability: Monitor for potential paradoxical response.

C. **Benzodiazepine class effects**:

1. Nausea and constipation, appetite changes, incontinence, urinary retention, menstrual irregularities, changes in libido, dry mouth, asthenia, hallucinations (rare), extrapyramidal symptoms, dystonia, sialorrhea, hypotension

D. **Serious reactions**:

1. Stevens-Johnson syndrome, angioedema, hypersensitivity reaction, anaphylactoid reaction: Monitor for skin changes, particularly during initiation and reintroduction, and titrate slowly.
2. Respiratory depression and CNS depression, dependency, abuse/misuse, depression with suicidality, hypoventilation (IM or IV use), withdrawal with possible seizures if abruptly discontinued: Use the lowest effective dosage for the shortest possible time; taper slowly to discontinue use.
3. Hepatic dysfunction with ALT/AST elevation, renal dysfunction, blood dyscrasias, agranulocytosis, leukopenia, pancytopenia, thrombocytopenia, lactate dehydrogenase elevation, jaundice: Monitor laboratory values at baseline and periodically.
4. Rare QTc prolongation with underlying arrhythmia: Consider checking ECG prior to initiation of treatment in at-risk patients.

E. **Risks in pregnancy and lactation**: Most benzodiazepines were designated Category D drugs in the prior FDA classification. See Table 3–2 ("Benzodiazepines in pregnancy") in the introduction to this chapter; see also Chapter 15 ("Women: Pregnancy, Postpartum, and Breastfeeding"). For current information on benzodiazepine use in lactation, readers are referred to the Drugs and Lactation Database (LactMed; www.ncbi.nlm.nih.gov/books/NBK501922/).

XIII. **Clinical Pearls/Prescribing Tips**

A. Lorazepam is one of the most popular benzodiazepines used, particularly in inpatient settings.
B. Use of lorazepam for longer than 4 months has not been assessed in safety trials.
C. Lorazepam may be the preferred benzodiazepine in delirium treatment because of its short half-life and metabolism outside of the liver; however, all benzodiazepines have potential to worsen delirium. Use with caution and consider combining with haloperidol.
D. Lorazepam may be preferred over other benzodiazepines for treatment of alcohol withdrawal, especially in patients with liver disease; it has no active metabolites, a shorter half-life, and less risk of accumulation.
E. Lorazepam is one of the few benzodiazepines available in liquid concentrate and injectable formulations.
F. Lorazepam can be used to treat anxiety associated with acute myocardial infarction.
G. Lorazepam may both cause and treat depression in different patient populations.
H. Lorazepam is possibly more sedating than other benzodiazepines used for anxiety, and thus is particularly useful in acute agitation.
I. Lorazepam is used as an adjunct to antipsychotics for treatment of acute mania and psychosis.
J. Lorazepam is commonly used as an adjunct to SSRIs and SNRIs for treatment of anxiety disorders and panic.
K. Lorazepam is often the benzodiazepine treatment of choice for catatonia, in part because of its flexible dosing formulations (PO, IM, IV).
L. Some severely ill patients may require dosages higher than 10 mg/day.
M. Some compounding pharmacies will make lorazepam cream/suppositories for hospice patients.
N. Benzodiazepine class use guidelines:

1. Use the lowest effective dosage for the shortest possible period of time. Regularly assess the need for continued treatment. Benzodiazepines are not recommended for long-term treatment of anxiety disorders; consider switching to an SSRI or SNRI for long-term maintenance. Consider augmenting with gabapentin or pregabalin for anxiety disorders to reduce benzodiazepine requirements.
2. When helping patients through the process of gradually tapering and discontinuing benzodiazepines, clinicians must be able to distinguish among reemergence of chronic anxiety disorder symptoms, rebound anxiety symptoms, and acute withdrawal symptoms.
3. **Caution**: Benzodiazepines can be fatal in overdose and withdrawal. Taper slowly. Protracted withdrawal can occur. Do not combine with other CNS depressants (e.g., other benzodiazepines, opioids). The benzodiazepine receptor antagonist flumazenil can be used in acute overdose but can precipitate seizures.

Further Reading

Ativan (lorazepam) [package insert]. U.S. Food and Drug Administration website. Revised September 2016. Available at: https://www.accessdata.fda.gov/drugsatfda_docs/label/2016/017794s044lbl.pdf. Accessed May 18, 2022.

Greenblatt DJ: Clinical pharmacokinetics of oxazepam and lorazepam. Clin Pharmacokinet 6(2):89–105, 1981 6111408

Stewart SA: The effects of benzodiazepines on cognition. J Clin Psychiatry 66(Suppl 2):9–13, 2005 15762814

References

Chung JY, Cho JY, Yu KS, et al: Pharmacokinetic and pharmacodynamic interaction of lorazepam and valproic acid in relation to UGT2B7 genetic polymorphism in healthy subjects. Clin Pharmacol Ther 83(4):595–600, 2008 17687269

Oxazepam

I. **Brand Names**: Serax (brand discontinued in U.S.)

II. **Therapeutic Class**: Benzodiazepine (short acting), anxiolytic

III. **Mechanism-Based Class**: GABA positive allosteric modulator (GABA PAM)

IV. **Mechanism(s) of Action**

A. Enhances GABA inhibition binding to stereo-specific benzodiazepine receptors on postsynaptic GABA neurons leading to hyperpolarization

V. **Indications**

A. FDA adult:

1. Anxiety disorders
2. Short-term relief of anxiety symptoms
3. Anxiety associated with depression
4. Anxiety, tension, agitation, and irritability in older patients
5. Alcohol use disorder with acute tremulousness, inebriation
6. Alcohol withdrawal

B. Evidence-based[1] off-label uses:

1. Catatonia
2. Confusional arousals
3. Sleep terrors

C. FDA pediatric: None

[1]Evidence strength varies; readers are referred to the literature for more detailed information.

VI. **Major Contraindications and When to Use Caution**

A. **Contraindications**:

1. Known hypersensitivity to medication or class
2. Acute-closure glaucoma
3. Oxazepam 15 mg tablets contain FD&C Yellow 5 (tartrazine), which may cause allergy-type reactions in some individuals.

B. **Use caution**: Substance use history, obstructive sleep apnea, elderly individuals or those with high fall risk, debilitated patients, concurrent use of other CNS depressant medications, concurrent use of opioids, severe respiratory disease, severe liver disease, renal impairment, seizure history, depression, porphyria, delirium, dementia.

C. **Avoid abrupt withdrawal**: Gradually taper to discontinue after long-term use, as abrupt discontinuation or rapid dosage reduction may cause acute withdrawal reactions, including increased risk of seizures, which may be life-threatening.

VII. **Dosage Formulations**

A. Generic capsule (10 mg, 15 mg, 30 mg)

VIII. **Dosage Ranges and Guidelines**

A. Dosage varies based on indication and tolerance (see Table 3–8 for usual dosage ranges).

B. Use a reduced dosage for elderly individuals and those with fall risk, hepatic or respiratory disease, or concurrent opioid use.

1. For elderly adults, start at 10 mg TID (increase cautiously to 15 mg TID–QID).

C. **Titration**: Start at dosages listed in Table 3–8. Increase in increments of 15–30 mg every 2–3 days to the usual maximum dosage range of 30–120 mg/day.

D. **Tapering**: Taper dosage by 25%–50% every 1–2 weeks based on response, tolerability, and patient factors. Reduce the dosage more slowly as the taper progresses. May require up to 6 months for full taper/discontinuation.

1. Taper by 15 mg every 3 days to reduce chance of withdrawal effects.
2. Some individuals may require a slower taper (e.g., 10 mg/week or 1% reduction every 3 days).

Table 3–8. Oxazepam indications and dosage ranges

Indications	Usual dosage ranges
Anxiety disorders	10–30 mg TID–QID
Mild to moderate anxiety	Mild/moderate anxiety: 15 mg TID–QID Severe anxiety/agitation: 15–30 mg TID–QID
Alcohol withdrawal	15–30 mg every 4–6 hours PRN or scheduled; it may be helpful to refer to established institutional protocols.
Parasomnias (off-label)	10–20 mg at bedtime

IX. Monitoring

A. Monitor baseline and periodic vital signs, complete blood count, creatinine, liver function tests, urinalysis, and physical and psychiatric evaluations.

1. Potential risk of hepatic dysfunction (aspartate transaminase [AST]/alanine aminotransferase [ALT] elevation), renal dysfunction, blood dyscrasias, jaundice
2. Leukopenia and elevated lactate dehydrogenase have been found in patients with long-term use of benzodiazepines.

B. Abuse/dependence/tolerance/withdrawal:

1. Oxazepam is a Schedule IV controlled substance. Routinely assess for use of other narcotics (boxed warning with opioids).
2. Consider periodic urine drug screens to monitor for other narcotic use.
3. Monitor for abuse, dependence, and tolerance.
4. Monitor for withdrawal symptoms; abrupt withdrawal can precipitate seizures and may be fatal.

C. Monitor for behavioral changes, alertness, and mental status (e.g., depression, suicidality).

D. Monitor for skin changes (Stevens-Johnson syndrome [SJS], toxic epidermal necrolysis [TEN]).

X. Relevant Pharmacokinetics/Pharmacodynamics

A. **Metabolism**: Hepatic glucuronidation, no active metabolites
B. **Time to peak plasma concentration**: 3 hours
C. **Half-life**: 8.2 hours (elimination 3–21 hours), short acting
D. **Hepatic impairment**: Not defined
E. **Renal impairment**: None

XI. Clinically Relevant Drug Interactions

A. Oxazepam has no known CYP interactions; remember the mnemonic "OTL": oxazepam, temazepam, and lorazepam are all metabolized "outside the liver."
B. Avoid concomitant use with opioids and other narcotics.
C. Avoid concomitant use with other CNS depressants. If used, dosage adjustments may be necessary.
D. Other sleep aids, including zolpidem and eszopiclone, should not be used with benzodiazepines.
E. Coadministration of benzodiazepines with antihypertensives or other medications that can lower blood pressure may result in additive hypotensive effects.

XII. Adverse Effects

A. **Boxed warnings**: See "Benzodiazepine Class Boxed Warnings" in the "Benzodiazepine Class Warnings and Precautions" section at the beginning of this chapter.

B. **Most common**:

1. Drowsiness, sedation, fatigue, ataxia, slurred speech, weakness, dizziness, syncope, diplopia, confusion, forgetfulness, euphoric mood, anterograde amnesia, impaired concentration, disinhibition, psychomotor impairment: Side effects are dosage dependent. Use the lowest effective dosage and titrate slowly to effect.

2. Nervousness, hyperexcitability, irritability: Monitor for potential paradoxical response.

C. **Benzodiazepine class effects**:

1. Nausea and constipation, appetite changes, incontinence, urinary retention, menstrual irregularities, changes in libido, dry mouth, asthenia, hallucinations (rare), extrapyramidal symptoms, dystonia, sialorrhea, hypotension

D. **Serious reactions**:

1. Stevens-Johnson syndrome, angioedema, hypersensitivity reaction, anaphylactoid reaction: Monitor for skin changes, particularly during initiation and reintroduction, and titrate slowly.
2. Respiratory depression and CNS depression, dependency, abuse, depression with suicidality, withdrawal with possible seizures if abruptly discontinued: Use lowest effective dosage for the shortest possible time; taper slowly to discontinuation.
3. Hepatic dysfunction with ALT/ AST elevation, renal dysfunction, blood dyscrasias, jaundice: Monitor laboratory values at baseline and periodically.

E. **Risks in pregnancy and lactation**: Most benzodiazepines were designated Category D drugs in the prior FDA classification. See Table 3–2 ("Benzodiazepines in pregnancy") in the introduction to this chapter; see also Chapter 15 ("Women: Pregnancy, Postpartum, and Breastfeeding"). For current information on benzodiazepine use in lactation, readers are referred to the Drugs and Lactation Database (LactMed; www.ncbi.nlm.nih.gov/books/NBK501922/).

XIII. **Clinical Pearls/Prescribing Tips**

A. Oxazepam has a rapid onset of action. Feelings of euphoria may lead to abuse, especially in patients with past or present substance use disorders.
B. Because of its short half-life and lack of active metabolites, oxazepam has a low risk of accumulation and may be preferred over other benzodiazepines for treatment of patients with liver disease.
C. Oxazepam may be preferred over other benzodiazepines in treatment of delirium.
D. Oxazepam's effectiveness has not been assessed for periods greater than 4 months. Prescribers should periodically reassess the usefulness of the drug.
E. Oxazepam can both cause and treat depression in different patients.
F. Benzodiazepine class use guidelines:

1. Use the lowest effective dosage for the shortest possible period of time. Regularly assess the need for continued treatment. Benzodiazepines are not recommended for long-term treatment of anxiety disorders; consider switching to an SSRI or SNRI for long-term maintenance. Consider augmenting with gabapentin or pregabalin for anxiety disorders to reduce benzodiazepine requirements.
2. When helping patients through the process of gradually tapering and discontinuing benzodiazepines, clinicians must be able to distinguish among reemergence of chronic anxiety disorder symptoms, rebound anxiety symptoms, and acute withdrawal symptoms.

3. **Caution** Benzodiazepines can be fatal in overdose and withdrawal. Taper slowly. Protracted withdrawal can occur. Do not combine with other CNS depressants (e.g., other benzodiazepines, opioids). The benzodiazepine receptor antagonist flumazenil can be used in acute overdose but can precipitate seizures.

Further Reading

Ansseau M, Papart P, Gérard MA, et al: Controlled comparison of buspirone and oxazepam in generalized anxiety. Neuropsychobiology 24(2):74–78, 1990–1991 2134114

Greenblatt DJ: Clinical pharmacokinetics of oxazepam and lorazepam. Clin Pharmacokinet 6(2):89–105, 1981 6111408

Griffin CE III, Kaye AM, Bueno FR, et al: Benzodiazepine pharmacology and central nervous system-mediated effects. Ochsner J 13(2):214–223, 2013 23789008

LiverTox: Oxazepam [updated June 22, 2023], in Clinical and Research Information on Drug-Induced Liver Injury [Internet]. Bethesda, MD, National Institute of Diabetes and Digestive and Kidney Diseases, 2012–. Available at: https://www.ncbi.nlm.nih.gov/books/NBK548104/. Accessed March 13, 2024.

Serax (oxazepam) [package insert]. U.S. Food and Drug Administration website. Revised June 2000. Available at: https://www.accessdata.fda.gov/drugsatfda_docs/label/2001/15539s52lbl.pdf. Accessed May 18, 2022.

Hypnotic Benzodiazepines

Estazolam

I. **Brand Names**: ProSom (discontinued in U.S.)
II. **Therapeutic Class**: Benzodiazepine (intermediate acting), hypnotic
III. **Mechanism-Based Class**: GABA positive allosteric modulator (GABA PAM)
IV. **Mechanism(s) of Action**

A. Enhances GABA inhibition binding to stereo-specific benzodiazepine receptors on postsynaptic GABA neurons leading to hyperpolarization.
B. Positive allosteric modulator of $GABA_A$ receptor, benzodiazepine site, causing increased permeability of neuronal membrane to chloride ions, results in hyperpolarization and depressed activity

V. **Indications**

A. FDA adult:

1. Insomnia, onset or maintenance

B. Evidence-based[1] off-label uses:

1. Catatonia
2. Can reduce comorbid anxiety when used to treat insomnia

C. FDA pediatric: None

VI. **Major Contraindications and When to Use Caution**

A. **Contraindications**:

1. Known hypersensitivity to medication or class
2. Angle-closure glaucoma
3. Use of itraconazole or ketoconazole (may increase serum concentration)

B. **Use caution**: Substance use history, obstructive sleep apnea, elderly individuals or those with high fall risk, debilitated patients, concurrent use of other CNS depressant medications, concurrent use of opioids, severe respiratory disease, severe liver disease, renal impairment, seizure history, depression, porphyria, delirium, dementia
C. **Avoid abrupt withdrawal**: Gradually taper to discontinue after long-term use, as abrupt discontinuation or rapid dosage reduction may cause acute withdrawal reactions, including increased risk of seizures, which may be life-threatening.

VII. **Dosage Formulations**

A. Generic tablet (1 mg, 2 mg [*both scored*])

---

[1]Evidence strength varies; readers are referred to the literature for more detailed information.

VIII. **Dosage Ranges and Guidelines**

A. Dosage varies greatly based on indication and tolerance. Usual dosage range is 1–2 mg at bedtime.
B. Use a reduced dosage for elderly individuals and those with fall risk, hepatic or respiratory disease, or concurrent opioid use.
C. Dosage may need to be adjusted if patient's smoking habits change.
D. **Titration**: Start at 1 mg and increase to 2 mg as needed based on response and tolerability.
E. **Tapering**: Taper dosage by 0.5 mg every 1–2 weeks. Some individuals may require a slower taper.

IX. **Monitoring**

A. Monitor baseline and periodic vital signs, complete blood count, creatinine, liver function tests, urinalysis, and physical and psychiatric evaluations.
   1. Potential risk of hepatic dysfunction (aspartate transaminase [AST]/alanine aminotransferase [ALT] elevation), renal dysfunction, blood dyscrasias, jaundice
   2. Leukopenia and elevated lactate dehydrogenase have been found in patients with long-term use of benzodiazepines.

B. Abuse/dependence/tolerance/withdrawal:
   1. Estazolam is a Schedule IV controlled substance. Routinely assess for use of other narcotics (boxed warning with opioids).
   2. Consider periodic urine drug screens to monitor for other narcotic use.
   3. Monitor for abuse, dependence, and tolerance.
   4. Monitor for withdrawal symptoms; abrupt withdrawal can precipitate seizures and may be fatal.

C. Monitor for behavioral changes, alertness, and mental status (e.g., depression, suicidality).
D. Monitor for skin changes (Stevens-Johnson syndrome [SJS], toxic epidermal necrolysis [TEN]).

X. **Relevant Pharmacokinetics/Pharmacodynamics**

A. **Metabolism**: Extensive hepatic metabolism into inactive metabolites, minor cytochrome P450 (CYP) 3A4 substrate
B. **Time to peak plasma concentration**: 0.5–6 hours
C. **Half-life**: 10–24 hours (intermediate acting)
D. **Hepatic impairment**: Caution advised.
E. **Renal impairment**: No adjustment needed. Accumulation of active metabolites can occur, so use with caution.

XI. **Clinically Relevant Drug Interactions**

A. Metabolized by CYP3A4
   1. Concurrent use of strong CYP3A4 inhibitors or inducers may change estazolam's serum concentration. Monitor therapy and consider adjustment as needed.
      a. Potent CYP3A4 inhibitors may decrease estazolam's clearance and increase its serum concentrations and effects. CYP3A4 inhibitors include nefazo-

done, fluvoxamine, fluoxetine, ketoconazole, itraconazole, isoniazid, and the HIV protease inhibitors ritonavir, indinavir, nelfinavir, saquinavir, and lopinavir, as well as grapefruit juice.

b. CYP3A4 inducers (e.g., carbamazepine, oxcarbazepine) and smoking may increase estazolam's clearance, resulting in decreased concentration and effect.

B. Avoid concomitant use with opioids and other narcotics.

C. Avoid concomitant use with other CNS depressants. If used, dosage adjustments may be necessary.

D. Other sleep aids, including zolpidem and eszopiclone, should not be used with benzodiazepines.

E. Coadministration of benzodiazepines with antihypertensives or other medications that can lower blood pressure may result in additive hypotensive effects.

XII. **Adverse Effects**

A. **Boxed warnings**: See "Benzodiazepine Class Boxed Warnings" in the "Benzodiazepine Class Warnings and Precautions" section at the beginning of this chapter.

B. **Most common**:

1. Drowsiness, sedation, fatigue, ataxia, slurred speech, weakness, dizziness, syncope, diplopia, confusion, forgetfulness, euphoric mood, anterograde amnesia, impaired concentration, disinhibition, psychomotor impairment: Side effects are dosage dependent. Use the lowest effective dosage and titrate slowly to effect.
2. Nervousness, hyperexcitability, irritability: Monitor for potential paradoxical response.

C. **Benzodiazepine class effects**:

1. Nausea and constipation, appetite changes, incontinence, urinary retention, menstrual irregularities, changes in libido, dry mouth, asthenia, hallucinations (rare), extrapyramidal symptoms, dystonia, sialorrhea, hypotension

D. **Serious reactions**:

1. Stevens-Johnson syndrome, angioedema, hypersensitivity reaction, anaphylactoid reaction: Monitor for skin changes, particularly during initiation and reintroduction, and titrate slowly.
2. Respiratory depression and CNS depression, dependency, abuse, depression with suicidality, withdrawal with possible seizures if abruptly discontinued: Use the lowest effective dosage for the shortest possible time; taper slowly to discontinue use.
3. Hepatic dysfunction with ALT/ AST elevation, renal dysfunction, blood dyscrasias, jaundice: Monitor laboratory values at baseline and periodically.

E. **Risks in pregnancy and lactation**: Most benzodiazepines were designated Category D drugs in the prior FDA classification. See Table 3–2 ("Benzodiazepines in pregnancy") in the introduction to this chapter; see also Chapter 15 ("Women: Pregnancy, Postpartum, and Breastfeeding"). For current information on benzodiazepine use in lactation, readers are referred to the Drugs and Lactation Database (LactMed; www.ncbi.nlm.nih.gov/books/NBK501922/).

XIII. **Clinical Pearls/Prescribing Tips**

A. Estazolam is generally prescribed for transient insomnia, for short-term use.

B. Estazolam has a narrow therapeutic index.

C. Estazolam can cause complex sleep behaviors, such as driving, cooking, making phone calls, or having sex while asleep. Individuals generally do not retain memories of these complex behaviors.

D. Recommend that patients lie down to sleep immediately after taking sleep medication.

E. Rebound insomnia may occur after stopping any sleep medication, including estazolam.

F. Smokers may require higher dosages (increased clearance leads to decreased levels).

G. Tolerance may develop; drug holidays can be used to restore effectiveness.

H. Benzodiazepine class use guidelines:

1. Use the lowest effective dosage for the shortest possible period of time. Regularly assess the need for continued treatment. Benzodiazepines are not recommended for long-term treatment of anxiety disorders; consider switching to an SSRI or SNRI for long-term maintenance. Consider augmenting with gabapentin or pregabalin for anxiety disorders to reduce benzodiazepine requirements.
2. When helping patients through the process of gradually tapering and discontinuing benzodiazepines, clinicians must be able to distinguish among reemergence of chronic anxiety disorder symptoms, rebound anxiety symptoms, and acute withdrawal symptoms.
3. **Caution**: Benzodiazepines can be fatal in overdose and withdrawal. Taper slowly. Protracted withdrawal can occur. Do not combine with other CNS depressants (e.g., other benzodiazepines, opioids). The benzodiazepine receptor antagonist flumazenil can be used in acute overdose but can precipitate seizures.

Further Reading

Estazolam package insert. U.S Food and Drug Administration, 2022. Available at: https://www.accessdata.fda.gov/spl/data/2a612458-8b9a-4125-a783-44327a8166d9/2a612458-8b9a-4125-a783-44327a8166d9.xml. Access March 13, 2024.

Rosenberg RP: Sleep maintenance insomnia: strengths and weaknesses of current pharmacologic therapies. Ann Clin Psychiatry 18(1):49–56, 200616517453

Stahl SM: Prescriber's Guide: Stahl's Essential Psychopharmacology, 7th Edition. Cambridge, UK, Cambridge University Press, 2020

Flurazepam

I. **Brand Names**: Dalmane (discontinued in U.S.)
II. **Therapeutic Class**: Benzodiazepine (long acting), hypnotic
III. **Mechanism-Based Class**: GABA positive allosteric modulator (GABA PAM)
IV. **Mechanism(s) of Action**

A. Enhances GABA inhibition binding to stereo-specific benzodiazepine receptors on postsynaptic GABA neurons leading to hyperpolarization

V. **Indications**

A. FDA adult:

1. Insomnia
2. Difficulty initiating sleep, frequent nighttime awakening, and/or early-morning awakening

B. Evidence-based[1] off-label uses:

1. Catatonia
2. Can reduce comorbid anxiety when used to treat insomnia

C. FDA pediatric: None

VI. **Major Contraindications and When to Use Caution**

A. **Contraindications**:

1. Known hypersensitivity to medication or class
2. Not indicated for patients younger than 15 years.

B. **Use caution**: Substance use history, obstructive sleep apnea, elderly individuals or those with high fall risk, debilitated patients, concurrent use of other CNS depressant medications, concurrent use of opioids, severe respiratory disease, severe liver disease, renal impairment, seizure history, depression, porphyria, delirium, dementia
C. **Avoid abrupt withdrawal**: Gradually taper to discontinue after long-term use, as abrupt discontinuation or rapid dosage reduction may cause acute withdrawal reactions, including increased risk of seizures, which may be life-threatening.

VII. **Dosage Formulations**

A. Generic capsule (15 mg, 30 mg)

VIII. **Dosage Ranges and Guidelines**

A. Dosage varies greatly based on indication and tolerance. Usual dosage range is 15–30 mg nightly.
B. Limit dosage to 15 mg/day in older adults due to the effects of sedation, dizziness, and confusion.
C. Use a reduced dosage for older individuals and those with fall risk, hepatic or respiratory disease, or concurrent opioid use.

---

[1]Evidence strength varies; readers are referred to the literature for more detailed information.

D. **Titration**: Start at 15 mg nightly and increase to 30 mg nightly as tolerated.
E. **Tapering**: Taper dosage by 25%–50% every 1–2 weeks based on response, tolerability, and patient factors. Reduce the dosage more slowly as the taper progresses. May require up to 6 months for full taper/discontinuation.

IX. **Monitoring**

A. Monitor baseline and periodic vital signs, complete blood count, creatinine, liver function tests, urinalysis, and physical and psychiatric evaluations.
   1. Potential risk of hepatic dysfunction (aspartate transaminase [AST]/alanine aminotransferase [ALT] elevation), renal dysfunction, blood dyscrasias, jaundice
   2. Leukopenia and elevated lactate dehydrogenase have been found in patients with long-term use of benzodiazepines.

B. Abuse/dependence/tolerance/withdrawal:
   1. Flurazepam is a Schedule IV controlled substance. Routinely assess for use of other narcotics (boxed warning with opioids).
   2. Consider periodic urine drug screens to monitor for other narcotic use.
   3. Monitor for abuse, dependence, and tolerance.
   4. Monitor for withdrawal symptoms; abrupt withdrawal can precipitate seizures and may be fatal.

C. Monitor for behavioral changes, alertness, and mental status (e.g., depression, suicidality).
D. Monitor for skin changes (Stevens-Johnson syndrome [SJS], toxic epidermal necrolysis [TEN]).

X. **Relevant Pharmacokinetics/Pharmacodynamics**

A. **Metabolism**: Hepatic cytochrome P450 (CYP) 3A4 partial substrate
B. **Time to peak plasma concentration**: 30–60 minutes
C. **Half-life**: 2–3 hours
   1. Active metabolites: 40–100 hours (long acting)

D. **Hepatic impairment**: Caution advised.
E. **Renal impairment**: No adjustment needed. Accumulation of active metabolites can occur, so use with caution.

XI. **Clinically Relevant Drug Interactions**

A. Partially metabolized by CYP3A4
   1. Concurrent use of strong CYP3A4 inhibitors or inducers may change flurazepam's serum concentrations; monitor therapy and consider adjustment as needed.
      a. Potent CYP3A4 inhibitors may decrease flurazepam's clearance and increase its serum concentrations and effects. CYP3A4 inhibitors include nefazodone, fluvoxamine, fluoxetine, ketoconazole, itraconazole, isoniazid, and the HIV protease inhibitors ritonavir, indinavir, nelfinavir, saquinavir, and lopinavir, as well as grapefruit juice.
      b. CYP3A4 inducers (e.g., carbamazepine, oxcarbazepine) and smoking may increase flurazepam's clearance, resulting in decreased concentration and effect.

B. Avoid concomitant use with opioids and other narcotics.
C. Avoid concomitant use with other CNS depressants. If used, dosage adjustments may be necessary.
D. Other sleep aids, including zolpidem and eszopiclone, should not be used with benzodiazepines
E. Coadministration of benzodiazepines with antihypertensives or other medications that can lower blood pressure may result in additive hypotensive effects.

XII. **Adverse Effects**

A. **Boxed warnings**: See "Benzodiazepine Class Boxed Warnings" in the "Benzodiazepine Class Warnings and Precautions" section at the beginning of this chapter.

B. **Most common**:

1. Drowsiness, sedation, fatigue, ataxia, slurred speech, weakness, dizziness, syncope, diplopia, confusion, forgetfulness, euphoric mood, anterograde amnesia, impaired concentration, disinhibition, psychomotor impairment: Use the lowest effective dosage and titrate slowly to effect.
2. Nervousness, hyperexcitability, irritability: Monitor for potential paradoxical response.

C. **Benzodiazepine class effects**:

1. Nausea and constipation, appetite changes, incontinence, urinary retention, menstrual irregularities, changes in libido, dry mouth, asthenia, hallucinations (rare), extrapyramidal symptoms, dystonia, sialorrhea, hypotension

D. **Serious reactions**:

1. Stevens-Johnson syndrome, angioedema, hypersensitivity reaction, anaphylactoid reaction: Monitor for skin changes, particularly during initiation and reintroduction, and titrate slowly.
2. Respiratory depression and CNS depression, dependency, abuse, depression with suicidality, withdrawal with possible seizures if abruptly discontinued: Use the lowest effective dosage for the shortest possible time; taper slowly to discontinue use.
3. Hepatic dysfunction with ALT/AST elevation, renal dysfunction, blood dyscrasias, jaundice: Monitor laboratory values at baseline and periodically.

E. **Risks in pregnancy and lactation**: Most benzodiazepines were designated Category D drugs in the prior FDA classification. See Table 3–2 ("Benzodiazepines in pregnancy") in the introduction to this chapter; see also Chapter 15 ("Women: Pregnancy, Postpartum, and Breastfeeding"). For current information on benzodiazepine use in lactation, readers are referred to the Drugs and Lactation Database (LactMed; www.ncbi.nlm.nih.gov/books/NBK501922/).

XIII. **Clinical Pearls/Prescribing Tips**

A. Sleep laboratory studies have objectively determined that flurazepam is effective for at least 28 consecutive nights of drug administration.
B. Flurazepam can cause complex sleep behaviors, such as driving, cooking, making phone calls, or having sex while asleep. Individuals generally do not retain memories of these complex behaviors.

C. Recommend that patients lie down to sleep immediately after taking sleep medication.
D. Flurazepam's longer half-life can lead to daytime sedation and impaired motor and cognitive functioning, which can increase over time (hangover effect). Use caution and taper dosage if accumulation is suspected.
E. Flurazepam's active metabolites may accumulate with long-term use, especially in elderly individuals. Limit use in this population because of fall risk/confusion.
F. Rebound insomnia and a discontinuation syndrome may occur after stopping any sleep medication; however, these effects may be less likely with flurazepam because of its longer half-life.
G. Benzodiazepine class use guidelines:
   1. Use the lowest effective dosage for the shortest possible period of time. Regularly assess the need for continued treatment. Benzodiazepines are not recommended for long-term treatment of anxiety disorders; consider switching to an SSRI or SNRI for long-term maintenance. Consider augmenting with gabapentin or pregabalin for anxiety disorders to reduce benzodiazepine requirements.
   2. When helping patients through the process of gradually tapering and discontinuing benzodiazepines, clinicians must be able to distinguish among reemergence of chronic anxiety disorder symptoms, rebound anxiety symptoms, and acute withdrawal symptoms.
   3. **Caution**: Benzodiazepines can be fatal in overdose and withdrawal. Taper slowly. Protracted withdrawal can occur. Do not combine with other CNS depressants (e.g., other benzodiazepines, opioids). The benzodiazepine receptor antagonist flumazenil can be used in acute overdose but can precipitate seizures.

Further Reading

Dalmane (flurazepam) [package insert]. U.S. Food and Drug Administration website. Revised April 2007. Available at: https://www.accessdata.fda.gov/drugsatfda_docs/label/2007/016721s076lbl.pdf. Accessed May 18, 2022.

Mahon WA, Inaba T, Stone RM: Metabolism of flurazepam by the small intestine. Clin Pharmacol Ther 22(2):228–233, 197718313

Quazepam

I. **Brand Names**: Doral

II. **Therapeutic Class**: Benzodiazepine (long acting), hypnotic

III. **Mechanism-Based Class**: GABA positive allosteric modulator (GABA PAM)

IV. **Mechanism(s) of Action**

A. Enhances GABA inhibition binding to stereo-specific benzodiazepine receptors on postsynaptic GABA neurons, leading to hyperpolarization

V. **Indications**

A. FDA adult:

1. Insomnia

B. Evidence-based[1] off-label uses:

1. Catatonia
2. Can reduce comorbid anxiety when used to treat insomnia

C. FDA pediatric: None

VI. **Major Contraindications and When to Use Caution**

A. **Contraindications**:

1. Known hypersensitivity to medication or class
2. Suspected/confirmed sleep apnea or pulmonary insufficiency
3. Angle-closure glaucoma

B. **Use caution**:

1. Substance use history, obstructive sleep apnea, elderly individuals or those with high fall risk, debilitated patients, concurrent use of other CNS depressant medications, concurrent use of opioids, severe respiratory disease, severe liver disease, renal impairment, seizure history, depression, porphyria, delirium, dementia.
2. Caution during daytime use due to sedative effects.

C. **Avoid abrupt withdrawal**: Gradually taper to discontinue after long-term use, as abrupt discontinuation or rapid dosage reduction may cause acute withdrawal reactions, including increased risk of seizures, which may be life-threatening.

VII. **Dosage Formulations**

A. Brand/generic tablet (15 mg [*scored*])

VIII. **Dosage Ranges and Guidelines**

A. Dosage varies greatly based on indication and tolerance. Usual dosage range is 7.5–15 mg at bedtime.

B. Use a reduced dosage for elderly individuals and those with fall risk, hepatic or respiratory disease, or concurrent opioid use.

---

[1]Evidence strength varies; readers are referred to the literature for more detailed information.

C. **Titration**: Start at 15 mg at bedtime. Can increase slowly to a maximum of 30 mg/day at bedtime.

D. **Tapering**: Taper by 7.5 mg every 1–2 weeks. Some individuals may require a slower taper.

IX. **Monitoring**

A. Monitor baseline and periodic vital signs, complete blood count, creatinine, liver function tests, urinalysis, and physical and psychiatric evaluations.

1. Potential risk of hepatic dysfunction (aspartate transaminase [AST]/alanine aminotransferase [ALT] elevation), renal dysfunction, blood dyscrasias, jaundice
2. Leukopenia and elevated lactate dehydrogenase have been found in patients with long-term use of benzodiazepines.

B. Abuse/dependence/tolerance/withdrawal:

1. Quazepam is a Schedule IV controlled substance. Routinely assess for use of other narcotics (boxed warning with opioids).
2. Consider periodic urine drug screens to monitor for other narcotic use.
3. Monitor for abuse, dependence, and tolerance.
4. Monitor for withdrawal symptoms—Abrupt withdrawal can precipitate seizures and may be fatal.

C. Monitor for behavioral changes, alertness, and mental status (e.g., depression, suicidality).

D. Monitor for skin changes (Stevens-Johnson syndrome [SJS], toxic epidermal necrolysis [TEN]).

X. **Relevant Pharmacokinetics/Pharmacodynamics**

A. **Metabolism**: Hepatic liver extensively; partial cytochrome P450 (CYP) 3A4

B. **Time to peak plasma concentration**: 2 hours

C. **Half-life**: 25–41 hours (long acting)

1. Active metabolites: 73 hours
2. Excretion: urine 31% (trace unchanged); feces 23%

D. **Hepatic impairment**: Decrease starting dosage to 7.5 mg. Caution advised; accumulation of active metabolites can occur.

E. **Renal impairment**: Decrease starting dosage to 7.5 mg. Caution advised; accumulation of active metabolites can occur.

XI. **Clinically Relevant Drug Interactions**

A. Metabolized by CYP3A4, CYP2C9, and CYP2C19

1. Concurrent use of strong CYP3A4 inhibitors or inducers may change quazepam's serum concentrations; monitor therapy and consider adjustment as needed.

   a. Potent CYP3A4 inhibitors may decrease quazepam's clearance and increase its serum concentrations and effects. CYP3A4 inhibitors include nefazodone, fluvoxamine, fluoxetine, ketoconazole, itraconazole, isoniazid, and the HIV protease inhibitors ritonavir, indinavir, nelfinavir, saquinavir, and lopinavir, as well as grapefruit juice.

b. CYP3A4 inducers (e.g., carbamazepine, oxcarbazepine) and smoking may increase quazepam's clearance, resulting in decreased concentration and effect.

B. Avoid concomitant use with opioids and other narcotics.
C. Avoid concomitant use with other CNS depressants. If used, dosage adjustments may be necessary.
D. Other sleep aids, including zolpidem and eszopiclone, should not be used with benzodiazepines
E. Coadministration of benzodiazepines with antihypertensives or other medications that can lower blood pressure may result in additive hypotensive effects.

XII. **Adverse Effects**

A. **Boxed warnings**: See "Benzodiazepine Class Boxed Warnings" in the "Benzodiazepine Class Warnings and Precautions" section at the beginning of this chapter.
B. **Most common**:

1. Drowsiness, sedation, fatigue, ataxia, slurred speech, weakness, dizziness, syncope, diplopia, confusion, forgetfulness, euphoric mood, anterograde amnesia, impaired concentration, disinhibition, psychomotor impairment: Side effects are dosage dependent. Use the lowest effective dosage and titrate slowly to effect.
2. Nervousness, hyperexcitability, irritability: Monitor for potential paradoxical response.
3. Complex sleep behaviors: Use the lowest effective dosage, limit to short-term use, take right before sleep, and lie down right after taking medication.

C. **Benzodiazepine class effects**:

1. Nausea and constipation, appetite changes, incontinence, urinary retention, menstrual irregularities, changes in libido, dry mouth, asthenia, hallucinations (rare), extrapyramidal symptoms, dystonia, sialorrhea, hypotension

D. **Serious reactions**:

1. Stevens-Johnson syndrome, angioedema, hypersensitivity reaction, anaphylactoid reaction: Monitor for skin changes, particularly during initiation and reintroduction, and titrate slowly.
2. Respiratory depression and CNS depression, dependency, abuse, depression with suicidality, withdrawal with possible seizures if abruptly discontinued: Use the lowest effective dosage for the shortest possible time; taper slowly to discontinue use.
3. Hepatic dysfunction with ALT/AST elevation, renal dysfunction, blood dyscrasias, jaundice: Monitor laboratory values at baseline and periodically.

E. **Risks in pregnancy and lactation**: Most benzodiazepines were designated Category D drugs in the prior FDA classification. See Table 3–2 ("Benzodiazepines in pregnancy") in the introduction to this chapter; see also Chapter 15 ("Women: Pregnancy, Postpartum, and Breastfeeding"). For current information on benzodiazepine use in lactation, readers are referred to the Drugs and Lactation Database (LactMed; www.ncbi.nlm.nih.gov/books/NBK501922/).

XIII. **Clinical Pearls/Prescribing Tips**

A. Quazepam is used primarily for insomnia. It is not recommended for use longer than 4 weeks.

B. Quazepam can cause complex sleep behaviors, such as driving, cooking, making phone calls, or having sex while asleep. Individuals generally do not retain memories of these complex behaviors.

C. Recommend that patients lie down to sleep right after taking sleep medication.

D. Quazepam is not recommended for long-term daily use because of the risk of metabolite accumulation.

E. Quazepam's longer half-life can lead to daytime sedation and impaired motor and cognitive functioning, which can increase over time (hangover effect). Use caution and taper dosage if accumulation is suspected.

F. Rebound insomnia may occur after stopping any sleep medication; however, this effect may be less severe with quazepam because of its longer half-life.

G. Avoid use in elderly individuals; long-term accumulation of active metabolites can lead to insidious onset of falls or confusion.

H. Benzodiazepine class use guidelines:

1. Use the lowest effective dosage for the shortest possible period of time. Regularly assess the need for continued treatment. Benzodiazepines are not recommended for long-term treatment of anxiety disorders; consider switching to an SSRI or SNRI for long-term maintenance. Consider augmenting with gabapentin or pregabalin for anxiety disorders to reduce benzodiazepine requirements.
2. When helping patients through the process of gradually tapering and discontinuing benzodiazepines, clinicians must be able to distinguish among reemergence of chronic anxiety disorder symptoms, rebound anxiety symptoms, and acute withdrawal symptoms.
3. **Caution**: Benzodiazepines can be fatal in overdose and withdrawal. Taper slowly. Protracted withdrawal can occur. Do not combine with other CNS depressants (e.g., other benzodiazepines, opioids). The benzodiazepine receptor antagonist flumazenil can be used in acute overdose but can precipitate seizures.

Further Reading

Ankier SI, Goa KL: Quazepam: a preliminary review of its pharmacodynamic and pharmacokinetic properties, and therapeutic efficacy in insomnia. Drugs 35(1):42–62, 1988 2894293

Doral (quazepam) [package insert]. U.S. Food and Drug Administration website. Revised October 2016. Available at: https://www.accessdata.fda.gov/drugsatfda_docs/label/2016/018708s023lbl.pdf. Accessed May 14, 2022.

Kales A, Bixler EO, Vela-Bueno A, et al: Comparison of short and long half-life benzodiazepine hypnotics: triazolam and quazepam. Clin Pharmacol Ther 40(4):378–386, 1986 3530586

Temazepam

I. **Brand Names**: Restoril
II. **Therapeutic Class**: Benzodiazepine (intermediate acting), hypnotic
III. **Mechanism-Based Class**: GABA positive allosteric modulator (GABA PAM)
IV. **Mechanism(s) of Action**

A. Enhances GABA inhibition binding to stereo-specific benzodiazepine receptors on postsynaptic GABA neurons, leading to hyperpolarization

V. **Indications**

A. FDA adult:

1. Short-term treatment of insomnia
2. For use in both early insomnia (difficulty falling asleep) and middle insomnia (nocturnal awakening)

B. Evidence-based[1] off-label uses:

1. Sleep terrors
2. Confusional arousals
3. Catatonia
4. Can reduce comorbid anxiety when used to treat insomnia

C. FDA pediatric: None

VI. **Major Contraindications and When to Use Caution**

A. **Contraindications**:

1. Known hypersensitivity to medication or class
2. Angle-closure glaucoma

B. **Use caution**: Substance use history, obstructive sleep apnea, elderly individuals or those with high fall risk, debilitated patients, concurrent use of other CNS depressant medications, concurrent use of opioids, severe respiratory disease, severe liver disease, renal impairment, seizure history, depression, porphyria, delirium, dementia.

C. **Avoid abrupt withdrawal**: Gradually taper to discontinue after long-term use, as abrupt discontinuation or rapid dosage reduction may cause acute withdrawal reactions, including increased risk of seizures, which may be life-threatening.

VII. **Dosage Formulations**

A. Brand/generic capsule (7.5 mg, 15 mg, 22.5 mg, 30 mg)

VIII. **Dosage Ranges and Guidelines**

A. Dosage varies greatly based on indication and tolerance. Usual dosage range is 7.5–30 mg nightly.

B. Use a reduced dosage for elderly individuals and those with fall risk, hepatic or respiratory disease, or concurrent opioid use.

---

[1]Evidence strength varies; readers are referred to the literature for more detailed information.

C. **Titration**: Start at 7.5 mg nightly. Increase slowly to a typical dosage of 15 mg at bedtime or a maximum of 30 mg at bedtime.

D. **Tapering**: Taper dosage by 7.5 mg every 1–2 weeks. Some individuals may require a slower taper.

IX. **Monitoring**

A. Monitor baseline and periodic vital signs, complete blood count, creatinine, liver function tests, urinalysis, and physical and psychiatric evaluations.

1. Potential risk of hepatic dysfunction (aspartate transaminase [AST]/alanine aminotransferase [ALT] elevation), renal dysfunction, blood dyscrasias, jaundice
2. Leukopenia and elevated lactate dehydrogenase have been found in patients with long-term use of benzodiazepines.

B. Abuse/dependence/tolerance/withdrawal:

1. Temazepam is a Schedule IV controlled substance. Routinely assess for use of other narcotics (boxed warning with opioids).
2. Consider periodic urine drug screens to monitor for other narcotic use.
3. Monitor for abuse, dependence, and tolerance.
4. Monitor for withdrawal symptoms; abrupt withdrawal can precipitate seizures and may be fatal.

C. Monitor for behavioral changes, alertness, and mental status (e.g., depression, suicidality).

D. Monitor for skin changes (Stevens-Johnson syndrome [SJS], toxic epidermal necrolysis [TEN]).

X. **Relevant Pharmacokinetics/Pharmacodynamics**

A. **Metabolism**: Hepatic
B. **Time to peak plasma concentration**: 1.5 hour
C. **Half-life**: 10 hours (intermediate acting)
D. **Hepatic impairment**: Not defined
E. **Renal impairment**: None

XI. **Clinically Relevant Drug Interactions**

A. Temazepam has no known CYP interactions; remember the mnemonic "OTL": oxazepam, temazepam, and lorazepam are all metabolized "outside the liver."

B. Avoid concomitant use with opioids and other narcotics.

C. Avoid concomitant use with other CNS depressants. If used, dosage adjustments may be necessary.

D. Other sleep aids, including zolpidem and eszopiclone, should not be used with benzodiazepines.

E. Coadministration of benzodiazepines with antihypertensives or other medications that can lower blood pressure may result in additive hypotensive effects.

XII. **Adverse Effects**

A. **Boxed warnings**: See "Benzodiazepine Class Boxed Warnings" in the "Benzodiazepine Class Warnings and Precautions" section at the beginning of this chapter.

B. **Most common**:

1. Drowsiness, sedation, fatigue, ataxia, slurred speech, weakness, dizziness, syncope, diplopia, confusion, forgetfulness, euphoric mood, anterograde amnesia, impaired concentration, disinhibition, psychomotor impairment: Side effects are dosage dependent. Use the lowest effective dosage and titrate slowly to effect.
2. Nervousness, hyperexcitability, irritability: Monitor for potential paradoxical response.

C. **Benzodiazepine class effects**:

1. Nausea and constipation, appetite changes, incontinence, urinary retention, menstrual irregularities, changes in libido, dry mouth, asthenia, hallucinations (rare), extrapyramidal symptoms, dystonia, sialorrhea, hypotension

D. **Serious reactions**:

1. Stevens-Johnson syndrome, angioedema, hypersensitivity reaction, anaphylactoid reaction: Monitor for skin changes, particularly during initiation and reintroduction, and titrate slowly.
2. Respiratory depression and CNS depression, dependency, abuse, depression with suicidality, withdrawal with possible seizures if abruptly discontinued: Use the lowest effective dosage for the shortest possible time; taper slowly to discontinue use.
3. Hepatic dysfunction with ALT/AST elevation, renal dysfunction, blood dyscrasias, jaundice: Monitor laboratory values at baseline and periodically.

E. **Risks in pregnancy and lactation**: Most benzodiazepines were designated Category D drugs in the prior FDA classification. See Table 3–2 ("Benzodiazepines in pregnancy") in the introduction to this chapter; see also Chapter 15 ("Women: Pregnancy, Postpartum, and Breastfeeding"). For current information on benzodiazepine use in lactation, readers are referred to the Drugs and Lactation Database (LactMed; www.ncbi.nlm.nih.gov/books/NBK501922/).

XIII. Clinical Pearls/Prescribing Tips

A. Temazepam is commonly prescribed for insomnia.
B. It is recommended that use of temazepam be limited to 7–10 days. Temazepam is not recommended for long-term daily use.
C. Rebound insomnia may occur after stopping any sleep medication, including temazepam.
D. Temazepam can cause complex sleep behaviors, such as driving, cooking, making phone calls, or having sex while asleep. Individuals generally do not retain memories of these complex behaviors.
E. Recommend that patients lie down to sleep immediately after taking sleep medication.
F. Avoid use of temazepam in elderly individuals; long-term accumulation of active metabolites can lead to insidious onset of falls or confusion.

G. Benzodiazepine class use guidelines:

1. Use the lowest effective dosage for the shortest possible period of time. Regularly assess the need for continued treatment. Benzodiazepines are not recommended for long-term treatment of anxiety disorders; consider switching to an SSRI or SNRI for long-term maintenance. Consider augmenting with gabapentin or pregabalin for anxiety disorders to reduce benzodiazepine requirements.
2. When helping patients through the process of gradually tapering and discontinuing benzodiazepines, clinicians must be able to distinguish among reemergence of chronic anxiety disorder symptoms, rebound anxiety symptoms, and acute withdrawal symptoms.
3. **Caution**: Benzodiazepines can be fatal in overdose and withdrawal. Taper slowly. Protracted withdrawal can occur. Do not combine with other CNS depressants (e.g., other benzodiazepines, opioids). The benzodiazepine receptor antagonist flumazenil can be used in acute overdose but can precipitate seizures.

Further Reading

Heel RC, Brogden RN, Speight TM, et al: Temazepam: a review of its pharmacological properties and therapeutic efficacy as an hypnotic. Drugs 21(5):321–340, 1981 6112127

Restoril (temazepam) [package insert]. U.S. Food and Drug Administration website. Revised September 2016. Available at: https://www.accessdata.fda.gov/drugsatfda_docs/label/2016/018163s064lbl.pdf. Accessed May 18 2022.

Triazolam

I. **Brand Names**: Halcion
II. **Therapeutic Class**: Benzodiazepine (short acting), hypnotic, sedative
III. **Mechanism-Based Class**: GABA positive allosteric modulator (GABA PAM)
IV. **Mechanism(s) of Action**

A. Enhances GABA inhibition binding to stereo-specific benzodiazepine receptors on postsynaptic GABA neurons leading to hyperpolarization

V. **Indications**

A. FDA adult:

1. Short-term treatment for insomnia

B. Evidence-based[1] off-label uses:

1. Catatonia
2. Procedural minimal sedation (dentistry)
3. Use limited due to potency, very short half-life, and addictive potential
4. Can reduce comorbid anxiety when used to treat insomnia

C. FDA pediatric: None

VI. **Major Contraindications and When to Use Caution**

A. **Contraindications**:

1. Known hypersensitivity to medication or class
2. Angle-closure glaucoma
3. Medications that significantly impair the metabolism by CYP3A4

B. **Use caution**: Substance use history, obstructive sleep apnea, elderly individuals or those with high fall risk, debilitated patients, concurrent use of other CNS depressant medications, concurrent use of opioids, severe respiratory disease, severe liver disease, renal impairment, seizure history, depression, porphyria, delirium, dementia.

C. **Avoid abrupt withdrawal**: Gradually taper to discontinue after long-term use, as abrupt discontinuation or rapid dosage reduction may cause acute withdrawal reactions, including increased risk of seizures, which may be life-threatening.

VII. **Dosage Formulations**

A. Brand tablet (0.25 mg [*scored*])
B. Generic tablet (0.125 mg, 0.25 mg)

VIII. **Dosage Ranges and Guidelines**

A. Dosage ranges vary greatly based on indication and tolerance. Usual dosage is 0.125–0.5 mg at bedtime.

---

[1]Evidence strength varies; readers are referred to the literature for more detailed information.

B. Use a reduced dosage for elderly individuals and those with fall risk, hepatic or respiratory disease, or concurrent opioid use. The recommended starting dosage for elderly adults is 0.125 mg taken at bedtime.

C. **Titration**: Start at 0.125–0.25 mg at bedtime and increase slowly to a maximum of 0.5 mg/day at bedtime. Overdosage may occur at 2 mg.

D. **Tapering**: Taper dosage by 0.125 mg every 1–2 weeks. Some individuals may require a slower taper.

IX. Monitoring

A. Monitor baseline and periodic vital signs, complete blood count, creatinine, liver function tests, urinalysis, and physical and psychiatric evaluations.

1. Potential risk of hepatic dysfunction (aspartate transaminase [AST]/alanine aminotransferase [ALT] elevation), renal dysfunction, blood dyscrasias, jaundice
2. Leukopenia and elevated lactate dehydrogenase have been found in patients with long-term use of benzodiazepines.

B. Abuse/dependence/tolerance/withdrawal:

1. Triazolam is a Schedule IV controlled substance. Routinely assess for use of other narcotics (boxed warning with opioids).
2. Consider periodic urine drug screens to monitor for other narcotic use.
3. Monitor for abuse, dependence, and tolerance.
4. Monitor for withdrawal symptoms; abrupt withdrawal can precipitate seizures and may be fatal.

C. Monitor for behavioral changes, alertness, and mental status (e.g., depression, suicidality).

D. Monitor for skin changes (Stevens-Johnson syndrome [SJS], toxic epidermal necrolysis [TEN]).

X. Relevant Pharmacokinetics/Pharmacodynamics

A. **Metabolism**: Hepatic cytochrome P450 (CYP) 3A4
B. **Time to peak plasma concentration**: 2 hours
C. **Half-life**: 1.5–5.5 hours (short acting)
D. **Hepatic impairment**: Use starting dosage of 0.125 mg/day.
E. **Renal impairment**: No adjustment needed.

XI. Clinically Relevant Drug Interactions

A. Metabolized by CYP3A4

1. Concurrent use of strong CYP3A4 inhibitors or inducers may change triazolam serum concentrations; monitor therapy and consider adjustment as needed.
   a. Potent CYP3A4 inhibitors may decrease triazolam's clearance and increase its serum concentrations and effects. CYP3A4 inhibitors include nefazodone, fluvoxamine, fluoxetine, ketoconazole, itraconazole, isoniazid, and the HIV protease inhibitors ritonavir, indinavir, nelfinavir, saquinavir, and lopinavir, as well as grapefruit juice.
   b. CYP3A4 inducers (e.g., carbamazepine, oxcarbazepine) and smoking may increase triazolam's clearance, resulting in decreased concentration and effect.

B. Avoid concomitant use with opioids and other narcotics.
C. Avoid concomitant use with other CNS depressants; dosage adjustments may be necessary.
D. Other sleep aids, including zolpidem and eszopiclone, should not be used with benzodiazepines.
E. Coadministration of benzodiazepines with antihypertensives or other medications that can lower blood pressure may result in additive hypotensive effects.
F. Triazolam is sensitive to fluctuations in gastric pH, which could affect blood levels.

XII. **Adverse Effects**

A. **Boxed warnings**: See "Benzodiazepine Class Boxed Warnings" in the "Benzodiazepine Class Warnings and Precautions" section at the beginning of this chapter.

B. **Most common**:

1. Drowsiness, sedation, fatigue, ataxia, slurred speech, weakness, dizziness, syncope, diplopia, confusion, forgetfulness, euphoric mood, anterograde amnesia, impaired concentration, disinhibition, psychomotor impairment: Side effects are dosage dependent. Use the lowest effective dosage and titrate slowly to effect.
2. Nervousness, hyperexcitability, irritability: Monitor for potential paradoxical response.
3. Complex sleep behaviors: Use the lowest effective dosage, limit to short-term use, take right before sleep, and lie down right after taking medication.

C. **Benzodiazepine class effects**:

1. Nausea and constipation, appetite changes, incontinence, urinary retention, menstrual irregularities, changes in libido, dry mouth, asthenia, hallucinations (rare), extrapyramidal symptoms, dystonia, sialorrhea, hypotension

D. **Serious reactions**:

1. Stevens-Johnson syndrome, angioedema, hypersensitivity reaction, anaphylactoid reaction: Monitor for skin changes, particularly during initiation and reintroduction, and titrate slowly.
2. Respiratory depression and CNS depression, dependency, abuse, depression with suicidality, withdrawal with possible seizures if abruptly discontinued: Use the lowest effective dosage for the shortest possible time; taper slowly to discontinue use.
3. Hepatic dysfunction with ALT/AST elevation, renal dysfunction, blood dyscrasias, jaundice: Monitor laboratory values at baseline and periodically.

E. **Risks in pregnancy and lactation**: Most benzodiazepines were designated Category D drugs in the prior FDA classification. See Table 3–2 ("Benzodiazepines in pregnancy") in the introduction to this chapter; see also Chapter 15 ("Women: Pregnancy, Postpartum, and Breastfeeding"). For current information on benzodiazepine use in lactation, readers are referred to the Drugs and Lactation Database (LactMed; www.ncbi.nlm.nih.gov/books/NBK501922/).

XIII. **Clinical Pearls/Prescribing Tips**

A. Triazolam is primarily used for insomnia but is banned in the United Kingdom because of a higher incidence of memory loss and depression compared with other benzodiazepines.

B. Insomnia that does not improve after 7–10 days of triazolam use may be indicative of insomnia secondary to an independent psychiatric or medical illness that requires further investigation.

C. Triazolam has been shown to cause complex sleep behaviors, such as driving, cooking, making phone calls, or having sex while asleep. Individuals generally do not retain memories of these complex behaviors.

D. Recommend that patients lie down to sleep immediately after taking sleep medication.

E. Rebound insomnia may occur after stopping any sleep medication, including triazolam.

F. Triazolam has a narrow therapeutic index.

G. Benzodiazepine class use guidelines:

1. Use the lowest effective dosage for the shortest possible period of time. Regularly assess the need for continued treatment. Benzodiazepines are not recommended for long-term treatment of anxiety disorders; consider switching to an SSRI or SNRI for long-term maintenance. Consider augmenting with gabapentin or pregabalin for anxiety disorders to reduce benzodiazepine requirements.
2. When helping patients through the process of gradually tapering and discontinuing benzodiazepines, clinicians must be able to distinguish among reemergence of chronic anxiety disorder symptoms, rebound anxiety symptoms, and acute withdrawal symptoms.
3. **Caution**: Benzodiazepines can be fatal in overdose and withdrawal. Taper slowly. Protracted withdrawal can occur. Do not combine with other CNS depressants (e.g., other benzodiazepines, opioids). The benzodiazepine receptor antagonist flumazenil can be used in acute overdose but can precipitate seizures.

Further Reading

Bélanger L, Belleville G, Morin C: Management of hypnotic discontinuation in chronic insomnia. Sleep Med Clin 4(4):583–592, 2009 20607118

Chouinard G: Issues in the clinical use of benzodiazepines: potency, withdrawal, and rebound. J Clin Psychiatry 65(Suppl 5):7–12, 2004 15078112

Halcion (triazolam) [package insert]. U.S. Food and Drug Administration website. Revised September 2016. Available at: https://www.accessdata.fda.gov/drugsatfda_docs/label/2016/017892s049lbl.pdf. Accessed May 14, 2022.

Kales A, Bixler EO, Vela-Bueno A, et al: Comparison of short and long half-life benzodiazepine hypnotics: triazolam and quazepam. Clin Pharmacol Ther 40(4):378–386, 1986 3530586

Other Benzodiazepines

Clobazam

I. **Brand Names**: Onfi, Sympazan
II. **Therapeutic Class**: Benzodiazepine (long acting), anticonvulsant
III. **Mechanism-Based Class**: GABA positive allosteric modulator (GABA PAM)
IV. **Mechanism(s) of Action**

A. Enhances GABA inhibition binding to stereospecific benzodiazepine receptors on postsynaptic GABA neurons leading to hyperpolarization
B. Positive allosteric modulator of $GABA_A$ receptor, benzodiazepine site, causing increased permeability of neuronal membrane to chloride ions, results in hyperpolarization and depressed activity

V. **Indications**

A. FDA adult:

1. Lennox-Gastaut syndrome
2. Seizure disorder (adjunctive)

B. Evidence-based[1] off-label uses:

1. Catamenial epilepsy
2. Treatment-refractory seizures (adjunctive)
3. Can reduce comorbid anxiety when used to treat insomnia.

C. FDA pediatric: None

VI. **Major Contraindications and When to Use Caution**

A. **Contraindications**:

1. Known hypersensitivity/allergy to medication or class
2. Myasthenia gravis
3. Angle-closure glaucoma

B. **Use caution**: Substance use history, obstructive sleep apnea, elderly individuals or those with high fall risk, debilitated patients, concurrent use of other CNS depressant medications, concurrent use of opioids, severe respiratory disease, severe liver disease, renal impairment, seizure history, depression, porphyria, delirium, dementia.
C. **Avoid abrupt withdrawal**: Gradually taper to discontinue after long-term use, as abrupt discontinuation or rapid dosage reduction may cause acute withdrawal reactions, including increased risk of seizures, which may be life-threatening.

---

[1]Evidence strength varies; readers are referred to the literature for more detailed information.

VII. **Dosage Formulations**

A. Brand: tablet (10 mg, 20 mg); concentrate (2.5 mg/mL); strip (5 mg, 10 mg, 20 mg)

1. Do not give strip with liquid.

B. Generic: tablet (10 mg, 20 mg); concentrate (2.5 mg/mL)

VIII. **Dosage Ranges and Guidelines**

A. Dosage varies greatly based on indication and tolerance. Usual dosage range is 5–40 mg/day (divided daily BID)

B. Use a reduced dosage for elderly individuals and those with fall risk, hepatic or respiratory disease, or concurrent opioid use.

C. **Titration**: Start at 5 mg/day BID. Increase by 5–10 mg per week.

D. **Tapering**: Taper dosage by no more than 5–10 mg per week. Some individuals may require a slower taper.

IX. **Monitoring**

A. Monitor baseline and periodic vital signs, complete blood count, creatinine, liver function tests, urinalysis, and physical and psychiatric evaluations.

1. Potential risk of hepatic dysfunction (aspartate transaminase [AST]/alanine aminotransferase [ALT] elevation), renal dysfunction, blood dyscrasias, jaundice
2. Leukopenia and elevated lactate dehydrogenase have been found in patients with long-term use of benzodiazepines.

B. Abuse/dependence/tolerance/withdrawal:

1. Clobazam is a Schedule IV controlled substance. Routinely assess for use of other narcotics (boxed warning with opioids).
2. Consider periodic urine drug screens to monitor for other narcotic use.
3. Monitor for abuse, dependence, and tolerance.
4. Monitor for withdrawal symptoms; abrupt withdrawal can precipitate seizures and may be fatal.

C. Monitor for behavioral changes, alertness, and mental status (e.g., depression, suicidality).

D. Monitor for skin changes (Stevens-Johnson syndrome [SJS], toxic epidermal necrolysis [TEN]).

X. **Relevant Pharmacokinetics/Pharmacodynamics**

A. **Metabolism**: Hepatic cytochrome P450 (CYP) 3A4, CYP2C19, and CYP2B6

1. Active metabolite: *N*-desmethylclobazam, half-life 71–82 hours; may accumulate in poor CYP2C19 metabolizers, requiring dosage adjustment.

B. **Time to peak plasma concentration**: Oral film strip: 0.33 to 4 hours; tablet: 0.5 to 4 hours; concentrate: 0.5–2 hours

C. **Half-life**: 16 hours in children, 36–42 hours in adults (long acting)

D. **Hepatic impairment**:

1. Child Pugh Class A or B: Start at 5 mg/day for 1 week; increase by 5 mg weekly.
2. Child Pugh Class C: Not defined.

E. **Renal impairment**: Not specified, except CrCl >30 mL/minute: No adjustment.

XI. Clinically Relevant Drug Interactions

A. Metabolized by CYP3A4, CYP2C19, CYP2B6, and P-glycoprotein/ABCB1.

1. Concomitant use of strong CYP2C19 and CYP3A4 inhibitors or inducers may change serum concentrations. Monitor therapy and consider adjustment as needed.

   a. Potent CYP3A4 inhibitors may decrease clearance and increase serum concentrations and effects. CYP3A4 inhibitors include nefazodone, fluvoxamine, fluoxetine, ketoconazole, itraconazole, isoniazid, and the HIV protease inhibitors ritonavir, indinavir, nelfinavir, saquinavir, and lopinavir.

      i. Grapefruit juice may also increase serum concentrations.

   b. CYP3A4 inducers (e.g., carbamazepine, oxcarbazepine) may increase clearance and decrease concentrations and effects.

      i. Smoking may also decrease serum concentrations.

2. Weak inducer of CYP3A4

B. Avoid concomitant use with opioids and other narcotics.

C. Avoid concomitant use with other CNS depressants. If used, dosage adjustments may be necessary.

D. Other sleep aids, including zolpidem and eszopiclone, should not be used with benzodiazepines.

E. Coadministration of benzodiazepines with antihypertensives or other medications that can lower blood pressure may result in additive hypotensive effects.

XII. Adverse Effects

A. **Boxed warnings**: See "Benzodiazepine Class Boxed Warnings" in the "Benzodiazepine Class Warnings and Precautions" section at the beginning of this chapter.

B. **Most common**:

1. Drowsiness, sedation, fatigue, ataxia, slurred speech, weakness, dizziness, syncope, diplopia, confusion, forgetfulness, euphoric mood, anterograde amnesia, impaired concentration, disinhibition, psychomotor impairment: Side effects are dosage dependent. Use the lowest effective dosage and titrate slowly to effect.
2. Nervousness, hyperexcitability, irritability: Monitor for potential paradoxical response.

C. **Benzodiazepine class effects**:

1. Nausea and constipation, appetite changes, fever, upper respiratory infection, cough, pneumonia, urinary tract infection, dysphagia, bronchitis, incontinence, urinary retention, menstrual irregularities, changes in libido, dry mouth, asthenia, hallucinations (rare), extrapyramidal symptoms, dystonia, sialorrhea, hypotension

D. **Serious reactions**:

1. Stevens-Johnson syndrome (SJS), toxic epidermal necrolysis (TEN) angioedema, hypersensitivity reaction, anaphylactoid reaction: Monitor for skin changes, particularly during initiation and reintroduction, and titrate slowly.
2. Respiratory depression and CNS depression, dependency, abuse, depression with suicidality, withdrawal with possible seizures if abruptly discontinued: Use the lowest effective dosage for the shortest possible time; taper slowly to discontinue use.
3. Hepatic dysfunction with ALT/ AST elevation, renal dysfunction, blood dyscrasias, leukopenia, thrombocytopenia, jaundice: Monitor laboratory values at baseline and periodically.

E. **Risks in pregnancy and lactation**: Most benzodiazepines were designated Category D drugs in the prior FDA classification. See Table 3–2 ("Benzodiazepines in pregnancy") in the introduction to this chapter; see also Chapter 15 ("Women: Pregnancy, Postpartum, and Breastfeeding"). For current information on benzodiazepine use in lactation, readers are referred to the Drugs and Lactation Database (LactMed; www.ncbi.nlm.nih.gov/books/NBK501922/).

XIII. **Clinical Pearls/Prescribing Tips**

A. Clobazam is widely used in Europe and Asia to treat anxiety.
B. In the United States, clobazam is typically used as a adjunctive agent with anticonvulsants to treat seizure disorders.
C. Clobazam has an atypical structure, with nitrogen at 1,5 positions on the aromatic ring (vs. the typical 1,4 benzodiazepine position) and targets different GABA subunits, which may make it less sedating.
D. Clinicians should educate patients regarding clobazam's withdrawal effects, avoid higher dosages, and closely monitor patients with seizure disorders.
E. Elderly patients, adolescent/pediatric patients, and patients with a substance use history should be carefully monitored.
F. Clobazam's longer half-life can lead to daytime sedation and impaired motor and cognitive functioning, which can increase over time. Use caution and taper dosage if accumulation is suspected.
G. Benzodiazepine class use guidelines:

1. Use the lowest effective dosage for the shortest possible period of time. Regularly assess the need for continued treatment. Benzodiazepines are not recommended for long-term treatment of anxiety disorders; consider switching to an SSRI or SNRI for long-term maintenance. Consider augmenting with gabapentin or pregabalin for anxiety disorders to reduce benzodiazepine requirements.
2. When helping patients through the process of gradually tapering and discontinuing benzodiazepines, clinicians must be able to distinguish among reemergence of chronic anxiety disorder symptoms, rebound anxiety symptoms, and acute withdrawal symptoms.
3. **Caution**: Benzodiazepines can be fatal in overdose and withdrawal. Taper slowly. Protracted withdrawal can occur. Do not combine with other CNS depressants (e.g., other benzodiazepines, opioids). The benzodiazepine receptor antagonist flumazenil can be used in acute overdose but can precipitate seizures.

Further Reading

Clobazam package insert. U.S Food and Drug Administration, 2021. Available at: https://www.accessdata.fda.gov/spl/data/a538029f-6387-4ea1-aa62-ecd14f31e0b6/a538029f-6387-4ea1-aa62-ecd14f31e0b6.xml. Accessed March 13, 2024.

Gauthier AC, Mattson RH: Clobazam: a safe, efficacious, and newly rediscovered therapeutic for epilepsy. CNS Neurosci Ther 21(7):543–548, 2015 25917225

Salpekar JA, Basu T, Thangaraj S, et al: The intersections of stress, anxiety and epilepsy. Int Rev Neurobiol 152:195–219, 2020 32450996

Tolbert D, Larsen F: A comprehensive overview of the clinical pharmacokinetics of clobazam. J Clin Pharmacol 59(1):7–19, 2019 30285275

Midazolam

I. **Brand Names**: Versed (brand discontinued), Seizalam, Nayzilam

II. **Therapeutic Class**: Benzodiazepine (short acting), sedative, anticonvulsant

III. **Mechanism-Based Class**: GABA positive allosteric modulator (GABA PAM)

IV. **Mechanism(s) of Action**

  A. Enhances GABA inhibition binding to stereo-specific benzodiazepine receptors on postsynaptic GABA neurons leading to hyperpolarization

V. **Indications**

  A. FDA adult:

    1. General anesthesia
    2. Sedation in mechanically ventilated patients in intensive care setting
    3. Procedural sedation (outside operating room)
    4. Sedation in pediatric patients
    5. Seizures
    6. Preoperative anxiolytic
    7. Drug-induced amnesia

  B. Evidence-based[1] off-label uses:

    1. Agitation (acute/severe)
    2. Intoxication (cocaine, methamphetamine, other sympathomimetics)
    3. Palliative and end-of-life sedation
    4. Refractory status epilepticus
    5. Catatonia
    6. Midazolam is generally not used specifically for anxiety alone, apart from perioperatively; however, it can reduce comorbid anxiety when used for other indications.

  C. FDA pediatric: None

---

[1]Evidence strength varies; readers are referred to the literature for more detailed information.

VI. **Major Contraindications and When to Use Caution**

A. **Contraindications**:

1. Known hypersensitivity to medication or class
2. Acute narrow-angle glaucoma

B. **Use caution**: Substance use history, obstructive sleep apnea, elderly individuals or those with high fall risk, debilitated patients, concurrent use of other CNS depressant medications, concurrent use of opioids, severe respiratory disease, severe liver disease, renal impairment, seizure history, depression, porphyria, delirium, dementia.

C. **Avoid abrupt withdrawal**: Gradually taper to discontinue after long-term use, as abrupt discontinuation or rapid dosage reduction may cause acute withdrawal reactions, including increased risk of seizures, which may be life-threatening.

VII. **Dosage Formulations**

A. Generic syrup (2 mg/mL)
B. Brand (Nayzilam) and generic nasal spray (5 mg/spray)
C. Generic injectable (1 mg/mL, 5 mg/mL)
D. Brand (Seizalam) injectable (IV/IM) (5 mg/mL)

VIII. **Dosage Ranges and Guidelines**

A. Dosage varies greatly based on indication and tolerance. Given the multiple formulations of midazolam, there are many dosage guidelines for different indications. For agitation, administer 2.5–5 mg every 3–5 minutes for IV and every 5–10 minutes for IM. The usual maximum dosage is 20 mg/day.

B. Use a reduced dosage for elderly individuals and those with fall risk, hepatic or respiratory disease, or concurrent opioid use.

C. Midazolam is usually not scheduled, but if so, taper slowly.

IX. **Monitoring**

A. Monitor baseline and periodic vital signs, complete blood count, creatinine, liver function tests, urinalysis, and physical and psychiatric evaluations.

1. Potential risk of hepatic dysfunction (aspartate transaminase [AST]/alanine aminotransferase [ALT] elevation), renal dysfunction, blood dyscrasias, jaundice
2. Leukopenia and elevated lactate dehydrogenase have been found in patients with long-term use of benzodiazepines.

B. Abuse/dependence/tolerance/withdrawal:

1. Midazolam is a Schedule IV controlled substance. Routinely assess for use of other narcotics (boxed warning with opioids).
2. Consider periodic urine drug screens to monitor for other narcotic use.
3. Monitor for abuse, dependence, and tolerance.
4. Monitor for withdrawal symptoms; abrupt withdrawal can precipitate seizures and may be fatal.

C. Monitor for behavioral changes, alertness, and mental status (e.g., depression, suicidality).
D. Monitor for skin changes (Stevens-Johnson syndrome [SJS], toxic epidermal necrolysis [TEN]).
E. Monitor for level of sedation.

X. **Relevant Pharmacokinetics/Pharmacodynamics**

A. **Metabolism**: Hepatic CYP 3A4
B. **Time to peak plasma concentration**:

1. IM: 30–60 minutes
2. IV: 3–5 minutes
3. Oral: 10–20 minutes
4. Intranasal (nasal spray): 10 minutes
5. Intranasal (solution, injection): 5 minutes

C. **Half-life**: 2–3 hours (very short acting)

1. Active metabolite: 1.8–6.4 hours

D. **Hepatic impairment**: Caution advised
E. **Renal impairment**: CrCl <10 mL/minute: Decrease the usual dosage by 50%.

XI. **Clinically Relevant Drug Interactions**

A. Metabolized primarily by CYP3A4 primarily and to a lesser extent by CYP2B6.

1. Concurrent use of strong CYP3A4 inhibitors or inducers may change triazolam serum concentrations; monitor therapy and consider adjustment as needed.

a. Potent CYP3A4 inhibitors may decrease triazolam's clearance and increase serum concentrations and effects. CYP3A4 inhibitors include nefazodone, fluvoxamine, fluoxetine, ketoconazole, itraconazole, isoniazid, and the HIV protease inhibitors ritonavir, indinavir, nelfinavir, saquinavir, and lopinavir, as well as grapefruit juice.
b. CYP3A4 inducers (e.g., carbamazepine, oxcarbazepine) and smoking may increase clearance, resulting in decreased concentration and effect.

B. Avoid concomitant use with opioids and other narcotics.
C. Avoid concomitant use with other CNS depressants. If used, dosage adjustments may be necessary.
D. Other sleep aids, including zolpidem and eszopiclone, should not be used with benzodiazepines.
E. Coadministration of benzodiazepines with antihypertensives or other medications that can lower blood pressure may result in additive hypotensive effects.

XII. **Adverse Effects**

A. **Boxed warnings**: See "Benzodiazepine Class Boxed Warnings" in the "Benzodiazepine Class Warnings and Precautions" section at the beginning of this chapter.

B. **Most common**:

1. Drowsiness, sedation, fatigue, ataxia, slurred speech, weakness, dizziness, syncope, diplopia, confusion, forgetfulness, euphoric mood, anterograde amnesia, impaired concentration, disinhibition, psychomotor impairment: Side effects are dosage dependent. Use the lowest effective dosage and titrate slowly to effect.
2. Nervousness, hyperexcitability, irritability: Monitor for potential paradoxical response.

C. **Benzodiazepine class effects**:

1. Nausea and constipation, appetite changes, incontinence, urinary retention, menstrual irregularities, changes in libido, dry mouth, asthenia, hallucinations (rare), extrapyramidal symptoms, dystonia, sialorrhea, hypotension

D. **Serious reactions**:

1. Stevens-Johnson syndrome, angioedema, hypersensitivity reaction, anaphylactoid reaction: Monitor for skin changes, particularly during initiation and reintroduction, and titrate slowly.
2. Respiratory depression and CNS depression, dependency, abuse, depression with suicidality, withdrawal with possible seizures if abrupt discontinuation: Use lowest effective dosage for shortest possible time; taper slowly to discontinue use.
3. Hepatic dysfunction with ALT/AST elevation, renal dysfunction, blood dyscrasias, jaundice: Monitor laboratory values at baseline and periodically.
4. Apnea, bradypnea, decreased respiratory tidal volume: Use only in closely monitored settings.

E. **Risks in pregnancy and lactation**: Most benzodiazepines were designated Category D drugs in the prior FDA classification. See Table 3–2 ("Benzodiazepines in pregnancy") in the introduction to this chapter; see also Chapter 15 ("Women: Pregnancy, Postpartum, and Breastfeeding"). For current information on benzodiazepine use in lactation, readers are referred to the Drugs and Lactation Database (LactMed; www.ncbi.nlm.nih.gov/books/NBK501922/).

XIII. **Clinical Pearls/Prescribing Tips**

A. There is no pill/tablet formulation of midazolam.
B. Midazolam is mostly used by anesthesiologists in inpatient, perioperative, and critical care settings.
C. Midazolam is sometimes given with IV ketamine to produce amnestic effects and prevent dysphoria during infusion.
D. Midazolam is very short acting.
E. Midazolam is not recommended for long-term use.
F. Protracted withdrawal can occur after prolonged use of midazolam with mechanical ventilation.
G. When discontinuing midazolam after prolonged use, especially in patients with chronic alcohol dependence, an alternative benzodiazepine may need to be used and tapered gradually.

H. Benzodiazepine class use guidelines:

1. Use the lowest effective dosage for the shortest possible period of time. Regularly assess the need for continued treatment. Benzodiazepines are not recommended for long-term treatment of anxiety disorders; consider switching to an SSRI or SNRI for long-term maintenance. Consider augmenting with gabapentin or pregabalin for anxiety disorders to reduce benzodiazepine requirements.
2. When helping patients through the process of gradually tapering and discontinuing benzodiazepines, clinicians must be able to distinguish among reemergence of chronic anxiety disorder symptoms, rebound anxiety symptoms, and acute withdrawal symptoms.
3. **Caution**: Benzodiazepines can be fatal in overdose and withdrawal. Taper slowly. Protracted withdrawal can occur. Do not combine with other CNS depressants (e.g., other benzodiazepines, opioids). The benzodiazepine receptor antagonist flumazenil can be used in acute overdose but can precipitate seizures.

Further Reading

Devlin JW, Skrobik Y, Gélinas C, et al: Clinical practice guidelines for the prevention and management of pain, agitation/sedation, delirium, immobility, and sleep disruption in adult patients in the ICU. Crit Care Med 46(9):e825–e873, 2018 30113379

Madsen BK, Zetner D, Møller AM, et al: Melatonin for preoperative and postoperative anxiety in adults. Cochrane Database Syst Rev (12):CD009861, 2020 33319916

Midazolam injection package insert. U.S. Food and Drug Administration, 2017. Available at: https://www.accessdata.fda.gov/drugsatfda_docs/label/2017/208878Orig1s000lbl.pdf. Accessed March 13, 2024.

Nonbenzodiazepine Medications With Anxiolytic Effects

Buspirone

I. **Brand Names**: BuSpar (brand discontinued in U.S.)
II. **Therapeutic Class**: Nonbenzodiazepine anxiolytic
III. **Mechanism-Based Class**: Serotonin-1A receptor partial agonist
IV. **Mechanism(s) of Action**

A. 5-HT_{1A} partial agonist at both pre- and postsynaptic receptors (Ki=3.98–214 nM), leading to anxiolytic and antidepressant effects
B. Weak/moderate antagonist of brain D_2 receptors (Ki=484 nM)
C. Major metabolites:

1. 6-Hydroxybuspirone: Circulates at levels 40 times higher than those of the parent molecule (Dockens et al. 2006\) (Ki=25 nM for 5-HT_{1A})
2. 1-Pyrimidinyl piperazine (1-PP) is a potent α_2-adrenergic receptor antagonist that increases norepinephrine and dopamine and may add to buspirone's potential antidepressant effect. The metabolite occurs at higher levels than the parent molecule.

V. **Indications**

A. FDA adult:

1. Generalized anxiety disorder (GAD)

B. Evidence-based[1] off-label uses:

1. Mixed anxiety and depression
2. Treatment-resistant depression (adjunctive)
3. Hypoactive sexual desire disorder in women
4. Bruxism induced by antidepressants

C. FDA pediatric: None

VI. **Major Contraindications and When to Use Caution**

A. Known allergy to buspirone
B. Use of buspirone within 14 days of taking an MAOI is associated with an increased risk of serotonin syndrome (2-week washout recommended).

[1]Evidence strength varies; readers are referred to the literature for more detailed information.

VII. **Dosage Formulations**

A. Generic tablet (5 mg [*scored*], 10 mg [*scored*], 15 mg [*multi-scored*], 30 mg [*multi-scored*])

VIII. **Dosage Ranges and Guidelines**

A. Dosage varies based on indication (see Table 3–9 for usual dosage ranges).
B. For generalized anxiety disorder, start at 10–15 mg/day (in 2–3 divided doses) and increase in 5-mg increments every 2–3 days to a maximum of 60 mg/day (2–3 divided doses). May require several weeks to show effects.
C. For off-label use to augment antidepressant treatment, start at 15–20 mg/day (2 divided doses) and increase to a maximum of 60 mg/day (2 divided doses).

Table 3–9. Buspirone indications and dosage ranges

Indications	Usual dosage ranges
Generalized anxiety disorder	10–15 mg/day → 60 mg/day (2–3 divided doses)
Depression augmentation (off-label)	15–20 mg/day → 60 mg/day (2 divided doses)

IX. **Monitoring**

A. Creatinine, liver function tests, physical and psychiatric evaluation at baseline.
B. Monitor vital signs, CBC, liver function tests, electrolytes, and urinalysis periodically during prolonged use.

X. **Relevant Pharmacokinetics/Pharmacodynamics**

A. **Metabolism**: Hepatic cytochrome P450 (CYP) 3A4 metabolism, several major metabolites, notably 6-hydroxy buspirone and 1-PP
B. **Time to peak plasma concentration**: <1 hour
C. **Half-life**: 2–3 hours
D. **Effect of food**: Absorption changes with food intake, so always take either with or without food for consistency.
E. **Hepatic impairment**: Caution advised; avoid use in patients with severe impairment.
F. **Renal impairment**: Mild to moderate impairment: Consider decreasing the usual dosage. Severe impairment: Avoid use.

XI. **Clinically Relevant Drug Interactions**

A. Metabolized by CYP3A4
   1. Concurrent use of strong CYP3A4 inhibitors or inducers may change serum concentration. Monitor therapy and consider adjustment as needed.
      a. Potent CYP3A4 inhibitors may decrease clearance and increase serum concentrations and effects. CYP3A4 inhibitors include nefazodone, fluvoxamine, fluoxetine, ketoconazole, itraconazole, isoniazid, and the HIV protease inhibitors ritonavir, indinavir, nelfinavir, saquinavir, and lopinavir, as well as grapefruit juice.

i. Patients receiving both buspirone and nefazodone experienced lightheadedness, asthenia, dizziness, and somnolence (Amneal Pharmaceuticals 2022).

b. CYP3A4 inducers (e.g., carbamazepine, oxcarbazepine) and smoking may increase clearance, resulting in decreased concentration and effect.

i. Rifampin has been shown to decrease plasma concentrations of buspirone.

XII. Adverse Effects

A. **Most common**:

1. Dizziness, headache, fatigue, dry mouth, impaired concentration, confusion, depression, lightheadedness. Management may involve medication discontinuation or dosage adjustment.
2. Paradoxical effects: insomnia, nervousness, excitement. Monitor for symptoms.

B. **Other effects**:

1. Nausea, diarrhea, abdominal pain, weakness, numbness, blurred vision. May improve over time.

C. **Extrapyramidal symptoms**:

1. A syndrome of restlessness (akathisia) occurring shortly after drug initiation has been noted in patients. This syndrome is thought to be related to the D_2 dopamine receptor binding.
2. Tardive dyskinesia is possible. Stop medication if this occurs.

D. **Serious reactions**:

1. Serotonin syndrome, cardiac symptoms (rare), acute dystonia, hostility. Stop medication and treat appropriately.

E. **Risks in pregnancy and lactation**: Buspirone was designated a Category B drug in the prior FDA classification (see Chapter 15, "Women: Pregnancy, Postpartum, and Breastfeeding"). For current information on buspirone's use in lactation, readers are referred to the Drugs and Lactation Database (LactMed; www.ncbi.nlm.nih.gov/books/NBK501922/).

XIII. Clinical Pearls/Prescribing Tips

A. Buspirone is often used in conjunction with SSRIs and SNRIs to augment anxiolytic effects, but is less potent than benzodiazepines and takes longer to work, so it may have better effects in patients who have never taken benzodiazepines.

B. Buspirone is more effective in GAD and ruminative anxiety than in OCD.

C. Buspirone may have some effect in depression.

D. Buspirone may be helpful in treating bruxism associated with SSRIs/SNRIs and may improve hypoactive sexual desire in women.

E. Some evidence supports off-label use of buspirone to treat sexual side effects associated with serotonergic antidepressants.

F. Buspirone requires twice-daily or three-times-a-day dosing for full effect.

G. Absorption of buspirone is affected by food.

H. Buspirone lacks the addictive potential and sexual side effects/weight gain often associated with other anxiolytic agents; overall, its side-effect profile is favorable. The most common side effect is dizziness. D_2 antagonism could lead to movement disorders, although this effect is rare.

I. Buspirone dosages greater than 20 mg/day have a higher likelihood of producing sedative effects.

J. Buspirone dosages may need to be adjusted for patients with renal or hepatic impairment. Buspirone use should be avoided in patients with severe impairment.

K. Buspirone hydrochloride has been shown to interfere with urinary metanephrine/catecholamine assays, potentially leading to false-positive results in pheochromocytoma testing.

Further Reading

Bristol-Myers Squibb: BuSpar (buspirone) [package insert]. U.S. Food and Drug Administration website. Revised November 2010. Available at: https://www.accessdata.fda.gov/drugsatfda_docs/label/2010/018731s051lbl.pdf. Accessed May 11, 2022.

Mahmood I, Sahajwalla C: Clinical pharmacokinetics and pharmacodynamics of buspirone, an anxiolytic drug. Clin Pharmacokinet 36(4):277–287, 1999 10320950

Petracca A, Nisita C, McNair D, et al: Treatment of generalized anxiety disorder: preliminary clinical experience with buspirone. J Clin Psychiatry 51(Suppl):31–39, 1990 2211564

References

Amneal Pharmaceuticals: Buspirone hydrochloride [package insert]. U.S. Food and Drug Administration website. Revised December 2022. Available at: https://www.accessdata.fda.gov/spl/data/f697167a-4d7c-42fb-91c0-7c1f877bf54a/f697167a-4d7c-42fb-91c0-7c1f877bf54a.xml. Accessed March 13, 2024.

Dockens RC, Salazar DE, Fulmor IE, et al: Pharmacokinetics of a newly identified active metabolite of buspirone after administration of buspirone over its therapeutic dose range. J Clin Pharmacol 46(11):1308–1312, 2006 17050795

Gabapentin[1]

I. **Brand Names**: Neurontin, Gralise, Horizant, Gabarone, Fanatrex

II. **Therapeutic Class**: Anticonvulsant

III. **Mechanism-Based Class**: Glutamate, voltage-gated calcium channel blocker

IV. **Mechanism(s) of Action**

A. Developed as a GABA analog.

B. High affinity for the $\alpha_2\delta$ auxiliary subunit of voltage-sensitive calcium channels in the CNS

C. Does not appear to interact with the GABA receptor.

D. Modulates excitatory neurotransmitter release.

V. **Indications**

A. FDA adult:

1. Adjunctive treatment of partial seizures
2. Postherpetic neuralgia
3. Restless legs syndrome (ER formulation)

B. Evidence-based[2] off-label uses:

1. Neuropathic pain
2. Fibromyalgia
3. Alcohol dependence and withdrawal
4. Bipolar disorder (adjunctive)
5. Anxiety disorders (adjunctive)
6. Perioperative anxiety
7. PTSD
8. Essential tremor
9. Cough, hiccups, pruritus
10. Vasomotor symptoms associated with menopause

C. FDA pediatric: None

VI. **Major Contraindications and When to Use Caution**

A. **Contraindications**:

1. Known hypersensitivity to medication or class

B. **Use caution**:

1. Patients with kidney disease (CrCl <60 mL/minute): Adjust dosage (see Table 3–10 ["Gabapentin dosage adjustment for patients with renal impairment"] under "Relevant Pharmacokinetics/Pharmacodynamics" later in chapter).
2. Individuals with a history of substance use disorder
3. Patients with respiratory impairment
4. Elderly patients

---

[1]Also see Chapter 10, "Treatment of Substance Use Disorders," for information regarding gabapentin's use for alcohol use disorder and opioid use disorder.

[2]Evidence strength varies; readers are referred to the literature for more detailed information.

5. Patients with depression
6. Concomitant CNS depressant use (additive effects)

C. Avoid abrupt withdrawal.

VII. **Dosage Formulations**

A. Generic: capsule (100 mg, 300 mg, 400 mg); tablet (600 mg, 800 mg); concentrate (50 mg/mL)

B. Brand: capsule (100 mg, 300 mg, 400 mg); tablet (600 mg, 800 mg); ER tablet (300 mg, 600 mg); concentrate (50 mg/mL)

1. Do not chew, break, or crush ER form. The ER tablet must be taken with food.

VIII. **Dosage Ranges and Guidelines**

A. Dosage varies greatly based on indication and tolerance (see Table 3–10 for usual dosage ranges). Usual dosage range is 100–1,800 mg/day (up to 3,600 mg/day for seizures).

B. Use a reduced dosage for elderly individuals and those with fall risk, hepatic or respiratory disease, or concurrent opioid use.

C. **Titration**: Varies depending on indication.

1. Off-label use for anxiety generally starts at 100–300 mg PO TID. Increase in 300-mg increments every 3 or more days, to a maximum of 2,400 mg/day (taken in 2–3 divided doses).

a. If patient is sensitive to side effects, consider starting at 100 mg/day and increasing from there.

2. For neuralgia, start at 300 mg once daily, then increase to BID, then TID; maximum dosage is 1,800 mg/day.

D. **Tapering**: Taper dosage gradually over 1 or more weeks to minimize risk of withdrawal effects, including seizures.

Table 3–10. Gabapentin indications and dosage ranges

Indications	Usual dosage ranges
Partial seizures	IR: 100–1,200 mg TID (total daily dosage of 2,400–3,600 mg divided)
Postherpetic neuralgia	IR: 300–600 mg TID (total daily dosage of 1,800 mg) ER: 300–1,800 mg/day
Restless legs syndrome (FDA approved for ER only)	ER: 600–1,200 mg/day (1–2 doses) IR: 100–2,400 mg 2 hours before bedtime. At dosages higher than 600 mg/day, consider taking 1/3 of dose at midday and 2/3 at bedtime.
Neuropathic pain (off-label)	IR: 100–1,200 mg TID (total daily dosage of 3,600 mg taken as a single dose or in 2–3 divided doses) ER: 300–3,600 mg/day

Table 3–10. Gabapentin indications and dosage ranges *(continued)*

Indications	Usual dosage ranges
Fibromyalgia (off-label)	IR: 100–800 mg TID (total daily dosage up to 2,400 mg taken as a single dose or in 2–3 divided doses)
Alcohol dependence or withdrawal (off-label)	Dependence: IR: 300–600 mg TID (total daily dosage of 1,800 mg divided) Withdrawal: IR: 300–400 TID for 1–3 days → 300–400 mg BID 1–3 days → discontinue
Anxiety disorders (off-label)	IR: 300–2,400 mg/day (in 2–3 divided doses)
Tremor (off-label)	600–1,200 mg TID (total daily dosage of 3,600 mg)

IX. **Monitoring**

A. Obtain creatinine levels at baseline and periodically.
B. Monitor for signs/symptoms of depression, behavior changes, suicidality.
C. Monitor for skin changes (Stevens-Johnson syndrome [SJS], toxic epidermal necrolysis [TEN]), particularly during initiation and reintroduction.

X. **Relevant Pharmacokinetics/Pharmacodynamics**

A. **Metabolism**: Gabapentin is cleared renally (100% unchanged); it has no hepatic metabolism.
   1. Gabapentin is highly lipid soluble, making it readily distributed across the blood-brain barrier.
B. **Time to peak plasma concentration**: IR: 2–4 hours; ER: 8 hours
C. **Half-life**: 5–7 hours
D. **Hepatic impairment**: No adjustment required.
E. **Renal impairment**: Adjust dosage according to Table 3–11. Gabapentin can be removed by hemodialysis.

Table 3–11. Gabapentin dosage adjustment for patients with renal impairment

CrCl (mL/minute)	Dosage
30–59	200–700 mg BID
16–29	200–700 mg once daily
15	100–300 mg once daily
<15	Decrease dosage proportionally from CrCl 15

Note. CrCl=creatinine clearance (volume of blood plasma cleared of creatinine per unit time).

XI. **Clinically Relevant Drug Interactions**

A. Gabapentin has few pharmacokinetic drug interactions.
B. Use caution with other CNS depressants (additive effects).
C. Gabapentin binds to polyvalent cations; absorption decreased by chelation (take 2 hours apart from calcium, magnesium, chromium, iron, zinc).
D. Do not take within 2 hours of administration of an antacid.
E. Naproxen may increase absorption.
F. Drugs that lower the seizure threshold may decrease gabapentin's antiseizure effects.

XII. **Adverse Effects**

A. **Common**:

1. Somnolence, dizziness, ataxia, fatigue, diplopia, tremor, abnormal thinking, depression, xerostomia, amblyopia, amnesia, euphoric mood, irritability: Sedative effects can wear off with time. Side effects are dosage dependent.

B. **Other effects**:

1. Nausea, vomiting, fever, peripheral edema, nystagmus, headache, constipation, dysarthria, weight gain, back pain, impotence, dyspepsia, asthenia, diarrhea, infection: Side effects are dosage dependent and usually wear off with time.
2. Hostility, emotional lability, hyperkinesia in children: Educate parents to watch for this potential paradoxical response.

C. **Serious reactions**:

1. Stevens-Johnson syndrome, angioedema, hypersensitivity reaction, anaphylactoid reaction, eosinophilic drug reaction, erythema multiforme, rhabdomyolysis: Monitor for skin changes, particularly during initiation and reintroduction, and titrate slowly.
2. Respiratory depression, suicidality, withdrawal with possible seizures if abruptly discontinued: Use the lowest effective dosage; taper slowly to discontinue use.

D. **Risks in pregnancy and lactation**

1. Gabapentin was designated a Category C drug in the prior FDA classification and is present in breast milk. A thorough risk/benefit discussion with the patient is recommended on continuing versus stopping the medication, including consultation with an OB/GYN specialist and/or lactation expert. See Chapter 15 ("Women: Pregnancy, Postpartum, and Breastfeeding") for more information.

XIII. **Clinical Pearls/Prescribing Tips**

A. Gabapentin is a Schedule V controlled substance. Routinely assess for use of other narcotics (boxed warning with opioids).
B. Most gabapentin use is off-label (such use may be justified for generalized anxiety disorder [GAD], panic disorder, and social anxiety disorder). Gabapentin is not FDA approved for anxiety disorders in the United States but is approved for GAD in Europe.

C. Gabapentin is often used in combination with SSRIs, SNRIs, or TCAs to treat anxiety and pain. It appears to be helpful for somatic and psychiatric symptoms of anxiety disorders and for patients with comorbid pain and anxiety disorders.
D. Some studies have reported mood-stabilizing effects. Gabapentin can be used as an augmenting agent; however, it has not demonstrated effectiveness as a monotherapy for bipolar disorder.
E. Notable benefits of gabapentin include the following: 1) it is not metabolized by the liver, and therefore can be used in patients with liver disease (100% unchanged urine excretion); 2) it is generally safe in long-term use; 3) it has a relatively mild side-effect profile and is generally well tolerated; 4) it has few pharmacokinetic drug interactions; 5) it enhances slow-wave delta sleep; and 6) discontinuation symptoms are less common with gabapentin than with other medications for anxiety.
F. Gabapentin can produce psychoactive effects and feelings of euphoria, and thus carries risk of psychological dependence and abuse potential (it is deemed a controlled substance in many states).
G. Gabapentin can cause rebound or paradoxical pain and can induce paradoxical reactions, including hyperactivity and agitation, especially in children.
H. In patients taking gabapentin for epilepsy, withdrawal from the drug, especially if abrupt, can lead to a rebound in or increased frequency of seizure activity.
I. Gabapentin can decrease concomitant opioid use.
J. Patients taking gabapentin should be monitored for suicidality.
K. Development of new or worsening tumors has been reported in humans taking gabapentin, although the causal relationship is unclear; however, recent analyses suggest that there is no link (Friedman et al. 2019).

Further Reading

Bockbrader HN, Wesche D, Miller R, et al: A comparison of the pharmacokinetics and pharmacodynamics of pregabalin and gabapentin. Clin Pharmacokinet 49(10):661–669, 2010 20818832

Neurontin (gabapentin) [package insert]. U.S Food and Drug Administration, 2022. Available at: https://www.accessdata.fda.gov/spl/data/20876c74-5c0b-472c-a19a-d79987402df2/20876c74-5c0b-472c-a19a-d79987402df2.xml. Accessed March 13, 2024.

Ondo W, Hunter C, Vuong KD, et al: Gabapentin for essential tremor: a multiple-dose, double-blind, placebo-controlled trial. Mov Disord 15(4):678–682, 2000 10928578

Stahl SM: Anticonvulsants as anxiolytics, part 2: pregabalin and gabapentin as alpha(2)delta ligands at voltage-gated calcium channels. J Clin Psychiatry 65(4):460–461, 2004 15119905

References

Friedman GD, Achacoso N, Habel LA: Gabapentin and cancer risk: updated findings from Kaiser Permanente Northern California. Perm J 23:18-040, 2019 30939265

Hydroxyzine[1]

I. **Brand Names**: Atarax (discontinued in U.S.), Vistaril

II. **Therapeutic Class**: Antihistamine (first-generation); anxiolytic, antiemetic, hypnotic

III. **Mechanism-Based Class**: Histamine receptor antagonist

IV. **Mechanism(s) of Action**

A. Nonselective central and peripheral histamine H_1 receptor antagonist (Ki=2.0–19 nM), leading to sedative and anti-nausea effects

B. Minor 5-HT_{2A} antagonist (Ki=170 nM), potentially contributing to anti-anxiety effects.

C. The antimuscarinic (anticholinergic) effect of hydroxyzine is much weaker than that of other first-generation antihistamines, such as diphenhydramine (Kubo et al. 1987); for example, hydroxyzine muscarinic acetylcholine (mACh) Ki=4,600 nM versus diphenhydramine M_3 Ki=84–229 nM. Thus, hydroxyzine is believed to be safer in elderly individuals than conventionally thought, although caution is still recommended in this population, especially at high dosages.

V. **Indications**

A. FDA adult and pediatric:

1. Anxiety
2. Pruritus/urticaria
3. Sedation (anesthesia adjunct)
4. Peripartum management: Reduce opioid dosage, control nausea

B. Evidence-based[2] off-label uses:

1. Insomnia
2. Muscle tension
3. Nausea/vomiting
4. Acute agitation

VI. **Major Contraindications and When to Use Caution**

A. **Contraindications**:

1. Known hypersensitivity to medication or class
2. Patients with prolonged QT interval

VII. **Dosage Formulations**

A. Generic: capsule (25 mg, 50 mg, 100 mg); tablet (10 mg, 25 mg, 50 mg); concentrate (10 mg/5 mL); injectable (25 mg/mL, 50 mg/mL; intramuscular only, not to be given intravenously or subcutaneously)

B. Brand: capsule (25 mg, 50 mg)

---

[1]Also see Chapter 4, "Nonbenzodiazepine Hypnotics," for information regarding hydroxyzine's off-label use for insomnia.

[2]Evidence strength varies; readers are referred to the literature for more detailed information.

VIII. **Dosage Ranges and Guidelines**

A. Dosage varies based on indication (see Table 3–12 for usual dosage ranges). Typical dosage range is 25–100 mg taken once daily to 4 times daily as needed (up to maximum dosage of 400 mg/day)

B. For pruritus/urticaria or patients sensitive to side effects, can start at lower dosages of 10–25 mg/day and increase as tolerated.

C. If too sedating, consider taking the daily dosage as a single dose at night. Use caution when combined with other sedative medications.

D. Divide dosage if higher than 100 mg/day.

Table 3–12. Hydroxyzine indications and dosage ranges

Indications	Usual dosage ranges
Anxiety	50–400 mg/day (e.g., 50–100 mg every 6 hours PRN) In children age <12 years: PO: 2 mg/kg/day in divided doses every 6 hours PRN IM: 0.5–1 mg/kg/dose IM every 4-6 hours PRN
Pruritus/urticaria	25–200 mg/day (e.g., 25 mg every 6–8 hours PRN) In children age <12 years: PO: 2 mg/kg/day in divided doses every 6 hours PRN IM: 0.5–1 mg/kg/dose IM every 4-6 hours PRN
Sedation with anesthesia	25–100 mg IM once PRN. Administer subsequent doses PO. In children age <12 years (may give prior to or after anesthesia): PO: 0.6 mg/kg/dose PO once PRN IM: 1.1 mg/kg/dose IM once PRN

Note. See manufacturer's prescribing information for further details on dosing (Pfizer Laboratories 2023).

IX. **Monitoring**

A. Creatinine, liver function tests, physical and psychiatric evaluation at baseline

B. Monitor vital signs, CBC, liver function tests, electrolytes, and urinalysis periodically during prolonged use.

X. **Relevant Pharmacokinetics/Pharmacodynamics**

A. **Metabolism**: Hepatic cytochrome P450 (CYP) unknown

B. **Active metabolite**: Cetirizine

C. **Time to peak plasma concentration**: 2–3 hours

D. **Half-life**: 20–25 hours

E. **Hepatic impairment**: Caution advised with severe impairment.

F. **Renal impairment**: CrCl <50 mL/minute: Decrease usual dosage by 50%; hydroxyzine is not significantly dialyzed.

XI. Clinically Relevant Drug Interactions

A. Caution with medications also known to have
   1. Anticholinergic effects.
   2. CNS depressant effects.
   3. Central histamine effects.

B. Caution with concomitant use of drugs known to prolong the QT interval, including certain antiarrhythmics (quinidine, procainamide, amiodarone, sotalol), antibiotics, methadone, ondansetron, droperidol, antipsychotics (haloperidol, ziprasidone, iloperidone, clozapine, quetiapine, chlorpromazine), and certain antidepressants (citalopram, fluoxetine).

C. May potentiate the actions of narcotics, CNS depressants, and anticholinergic medications, particularly meperidine (Demerol) and barbiturates.

D. May reverse the vasopressor effect of epinephrine. Use norepinephrine or metaraminol instead if necessary.

XII. Adverse Effects

A. **Most common**:
   1. Dizziness, drowsiness, xerostomia, ataxia, weakness, headache, nausea, slurred speech, bitter taste, agitation, hallucinations, tremor
   2. Children can have paradoxical effects and hyperactivity.

B. **Severe reactions**:
   1. Dyspnea, seizure, heat stroke, torsades de pointes, QT prolongation, respiratory depression (rare), bronchodilation

C. **Risks in pregnancy and lactation**:
   1. Pregnancy: Hydroxyzine should not be taken in early pregnancy. However, in late pregnancy and prepartum, IM injection can be used for anxiety and can reduce narcotic requirements by up to 50%, thus reducing neonatal narcotic effects.
   2. Lactation: For current information on benzodiazepine use in lactation, readers are referred to the Drugs and Lactation Database (LactMed; www.ncbi.nlm.nih.gov/books/NBK501922/).

XIII. Clinical Pearls/Prescribing Tips

A. Hydroxyzine's anti-anxiety effects could be related to minor 5-HT_{2A} antagonism (Lader and Scotto 1998) and also to the tranquilizing effects of H_1 antagonism.

B. Hydroxyzine is often used in conjunction with SSRIs and SNRIs for anxiety, especially for more severe anxiety.

C. Hydroxyzine is commonly used in inpatient psychiatric hospitals and for outpatients on an as-needed basis for anxiety disorders; it can also be given as an IM injection in an emergency.

D. Hydroxyzine has no dependence, tolerance, or abuse liability and no withdrawal effects; it is a non-habit-forming, practical, and effective treatment for anxiety.

E. Use caution when prescribing hydroxyzine in elderly individuals, particularly those with risk for falls. If hydroxyzine is used in conjunction with other CNS depressants, consider reducing the other CNS depressant dosage by half. Hydroxyzine is useful in peripartum and preoperative anxiety.
F. Hydroxyzine has very little affinity for muscarinic receptors compared with diphenhydramine, and thus is relatively much less likely to cause anticholinergic effects (although such effects are possible; use caution with elderly patients).
G. When used adjunctively to treat substance use disorder, hydroxyzine can effectively reduce narcotic dosages.
H. Hydroxyzine overdose can cause severe hypotension and QT prolongation/torsades de pointes (epinephrine is ineffective in resuscitation).
I. Hydroxyzine is metabolized in the liver to its main metabolite. cetirizine. Use caution in patients with hepatic dysfunction or severe kidney dysfunction.

References

Kubo N, Shirakawa O, Kuno T, Tanaka C: Antimuscarinic effects of antihistamines: quantitative evaluation by receptor-binding assay. Jpn J Pharmacol 43(3):277–282, 1987 2884340

Lader M, Scotto JC: A multicentre double-blind comparison of hydroxyzine, buspirone and placebo in patients with generalized anxiety disorder. Psychopharmacology (Berl) 139(4):402–406, 1998 9809861

Pfizer Laboratories: Vistaril (hydroxyzine pamoate) capsules and oral suspension [package insert]. Revised May 2023. Available at: https://dailymed.nlm.nih.gov/dailymed/fda/fdaDrugXsl.cfm?setid=c271f97f-040e-492b-9194-2c8b74675a95&type=display. Accessed September 9, 2024.

Pregabalin

I. **Brand Names**: Lyrica, Lyrica CR
II. **Therapeutic Class**: Anticonvulsant
III. **Mechanism-Based Class**: Glutamate, voltage gated calcium channel blocker
IV. **Mechanism(s) of Action**

A. Developed as a GABA analog.
B. High affinity for alpha-2/delta auxiliary subunit of voltage-sensitive calcium channels in CNS.
C. Does not appear to interact with the GABA receptor.
D. Modulates excitatory neurotransmitter release.

V. **Indications**

A. FDA adult:

1. Adjunctive treatment of partial seizures in adults and children (IR)
2. Postherpetic neuralgia (IR and CR)
3. Diabetic peripheral neuropathy (IR and CR)
4. Neuropathic pain associated with spinal cord injury (IR)
5. Fibromyalgia (IR)

B. Evidence-based[1] off-label uses:

1. Generalized anxiety disorder (GAD)
2. Peripheral neuropathic pain
3. Panic disorder
4. Social anxiety disorder
5. Pruritus
6. Vasomotor symptoms associated with menopause

C. FDA pediatric: None

VI. **Major Contraindications and When to Use Caution**

A. **Contraindications**:

1. Known hypersensitivity to medication or class

B. **Use caution**:

1. Kidney disease (CrCl <60 mL/minute): Adjust dosage (see Table 3–13 ["Pregabalin dosage conversion for patients with renal impairment"] in the "Relevant Pharmacokinetics/Pharmacodynamics" section later in this chapter).
2. Drug abuse history
3. Angioedema history
4. Respiratory impairment
5. Elderly individuals (sensitive to sedation effects, risk of falls)
6. Chronic heart failure (New York Heart Association [NYHA] Class III–IV)
7. Depression
8. Lactose intolerance (Lapp lactase deficiency or glucose-galactose malabsorption)
9. Concomitant CNS depressant use (additive effects)

C. Avoid abrupt withdrawal.

VII. **Dosage Formulations**

A. Brand/generic: IR capsule (25 mg, 50 mg, 75 mg, 100 mg, 150 mg, 200 mg, 225 mg, 300 mg); concentrate (20 mg/mL)

B. Brand/generic ER/CR tablet (82.5 mg, 165 mg, 247.5 mg, 330 mg)

1. Do not chew, break, or crush ER form. The ER tablet must be taken with food.

C. Conversion from IR to ER:

1. IR 75 mg=ER 82.5 mg
2. IR 150 mg=ER 165 mg
3. IR 225 mg=ER 247.5 mg
4. IR 300 mg=ER 330 mg
5. IR 450 mg=ER 495 mg
6. IR 600 mg=ER 660 mg

---

[1]Evidence strength varies; readers are referred to the literature for more detailed information.

VIII. **Dosage Ranges and Guidelines**

A. Dosage varies greatly based on indication and tolerance (see Table 3–13 for usual dosage ranges).
B. Typical dosage range for IR formulation is 150–600 mg/day taken in 2–3 divided doses (Baldwin et al. 2013); for CR formulation, typical dosage is 330 mg/day.
C. In general, give one-third to one-sixth of the dosage of gabapentin.
D. Use a reduced dosage for elderly individuals and those with fall risk, hepatic or respiratory disease, or concurrent opioid use.
E. **Titration**:
   1. For neuropathic pain, generally start at 25–150 mg/day (in 2–3 divided doses) and increase by 25–150 mg at weekly intervals to a maximum of 600 mg/day (in 2–3 divided doses).
   2. For anxiety, generally start at 150 mg/day (in 2–3 divided doses) and increase by 150 mg at weekly intervals to a maximum of 600 mg/day (in 2–3 divided doses).
F. **Tapering**: Taper dosage slowly over 1 or more weeks to minimize risk of withdrawal effects, including seizures.

Table 3–13. Pregabalin indications and dosage ranges

Indications	Usual dosage ranges
Partial seizures, adjunct	IR: 150–600 mg/day (in 2–3 divided doses) (75–300 mg BID or 50–200 mg TID)
General neuropathic pain	IR: 300–600 mg/day (in 2–3 divided doses)
Diabetic neuropathic pain	IR: 50–100 mg TID; maximum 450 mg/day (in 2–3 divided doses) ER/CR: 165–330 mg/day
Postherpetic neuralgia	IR: 150–300 mg/day (in 2–3 divided doses; 75–150 mg BID or 50–100 mg TID) ER/CR: 165–660 mg/day
Spinal cord injury–associated neuropathic pain	IR (oral): 75–300 mg BID Start with 75 mg BID; may increase within 1 week (based on response and tolerability) to 150 mg BID. After 2–3 weeks, may further increase, up to a maximum of 600 mg/day.
Fibromyalgia	IR: 75–225 mg BID; maximum dosage: 450 mg/day
Anxiety disorders (off-label)	IR: 150–600 mg/day (in 2–3 divided doses; 75–300 mg BID or 50–200 mg TID) Daily dosages lower than 150 mg may be suboptimal.
Restless legs syndrome (off-label)	IR: 150–450 mg 1–3 hours prior to bedtime

IX. Monitoring

A. Obtain creatinine levels at baseline and periodically.
B. Monitor for signs/symptoms of depression, behavior changes, suicidality.
C. Monitor for skin changes (Stevens-Johnson syndrome [SJS], toxic epidermal necrolysis [TEN]), particularly during initiation and reintroduction.

X. Relevant Pharmacokinetics/Pharmacodynamics

A. **Metabolism**: Renal (90% unchanged); minimal to no hepatic metabolism
B. **Time to peak plasma concentration**: Affected by food intake (IR: 1.5 hours fasting/3 hours with food; ER: 8 hours with food)
C. **Half-life**: 5–7 hours (adults); 3–6 hours (pediatric patients)
D. **Hepatic impairment**: No adjustment required.
E. **Renal impairment**: Adjust dosage according to creatinine clearance (see Table 3–14 for dosage conversions for renally impaired patients). Pregabalin can be removed by hemodialysis (see Table 3–15 for dosage conversions for patients undergoing hemodialysis).

Table 3–14. Pregabalin dosage conversion for patients with renal impairment

Normal dosage	CrCl 30–60	CrCl 15–29	CrCl <15
150 mg/day	75 mg/day (BID–TID)	25–50 mg/day (QD–BID)	25 mg/day
300 mg/day	150 mg/day (BID–TID)	75 mg/day (QD–BID)	25–50 mg/day
450 mg/day	225 mg/day (BID–TID)	100–150 mg/day (QD–BID)	50–75 mg/day
600 mg/day	300 mg/day (BID–TID)	150 mg/day (QD–BID)	75 mg/day

Note. CrCl=creatinine clearance (mL/minute). BID=twice daily; QD=once daily; TID=three times daily.

Table 3–15. Pregabalin dosage conversion for patients undergoing hemodialysis

Normal dosage	Converted dosage
150 mg/day	25 mg once daily (25–50 mg*)
300 mg/day	25–50 mg once daily (50–75 mg*)
450 mg/day	50–75 mg once daily (75–100 mg*)
600 mg/day	75 mg once daily (100–150 mg*)

*Given as supplement after dialysis if next dose is not due directly after dialysis.

XI. Clinically Relevant Drug Interactions

A. Use caution with other CNS depressants (additive effects).
B. Few pharmacokinetic drug interactions.
C. Drugs that lower seizure threshold may decrease pregabalin's antiseizure effects.
D. Use caution with other drugs that can cause angioedema.

XII. Adverse Effects

A. **Most common**:

1. Sedation, impaired attention, confusion, blurred vision, diplopia, dizziness, ataxia, fatigue, tremor, dysarthria, paresthesia, memory impairment, poor coordination, euphoric mood, irritability; Sedative effects can wear off with time. Side effects are dosage dependent.

B. **Other effects**:

1. Vomiting, dry mouth, constipation, flatulence, weight gain, increased appetite, peripheral edema, libido decreased, erectile dysfunction. Side effects are dosage dependent. Food affects absorption.

C. **Serious reactions**:

1. Stevens-Johnson syndrome, angioedema, hypersensitivity reaction, anaphylactoid reaction, exfoliative dermatitis, rhabdomyolysis, thrombocytopenia: monitor for skin changes, particularly during initiation and reintroduction, and titrate slowly.
2. Respiratory depression, suicidality, withdrawal with possible seizures if abruptly discontinued: use lowest effective dosage; taper slowly to discontinue use.

D. **Risks in pregnancy and lactation**:

1. Pregabalin has not been studied in pregnant women. It was designated a Category C drug in the prior FDA classification and is present in breast milk. A thorough risk/benefit discussion with the patient is recommended on continuing versus stopping the medication, including consultation with an OB/GYN specialist and/or lactation expert. See Chapter 15 ("Women: Pregnancy, Postpartum, and Breastfeeding") for more information.

XIII. Clinical Pearls/Prescribing Tips

A. Pregabalin is not FDA approved for anxiety disorders in the United States, although it is approved for GAD in Europe.

B. Most use of pregabalin is off-label (use may be justified for generalized anxiety disorder, panic disorder, and social anxiety disorder). Off-label use of pregabalin for bipolar disorder may not be justified.

C. Pregabalin is often used in combination with SSRIs, SNRIs, and TCAs for anxiety and pain. In addition, it is helpful for somatic and psychiatric symptoms of anxiety disorders and for patients with comorbid pain and anxiety disorders.

D. Pregabalin is more potent and possibly better tolerated than gabapentin.

E. Notable benefits of pregabalin include the following: 1) it is not metabolized by the liver, and therefore can be used in patients with liver disease (100% unchanged urine excretion); 2) it is generally safe in long-term use; 3) it has a relatively mild side-effect profile and is generally well tolerated; 4) it has few pharmacokinetic drug interactions; 5) it enhances slow-wave delta sleep; and 6) discontinuation symptoms are less common with pregabalin than with other medications for anxiety.

F. Pregabalin can produce psychoactive effects and feelings of euphoria, and thus carries risk for psychological dependence and abuse potential (Schedule V controlled substance).

G. Pregabalin can cause rebound or paradoxical pain and can induce paradoxical reactions, including hyperactivity and agitation, especially in children.
H. In patients taking pregabalin for epilepsy, withdrawal from the drug, especially if abrupt, can lead to a rebound in or increased frequency of seizure activity.
I. Pregabalin can reduce concomitant opioid use.
J. Individuals taking pregabalin should be monitored for suicidality.
K. Pregabalin was found to induce hemangiosarcomas in mice models; however, no evidence in humans is available (Pfizer Inc 2020).

Further Reading

Bockbrader HN, Wesche D, Miller R, et al: A comparison of the pharmacokinetics and pharmacodynamics of pregabalin and gabapentin. Clin Pharmacokinet 49(10):661–669, 2010 20818832

Lauria-Horner BA, Pohl RB: Pregabalin: a new anxiolytic. Expert Opin Investig Drugs 12(4):663–672, 2003 12665421

Montgomery S, Emir B, Haswell H, et al: Long-term treatment of anxiety disorders with pregabalin: a 1 year open-label study of safety and tolerability. Curr Med Res Opin 29(10):1223–1230, 2013 23808960

Moore RA, Straube S, Wiffen PJ, et al: Pregabalin for acute and chronic pain in adults. Cochrane Database Syst Rev (3):CD007076, 2009 19588419

Stahl SM: Anticonvulsants and the relief of chronic pain: pregabalin and gabapentin as alpha(2)delta ligands at voltage-gated calcium channels. J Clin Psychiatry 65(5):596–597, 2004 15163243

References

Baldwin DS, Ajel K, Masdrakis VG, et al: Pregabalin for the treatment of generalized anxiety disorder: an update. Neuropsychiatr Dis Treat 9:883–892, 2013 23836974

Pfizer Inc: Lyrica (pregabalin capsule, solution) [package insert]. U.S Food and Drug Administration website. Revised May 2020. Available at: https://www.accessdata.fda.gov/spl/data/b9b1285a-2cb3-4789-8b0e-8d5e1b253534/b9b1285a-2cb3-4789-8b0e-8d5e1b253534.xml. Accessed March 13, 2024.

Propranolol

I. **Brand Names**: Inderal, Inderal LA, Inderal XL, Hemangeol, InnoPran XL
II. **Therapeutic Class**: Antihypertensive
III. **Mechanism-Based Class**: Competitive nonselective beta-blocker
IV. **Mechanism(s) of Action**

A. Adrenergic inhibition: Competitively inhibits the binding of catecholamines, thus blocking sympathetic stimulation of β_1-adrenergic receptors in the vascular smooth muscle and cardiac myocytes.
B. For tremor, competitive inhibition of peripheral β_2-adrenergic receptors (also in bronchial smooth muscle leading to bronchial vasospasm)
C. Serotonergic activity: Via 5-HT_{1A} and 5-HT_{1B}, possible role in treating migraine
D. $Beta_1$-adrenergic receptor blockade may potentially prevent fear conditioning and autonomic hyperactivity in PTSD.
E. Inhibition of nitric oxide synthesis.

V. **Indications**

A. FDA adult:

1. Migraine prophylaxis
2. Essential tremor
3. Pheochromocytoma
4. Chronic stable angina
5. Atrial fibrillation/ flutter
6. Cardiac arrhythmias
7. Post–myocardial infarction risk reduction
8. Idiopathic hypertrophic subaortic stenosis (IHSS)
9. Hypertension

B. Evidence-based[1] off-label uses:

1. Performance anxiety
2. Panic disorder
3. Antipsychotic-induced akathisia
4. Parkinsonian tremor
5. Violence, aggression
6. Generalized anxiety disorder
7. PTSD, prophylactic

C. FDA pediatric: None

VI. **Major Contraindications and When to Use Caution**

A. **Contraindications**:

1. Known allergy to medication or class
2. Concomitant use of alpha-agonists, which can lead to unopposed alpha-activation, resulting in malignant hypertension.

---

[1]Evidence strength varies; readers are referred to the literature for more detailed information.

3. Bradycardia, heart block, cardiogenic shock
4. Severe chronic obstructive pulmonary disease or bronchial asthma

VII. **Dosage Formulations**

A. Brand: LA capsule (60 mg, 80 mg, 120 mg, 160 mg); XL capsule (80 mg, 120 mg)
B. Generic: tablet (10 mg, 20 mg, 40 mg, 60 mg, 80 mg); capsule (60 mg, 80 mg, 120 mg, 160 mg); ER capsule (60 mg, 80 mg, 120 mg, 160 mg); concentrate (20 mg/5 mL, 40 mg/5 mL); injection—various (1 mg/1 mL)

VIII. **Dosage Ranges and Guidelines**

A. Dosage varies greatly based on indication and tolerance (see Table 3–16 for usual dosage ranges).
B. **Titration**:
   1. For performance anxiety, start at a dose of 10–20 mg taken 1 hour prior to the anxiety-producing event. If ineffective, can increase dose by 10–20 mg up to a maximum of 80 mg/day.
   2. For other indications, dosages can vary greatly. Dosages of up to 240 mg/day have been used for PTSD and of up to 400 mg/day for aggression or migraine.
C. **Tapering**: Taper over 1–2 weeks.
   1. Boxed warning: Rapid cessation of propranolol is associated with a boxed warning for severe angina exacerbation, myocardial infarction, or ventricular arrhythmias in patients with preexisting angina (Fresenius Kabi USA 2023).

Table 3–16. Propranolol indications and dosage ranges

Indications	Usual dosage ranges
Migraine	IR/ER: 40–400 mg (in 2–3 divided doses) Manufacturer's labeling lists 240 mg/day as the maximum dosage
Essential tremor	IR/ER: 60–320 mg (in 2–3 divided doses)
PTSD (off-label)	40–240 mg (in 2–3 divided doses)
Aggression (off-label)	40–400 mg (in 2–3 divided doses) 20–120 mg (divided doses BID–TID)
Performance anxiety (off-label)	10–80 mg taken 30 minutes to 1 hour prior to event
Akathisia due to antipsychotics (off-label)	10–120 mg/day (taken as a single dose or in 2 divided doses)
Lithium-induced tremor (off-label)	10–80 mg/day (in 3–4 divided doses)

IX. **Monitoring**

A. Blood pressure and heart rate should be monitored.

X. **Relevant Pharmacokinetics/Pharmacodynamics**

A. **Metabolism**: Hepatic extensively; cytochrome P450 (CYP) 1A2, CYP2C19, CYP2D6 (primary)

B. **Time to peak plasma concentration**: 1–4 hours (IR); 12–14 hours (ER); 6 hours (long acting)

C. **Half-life**: 3–5 hours (IR); 8–11 hours (ER)

D. **Hepatic impairment**: Caution advised; consider decreasing IV dosage.

E. **Renal impairment**: Not defined, caution advised.

XI. **Clinically Relevant Drug Interactions**

A. Metabolized by CYP1A2, CYP2D6, and to a lesser extent CYP2C19

1. Propranolol levels can be increased by drugs that inhibit CYP2D6 metabolism, such as oral contraceptives, cimetidine, ciprofloxacin, hydralazine, hydroxychloroquine, phenothiazines, loop diuretics, and SSRIs.

B. Weak inhibitor of CYP1A2

C. Selective inhibitor of monoamine oxidase A (MAO-A)

D. Concomitant use with other antihypertensive agents can worsen hypotension, bradycardia, QTc prolongation, arrhythmias, orthostasis, and slow atrioventricular conduction.

E. Use caution with calcium channel blockers (additive effects).

F. Increased risk of orthostatic hypotension when combined with prazosin.

G. Can increase adverse effects of gabapentin and benzodiazepines.

H. Can increase anticoagulant effect of warfarin.

I. Thyroid hormone, penicillins, barbiturates, cholestyramine, and calcium and aluminum salts can all decrease the effects of propranolol.

XII. **Adverse Effects**

A. **Most common**:

1. Bradycardia, hypotension, vertigo, fatigue, dizziness, depression, sleep disturbances
2. Sexual dysfunction, decreased libido, urinary retention
3. Exacerbation of Raynaud's phenomenon, joint pain, peripheral vascular disease
4. Changes in glucose, weight gain
5. Rebound hypertension (when discontinued)
6. Sinusitis, pneumonia, bronchospasm, upper respiratory infection symptoms

B. **Boxed warning**: Rapid cessation of propranolol can lead to severe angina exacerbation, myocardial infarction, and ventricular arrhythmias in patients with preexisting angina. To avoid these effects, a gradual taper of 1–2 weeks is recommended if propranolol needs to be discontinued (Fresenius Kabi USA 2023).

C. **Risks in pregnancy and lactation**: Propranolol was designated a Category C drug in the prior FDA classification and is present in breast milk. A thorough risk/benefit discussion with the patient is recommended on continuing versus stopping the medication, including consultation with an OB/GYN specialist and/or lactation expert. See Chapter 15 ("Women: Pregnancy, Postpartum, and Breastfeeding") for more information.

XIII. **Clinical Pearls/Prescribing Tips**

A. Propranolol is often used in combination with other medications.
B. Propranolol is an effective adjunctive treatment for situational and generalized anxiety.
C. Propranolol is not habit forming and does not affect the sensorium at lower dosages; thus, it is particularly useful in situations where use of other sedating anxiolytic medications is not advisable (e.g., test-taking, performance, or work-related anxiety; history of substance use disorder)
D. Use of propranolol should be avoided in patients with severe asthma or chronic obstructive pulmonary disease.

Further Reading

Glennon R, Dukat M, Westkaemper RB: Serotonin receptor subtypes and ligands, in Psychopharmacology: The Fourth Generation of Progress. Edited by Bloom FE, Kupfer DJ. New York, Raven Press, 2000, pp 415–429

Sprouse JS, Aghajanian GK: (-)-Propranolol blocks the inhibition of serotonergic dorsal raphe cell firing by 5-HT1A selective agonists. Eur J Pharmacol 128(3):295–298, 1986 2878817

References

Fresenius Kabi USA: Propranolol (propranolol hydrochloride injection, solution) [package insert]. U.S Food and Drug Administration website. Revised January 2023. Available at: https://www.accessdata.fda.gov/spl/data/505851c4-b18c-4cd7-805c-4e923cc1fa7e/505851c4-b18c-4cd7-805c-4e923cc1fa7e.xml. Accessed March 13, 2024.

4

Nonbenzodiazepine Hypnotics

Richard C. Shelton, M.D.

Overview

- Several classes of nonbenzodiazepine medications are used for sleep disorders (insomnia or nightmares), including $GABA_A$ receptor–positive allosteric modulators ($GABA_A$ PAMs), melatonin and melatonin receptor agonists, orexin receptor antagonists, antihistamines, and sedating antidepressants. Norepinephrine α_1 receptor antagonist antihypertensives are used for treatment of nightmares, particularly in the context of PTSD.
- Patient education on sleep hygiene should be provided for all patients with insomnia. Cognitive-behavioral therapy for insomnia (CBT-i) is equally effective as medications and should be used prior to medication management whenever possible. Among medications for insomnia, melatonin and the melatonin receptor agonist ramelteon, sedating antidepressants, and orexin receptor antagonists should be tried before using $GABA_A$ PAMs.
- Prazosin is the most commonly used α_1 receptor antagonist for nightmares. However, doxazosin has a much longer half-life and can provide some relief for hyperarousal symptoms of PTSD during the day.

GABA-A Receptor Positive Allosteric Modulators (PAMs)

Eszopiclone

I. **Brand Name**: Lunesta

II. **Therapeutic Class**: Nonbenzodiazepine hypnotic

III. **Mechanism-Based Class**: $GABA_A$ receptor positive allosteric modulator

IV. **Mechanism(s) of Action**

A. Positive allosteric modulator of $GABA_A$ receptors at the benzodiazepine binding site; enhances activity of $GABA_A$ receptors.

B. Binds to $GABA_A$ receptor α_1, α_2, α_3, and α_5 subunits with approximately equal affinity.

V. **Indications**

A. FDA adult: Insomnia (decreases sleep latency, improves sleep maintenance)

B. Evidence-based[1] off-label uses: Antidepressant adjunctive therapy for treatment-resistant depression (two positive, two negative trials [Aiken and Newsome 2021])

C. FDA pediatric: None

VI. **Major Contraindications and When to Use Caution**

A. **Major contraindications**:

1. Known allergy to eszopiclone or zopiclone

B. **Use caution**:

1. Recent history of sedative-hypnotic or alcohol use disorders.
2. Older adult patients (risk of accidents).

VII. **Dosage Formulations**

A. Brand tablet (1 mg, 2 mg, 3 mg [*not scored*])

B. Generic tablet (1 mg, 2 mg, 3 mg [*not scored*])

VIII. **Dosage Ranges and Guidelines**

A. Refer to Table 4–1 for dosage ranges and guidelines.

B. Start at 1 mg taken about 60 minutes before bedtime (T_{max}=90 minutes).

C. May increase to 2 mg or 3 mg if needed.

D. Consider lower starting doses in elderly adult patients (1/2 of 1-mg tablet).

---

[1]Evidence strength varies; readers are referred to the literature for more detailed information.

Table 4–1. Eszopiclone indications and dosage ranges

Indications	Usual dosage ranges
Insomnia	1–3 mg/day
Treatment-resistant major depressive disorder	1–3 mg/day

IX. **Monitoring**: None

X. **Relevant Pharmacokinetics/Pharmacodynamics**

A. **Metabolism**: Hepatic (cytochrome P450 [CYP] 3A4 and CYP2E1)

B. **Time to peak plasma concentration**: 1 hour

C. **Half-life**: 6 hours

D. **Hepatic impairment**: No dosage adjustment needed except for severe hepatic impairment.

E. **Renal impairment**: No dosage adjustment necessary (only 10% renal elimination).

XI. **Clinically Relevant Drug Interactions**

A. Metabolized by CYP3A4

1. Dosage adjustment is required with CYP3A4 inhibitors or inducers.

B. Use with caution in combination with other sedative-hypnotics (e.g., benzodiazepines), which may increase risk for oversedation and accidents.

XII. **Adverse Effects**

A. **Most common**:

1. CNS: Daytime somnolence ("hangover" effect), dizziness, lightheadedness, discoordination
2. Other: Dry mouth, dysgeusia (bad taste)

B. **Uncommon**: Anxiety, confusion, disinhibition, discoordination/ataxia, memory problems, rash or other allergic reaction

C. **Risks in pregnancy and lactation**:

1. Eszopiclone was designated a Category C drug in the prior FDA classification and is present in breast milk. A thorough risk/benefit discussion with the patient is recommended on continuing versus stopping the medication, including consultation with an OB/GYN specialist and/or lactation expert. See Chapter 15 ("Women: Pregnancy, Postpartum, and Breastfeeding") for more information.

XIII. **Clinical Pearls/Prescribing Tips**

A. Use in elderly adults is not recommended, given that eszopiclone increases risk for discoordination and falls in these patients. Limit dosage in older adults (age ≥65 years) to a maximum of 3 mg/day.

B. Eszopiclone and zopiclone (half-life 6 hours) may provide greater improvement in sleep maintenance relative to zolpidem (half-life 3 hours) or zaleplon (half-life 1 hour). In particular, eszopiclone and zopiclone, because of their relatively longer half-life, may have utility in middle as well as initial insomnia.

C. Approximate comparative half-lives of the "Z drugs" are as follows: zaleplon (1 hour) < zolpidem IR (2.5 hours) < zolpidem CR (5 hours) < eszopiclone (6 hours).
D. Cognitive-behavioral therapy for insomnia (CBT-i) is an effective alternative to medication management.

Further Reading

American Academy of Sleep Medicine Clinical Practice Guidelines. Available at: https://aasm.org/clinical-resources/practice-standards/practice-guidelines/. Accessed May 2022.

Bhandari P, Sapra A: Zaleplon [updated June 21, 2023], in StatPearls [internet]. Treasure Island, FL, StatPearls Publishing, 2024 January–. Available at: https://www.ncbi.nlm.nih.gov/books/NBK551571/. Accessed June 21, 2024.

Eszopiclone product information: U.S. Food and Drug Administration, 2008. Available at: https://www.accessdata.fda.gov/drugsatfda_docs/label/2009/021476s012lbl.pdf. Accessed May 2022.

U.S. Food and Drug Administration: Clinical pharmacology review, eszopiclone. Available at: https://www.fda.gov/files/drugs/published/Eszopiclone-21476-Clinpharm-BPCA.pdf. Accessed May 2022.

References

Aiken C, Newsome K: Can Eszopiclone Augment Antidepressants? (Podcast). Newburyport, MA, Carlat Publishing, 2021. Available at: https://www.thecarlatreport.com/blogs/2-the-carlat-psychiatry-podcast/post/3428-can-eszopiclone-augment-antidepressants-#:~:text=Kellie%20Newsome%3A%20So%20far%20eszopiclone,helped%20sleep%20but%20not%20depression. Accessed July 15, 2024.

Zaleplon

I. **Brand Name**: Sonata
II. **Therapeutic Class**: Nonbenzodiazepine hypnotic
III. **Mechanism-Based Class**: $GABA_A$ receptor positive allosteric modulator
IV. **Mechanism(s) of Action**

A. Positive allosteric modulator of $GABA_A$ receptors at the benzodiazepine binding site; enhances activity of $GABA_A$ receptors.
B. Zaleplon has higher affinity for $GABA_A$ receptor α_1 subunits than for α_2 or α_3 subunits. It also has greater binding at γ_3 than at γ_2 subunit–containing receptors.

V. **Indications**

A. FDA adult: Insomnia (decreases sleep latency)
B. Off-label uses: None
C. FDA pediatric: None

VI. **Major Contraindications and When to Use Caution**

A. **Major contraindications**:

1. Known allergy to zaleplon

B. **Use caution**:

1. Recent history of sedative-hypnotic or alcohol use disorders
2. Elderly patients (risk of accidents)

VII. **Dosage Formulations**

A. Brand capsule (5 mg, 10 mg)
B. Generic capsule (5 mg, 10 mg)

VIII. **Dosage Ranges and Guidelines**

A. Start at 5 mg taken about 60 minutes before bedtime (T_{max}=90 minutes).
B. May increase to 10 mg if needed. Occasionally patients may benefit from a 20-mg dose if they do not see benefit at lower doses.
C. Limit dosage to 5 mg/day in older adult patients.

IX. **Monitoring**: None
X. **Relevant Pharmacokinetics/Pharmacodynamics**

A. **Metabolism**: Hepatic (cytochrome P450 [CYP] 3A4 and CYP1A2)
B. **Time to peak plasma concentration**: 1 hour
C. **Half-life**: 1 hour
D. **Hepatic impairment**: No adjustment needed except for severe hepatic impairment.
E. **Renal impairment**: No dosage adjustment necessary (only 10% renal elimination).

XI. **Clinically Relevant Drug Interactions**

A. Metabolized by CYP3A4.

1. Dosage adjustment is required with CYP3A4 inhibitors or inducers.

B. Use with caution in combination with other sedative-hypnotics (e.g., benzodiazepines), which may increase risk for oversedation and accidents.

XII. **Adverse Effects**

A. **Most common**:

1. CNS: Daytime somnolence ("hangover" effect), dizziness, lightheadedness, discoordination
2. Other: Dry mouth, dysgeusia (bad taste)

B. **Uncommon**: Anxiety, confusion, disinhibition, discoordination/ataxia, memory problems, rash or other allergic reaction

C. **Risks in pregnancy and lactation**:

1. Zaleplon was designated a Category C drug in the prior FDA classification and is present in breast milk. A thorough risk/benefit discussion with the patient is recommended on continuing versus stopping the medication, including consultation with an OB/GYN specialist and/or lactation expert. See Chapter 15 ("Women: Pregnancy, Postpartum, and Breastfeeding") for more information.

XIII. **Clinical Pearls/Prescribing Tips**

A. Limit dosage in older adults (age ≥65 years) to a maximum of 5 mg/day.

B. Because of its relatively short half-life (1 hour), zaleplon may be a preferred agent in patients with only initial insomnia.

C. Approximate comparative half-lives of the "Z drugs" are as follows: zaleplon (1 hour) < zolpidem IR (2.5 hours) < zolpidem CR (5 hours) < eszopiclone (6 hours).

D. Cognitive-behavioral therapy for insomnia (CBT-i) is an effective alternative to medication management.

Further Reading

American Academy of Sleep Medicine Clinical Practice Guidelines. Available at: https://aasm.org/clinical-resources/practice-standards/practice-guidelines/. Accessed May 2022.

Bhandari P, Sapra A: Zaleplon, in StatPearls. Treasure Island, FL, StatPearls Publishing, 2021

Zaleplon Clinical Pharmacology Review. Center for Drug Evaluation and Research, 1998. Available at: https://www.accessdata.fda.gov/drugsatfda_docs/nda/99/20859_Sonata_clinphrmr.pdf. Accessed May 2022.

Zaleplon prescribing information. U.S. Food and Drug Administration, 2007. Available at: https://www.accessdata.fda.gov/drugsatfda_docs/label/2007/020859s011lbl.pdf. Accessed May 2022.

Zolpidem

I. **Brand Names**: Ambien, Ambien CR, Intermezzo (sublingual), ZolpiMist (oral mucosal spray)
II. **Therapeutic Class**: Nonbenzodiazepine hypnotic
III. **Mechanism-Based Class**: $GABA_A$ receptor positive allosteric modulator
IV. **Mechanism(s) of Action**

A. Positive allosteric modulator of $GABA_A$ receptors at the benzodiazepine binding site; enhances activity of $GABA_A$ receptors.
B. Predominantly a $GABA_A$ receptor α_1 subunit modulator, with much lower activity at α_2 and α_3 subunits.

V. **Indications**

A. FDA adult: Short-term treatment of insomnia
B. Off-label uses: None
C. FDA pediatric: None

VI. **Major Contraindications and When to Use Caution**

A. **Major contraindication**:

1. Known allergy to zolpidem

B. **Use caution**:

1. Recent history of sedative-hypnotic or alcohol use disorders
2. Older adult patients (risk of accidents)

VII. **Dosage Formulations**

A. Brand: Immediate-release (IR) tablet (5, 10 mg [*scored*]), controlled-release (CR) tablet (6.25 mg, 12.5 mg), sublingual tablet (1.75 mg, 3.5 mg), oral mucosal spray (5 mg, 10 mg)
B. Generic: IR tablet (5 mg, 10 mg [*scored*]), CR tablet (6.25 mg, 12.5 mg)

VIII. **Dosage Ranges and Guidelines**

A. Refer to Table 4–2 for dosage ranges and guidelines.
B. IR: Start at 2.5 mg or 5 mg taken about 60 minutes before bedtime (Tmax = 60 minutes). Raise to 10 mg if needed. For women, a dosage no higher than 5 mg/day taken at bedtime is recommended because of the risk of adverse effects (see "Gender difference in pharmacokinetics" in "Relevant Pharmacokinetics/Pharmacodynamics" section below). For adults older than 65 years, limit the IR dosage to 5 mg/day.
C. CR: Start at 6.25 mg. Increase to 12.5 mg as needed. For women, the dosage should not exceed 6.25 mg/day taken at bedtime (see "Gender difference in pharmacokinetics" in "Relevant Pharmacokinetics/Pharmacodynamics" section below). For adults older than 65 years, limit the CR dosage to 6.5 mg/day.
D. Sublingual tablet: 1.75 mg for women and 3.5 mg for men taken once nightly for middle-of-the-night awakening.

Table 4–2. Zolpidem dosage ranges for insomnia

Formulation	Usual dosage range
Immediate release	2.5–10 mg/day
Controlled release	6.25–12.5 mg/day
Sublingual tablet	1.75 mg/day (women), 3.5 mg/day (men) for middle-of-the-night awakening
Oral mucosal spray	5–10 mg/day

IX. **Monitoring**: None

X. **Relevant Pharmacokinetics/Pharmacodynamics**

A. **Metabolism**: Hepatic (cytochrome P450 [CYP] 3A4 and CYP1A2)

B. **Time to peak plasma concentration**:

1. IR: 1 hour
2. CR: 1 hour
3. Sublingual: 40 minutes
4. Oral mucosal spray: 30 minutes

C. **Half-life**: 3 hours

D. **Hepatic impairment**: Reduce dosage by 50% in moderate to severe hepatic impairment.

E. **Renal impairment**: No dosage adjustment necessary (limited renal elimination).

F. **Gender difference in pharmacokinetics**: Non-elderly women clear zolpidem tartrate from the body at a lower rate than non-elderly men. Given the higher blood levels of zolpidem tartrate in women than men at a given dose, the recommended initial dose for adult women is 5 mg, and the recommended dose for adult men is 5 or 10 mg (AvKARE 2024).

XI. **Clinically Relevant Drug Interactions**

A. Metabolized by CYP3A4.

1. Dosage adjustment required with CYP3A4 inhibitors or inducers.

B. Use with caution in combination with other sedative-hypnotics (e.g., benzodiazepines), which may increase the risk for oversedation and accidents. Do not combine with alcohol.

XII. **Adverse Effects**

A. **Most common**:

1. CNS: Daytime somnolence ("hangover" effect), dizziness, lightheadedness
2. Other: Dry mouth, dysgeusia (bad taste)

B. **Uncommon**: Anxiety, complex sleep behavior (e.g., sleepwalking), confusion, disinhibition, discoordination/ataxia, lethargy, memory problems, rash or other allergic reaction

C. **Risks in pregnancy and lactation:**
   1. Zolpidem was designated a Category C drug in the prior FDA classification. Use with caution during pregnancy. Zolpidem use is generally not recommended while breastfeeding.

XIII. **Clinical Pearls/Prescribing Tips**

A. Limit dosage in older adults (age ≥65 years) to a maximum of 5 mg/day (IR) or 6.5 mg/day (CR).
B. Complex sleep behavior may occur more commonly with zolpidem than with other Z drugs. Behaviors can include sleep walking, eating, or driving and can be dangerous. Patients usually have amnesia for these behaviors.
C. Eszopiclone (half-life 6 hours) may provide greater improvement in sleep maintenance relative to zaleplon (half-life 1 hour) of zolpidem (half-life 3 hours).
D. Approximate comparative half-lives of the "Z drugs" are as follows: zaleplon (1 hour) < zolpidem IR (2.5 hours) < zolpidem CR (5 hours) < eszopiclone (6 hours).
E. Cognitive-behavioral therapy for insomnia (CBT-i) is an effective alternative to medication management.

Further Reading

American Academy of Sleep Medicine Clinical Practice Guidelines. Available at: https://aasm.org/clinical-resources/practice-standards/practice-guidelines/. Accessed May 2022.

Bouchette D, Akhondi H, Quick J: Zolpidem, in StatPearls. Treasure Island, FL, StatPearls Publishing, 2022

Neubauer DN: ZolpiMist a new formulation of zolpidem tartrate for the short-term treatment of insomnia in the US. Nat Sci Sleep 2:79–84, 2010 23616700

Zolpidem (controlled release) product information. U.S. Food and Drug Administration, 2014. Available at: https://www.accessdata.fda.gov/drugsatfda_docs/label/2016/021774s018lbl.pdf. Accessed May 2022.

Zolpidem (controlled release) Clinical Pharmacology and Biopharmaceutics Review. Center for Drug Evaluation and Research, 2005. Available at: https://www.accessdata.fda.gov/drugsatfda_docs/nda/2005/021774s000_BioPharmR.pdf. Accessed May 2022.

Zolpidem (immediate release) product information. U.S. Food and Drug Administration, 2004. Available at: https://www.accessdata.fda.gov/drugsatfda_docs/label/2016/021774s018lbl.pdf. Accessed May 2022.

Zolpidem (immediate release) Clinical Pharmacology and Biopharmaceutics Review. Center for Drug Evaluation and Research, 2004. Available at: https://www.accessdata.fda.gov/drugsatfda_docs/nda/2007/021412s000_ClinPharmR.pdf. Accessed May 2022.

Zolpidem (sublingual) Clinical Pharmacology and Biopharmaceutics Review. Center for Drug Evaluation and Research, 2011. Available at: https://www.accessdata.fda.gov/drugsatfda_docs/nda/2011/022328Orig1s000ClinPharmR.pdf. Accessed May 2022.

References

AvKARE: Zolpidem tartrate [package insert]. U.S. Food and Drug Administration website. Revised January 2024. Available at: https://dailymed.nlm.nih.gov/dailymed/fda/fdaDrugXsl.cfm?setid=8247ff5c-c3da-f800-e053-2991aa0a9c48&type=display. Accessed July 2, 2024.

Zopiclone

I. **Brand Name**: Imovane (not currently available in the United States)

II. **Therapeutic Class**: Nonbenzodiazepine hypnotic

III. **Mechanism-Based Class**: $GABA_A$ receptor positive allosteric modulator

IV. **Mechanism(s) of Action**

A. Positive allosteric modulator of $GABA_A$ receptors at the benzodiazepine binding site; enhances activity of $GABA_A$ receptors.

B. Binds to $GABA_A$ receptor α_1, α_2, α_3, and α_5 subunits with approximately equal affinity.

V. **Indications**

A. FDA adult: None

B. Evidence-based[1] off-label uses: Insomnia (decreases sleep latency, improves sleep maintenance)

C. FDA pediatric: None

VI. **Major Contraindications and When to Use Caution**

A. **Major contraindications**:

1. Known allergy to zopiclone or eszopiclone

B. **Use caution**:

1. Recent history of sedative-hypnotic or alcohol use disorders
2. Elderly patients (risk of accidents)

VII. **Dosage Formulations**

A. Brand tablet (3.75, 7.5 mg [*scored*])

B. Generic tablet (3.75, 7.5 mg [*scored*])

VIII. **Dosage Ranges and Guidelines**

A. Start at 3.75 mg taken ~60 minutes before bedtime (Tmax=90 minutes).

B. May increase to 7.5 mg if needed.

C. Consider using lower starting doses (e.g., 1/2 tablet) in older adult patients.

IX. **Monitoring**: None

X. **Relevant Pharmacokinetics/Pharmacodynamics**

A. **Metabolism**: Hepatic (cytochrome P450 [CYP] 3A4 and CYP2E1)

B. **Time to peak plasma concentration**: 1 hour

C. **Half-life**: 6 hours

D. **Hepatic impairment**: No adjustment except for severe hepatic impairment.

E. **Renal impairment**: No dosage adjustment necessary (only 10% renal elimination).

XI. **Clinically Relevant Drug Interactions**

A. Metabolized by CYP3A4

1. Dosage adjustment is required with CYP3A4 inhibitors or inducers.

---

[1]Evidence strength varies; readers are referred to the literature for more detailed information.

B. Use with caution in combination with other sedative-hypnotics (e.g., benzodiazepines), which may increase risk for oversedation and accidents.

XII. **Adverse Effects**

A. **Most common**:

1. CNS: Daytime somnolence ("hangover" effect), dizziness, lightheadedness, discoordination
2. Other: Dry mouth, dysgeusia (bad taste)

B. **Uncommon**: Anxiety, confusion, disinhibition, discoordination/ataxia, memory problems, rash or other allergic reaction

C. **Risks in pregnancy and lactation**:

1. Zopiclone was designated a Category C drug in the prior FDA classification and is present in breast milk. A thorough risk/benefit discussion with the patient is recommended on continuing versus stopping the medication, including consultation with an OB/GYN specialist and/or lactation expert. See Chapter 15 ("Women: Pregnancy, Postpartum, and Breastfeeding") for more information.

XIII. **Clinical Pearls/Prescribing Tips**

A. Zopiclone is not currently available in the United States.
B. Clinical trials showed no evidence of significant tolerance over 6 months.
C. Limit dosage in older adults (age ≥65 years) to a maximum of 3.75 mg/day.
D. Zopiclone and eszopiclone (half-life 6 hours) may provide greater improvement in sleep maintenance relative to zolpidem (half-life 3 hours) or zaleplon (half-life 1 hour). In particular, zopiclone and eszopiclone, because of their relatively longer half-life, may have utility in middle as well as initial insomnia.
E. Approximate comparative half-lives of the "Z drugs" are as follows: zaleplon (1 hour) < zolpidem IR (2.5 hours) < zolpidem CR (5 hours) < eszopiclone (6 hours).
F. Cognitive-behavioral therapy for insomnia (CBT-i) is an effective alternative to medication management. One study showed superior benefit of CBT-i relative to zopiclone for insomnia in older patients (Sivertsen et al. 2006).

Further Reading

American Academy of Sleep Medicine Clinical Practice Guidelines: https://aasm.org/clinical-resources/practice-standards/practice-guidelines/. Accessed May 2022

Electronic Medicines Compendium review: Zaleplon. April 2022. https://www.medicines.org.uk/emc/medicine/26364/SPC/Zopiclone+7.5mg+Tablets/#gref. Accessed May 2022.

Noble S, Langtry HD, Lamb HM: Zopiclone: an update of its pharmacology, clinical efficacy and tolerability in the treatment of insomnia. Drugs 55(2):277–302, 1998 9506247

References

Sivertsen B, Omvik S, Pallesen S, et al: Cognitive behavioral therapy vs zopiclone for treatment of chronic primary insomnia in older adults: a randomized controlled trial. JAMA 295(24):2851–2858, 2006 16804151

Melatonin and Melatonin Receptor Agonists

Melatonin

I. **Brand Names**: ZzzQuil Zzzs, Olly, Unisom

II. **Therapeutic Class**: Insomnia treatment

III. **Mechanism-Based Class**: Natural melatonin receptor agonist extracted from animal products or made by microorganisms

IV. **Mechanism(s) of Action**

A. Activation of melatonin MT_1 (*MTR1A*) and MT_2 (*MTR1B*) receptors.

B. Melatonin receptors promote sleep and set circadian rhythm.

V. **Indications**

A. FDA adult: None

B. Evidence-based[1] off-label uses:

1. Insomnia
2. Delayed sleep-wake phase disorder
3. Non-24-hour sleep-wake rhythm disorder in individuals with blindness

C. FDA pediatric: None. There is weak evidence in support of melatonin for delayed sleep-wake phase disorder and irregular sleep-wake rhythm disorder.

VI. **Major Contraindications and When to Use Caution**

D. **Major contraindications**: Older adults with major neurocognitive disorder (McCleery and Sharpley 2020)

E. **Use caution**: Older adults with mild neurocognitive disorder (McCleery and Sharpley 2020)

VII. **Dosage Formulations**

A. Brand and generic immediate-release (IR) tablet and capsule (0.5 mg, 1 mg, 2.5 mg, 5 mg, 10 mg, 20 mg, 30 mg, 60 mg)

B. Brand and generic extended-release (ER) table and capsule (1.5 mg, 2 mg, 3 mg, 4 mg, 5 mg, 6 mg, 7.5 mg, 10 mg)

C. Brand and generic gummies (0.3 mg, 1 mg, 5 mg, 6 mg, 10 mg)

D. Brand and generic liquid (0.05 mg/mL, 0.25 mg/mL, 1 mg/mL, 3 mg/mL, 4 mg/mL, 5 mg/mL, 10 mg/mL)

E. Other forms: Orally dissolving tablet (ODT), dissolving strip, sublingual tablet, oral spray, various combination products (e.g., ashwagandha root, chamomile, curcumin, lavender, L-threonine, turmeric, valerian root, 5-hydroxytryptophan [5-HTP])

---

[1]Evidence strength varies; readers are referred to the literature for more detailed information.

VIII. **Dosage Ranges and Guidelines**

A. Refer to Table 4–3 for dosage ranges and guidelines.
B. Insomnia: Start at 3 mg about 1 hour before bedtime. Raise dose to 5 mg, 7.5 mg, or 10 mg as needed. The dose may also be lowered if excessive sedation occurs.
C. Delayed sleep-wake phase disorder (pediatric and adult): Start at 3–5 mg taken 2 hours ahead of bedtime. Dose may be lowered if adverse effects occur. Also consider shifting the timing of dosing to earlier before bedtime if later dosing is ineffective. Morning bright light therapy (10,000 lux for 30 minutes) may also be helpful.
D. Non-24-hour sleep-wake rhythm disorder (blind patients): 0.3–10 mg taken 1–5 hours before bedtime.
E. Irregular sleep-wake rhythm disorder (pediatric): Start at 2–3 mg taken 30–40 minutes before bedtime. Raise the dosage to 5 mg, 7.5 mg, or 10 mg if needed.

Table 4–3. Melatonin indications and dosage ranges

Indications	Usual dosage range
Insomnia	0.1–10 mg/day
Delayed sleep-wake phase disorder (pediatric and adult)	3–5 mg/day
Non-24-hour sleep-wake rhythm disorder	0.3–10 mg/day
Irregular sleep-wake rhythm disorder (pediatric)	2–10 mg/day

IX. **Monitoring**: None

X. **Relevant Pharmacokinetics/Pharmacodynamics**

A. **Metabolism**: Hepatic and extrahepatic (cytochrome P450 [CYP] 1A2, CYP1A1, CYP1B1, CYP2C19).
B. **Time to peak plasma concentration**: 1 hour (IR tablet). Other forms vary depending on preparation (more rapid for ODT, sublingual, liquid, oral film, spray; slower for ER preparations).
C. **Half-life**: 30 minutes (range 20–50 minutes)
D. **Hepatic impairment**: Impairment leads to a significantly longer half-life and higher blood levels. However, given melatonin's tolerability and short half-life, its use in individuals with hepatic impairment is unlikely to have adverse consequences.
E. **Renal impairment**: No dosage adjustment necessary.

XI. **Clinically Relevant Drug Interactions**: None

XII. **Adverse Effects**

A. Morning somnolence
B. Headaches, hypotension, hypertension, indigestion, decreased semen quality, and exacerbation of alopecia areata have been reported with higher doses of melatonin (>5 mg/day), although the frequency of these effects is not known.

XIII. **Clinical Pearls/Prescribing Tips**

A. Orally administered melatonin has a high hepatic first-past extraction ratio.

B. Concerns have been raised about the accuracy of the labeled (mg) strengths in OTC products. Use of products that are United States Pharmacopeia (USP) Convention Verified is recommended.

C. The American Academy of Sleep Medicine (Auger et al. 2015) also recommends morning bright light therapy for advanced sleep-wake phase disorder and irregular sleep-wake rhythm disorder.

D. Higher melatonin doses (e.g., 10 mg or more) are usually not more effective and may cause more side effects.

E. Dosing recommendations are not well established and are based on the available research literature and guidelines. Adequate dose-ranging studies have not been conducted.

Further Reading

American Academy of Sleep Medicine Clinical Practice Guidelines. Available at: https://aasm.org/clinical-resources/practice-standards/practice-guidelines/. Accessed May 2022.

Kaur H, Spurling BC, Bollu PC: Chronic insomnia, in StatPearls. Treasure Island, FL, StatPearls Publishing, 2022

Savage RA, Zafar N, Yohannan S, et al: Melatonin, in StatPearls. Treasure Island, FL, StatPearls Publishing, 2021

References

Auger RR, Burgess HJ, Emens JS, et al: Clinical practice guideline for the treatment of intrinsic circadian rhythm sleep-wake disorders: an update for 2015. An American Academy of Sleep Medicine Clinical Practice Guideline. J Clin Sleep Med 11(10):1199–1236, 2015 26414986

McCleery J, Sharpley AL: Pharmacotherapies for sleep disturbances in dementia. Cochrane Database Syst Rev (11):CD009178, 2020 33189083

Ramelteon

I. **Brand Name**: Rozerem

II. **Therapeutic Class**: Insomnia treatment

III. **Mechanism-Based Class**: Melatonin receptor agonist

IV. **Mechanism(s) of Action**

A. Activation of melatonin MT_1 (*MTNR1A)* and MT_2 (*MTNR1B*) receptors.

B. Melatonin receptors promote sleep and set circadian rhythm.

C. One active metabolite (M-II)

V. **Indications**

A. FDA adult: Insomnia

B. Evidence-based[1] off-label uses:

1. Delayed sleep-wake phase disorder
2. Non-24-hour sleep-wake rhythm disorder in individuals with blindness

C. FDA pediatric: None

VI. **Major Contraindications and When to Use Caution**

A. **Use caution**:

1. Patients who develop angioedema should not be rechallenged. Do not use in combination with strong CYP1A2 inhibitors (e.g., fluvoxamine).
2. Older adults with neurocognitive disorder

VII. **Dosage Formulations**

A. Brand and generic immediate-release (IR) tablet (8 mg)

VIII. **Dosage Ranges and Guidelines**

A. **Insomnia**: 8 mg taken ~1 hour before bedtime. If excessive sedation occurs, the dose may be lowered by splitting the tablet.

B. **Delayed sleep-wake phase disorder** (adult): 8 mg taken 2 hours before bedtime. If adverse effects occur, the dose may be lowered by splitting the tablet. Consider shifting the timing of the dose to earlier if later dosing is ineffective. Morning bright light therapy (10,000 lux for 30 minutes) may also be helpful.

C. **Non-24-hour sleep-wake rhythm disorder** (individuals with blindness): 8 mg taken 1–5 hours before bedtime

IX. **Monitoring**: None

X. **Relevant Pharmacokinetics/Pharmacodynamics**

A. **Metabolism**: Hepatic (cytochrome P450 [CYP] 1A2 [major], CYP2C19, CYP3A4)

B. **Time to peak plasma concentration**: 45 minutes

C. **Half-life**:

1. 1–2.5 hours
2. M-II (primary active metabolite): 2–5 hours

---

[1]Evidence strength varies; readers are referred to the literature for more detailed information.

D. **Hepatic impairment**: Impairment leads to significantly higher blood levels and may prolong the therapeutic and adverse effects.
E. **Renal impairment**: No dosage adjustment necessary.
F. **Effect of food**: Time to maximum concentration is delayed by 45 minutes.

XI. Clinically Relevant Drug Interactions

A. Metabolized primarily by CYP1A2 and to a minor extent by CYP3A4 and CYP2C19.
  1. Blood levels are increased by CYP1A2 and (to a lesser extent) CYP3A4 inhibitors.
  2. Blood levels are decreased by CYP3A4 inducers.

B. Do not use with alcohol (increased effect).

XII. Adverse Effects

A. Daytime somnolence, fatigue, dizziness, nausea, insomnia exacerbation.
B. Complex sleep behaviors (e.g., sleepwalking, eating, dangerous behaviors) can occur but are rare.
C. Overall, the rate of side effects is very low. Only about 1% of participants in clinical trials discontinued because of adverse events (Takeda Pharmaceuticals America 2018).
D. Ramelteon has in rare cases been associated with anaphylaxis.
E. Worsening of depression or suicidal ideation can in rare cases occur in depressed patients.
F. Ramelteon raises prolactin levels in women and can lead to gynecomastia and galactorrhea.
G. **Risks in pregnancy and lactation**:
  1. Extremely high-dose ramelteon caused major malformations in animal studies (Takeda Pharmaceuticals America 2018). No risk to humans has been shown in postmarketing surveillance, but absolute pregnancy risks are unknown. Consider consultation with an OB/GYN specialist.
  2. Transmission in breast milk was shown in animal studies (Takeda Pharmaceuticals America 2018); transmission in humans is unknown. Infants fed breast milk from mothers using ramelteon should be monitored for sedation. Consider consultation with an OB/GYN specialist or lactation expert.

XIII. Clinical Pearls/Prescribing Tips

A. Ramelteon has no risk of abuse or dependency.
B. The American Academy of Sleep Medicine (Auger et al. 2015) also recommends morning bright light therapy for advanced sleep-wake phase disorder and irregular sleep-wake rhythm disorder.
C. There is evidence that administration of ramelteon (either alone or in combination with suvorexant) in the intensive care setting may reduce the risk of delirium in vulnerable patients.
D. Ramelteon should be taken only if the patient has a full 7 hours available/devoted to sleep.

Further Reading

American Academy of Sleep Medicine Clinical Practice Guidelines. Available at: https://aasm.org/clinical-resources/practice-standards/practice-guidelines/. Accessed May 2022.

Kaur H, Spurling BC, Bollu PC: Chronic insomnia, in StatPearls. Treasure Island, FL, StatPearls Publishing, 2022

Zammit GK: Ramelteon: a novel hypnotic indicated for the treatment of insomnia. Psychiatry (Edgmont) 4(9):36–42, 2007 20532119

References

Auger RR, Burgess HJ, Emens JS, et al: Clinical practice guideline for the treatment of intrinsic circadian rhythm sleep-wake disorders: an update for 2015. An American Academy of Sleep Medicine Clinical Practice Guideline. J Clin Sleep Med 11(10):1199–1236, 2015 26414986

Takeda Pharmaceuticals America: Rozerem (ramelteon) prescribing information. Revised December 2018. Available at: https://www.accessdata.fda.gov/drugsatfda_docs/label/2018/021782s021lbl.pdf. Accessed July 19, 2024.

Orexin Receptor Antagonists

Daridorexant

I. **Brand Name**: Quviviq

II. **Therapeutic Class**: Insomnia treatment

III. **Mechanism-Based Class**: Dual orexin (OX_1, OX_2) receptor antagonist

IV. **Mechanism(s) of Action**

A. Blockade of orexin OX_1 and OX_2 receptors

1. Orexin enhances wakefulness via OX_1 and OX_2.
2. Note that orexin is also referred to as ***hypocretin***, especially in the sleep literature.

V. **Indications**

A. FDA adult: Insomnia (decreases sleep latency, improves sleep maintenance)

B. Off-label uses: None

C. FDA pediatric: None

VI. **Major Contraindications and When to Use Caution**

A. **Major contraindications**:

1. Known allergy to daridorexant
2. Narcolepsy (daridorexant can worsen symptoms)
3. Use by patients with sedative-hypnotic or other substance use disorder history
4. Use in older adult patients (risk of falls or other accidents)
5. Concomitant use with strong CYP3A4 inhibitors or with moderate or strong CYP3A4 inducers
   a. The package insert recommends avoidance of doses higher than 25 mg at bedtime when taken concomitantly with moderate CYP3A4 inhibitors (Idorsia Pharmaceuticals US 2022).
   b. The package insert recommends avoiding concomitant use of moderate or strong CYP3A4 inducers.

B. **Use caution**:

1. Daridorexant may impair driving ability on the day following dosing, especially early in treatment. Use caution or avoid driving if necessary.
2. In patients with depression, hypnotics can worsen depression/suicidal ideation.
3. Daridorexant's effect on respiratory function should be carefully considered.
4. If insomnia persists after 7–10 days of treatment, the diagnosis should be reevaluated.

VII. **Dosage Formulations**

A. Brand film-coated tablet (25 mg, 50 mg [*not scored*])

B. Generic: None

VIII. **Dosage Ranges and Guidelines**

A. Start at 50 mg taken ~30 minutes before bedtime (Tmax=90 minutes). The dose may be decreased to 25 mg taken 30 minutes before bedtime as clinically indicated.
B. No dosage adjustment is required in older adults.
C. Take only once per night. Daridorexant should be taken only if the patient has at least 7 hours remaining/available to sleep.
D. Safety data on daridorexant in pediatric populations are not yet available.

IX. **Monitoring**: None

X. **Relevant Pharmacokinetics/Pharmacodynamics**

A. **Metabolism**: Hepatic (predominantly cytochrome P450 [CYP] 3A4 and to a much lesser extent CYP3A5)
B. **Time to peak plasma concentration**: 1–2 hours
C. **Half-life**: 8 hours (The half-life is variable and depends on the patient's CYP3A4 metabolizer status; see "Clinically Relevant Drug Interactions" below.)
D. **Effect of food**: Slows absorption, lowers peak concentration, and delays time to peak plasma concentration by 2 hours. The solubility of daridorexant is pH dependent.
    1. Coadministration with the antacid medication famotidine decreases the Cmax by 39% without affecting bioavailability.
E. **Hepatic impairment**: Daridorexant has not been tested—and should not be used—in patients with severe hepatic impairment. Keep dosage at 25 mg/day in patients with moderate hepatic impairment.
F. **Renal impairment**: No dosage adjustment necessary.

XI. **Clinically Relevant Drug Interactions**

A. Metabolized by CYP3A4
    1. Dosage adjustment is required when used in combination with CYP3A4 inhibitors or inducers (lower and higher dosages, respectively).
    2. Dosage adjustment may be required if the dosage of a CYP3A4 inhibitor or inducer is changed or the medication is discontinued.
    3. The duration of the sedative effect depends on the patient's CYP3A4 metabolizer status.
        a. Daridorexant's half-life is increased when used concomitantly with CYP3A4 inhibitors, and shortened when used with inducers.
    4. CYP3A4 inhibitors:
        a. Commonly used strong inhibitors: Several protease inhibitors (e.g., indinavir, ritonavir), clarithromycin, ketoconazole
        b. Moderate inhibitors: Ciprofloxacin, diltiazem, erythromycin, fluconazole, fluvoxamine, grapefruit and juice, verapamil
            i. The package insert recommends avoidance of dosages higher than 25 mg nightly when taken concomitantly with moderate CYP3A4 inhibitors (Idorsia Pharmaceuticals US 2022).

5. CYP3A4 inducers: Apalutamide, carbamazepine, efavirenz, enzalutamide, phenytoin, rifampin, St. John's wort

B. Daridorexant itself is a CYP2C9 inducer and should be used with caution in combination with CYP2C9 substrates. The potential for interaction should be evaluated on a case-by-case basis.

C. Use with caution in combination with other sedative-hypnotics (e.g., benzodiazepines), which may increase the risk for oversedation and accidents.

XII. **Adverse Effects**

A. **Most common**:

1. CNS: Daytime somnolence ("hangover" effect)
2. Other: Dizziness, fatigue, nausea

B. **Uncommon**: Sleep paralysis, hypnagogic and hypnopompic hallucinations, complex sleep behavior (e.g., sleepwalking, sleep driving), cataplexy (rare), dizziness, diarrhea, new onset or worsening of suicidal ideation (rare).

C. **Risks in pregnancy and lactation**:

1. Effects on the human fetus are unknown, and caution should be used, including possible consultation with an OB/GYN specialist.
2. No information is available on using daridorexant while breastfeeding. However, because daridorexant is highly protein bound, it seems unlikely to be excreted in human breast milk. When in doubt, consult with an OB/GYN specialist or lactation expert.

XIII. **Clinical Pearls/Prescribing Tips**

A. Dual orexin receptors have modest benefits for sleep. Daridorexant has demonstrated greater improvement of both subjective and objective measures of sleep onset and maintenance in comparison with placebo.

B. No benzodiazepine-like withdrawal effects have been reported with abrupt discontinuation of daridorexant after long-term administration.

C. Although all dual orexin receptor antagonists are Schedule IV drugs, they seem to have relatively low abuse potential. However, they should be used with caution.

D. Cognitive-behavioral therapy for insomnia (CBT-i) is an effective alternative to medication management.

Further Reading

American Academy of Sleep Medicine Clinical Practice Guidelines. Available at: https://aasm.org/clinical-resources/practice-standards/practice-guidelines/. Accessed May 2022.

Gehin M, Wierdak J, Sabattini G, et al: Effect of gastric pH and of a moderate CYP3A4 inducer on the pharmacokinetics of daridorexant, a dual orexin receptor antagonist. Br J Clin Pharmacol 88(2):810–819, 2022 34371524

Jacobson LH, Hoyer D, de Lecea L: Hypocretins (orexins): the ultimate translational neuropeptides. J Intern Med 291(5):533–556, 2022 35043499

Kaur H, Spurling BC, Bollu PC: Chronic insomnia, in StatPearls. Treasure Island, FL, StatPearls Publishing, 2022

References

Idorsia Pharmaceuticals US: Quviviq (daridorexant) tablets, for oral use [package insert]. U.S. Food and Drug Administration website. Revised January 2022. Available at: https://www.accessdata.fda.gov/drugsatfda_docs/label/2022/214985s000lbl.pdf. Accessed June 21, 2024.

Lemborexant

I. **Brand Name**: Dayvigo

II. **Therapeutic Class**: Insomnia treatment

III. **Mechanism-Based Class**: Dual orexin (OX_1, OX_2) receptor antagonist

IV. **Mechanism(s) of Action**

A. Blockade of orexin OX_1 and OX_2 receptors.

B. Orexin enhances wakefulness via OX_1 and OX_2.

C. Note that orexin is also referred to as *hypocretin*, especially in the sleep literature.

V. **Indications**

A. FDA adult: Insomnia (decreases sleep latency, improves sleep maintenance)

B. Off-label uses: None

C. FDA pediatric: None

VI. **Major Contraindications and When to Use Caution**

A. **Major contraindications**:

1. Known allergy to lemborexant
2. Narcolepsy (lemborexant can worsen symptoms)
3. Concomitant use with strong cytochrome P450 (CYP) 3A4 inhibitors
4. Use by individuals who are CYP3A4 poor metabolizers (the duration of effect is substantially increased)

B. **Use caution**:

1. Concomitant use with moderate CYP3A4 inhibitors.
2. Use by patients with sedative-hypnotic or other substance use disorder history
3. Use in older adult patients (risk of falls or other accidents)

C. Lemborexant may impair driving ability on the day following dosing, especially early in treatment. Use caution.

VII. **Dosage Formulations**

A. Brand tablet (5 mg, 10 mg [*not scored*])

B. Generic: None

VIII. **Dosage Ranges and Guidelines**

A. Start at 5 mg about 30 minutes before bedtime (Tmax=90 minutes). Raise dosage to 10 mg/day if needed.

B. Keep dosage at 5 mg/day in patients older than 65 years.

C. Take only once per night. Lemborexant should be taken only if the patient has at least 7 hours remaining/available to sleep.

IX. **Monitoring**: None

X. **Relevant Pharmacokinetics/Pharmacodynamics**

A. **Metabolism**: Hepatic (predominantly cytochrome P450 [CYP] 3A4 and to a much lesser extent CYP3A5).

B. **Time to peak plasma concentration**: 2 hours

C. **Half-life**: 18 hours (The half-life is variable and depends on the patient's CYP3A4 metabolizer status; see "Clinically Relevant Drug Interactions" below.)

D. **Effect of food**: Slows absorption, lowers peak concentration, delays time to peak plasma concentration by 2 hours.

E. **Hepatic impairment**: Lemborexant has not been tested—and should not be used—in patients with severe hepatic impairment. Keep dose at 5 mg in patients with moderate impairment.

F. **Renal impairment**: No dosage adjustment necessary.

XI. **Clinically Relevant Drug Interactions**

A. Metabolized by CYP3A4

1. Dosage adjustment is required with concomitant use of CYP3A4 inhibitors or inducers (lower or higher dosages, respectively).
2. Dosage adjustment may be required if a concomitant CYP3A4 inhibitor or inducer is added to or removed from the patient's medication list or the dosage of the concomitant inhibitor or inducer is changed.
3. The duration of the sedative effect depends on the patient's CYP3A4 metabolizer status.

   a. Lemborexant's half-life is increased when used concomitantly with CYP3A4 inhibitors, and shortened when used with inducers.

4. CYP3A4 inhibitors:

   a. Commonly used strong inhibitors: Several protease inhibitors (e.g., indinavir, ritonavir), clarithromycin, ketoconazole
   b. Moderate inhibitors: Ciprofloxacin, diltiazem, erythromycin, fluconazole, fluvoxamine, grapefruit and juice, verapamil.

      i. Keep dosage at 25 mg/day for patients taking moderate CYP3A4 inhibitors.

5. CYP3A4 inducers: Apalutamide, carbamazepine, efavirenz, enzalutamide, phenytoin, rifampin, St. John's wort

B. Use with caution in combination with other sedative-hypnotics (e.g., benzodiazepines), which may increase risk for oversedation and accidents.

XII. **Adverse Effects**

A. **Most common**:

1. CNS: Daytime somnolence ("hangover" effect)
2. Other: Dizziness, fatigue, nausea

B. **Uncommon**: Sleep paralysis, hypnagogic and hypnopompic hallucinations, complex sleep behavior (e.g., sleepwalking, sleep driving), cataplexy (rare), dizziness, diarrhea, new onset or worsening of suicidal ideation (rare).

C. **Risks in pregnancy and lactation**:

1. Lemborexant was associated with fetal malformations in animal studies only at very high doses. Effects on the human fetus are unknown.
2. Lemborexant was present in breast milk in animal studies, and it is likely to be present in human breast milk, which may lead to infant sedation.

XIII. **Clinical Pearls/Prescribing Tips**

A. Dual orexin receptors have shown modest benefits for sleep in clinical trials (Esai 2019):

1. Latency to sleep onset for lemborexant was improved with the 5 mg and 10 mg doses by 4.5 and 5.5 minutes, respectively, at the end of 1 month and by 7.3 and 8.1 minutes at the end of 6 months relative to change with placebo.
2. Subjective sleep efficiency was improved with the 5 mg and 10 mg doses by 6.1% and 8.1%, respectively, at the end of 1 month and by 4.5% with both doses at the end of 6 months relative to placebo.
3. The subjective wake time after sleep onset was improved with the 5 mg and 10 mg doses by 23.9 and 25.3 minutes, respectively, at the end of 1 month and by 17.4 and 12.6 minutes at the end of 6 months relative to placebo.

B. No benzodiazepine-like withdrawal effects have been reported with abrupt discontinuation of lemborexant after long-term administration.

C. Lemborexant has a very long half-life (18 hours), which may lead to problematic side effects the day after dosing. The dual orexin inhibitor daridorexant has a shorter half-life (8 hours).

D. Cognitive-behavioral therapy for insomnia (CBT-i) is an effective alternative to medication management.

Further Reading

American Academy of Sleep Medicine Clinical Practice Guidelines. Available at: https://aasm.org/clinical-resources/practice-standards/practice-guidelines/. Accessed May 2022.

Jacobson LH, Hoyer D, de Lecea L: Hypocretins (orexins): the ultimate translational neuropeptides. J Intern Med 291(5):533–556, 2022 35043499

Kaur H, Spurling BC, Bollu PC: Chronic Insomnia, in StatPearls. Treasure Island, FL, StatPearls Publishing, 2022

Lemborexant, Multi-Discipline Review. Center for Drug Evaluation and Research, 2018. https://www.accessdata.fda.gov/drugsatfda_docs/nda/2019/212028Orig1s000MultidisciplineR.pdf. Accessed May 2022.

References

Esai: Dayvigo (lemborexant) prescribing information. Revised December 2019. Available at: https://www.accessdata.fda.gov/drugsatfda_docs/label/2019/212028s000lbl.pdf. Accessed July 19, 2024.

Suvorexant

I. **Brand Name**: Belsomra

II. **Therapeutic Class**: Insomnia treatment

III. **Mechanism-Based Class**: Dual orexin (OX_1, OX_2) receptor antagonist

IV. **Mechanism(s) of Action**

A. Blockade of orexin OX_1 and OX_2 receptors.

B. Orexin enhances wakefulness via OX_1 and OX_2.

C. Note that orexin is also referred to as *hypocretin*, especially in the sleep literature.

V. **Indications**

A. FDA adult: Insomnia (decreases sleep latency, improves sleep maintenance)

B. Off-label uses: None

C. FDA pediatric: None

VI. **Major Contraindications and When to Use Caution**

A. **Major contraindications**:

1. Known allergy to suvorexant
2. Narcolepsy (suvorexant can worsen symptoms).
3. CYP3A4 poor metabolizer status (the duration of effect is substantially increased)

B. **Use caution:**

1. Patients with sedative-hypnotic or other substance use disorder history
2. Suvorexant may impair driving ability on the day following dosing.

VII. **Dosage Formulations**

A. Brand tablet (5 mg, 10 mg, 15 mg, 20 mg [*not scored*])

B. Generic: None

VIII. **Dosage Ranges and Guidelines**

A. Start at 10 mg taken about 30 minutes before bedtime (Tmax=120 minutes).

B. May reduce to 5 mg or increase to 15 or 20 mg if needed.

C. Start at 5 mg in older adult patients.

D. Take only once per night. Suvorexant should be taken only if the patient has at least 7 hours remaining/devoted to sleep.

IX. **Monitoring**: None

X. **Relevant Pharmacokinetics/Pharmacodynamics**

A. **Metabolism**: Hepatic (predominantly cytochrome P450 [CYP] 3A4 with a minor contribution by CYP2C19).

B. **Time to peak plasma concentration**: 2 hours

C. **Half-life**: 12 hours (The half-life is variable and depends on the patient's CYP3A4 metabolizer status; see "Clinically Relevant Drug Interactions" below.)

D. **Hepatic impairment**: No adjustment is needed for mild to moderate hepatic impairment. Lower dosages should be used in severe impairment.

E. **Renal impairment**: No dosage adjustment necessary.

XI. Clinically Relevant Drug Interactions

A. Metabolized by CYP3A4

1. Dosage adjustment is required with concomitant use of CYP3A4 inhibitors or inducers (lower or higher dosages, respectively).
2. Dosage adjustment may be required if a concomitant CYP3A4 inhibitor or inducer is added to or removed from the patient's medication list or the dosage of the concomitant inhibitor or inducer is changed.
3. The duration of the sedative effect depends on the patient's CYP3A4 metabolizer status.
   a. Suvorexant's half-life is increased when it is used concomitantly with CYP3A4 inhibitors, and shortened when used with inducers; for example, with ketoconazole (a strong CYP3A4 inhibitor), it is 19.4 hours, and with rifampin (a CYP3A4 inducer), it is 7.7 hours.
4. CYP3A4 inhibitors:
   a. Commonly used strong inhibitors: Several protease inhibitors (e.g., indinavir, ritonavir), clarithromycin, ketoconazole
      i. Avoid concomitant use with strong CYP3A4 inhibitors.
   b. Moderate inhibitors: Ciprofloxacin, diltiazem, erythromycin, fluconazole, fluvoxamine, grapefruit and juice, verapamil.
      i. Keep dosage at 25 mg/day for patients taking moderate CYP3A4 inhibitors.
5. CYP3A4 inducers: Apalutamide, carbamazepine, efavirenz, enzalutamide, phenytoin, rifampin, St. John's wort

B. Use with caution in combination with other sedative-hypnotics (e.g., benzodiazepines), which may increase risk for oversedation and accidents.

XII. Adverse Effects

A. **Most common**:

1. CNS: Daytime somnolence ("hangover" effect)
2. Other: Dizziness

B. **Uncommon**: Sleep paralysis, abnormal dreams, hypnagogic and hypnopompic hallucinations, complex sleep behavior (e.g., sleepwalking, sleep driving), cataplexy (rare), dizziness, nausea, diarrhea, new onset or worsening of suicidal ideation (10 mg: 0%, 20 mg: 1.6% [Sutton 2015]).

1. Balance or memory problems do not appear to occur at dosages up to 20 mg/day but may occur at higher dosages.

C. **Risks in pregnancy and lactation**:

1. Suvorexant was designated a Category C drug in the prior FDA classification and is present in breast milk. A thorough risk/benefit discussion with the patient is recommended on continuing versus stopping the medication, including consultation with an OB/GYN specialist and/or lactation expert. See Chapter 15 ("Women: Pregnancy, Postpartum, and Breastfeeding") for more information.

XIII. **Clinical Pearls/Prescribing Tips**

A. Suvorexant has shown modest benefit for sleep in two pivotal trials (Merck Sharp & Dohme LLC 2023):

1. Sleep onset was improved by about 8–10 minutes at the end of 1 month and by 0–8 minutes after 3 months relative to placebo .
2. Sleep maintenance was improved by 24–26 minutes and 17–31 minutes at 1 month and 3 months, respectively.
3. Total sleep time was increased by 16–21 and 11–22 minutes at 1 month and 3 months, respectively.

B. Suvorexant was beneficial for sleep onset and maintenance in a study in older adult patients with Alzheimer's disease (Herring et al. 2020).

C. No rebound insomnia has been reported with abrupt discontinuation of suvorexant after long-term administration.

D. Suvorexant has a long half-life and a broad half-life range (about 8–19 hours). Daridorexant has a shorter half-life (8 hours) and a more narrow half-life range (6–10 hours).

E. Cognitive-behavioral therapy for insomnia (CBT-i) is an effective alternative to medication management.

Further Reading

American Academy of Sleep Medicine Clinical Practice Guidelines. Available at: https://aasm.org/clinical-resources/practice-standards/practice-guidelines/. Accessed May 2022.

Jacobson LH, Hoyer D, de Lecea L: Hypocretins (orexins): the ultimate translational neuropeptides. J Intern Med 291(5):533–556, 2022 35043499

References

Herring WJ, Ceesay P, Snyder E, et al: Polysomnographic assessment of suvorexant in patients with probable Alzheimer's disease dementia and insomnia: a randomized trial. Alzheimers Dement 16(3):541-551, 2020 31944580

Merck Sharp & Dohme LLC: Belsomra (suvorexant) [package insert]. U.S. Food and Drug Administration website. Revised February 2023. Available at: https://www.merck.com/product/usa/pi_circulars/b/belsomra/belsomra_pi.pdf. Accessed June 21, 2024.

Sutton EL: Profile of suvorexant in the management of insomnia. Drug Des Devel Ther 9:6035-6042, 2015 26648692

Antihistamines

Diphenhydramine (Insomnia)

I. **Brand Names**: Benadryl, Simply Sleep

II. **Therapeutic Class**: Antihistamine (first-generation)

III. **Mechanism-Based Class**: Histamine-1 (H_1) antagonist

IV. **Mechanism of Action (Insomnia)**

A. Blockade of H_1 receptors

V. **Indications**

A. FDA adult:

1. Allergies
2. Insomnia

B. Evidence-based[1] off-label uses:

1. Extrapyramidal symptoms (anticholinergic)
2. Nausea

C. FDA pediatric: Allergies

VI. **Major Contraindications and When to Use Caution**

A. **Major contraindications**:

1. Known allergy to diphenhydramine
2. Cognitive disorder

B. **Use caution**:

1. Elderly patients (risk of oversedation and falls)
2. People with narrow-angle glaucoma, stenosing peptic ulcer, pyloroduodenal obstruction, symptomatic prostatic hypertrophy, or bladder-neck obstruction

VII. **Dosage Formulations**

A. Generic and brand immediate-release (IR) tablet or capsule (12.5 mg, 19 mg, 25 mg, 50 mg)

B. Generic and brand liquid (6.25 mg/mL, 6.25 mg/5 mL, 10 mg/mL, 12.5 mg/5 mL; 25 mg/5 mL, 50 mg/30 mL, 50 mg/mL)

C. Generic and brand cream (1%, 2%)

D. Other dosage forms: Chewables, gummies, mucosal strip, orally dissolving tablet, gel, various combination products

VIII. **Dosage Ranges and Guidelines (Insomnia)**

A. Refer to Table 4–4 for dosage ranges and guidelines.

B. Start at 25 mg taken ~1 hour before bedtime (Tmax=3 hours).

---

[1]Evidence strength varies; readers are referred to the literature for more detailed information.

C. May be increased to 50 mg/day as needed. The dose can be lowered to as little as 12.5 mg with a pill splitter. Doses can be adjusted in 12.5-mg increments by splitting 25-mg tablets.
D. Lower dosages are typically required in older adult patients.

Table 4–4. Diphenhydramine indications and dosage ranges

Indications	Usual dosage ranges
Allergies	12.5–50 mg/day
Insomnia	12.5–50 mg/day

IX. **Monitoring**: None

X. **Relevant Pharmacokinetics/Pharmacodynamics**

A. **Metabolism**: Hepatic (cytochrome P450 [CYP] 2D6 [primary pathway], CYP1A2, CYP2C9, CYP2C19)
B. **Time to peak plasma concentration**: 1.5 hours
C. **Half-life**: 4 hours (range 3.4–9.5 hours)
D. **Hepatic impairment**: Impairment lengthens half-life and increases diphenhydramine blood levels; dosages should be adjusted accordingly. Because of the longer half-life in hepatically impaired individuals, diphenhydramine may not be an appropriate choice for treating insomnia in people with moderate to severe hepatic impairment.
E. **Renal impairment**: No significant effects on diphenhydramine levels.
F. **Age-related reduction in drug clearance**: Clearance may be reduced in elderly adults. However, typical dosages used for insomnia are usually well tolerated.

XI. **Clinically Relevant Drug Interactions**

A. Metabolized by CYP2D6 (primarily)
1. Dosage adjustment/decrease may be required if coadministered with concomitant CYP2D6 inhibitors.
2. Dosage may need to be adjusted after a change in dose or discontinuation of a concomitantly used CYP2D6 inhibitor.
3. Commonly used CYP2D6 strong inhibitors: Fluoxetine, paroxetine, bupropion, ritonavir, cannabidiol. Moderate inhibitors: Duloxetine, terbinafine.
4. Diphenhydramine dosages will need to be adjusted for patients who are intermediate, poor, rapid, or ultrarapid metabolizers of CYP2D6.

XII. **Adverse Effects**

A. **Most common**:
1. CNS: Oversedation, daytime somnolence.
2. Other: Blurred vision, constipation, dry mouth and other mucous membranes, dysgeusia (bad taste), fatigue, increased appetite and weight gain, indigestion, increased body temperature, orthostatic hypotension, pupil dilation with light sensitivity, tachycardia, tremor, urinary hesitancy or retention.

B. **Uncommon**: Agitation, ataxia, elevated transaminases (usually mild), confusion, diaphoresis, disorientation, distorted vision, dizziness, erectile dysfunction, hallucinations (very rare), irritability, memory problems, nauseas and vomiting (usually at higher dosages), rash or other allergic reaction, rebound insomnia, restlessness, worsening of restless legs.

1. Some patients can become paradoxically anxious or agitated after taking diphenhydramine.
2. Confusion and memory problems are more common in older adults, although they occur less frequently when lower doses are used.

C. **Risks in pregnancy and lactation**:

1. An increase in major malformations was not demonstrated in animal studies. Risks in humans are unclear but are probably low. Anecdotally, diphenhydramine seems to be commonly used on OB/GYN inpatient wards in pregnant patients. Always consider consultation with an OB/GYN specialist if in doubt.
2. Diphenhydramine is excreted into breast milk and may cause infant somnolence or constipation.

XIII. **Clinical Pearls/Prescribing Tips**

A. CYP2D6 is the primary metabolic pathway for diphenhydramine. Therefore, the duration of action is highly variable, which means that some people will awaken too early and others will experience prolonged daytime sedation.

B. Patients who are intermediate or poor CYP2D6 metabolizers will have more side effects.

C. Because of its less variable half-life and fewer side effects (in most patients), trazodone may be a better first choice for insomnia than diphenhydramine.

D. Diphenhydramine has potent anticholinergic effects. If an H_1 antihistamine is needed, consider hydroxyzine, given its relatively weaker anticholinergic activity (Kubo et al. 1987).

E. Unlike the "Z drugs," diphenhydramine has limited abuse potential.

F. Cognitive-behavioral therapy for insomnia (CBT-i) is an effective alternative to medication management.

Further Reading

American Academy of Sleep Medicine Clinical Practice Guidelines. Available at: https://aasm.org/clinical-resources/practice-standards/practice-guidelines/. Accessed May 2022.

Benadryl prescribing information. U.S. Food and Drug Administration, 2022. Available at: https://www.accessdata.fda.gov/spl/data/5e630d0e-4bc2-4f90-ac6a-e5e297d94cb8/5e630d0e-4bc2-4f90-ac6a-e5e297d94cb8.xml. Accessed March 13, 2024.

Everitt H, Baldwin DS, Stuart B, et al: Antidepressants for insomnia in adults. Cochrane Database Syst Rev (5):CD010753, 2018 29761479

References

Kubo N, Shirakawa O, Kuno T, et al: Antimuscarinic effects of antihistamines: quantitative evaluation by receptor-binding assay. Jpn J Pharmacol 43(3):277–282, 1987 2884340

Doxylamine (Insomnia)

I. **Brand Names**: Unisom, Aldex AN, Doxytex, NyQuil, Ultra Sleep, Diclegis and Bonjesta (with vitamin B_6), others

II. **Therapeutic Class**: Antihistamine (first-generation)

III. **Mechanism-Based Class**: Histamine-1 (H_1) antagonist

IV. **Mechanism of Action (Insomnia)**: Blockade of H_1 receptors

V. **Indications**

A. FDA adult: Insomnia, morning sickness (doxylamine plus vitamin B_6), allergies
B. Off-label uses: None
C. FDA pediatric: Insomnia, allergies

VI. **Major Contraindications and When to Use Caution**

A. **Major contraindications**:

1. Known allergy to doxylamine or diphenhydramine
2. Concurrent use of a monoamine oxidase inhibitor (MAOI)
3. Current alcohol use

B. **Use caution**:

1. Older adult patients (risk of oversedation and falls)
2. People with closed-angle glaucoma, stenosing peptic ulcer, pyloroduodenal stenosis, symptomatic prostatic hypertrophy, or bladder-neck obstruction
3. Patients with neurocognitive disorders
4. Individuals with severe asthma or chronic obstructive pulmonary disease

VII. **Dosage Formulations**

A. Generic and brand immediate-release (IR) tablet (25 mg)
B. Generic and brand oral suspension (5 mg/5 mL)
C. Brand chewable tablet (5 mg)
D. Doxylamine 10 mg/vitamin B_6 10 mg sustained-release (SR) tablet (morning sickness)

VIII. **Dosage Ranges and Guidelines**

E. Insomnia (adults and children age 12 years and older): 25 mg taken 30 minutes before bedtime
F. Morning sickness (doxylamine 10 mg/vitamin B_6 10 mg):
10 mg/10 mg → 20 mg/20 mg at bedtime
G. Allergy (1 dose every 4–6 hours; maximum of 6 doses/day)

1. Adults; children age 12 years and older: 10 mg
2. Children age 6–11 years: 5 mg
3. Children age 2–5 years: 2.5 mg

IX. **Monitoring**: None

X. Relevant Pharmacokinetics/Pharmacodynamics

A. **Metabolism**: Hepatic (cytochrome P450 [CYP] 2D6, CYP1A2, CYP2C9)
B. **Time to peak plasma concentration**: 2 hours (immediate-release), 7 hours (sustained-release).
C. **Half-life**: 10 hours (range 7–13 hours)
D. **Hepatic impairment**: Lengthens half-life and increases blood levels of doxylamine. Dosage reduction may be warranted. Use caution.
E. **Renal impairment**: Unknown
F. **Age-related reduction in drug clearance**: Clearance may be reduced in elderly adults. However, typical dosages used for insomnia are usually well tolerated. Use with caution.

XI. Clinically Relevant Drug Interactions

A. May cause oversedation when combined with other sedative medications.
B. Avoid combining with other anticholinergic medications (e.g., tricyclic antidepressants).

XII. Adverse Effects

A. **Most common**:
   1. CNS: Oversedation, daytime somnolence
   2. Other: Dry mouth, fatigue, urinary retention (related to anticholinergic effects)

B. **Uncommon**: Agitation, ataxia, attention and memory problems, confusion, constipation, delusions (very rare), diarrhea, hallucinations (very rare), irritability, rash or other allergic reaction, rebound insomnia, rhabdomyolysis (very rare), seizures, tachycardia, weight gain, vertigo, vivid dreams.
   1. Confusion and memory problems are more common in older adults.
   2. Agitation and psychosis are more common in overdose, which can also cause rhabdomyolysis, delirium, coma, and cardiorespiratory arrest.

C. **Risks in pregnancy and lactation**:
   1. Doxylamine is generally considered safe in pregnancy and is used for morning sickness.
   2. Doxylamine is excreted into breast milk and may cause infant somnolence or constipation. Use in breastfeeding women is not recommended.

XIII. Clinical Pearls/Prescribing Tips

A. Unlike the "Z drugs," doxylamine has limited abuse potential.
B. Long-term use of doxylamine is not recommended.
C. Cognitive-behavioral therapy for insomnia (CBT-i) is an effective alternative to medication management and is often considered the first-line treatment for insomnia.
D. Anticholinergic effects may occur, but these are less common with doxylamine than with diphenhydramine.

Further Reading

American Academy of Sleep Medicine Clinical Practice Guidelines. Available at: https://aasm.org/clinical-resources/practice-standards/practice-guidelines/. Accessed May 2022.

Brott NR, Reddivari AKR: Doxylamine, in StatPearls. Treasure Island, FL, StatPearls Publishing, 2022

Doxylamine plus B6 prescribing information. U.S. Food and Drug Administration, 2015. Available at: https://www.accessdata.fda.gov/drugsatfda_docs/label/2016/205811Orig1s000lbl.pdf. Accessed June 2022.

Unisom prescribing information. U.S. Food and Drug Administration, 2013. Available at: https://www.accessdata.fda.gov/drugsatfda_docs/label/2013/018066Orig1s020lbl.pdf. Accessed June 2022.

Hydroxyzine (Insomnia)

I. **Brand Names**: Vistaril (hydroxyzine pamoate), Atarax (discontinued in U.S.)

II. **Therapeutic Class**: Antihistamine (first-generation), hypnotic, antiemetic, anxiolytic

III. **Mechanism-Based Class**: Histamine-1 (H_1) receptor antagonist; weak serotonin-2A (5-HT_{2A}) receptor antagonist

IV. **Mechanism of Action (Insomnia)**

A. Blockade of H_1 receptors

V. **Indications**

A. FDA adult and pediatric:

1. Anxiety
2. Pruritus/urticaria
3. Presurgical sedation

B. Evidence-based[1] off-label uses:

1. Insomnia
2. Extrapyramidal symptoms (anticholinergic)
3. Nausea (especially due to motion sickness)

VI. **Major Contraindications and When to Use Caution**

A. **Major contraindications**:

1. Known allergy to hydroxyzine, cetirizine, or levocetirizine
2. Long QTc interval or concomitant use with drugs that prolong QTc

[1]Evidence strength varies; readers are referred to the literature for more detailed information.

B. **Use caution**:

1. Older adult patients (risk of oversedation and falls)
2. People with narrow-angle glaucoma, stenosing peptic ulcer, pyloroduodenal obstruction, symptomatic prostatic hypertrophy, or bladder-neck obstruction
3. Patients with neurocognitive disorders

VII. **Dosage Formulations**

A. Generic and brand hydroxyzine pamoate immediate-release (IR) capsule (25 mg, 50 mg)
B. Generic and brand hydroxyzine pamoate oral suspension (equivalent to 25 mg hydroxyzine/5 mL)
C. Generic and brand hydroxyzine HCl IR tablet (10 mg, 25 mg, 50 mg)
D. Generic and brand hydroxyzine HCl solution for IM injection (25 mg/mL, 50 mg/mL) (Do not administer intravenously.)

VIII. **Dosage Ranges and Guidelines**

A. Refer to Table 4–5 for dosage ranges and guidelines.
B. Anxiety (adults): 25–100 mg taken up to 4 times per day. The dose can be reduced to 25 mg in the event of side effects.
C. Insomnia (off-label) (adults): 25–100 mg taken 60–90 minutes before bedtime.
D. Pruritus:

1. Adults: 25 mg taken up to 4 times per day
2. Children age <6 years): 25 mg BID
3. Children age ≥6 years): 25 mg taken 2–4 times per day

Table 4–5. Hydroxyzine indications and dosage ranges

Indications	Usual dosage ranges
Anxiety (adults)	25–100 mg/day
Pruritus due to allergy (adults)	25–50 mg/day
Insomnia (off-label) (adults)	12.5–50 mg/day

Note. See manufacturer's prescribing information for further details on dosing (Pfizer Laboratories 2023).

IX. **Monitoring**: None

X. **Relevant Pharmacokinetics/Pharmacodynamics**

A. **Metabolism**: Hepatic (cytochrome P450 [CYP] 3A4, CYP3A5)
B. **Time to peak plasma concentration**: 2 hours (pamoate capsule)
C. **Half-life**:

1. Adults: 20 hours
2. Elderly adults: 29 hours
3. Children: 7 hours

D. **Hepatic impairment**: Hydroxyzine lengthens half-life and increases blood levels. Doses should be adjusted accordingly. Use with caution.
E. **Renal impairment**: No significant effects on hydroxyzine levels.
F. **Age-related reduction in drug clearance**: Clearance may be reduced in elderly adults. However, typical dosages used for insomnia are usually well tolerated.

XI. **Clinically Relevant Drug Interactions**

A. Avoid using with drugs that prolong QTc interval (e.g., amiodarone, asenapine, chloroquine, chlorpromazine, clozapine, citalopram (at higher dosages), iloperidone, thioridazine, tricyclic antidepressants, ziprasidone)
B. May cause oversedation when combined with other sedating medications. Use caution.

XII. **Adverse Effects**

A. **Most common**:

1. CNS: Oversedation, daytime somnolence
2. Other: Constipation, dizziness, dry mouth, discoordination

B. **Uncommon**: Agitation, confusion, hallucinations (very rare), memory problems, nausea, rash or other allergic reaction, rebound insomnia, weight gain, vivid dreams.

1. Confusion and memory problems are more common in older adults, although they occur less frequently when lower dosages are used.

C. **Risks in pregnancy and lactation**:

1. An increase in major malformations has not been demonstrated in animal studies. Risks in humans are unclear but are probably low. When in doubt, consider consultation with an OB/GYN specialist.
2. Hydroxyzine is excreted into breast milk and may cause infant somnolence or constipation. Use in breastfeeding is not recommended.

XIII. **Clinical Pearls/Prescribing Tips**

A. Hydroxyzine pamoate is the preferred form for anxiety and insomnia.
B. Unlike the "Z drugs," hydroxyzine has limited abuse potential.
C. Cognitive-behavioral therapy for insomnia (CBT-i) is an effective alternative to medication management.
D. Compared with certain other H_1 receptor antagonists (e.g., diphenhydramine), hydroxyzine has weaker affinity for muscarinic receptors, which makes anticholinergic side effects less likely (Kubo et al. 1987).

Further Reading

American Academy of Sleep Medicine Clinical Practice Guidelines. Available at: https://aasm.org/clinical-resources/practice-standards/practice-guidelines/. Accessed May 2022.

Hydroxyzine HCl (tablet and oral suspension) prescribing information. U.S. Food and Drug Administration, 2019. Available at: https://gskpro.com/content/dam/global/hcpportal/en_SG/products/PDF/atarax/pdf/atarax_pi_ncds06si_approved_17sep19.pdf. Accessed June 2022.

Hydroxyzine pamoate (capsule and oral suspension) prescribing information. U.S. Food and Drug Administration, 2014. Available at: https://www.accessdata.fda.gov/drugsatfda_docs/label/2014/011459s048%2C011795s025lbl.pdf. Accessed June 2022.

References

Kubo N, Shirakawa O, Kuno T, et al: Antimuscarinic effects of antihistamines: quantitative evaluation by receptor-binding assay. Jpn J Pharmacol 43(3):277–282, 1987 2884340

Pfizer Laboratories: Vistaril (hydroxyzine pamoate) capsules and oral suspension [package insert]. Revised May 2023. Available at: https://dailymed.nlm.nih.gov/dailymed/fda/fdaDrugXsl.cfm?setid=c271f97f-040e-492b-9194-2c8b74675a95&type=display. Accessed September 9, 2024.

Antidepressants

Amitriptyline[1] (Insomnia)

I. **Brand Names**: Elavil, Endep, Vanatrip, Amitid, Amitril (all branded products discontinued)

II. **Therapeutic Class**: Tricyclic antidepressant (TCA)

III. **Mechanism-Based Class**

A. Serotonin transporter (SERT) and norepinephrine transporter (NET) reuptake inhibitor (parent amitriptyline, SERT > NET, primary metabolite, NET > SERT)

B. Histamine-1 (H_1) and serotonin-2A (5-HT_{2A}) receptor antagonist

C. Sodium channel antagonist (Na_v1 voltage-gated sodium channel [VGSC] isoforms $Na_v1.3$, $Na_v1.5$, $Na_v1.6$, $Na_v1.7$, $Na_v1.8$)

IV. **Mechanism of Action (Insomnia)**

A. Blockade of H_1 and 5-HT_{2A} receptors

V. **Indications**

A. FDA adult: Major depressive disorder

B. Evidence-based[2] off-label uses:

1. Insomnia
2. Pain: Musculoskeletal, fibromyalgia, headache (including migraine), burning mouth syndrome
3. Irritable bowel syndrome

C. Other off-label uses (with limited supporting data/evidence):

1. Generalized anxiety disorder
2. OCD
3. PTSD
4. Urinary incontinence

D. FDA pediatric: None

VI. **Major Contraindications and When to Use Caution**

A. **Major contraindications**:

1. Known allergy to amitriptyline or nortriptyline
2. Prior QTc prolongation

[1]See Chapter 2, "Antidepressants," for more information regarding amitriptyline.

[2]Evidence strength varies; readers are referred to the literature for more detailed information.

B. **Use caution**:

1. Older adult patients (risk of oversedation and falls)
2. Patients with prior cardiovascular disease (especially unstable angina or recent myocardial infarction)

VII. **Dosage Formulations**

A. Generic immediate-release (IR) tablet (10 mg, 25 mg, 50 mg, 75 mg, 100 mg, 150 mg [*scored*])

B. Generic liquid (10 mg/5 mL, 25 mg/5 mL, 50 mg/5 mL)

VIII. **Dosage Ranges and Guidelines (Insomnia)**

A. Refer to Table 4–6 for dosage ranges and guidelines.

B. Start at 10 mg taken about 1–3 hours before bedtime (Tmax=4 hours).

C. May be increased to 25, 50, 75, or 100 mg/day as needed. The dose can be lowered to as little as 5 mg using a pill splitter. Doses can be adjusted in 5-mg or 12.5-mg increments by splitting 10-mg or 25-mg tablets.

D. Lower dosages are typically required in older adult patients.

Table 4–6. Amitriptyline indications and dosage ranges

Indications	Usual dosage ranges
Depression	75–200 mg/day
Insomnia	10–100 mg/day

IX. **Monitoring**: None

X. **Relevant Pharmacokinetics/Pharmacodynamics**

A. **Metabolism**: Hepatic (cytochrome P450 [CYP] 2D6, CYP2C19)

B. **Time to peak plasma concentration**: 4 hours

C. **Half-life**:

1. Amitriptyline: 21 hours
2. Nortriptyline (primary metabolite): About 30 hours (range 18–44 hours)

D. **Effect of food**: The time to maximum concentration (Tmax) is increased by about 1 hour if dose is administered with a meal. Total absorption is unchanged.

E. **Hepatic impairment**: Increases amitriptyline and nortriptyline blood levels. Dosages should be adjusted accordingly.

F. **Renal impairment**: No significant effects on amitriptyline or nortriptyline levels.

G. **Age-related reduction in drug clearance**: Clearance may be reduced in elderly adults. Half-life is slightly increased in older patients, but there is usually very little difference in blood levels.

XI. Clinically Relevant Drug Interactions

A. Metabolized by CYP2D6 and CYP2C19

1. Amitriptyline dosage adjustments may be required if coadministered with CYP2D6 inhibitors.
2. Amitriptyline dosages will need to be adjusted for patients who are intermediate, poor, rapid, or ultrarapid metabolizers of CYP2D6.
3. Amitriptyline dosages may need to be adjusted after a change in dosage or discontinuation of a concomitantly used CYP2D6 inhibitor.
4. Commonly used CYP2D6 strong inhibitors: Fluoxetine, paroxetine, bupropion, ritonavir, cannabidiol. Moderate inhibitors: Duloxetine, terbinafine
5. CYP2C19 strong inhibitors can increase amitriptyline blood levels up to twofold.

B. Avoid use with monoamine oxidase inhibitors (MAOIs) (risk of serotonin syndrome).

XII. Adverse Effects

A. **Most common**:

1. CNS: Anxiety, dizziness, somnolence
2. Other: Blurred vision, constipation, dizziness, dry mouth, fatigue, impotence and anorgasmia, increased appetite and weight gain, indigestion, orthostatic hypotension, reduced libido, tachycardia, tremor, urinary hesitancy or retention

B. **Uncommon**: Elevated transaminases (usually mild), confusion, dyskinesias, hepatotoxicity (rare), memory problems, QTc prolongation, rash or other allergic reactions, restless legs, stuttering

1. New onset or worsening of suicidal ideation or self-injury in adolescents or young adults (i.e., antidepressant class effect)
2. Confusion and memory problems are more common in older adults, although they occur less frequently when lower dosages are used.

C. **Risks in pregnancy and lactation**:

1. Tricyclic antidepressants as a class were found to be associated with an increased risk of gastrointestinal malformations following pregnancy exposure in one study (Bérard et al. 2017).
2. Withdrawal symptoms, arrhythmias, irritability, respiratory distress, muscle spasms, seizures, and urinary retention have been reported in infants exposed to TCAs just before delivery (ACOG Practice Bulletin 2008).
3. Amitriptyline is excreted into breast milk and may cause infant somnolence or constipation. The World Health Organization (2002) has stated that the use of amitriptyline is compatible with breastfeeding at dosages up to 150 mg/day (barring infant adverse effects).

XIII. **Clinical Pearls/Prescribing Tips**

A. Because of the long half-life of amitriptyline and its primary metabolite nortriptyline, daytime sedation is common. Lowering the dosage is the only effective means of managing this problem.
B. Given its shorter half-life and fewer side effects, trazodone may be a better first choice for insomnia than amitriptyline among the sedating antidepressants.
C. Unlike the "Z drugs," amitriptyline has no (or extremely limited) abuse potential.
D. Cognitive-behavioral therapy for insomnia (CBT-i) is an effective alternative to medication management.

Further Reading

American Academy of Sleep Medicine Clinical Practice Guidelines. American Academy of Sleep Medicine. Available at: https://aasm.org/clinical-resources/practice-standards/practice-guidelines/. Accessed May 2022.

Amitriptyline. FDA prescribing information, May 2014. Available at: https://www.accessdata.fda.gov/drugsatfda_docs/label/2014/085966s095,085969s084,085968s096,085971s075,085967s076,085970s072lbl.pdf. Accessed May 2022.

Everitt H, Baldwin DS, Stuart B, et al: Antidepressants for insomnia in adults. Cochrane Database Syst Rev (5):CD010753, 2018 29761479

Thour A, Marwaha R: Amitriptyline, in StatPearls. Treasure Island, FL, StatPearls Publishing, 2022

References

ACOG Practice Bulletin: Clinical management guidelines for obstetrician-gynecologists number 92, April 2008 (replaces practice bulletin number 87, November 2007). Use of psychiatric medications during pregnancy and lactation. ACOG Committee on Practice Bulletins—Obstetrics. Obstet Gynecol 111(4):1001–1020, 2008 18378767

Bérard A, Zhao JP, Sheehy O: Antidepressant use during pregnancy and the risk of major congenital malformations in a cohort of depressed pregnant women: an updated analysis of the Quebec Pregnancy Cohort. BMJ Open 7(1):e013372, 2017 28082367

World Health Organization: Breast Feeding and Maternal Medication. Recommendations for Drugs in the Eleventh WHO Model List of Essential Drugs. Geneva, Switzerland, World Health Organization, February 2002. Available at: https://www.who.int/publications/i/item/55732. Accessed July 15, 2024.

Doxepin[1] (Insomnia)

I. **Brand Names**: Sinequan (discontinued), Adapin (discontinued), Prodoxin, Silenor, Zonalon

II. **Therapeutic Class**: Tricyclic antidepressant (TCA); antihistamine

III. **Mechanism-Based Class**

A. Histamine-1 (H_1) and serotonin-2A (5-HT_{2A}) receptor antagonist

B. Serotonin transporter (SERT) and norepinephrine transporter (NET) reuptake inhibitor

IV. **Mechanism of Action (insomnia)**

A. Blockade of H_1 and 5-HT_{2A} receptors

V. **Indications**

A. FDA adult:

1. Major depressive disorder
2. Insomnia
3. Dermatological allergies

B. Evidence-based[2] off-label uses: A variety of allergic and hypersensitivity reactions (e.g., urticaria, atopic dermatitis, lichen simplex)

C. FDA pediatric: None

VI. **Major Contraindications and When to Use Caution**

A. **Major contraindications**:

1. Known allergy to doxepin
2. Prior QTc prolongation

B. **Use caution**:

1. Elderly patients (risk of oversedation and falls)
2. Patients with prior cardiovascular disease (especially unstable angina or recent myocardial infarction)

VII. **Dosage Formulations**

A. Generic and brand immediate-release (IR) capsule (10 mg, 25 mg, 50 mg, 75 mg, 100 mg, 150 mg)

B. Generic and brand tablet (3 mg, 6 mg)

C. Generic liquid (10 mg/mL)

D. Generic cream (5%; each gram of cream contains 50 mg of doxepin hydrochloride—equivalent to 44.3 mg of doxepin)

VIII. **Dosage Ranges and Guidelines (insomnia)**

A. Refer to Table 4–7 for dosage ranges and guidelines.

B. Start at 3 mg taken about 1–2 hours before bedtime (T_{max}=3 hours).

---

[1]See Chapter 2, "Antidepressants," for more information regarding doxepin.

[2]Evidence strength varies; readers are referred to the literature for more detailed information.

C. May be increased to 6, 10, 25, or 50 mg as needed. The dose can be reduced to as little as 1.5 mg with a pill splitter. Doses can be adjusted in 1.5-mg increments by splitting 3-mg tablets.
D. Lower dosages are typically required in older adult patients.
E. Dosages will need to be adjusted for CYP2D6 intermediate, poor, rapid, and ultrarapid metabolizers.

Table 4–7. Doxepin indications and dosage ranges

Indications	**Usual dosage ranges**
Depression	75–150 mg/day
Insomnia	3–50 mg/day

IX. **Monitoring**: For depression, blood levels should be 150-250 ng/mL. There are no relevant blood levels for insomnia treatment.

X. **Relevant Pharmacokinetics/Pharmacodynamics**

A. **Metabolism**: Hepatic (cytochrome P450 [CYP] 2D6 [primary pathway], CYP2C19, CYP1A2, CYP3A4).
B. **Time to peak plasma concentration**: 4 hours
C. **Half-life**: 17 hours (range 8–24 hours)
D. **Hepatic impairment**: Increases doxepin blood levels. Dosages should be adjusted accordingly.
E. **Renal impairment**: No significant effects on doxepin levels.
F. **Age-related reduction in drug clearance**: Clearance may be reduced in elderly adults. However, typical dosages used for insomnia are usually well tolerated.

XI. **Clinically Relevant Drug Interactions**

A. Metabolized primarily by CYP2D6 and (to a lesser extent) by CYP2C19 and CYP3A4
1. Doxepin dosage adjustments may be required if coadministered with a CYP2D6 inhibitor (decreased).
2. The doxepin dosage may need to be adjusted after discontinuation of a CYP2D6 inhibitor or a change in the CYP2D6 inhibitor's dosage.
3. Doxepin dosages will need to be adjusted for patients who are poor, intermediate, rapid, or ultrarapid metabolizers of CYP2D6.
4. Commonly used CYP2D6 strong inhibitors include fluoxetine, paroxetine, bupropion, ritonavir, and cannabidiol; moderate inhibitors include duloxetine and terbinafine.
5. CYP2C19 strong inhibitors can increase blood levels up to twofold. (Strong inhibitors include fluconazole, ticlopidine, fluvoxamine, and fluoxetine.)

B. Avoid concomitant use with monoamine oxidase inhibitors (MAOIs) (risk of serotonin syndrome).

XII. Adverse Effects

A. **Most common**:

1. CNS: Anxiety, dizziness, oversedation, daytime somnolence.
2. Other: Blurred vision, constipation, dizziness, dry mouth, dysgeusia (bad taste), fatigue, increased appetite and weight gain, indigestion, orthostatic hypotension, reduced libido, tachycardia, tremor, urinary hesitancy or retention.

B. **Uncommon**: Elevated transaminases (usually mild), bowel obstruction (rare), confusion, diaphoresis, disorientation, edema, hepatotoxicity (rare), hypertension, nausea, memory problems, photosensitivity, QTc prolongation, rash or other allergic reactions, rebound insomnia, syndrome of inappropriate antidiuretic hormone secretion, vomiting

1. New onset or worsening of suicidal ideation or self-injury in adolescents or young adults (i.e., antidepressant class effect)
2. Confusion and memory problems are more common in older adults, although they occur less frequently when lower dosages are used.

C. **Risks in pregnancy and lactation**:

1. An increase in major malformations was not demonstrated in animal studies. Risks in humans are unclear but are probably low. Always consider consultation with an OB/GYN specialist.
2. Tricyclic antidepressants as a class were associated with an increased risk of gastrointestinal malformations following pregnancy exposure in one study (Bérard et al. 2017).
3. Doxepin is excreted into breast milk and may cause infant somnolence or constipation. This is seldom a problem with low doses. Always consider consultation with an OB/GYN specialist or lactation expert.

XIII. Clinical Pearls/Prescribing Tips

A. Because of doxepin's long half-life, daytime sedation is common. Lowering the dosage is the only effective means of managing this problem.

B. Because of its shorter half-life and fewer side effects, trazodone may be a better first choice for insomnia than doxepin among the sedating antidepressants.

C. Unlike the "Z drugs," doxepin has no (or extremely limited) abuse potential.

D. Cognitive-behavioral therapy for insomnia (CBT-i) is an effective alternative to medication management.

Further Reading

Almasi A, Meza CE: Doxepin, in StatPearls. Treasure Island, FL, StatPearls Publishing, 2022

American Academy of Sleep Medicine Clinical Practice Guidelines. Available at: https://aasm.org/clinical-resources/practice-standards/practice-guidelines/. Accessed May 2022.

Doxepin (depression) prescribing information. U.S. Food and Drug Administration, 2007. Available at: https://www.accessdata.fda.gov/drugsatfda_docs/label/2007/016798s054,017516s023lbl.pdf. Accessed May 2022.

Doxepin (insomnia) prescribing information. U.S. Food and Drug Administration, 2010. Available at: https://www.accessdata.fda.gov/drugsatfda_docs/label/2010/022036lbl.pdf. Accessed May 2022.
Everitt H, Baldwin DS, Stuart B, et al: Antidepressants for insomnia in adults. Cochrane Database Syst Rev (5):CD010753, 2018 29761479

References

Bérard A, Zhao JP, Sheehy O: Antidepressant use during pregnancy and the risk of major congenital malformations in a cohort of depressed pregnant women: an updated analysis of the Quebec Pregnancy Cohort. BMJ Open 7(1):e013372, 2017 28082367

Mirtazapine[1] (Insomnia)

I. **Brand Names**: Remeron, Remeron Soltab
II. **Therapeutic Class**: Tetracyclic antidepressant
III. **Mechanism-Based Class**: Histamine, norepinephrine, and serotonin receptor modulator
IV. **Mechanism of Action (Insomnia)**
  A. Blockade of H_1 and 5-HT_{2A} receptors (improvements in sleep are likely the result of this blockade)
  B. Inhibition of histamine (H_1), norepinephrine α_2, and serotonin 5-HT_{2A}, 5-HT_{2C}, 5-HT_3, and 5-HT_{2B} receptors.
V. **Indications**
  A. FDA adult:
    1. Major depressive disorder
  B. Evidence-based[2] off-label uses:
    1. Insomnia
    2. Low appetite/weight loss (especially in older adult patients, particularly in the context of depression)
  C. Other off-label uses (with very limited supporting data):
    1. Generalized anxiety disorder
    2. OCD
    3. Social anxiety disorder
    4. Panic disorder
    5. PTSD
    6. Nausea
    7. Pruritis

---

[1]See Chapter 2, "Antidepressants," for more information regarding mirtazapine.
[2]Evidence strength varies; readers are referred to the literature for more detailed information.

D. FDA pediatric: None

VI. **Major Contraindications and When to Use Caution**

A. **Major contraindications**:

1. Known allergy to mirtazapine

B. **Use caution**:

1. Older adult patients (risk of oversedation and falls).

C. **Avoid abrupt withdrawal**: Abruptly stopping mirtazapine may cause discontinuation effects (e.g., depression, anxiety, dizziness, paresthesias, diarrhea, nausea, flu-like symptoms).

VII. **Dosage Formulations**

A. Brand and generic immediate-release (IR) tablet (7.5 mg, 15 mg, 30 mg, 45 mg [*scored*])
B. Brand (Remeron Soltab) orally dissolving tablet (15 mg, 30 mg, 45 mg)

VIII. **Dosage Ranges and Guidelines (Insomnia)**

A. Refer to Table 4–8 for dosage ranges and guidelines.
B. Start at 7.5 mg taken about 60–90 minutes before bedtime (Tmax=90 minutes).
C. May increase or decrease in 7.5-mg increments as needed. The typical dosage range is 7.5–30 mg nightly, although some patients may require higher dosages. Note that higher dosages may also produce activation and worsen insomnia.
D. Lower dosages are typically required in older adult patients, especially men.

Table 4–8. Mirtazapine indications and dosage ranges

Indications	Usual dosage ranges
Depression	15–45 mg/day
Insomnia	7.5–30 mg/day

IX. **Monitoring**: None

X. **Relevant Pharmacokinetics/Pharmacodynamics**

A. **Metabolism**: Hepatic (cytochrome P450 [CYP] 1A2, CYP2D6, and CYP3A4)
B. **Time to peak plasma concentration**: About 100 minutes
C. **Half-life**: About 30 hours (range 20–40 hours). Half-life is variable based in part on patient CYP2D6 and CYP3A4 genotypes. Mirtazapine's half-life is affected by CYP3A4 inhibitors and inducers (increased and decreased, respectively) and CYP2D6 inhibitors (increased).
D. **Effect of food**: The time to maximum concentration (Tmax) is increased by about 1 hour if administered with a meal. Total absorption is unchanged.
E. **Hepatic impairment**: Mirtazapine levels are increased about 30% in patients with hepatic impairment. Dosages should be adjusted accordingly.

F. **Renal impairment**: Blood levels of mirtazapine are increased about 30% in patients with moderate renal impairment (creatinine clearance [CrCl] = 11–39 mL/min/1.73 m^2) and about 50% in severe impairment (CrCl < 10 mL/min/1.73 m^2). Dosages should be adjusted in patients with significant impairment.

G. **Age-related reduction in drug clearance**: Clearance may be reduced in elderly adults. Clearance may be reduced in elderly males by 30% and females by 10%.

XI. **Clinically Relevant Drug Interactions**

A. Metabolized by CYP3A4 (major) as well as by CYP1A2, CYP2C9, and CYP2D6 (to a lesser extent).

1. Mirtazapine dosage adjustments may be required if coadministered with CYP3A4 inhibitors or inducers (decrease or increase, respectively) or with CYP2D6 inhibitors (decreased). Dosages may need to be adjusted after a change in dosage or discontinuation of a concomitantly used inducer or inhibitor.

   a. Commonly used CYP3A4 strong inhibitors: Several protease inhibitors (e.g., indinavir, ritonavir), clarithromycin, ketoconazole. Moderate inhibitors: Ciprofloxacin, diltiazem, erythromycin, fluconazole, fluvoxamine, grapefruit and juice, verapamil.
   b. CYP3A4 inducers: Apalutamide, carbamazepine, efavirenz, enzalutamide, phenytoin, rifampin, St. John's wort.
   c. Commonly used CYP2D6 strong inhibitors: Fluoxetine, paroxetine, bupropion, ritonavir, cannabidiol. Moderate inhibitors: duloxetine, terbinafine.

B. Use with caution in combination with other sedative-hypnotics (e.g., benzodiazepines) or alcohol, which may increase risk for oversedation and accidents.

C. Avoid use with monoamine oxidase inhibitors (MAOIs) (risk of serotonin syndrome).

XII. **Adverse Effects**

A. **Most common**:

1. CNS: Daytime somnolence ("hangover" effect), dizziness
2. Other: Increased appetite, weight gain, constipation, dry mouth

B. **Uncommon**: Elevated transaminases (usually mild), elevated triglycerides and cholesterol (which may be associated with weight gain), confusion, discoordination/ataxia, rash or other allergic reaction, arthralgias

1. New onset or worsening of suicidal ideation or self-injury in adolescents or young adults (i.e., antidepressant class effect)

C. **Rare**: Severe neutropenia was reported in an extremely small number of people in the clinical trials (3 of 2,796; 1.1 per 1,000 patients). All recovered after mirtazapine was discontinued (Organon 2021). If a patient develops sore throat, fever, stomatitis, or other signs of infection along with a low white blood cell (WBC) count, mirtazapine should be discontinued, and the WBC count should be monitored until it recovers (absolute neutrophil count > 1,000/mm^3).

D. **Risks in pregnancy and lactation:**

1. Mirtazapine has not been shown to increase fetal malformations, but it is associated with fetal loss in animal studies. Risks in human pregnancy are unknown.
2. Mirtazapine may be transmitted in breast milk and might cause oversedation of infants, although the absolute transmission is low.

XIII. **Clinical Pearls/Prescribing Tips**

A. Because of its long (30-hour) half-life, daytime sedation is common with mirtazapine, and dosage adjustment is the only effective means of managing this problem. The reader is referred to comprehensive texts and other sources for more detail (e.g., Schatzberg and Nemeroff 2024).

B. Unlike the "Z drugs," mirtazapine has no (or extremely limited) abuse potential.

C. Mirtazapine is generally well tolerated in older patients, and it can be a good choice for treatment of insomnia, especially in patients with low appetite.

D. Cognitive-behavioral therapy for insomnia (CBT-i) is an effective alternative to medication management.

Further Reading

American Academy of Sleep Medicine Clinical Practice Guidelines. Available at: https://aasm.org/clinical-resources/practice-standards/practice-guidelines/. Accessed May 2022.

Jilani TN, Gibbons JR, Faizy RM, et al: Mirtazapine, in StatPearls. Treasure Island, FL, StatPearls Publishing, 2022

Center for Drug Evaluation and Research: Mirtazapine Clinical Pharmacology/Biopharmaceutics Review. 1997. Available at: https://www.accessdata.fda.gov/drugsatfda_docs/nda/97/20-415S003_Remeron_BioPharmr.pdf. Accessed June 21, 2024.

Schering Corporation: Remeron (mirtazapine) [package insert]. U.S. Food and Drug Administration website. 2009. Available at: https://www.accessdata.fda.gov/drugsatfda_docs/label/2010/020415s023s024.pdf. Accessed May 2022.

References

Organon: Remeron (mirtazapine) tablets [package insert]. Jersey City, NJ, Organon, revised November 2021. Available at: https://www.organon.com/product/usa/pi_circulars/r/remeron/remeron_tablets_pi.pdf. Accessed June 21, 2024.

Schatzberg AF, Nemeroff CB (eds): The American Psychiatric Association Publishing Textbook of Psychopharmacology, 6th Edition. Washington, DC, American Psychiatric Association Publishing, 2024

Trazodone[1] (Insomnia)

I. **Brand Names**: Desyrel (discontinued), Desyrel Dividose (discontinued), Oleptro extended release (discontinued)

II. **Therapeutic Class**: Antidepressant

III. **Mechanism-Based Class:** Serotonin receptor antagonist and reuptake inhibitor (SARI)

IV. **Mechanism(s) of Action**

A. Blockade of 5-HT_{2A} and 5-HT_{2B} receptors
B. Moderately potent inhibition of the serotonin transporter (SERT); dosage-dependent weak to moderate effects
C. Potent α_1 receptor blockade

V. **Indications**

A. FDA adult:

1. Major depressive disorder

B. Evidence-based[2] off-label uses:

1. Insomnia

C. Other off-label uses (with very limited supporting data):

1. Generalized anxiety disorder
2. Other anxiety disorders
3. PTSD

D. FDA pediatric: None

VI. **Major Contraindications and When to Use Caution**

A. **Major contraindications**:

1. Known allergy to trazodone

B. **Use caution**:

1. Older adult patients (risk of oversedation and falls)

VII. **Dosage Formulations**

A. Generic immediate-release (IR) tablet (50, 100, 150, 300 mg [*scored*])
B. Brand formulations are no longer available.

VIII. **Dosage Ranges and Guidelines (Insomnia)**

A. Refer to Table 4–9 for dosage ranges and guidelines.
B. Start at 50 mg taken about 60–90 minutes before bedtime (Tmax=90 minutes). In clinical practice, the dose is commonly repeated after 1 hour if no effect is seen, while remaining mindful of the total daily dose.

---

[1]See Chapter 2, "Antidepressants," for more information regarding trazodone.
[2]Evidence strength varies; readers are referred to the literature for more detailed information.

C. May increase or decrease the dosage in 25-mg increments (1/2 of a 50-mg tablet). The typical dosage range is 25–300 nightly as needed.
D. Consider lower starting dosages in older adult patients (25 mg/day).

Table 4–9. Trazodone indications and dosage ranges

Indications	Usual dosage ranges
Depression	150–400 mg/day
Insomnia	25–300 mg/day

IX. **Monitoring**: None

X. **Relevant Pharmacokinetics/Pharmacodynamics**

A. **Metabolism**: Hepatic (cytochrome P450 [CYP] 3A4, CYP2D6, and CYP1A2)
B. **Time to peak plasma concentration**: 90 minutes
C. **Half-life**:
   1. Trazodone: about 6 hours (variable based on CYP genotypes)
   2. Primary metabolite meta-chlorophenylpiperazine (mCPP): 6 hours (also variable)
D. **Hepatic impairment**: Trazodone has not been systematically studied in patients with hepatic impairment. It has exclusive hepatic clearance, so impairment is expected to affect metabolism.
E. **Renal impairment**: Trazodone has not been systematically studied in patients with renal impairment. However, there is little if any direct renal clearance.

XI. **Clinically Relevant Drug Interactions**

A. Metabolized by CYP34
   1. Dosage adjustment may be required with CYP3A4 inhibitors or inducers (decrease or increase, respectively). Dosage may need to be adjusted after a change in dose or discontinuation of an inducer or inhibitor.
B. Trazodone's primary metabolite, meta-chlorophenylpiperazine (mCPP), can be very anxiogenic (e.g., can cause panic attacks), stimulating, and (in rare cases) hallucinogenic. mCPP is a CYP2D6 substrate and can accumulate in intermediate and (especially) poor metabolizers of CYP2D6. The effects of mCPP accumulation include worsening of insomnia and anxiety, and clinicians should be able to recognize these effects as potentially attributable to this cause.
C. Use with caution in combination with other sedative-hypnotics (e.g., benzodiazepines) or alcohol, which may increase the risk of oversedation and accidents.
D. Avoid use with monoamine oxidase inhibitors (MAOIs), especially at dosages higher than 100 mg/day (risk of serotonin syndrome).
E. Trazodone prolongs the QTc interval and should be avoided in patients with known QTc prolongation or in combination with drugs that also increase the QTc.
F. Trazodone may increase the effects of anticoagulants.

XII. **Adverse Effects**

A. **Most common**:

1. CNS: Daytime somnolence ("hangover" effect), dizziness/lightheadedness (α_1 receptor blockade)
2. Other: Dry mouth, blurred vision, dizziness, fatigue, nausea and vomiting

B. **Uncommon**: Anxiety, confusion, drug-associated spontaneous orgasm (very rare), discoordination/ataxia, exacerbation of angle-closure glaucoma, hyponatremia, nasal congestion, orthostatic hypotension, penile or clitoral priapism (rare), syncope, rash or other allergic reaction

1. New onset or worsening of suicidal ideation or self-injury in adolescents or young adults (i.e., antidepressant class effect)

C. **Risks in pregnancy and lactation**:

1. Trazodone was not shown to increase fetal malformations in animal studies. Risks in human pregnancy are unknown.
2. Trazodone is transmitted in breast milk and can cause oversedation in infants.

XIII. **Clinical Pearls/Prescribing Tips**

A. Trazodone is often underdosed. Dosages higher than 50 or 100 mg nightly may be needed to produce adequate sleep in some patients. The author has used dosages up to 300 mg nightly in some patients with caution.

B. Oversedation, especially morning somnolence, can be managed in two ways:

1. Lowering the dose (including using 1/2 or 1/4 of a 50-mg tablet).
2. Dosing earlier in the evening (e.g., back up the dosing time in 15- or 30-minute increments to produce optimal results).

C. Trazodone has relatively potent α_1 blockade (Ki=12–42 nM), so monitor for orthostatic hypotension, dizziness, and falls, especially in elderly adults.

D. Unlike the "Z-drugs," trazodone has no (or extremely limited) abuse potential.

E. Cognitive-behavioral therapy for insomnia (CBT-i) is an effective alternative to medication management.

Further Reading

Shin JJ, Saadabadi A: Trazodone, in StatPearls. Treasure Island, FL, StatPearls Publishing, 2022

Trazodone (extended-release) Medical Review(s). Center for Drug Evaluation and Research, 2019. Available at: https://www.accessdata.fda.gov/drugsatfda_docs/nda/2010/022411s000MedR.pdf. Accessed May 2022.

Trazodone prescribing information. U.S. Food and Drug Administration, 2017. Available at: https://www.accessdata.fda.gov/drugsatfda_docs/label/2017/018207s032lbl.pdf. Accessed May 2022.

Yi XY, Ni SF, Ghadami MR, et al: Trazodone for the treatment of insomnia: a meta-analysis of randomized placebo-controlled trials. Sleep Med 45:25–32, 2018 29680424

Antihypertensives

Clonidine[1] (Nightmares)

I. **Brand Names**: Catapres, Catapres-TTS (transdermal therapeutic system), Duraclon (IV formulation), Jenloga (extended-release), Kapvay (extended-release), Nexiclon XR (extended-release)

II. **Therapeutic Class**: Antihypertensive

III. **Mechanism-Based Class**: Centrally acting α_2-adrenergic receptor agonist

IV. **Mechanism(s) of Action**

A. Blockade/activation of norepinephrine α_1 and α_2 receptors

V. **Indications**

A. FDA adult:

1. ADHD
2. Hypertension

B. Evidence-based off-label uses:

1. Trauma-related nightmares
2. Tics associated with Tourette syndrome

C. Other off-label uses (with limited supporting data/evidence):

1. Insomnia, borderline personality disorder, anxiety disorders, restless legs syndrome, rosacea, migraines, perimenopausal hot flashes, diarrhea associated with irritable bowel syndrome, perioperative treatment of pheochromocytoma, hallucinogen persisting perception disorder, PTSD symptoms

D. FDA pediatric: ADHD

VI. **Major Contraindications and When to Use Caution**

A. **Major contraindications**:

1. Known hypersensitivity to clonidine
2. Stop clonidine before cataract surgery to reduce the incidence of intraoperative floppy iris syndrome (IFIS).

B. **Use caution**:

1. People with low blood pressure or who are taking other antihypertensives, which may require dosage adjustment when coadministered with clonidine
2. Older adult patients
3. Concomitant use with sedatives or drugs that induce atrioventricular (AV) conduction delays (e.g., tricyclic antidepressants)

---

[1]Also see Chapter 7, "Stimulants," and Chapter 10, "Treatment of Substance Use Disorders" for more information regarding clonidine's use for other indications and conditions.

VII. Dosage Formulations

A. Generic immediate-release (IR) tablet (0.1 mg, 0.2 mg, 0.3 mg)
B. Brand (Kapvay) or generic 12-hour extended-release (ER) tablet (0.1 mg)
C. Brand (Nexiclon XR) or generic 24-hour ER tablet (0.17 mg)
D. Catapres-TTS is a weekly transdermal patch system available in three patch sizes/dose strengths. A generic patch is available in the same doses.

1. Formulations: Catapres-TTS-1 (3.5 cm^2 [0.1 mg/day]; Catapres-TTS-2: 7.0 cm^2 [0.2 mg/day]; Catapres-TTS-3: 10.5 cm^2 [0.3 mg/day])
2. Apply once every 7 days to a hairless area of intact skin on the upper outer arm or chest. Each new application should be on a different skin site from the previous location.

VIII. Dosage Ranges and Guidelines

A. ADHD (children age 6–17 years): Start at 0.1 mg/day. Adjust in 0.1-mg increments to a maximum of 0.4 mg/day as needed. Dosages higher than 0.1 mg/day should be divided between morning and bedtime.
B. Trauma-related nightmares (adults): Start at 0.1 mg taken at bedtime. Advance as needed to 0.4 mg/day in 0.1-mg increments.
C. Hypertension: Start at 0.1 mg twice per day. Advance in 0.1-mg to 0.2-mg increments as required. Maximum dosage is 0.6 mg/day divided into 2 doses. A larger portion of the daily dosage may need to be taken at bedtime to prevent daytime somnolence.

IX. **Monitoring**: None

X. Relevant Pharmacokinetics/Pharmacodynamics

A. **Metabolism**: Hepatic (cytochrome P450 [CYP] 2D6, CYP1A1, CYP1A2, CYP3A4, and CYP3A5).
B. **Time to peak plasma concentration**:

1. IR: About 2 hours
2. ER: About 5.5 hours (range: 4–7 hours)

C. **Half-life**: 13 hours
D. **Hepatic impairment**: Clonidine is hepatically metabolized, and impairment leads to increased blood levels and half-life.
E. **Renal impairment**: Fifty percent of clonidine is eliminated unchanged in urine. Renal impairment results in a substantial increase in half-life and blood levels. Use in patients with moderate to severe renal impairment is not recommended.

XI. Clinically Relevant Drug Interactions

A. Use with caution with other antihypertensives, sedatives, or drugs that induce atrioventricular conduction delays (e.g., tricyclic antidepressants).

XII. Adverse Effects

A. **Most common**: Orthostatic hypotension, anxiety, constipation, dizziness, dry mouth, erectile dysfunction, fatigue, headache, nausea, rash, salivary gland pain, somnolence. Most side effects improve with continued use and can be reduced by starting at a low dosage and titrating slowly.

B. **Uncommon**: Angioedema, allergy (including urticaria), bradycardia, delusions (rare), elevated transaminases, hallucinations (rare), nightmares, paresthesias, pruritus, syncope.

C. Catapres-TTS: In addition to the side effects listed above, about half of patients using the transdermal patch will develop local erythema related to the patch itself. Other possible skin reactions include hyperpigmentation, localized edema, papules, and vesiculation.

D. **Risks in pregnancy and lactation:**

1. Fetal loss was shown in animal studies at both low and high dosages. Fetal malformations were not shown in animal studies. However, risk in pregnancy in humans is unknown. Clonidine's use in pregnant women is not recommended.
2. A relatively high amount of clonidine is transmitted in breast milk and may result in adverse reactions in infants. Use while breastfeeding is not recommended.

XIII. **Clinical Pearls/Prescribing Tips**

A. Patients taking clonidine should be warned to get up slowly when rising from a seated or lying position to reduce the risk of dizziness and fainting, especially early in treatment.

B. For older adult patients, use lower dosages and increase in small increments.

C. There are very few data supporting the use of clonidine in the management of PTSD or trauma-related nightmares.

D. For ADHD, clonidine is less effective than classic CNS stimulants in improving focus and distractibility. It is more effective for impulsivity, emotion regulation problems, and insomnia. Clonidine is often used in combination with stimulant medications.

E. When discontinuing clonidine, taper dosages to prevent rebound hypertension.

Further Reading

Catapres-TTS prescribing information. U.S. Food and Drug Administration, October 2011. Available at: https://www.accessdata.fda.gov/drugsatfda_docs/label/2012/018891s028lbl.pdf. Accessed March 13, 2024.

Clonidine ER prescribing information. U.S. Food and Drug Administration, 2010. Available at: https://www.accessdata.fda.gov/drugsatfda_docs/label/2010/022331s001s002lbl.pdf. Accessed March 13, 2024.

Clonidine prescribing information. U.S. Food and Drug Administration, 2005. Available at: https://www.accessdata.fda.gov/drugsatfda_docs/label/2009/017407s034lbl.pdf. Accessed March 13, 2024.

Detweiler MB, Pagadala B, Candelario J, et al: Treatment of post-traumatic stress disorder nightmares at a veterans affairs medical center. J Clin Med 5(12):117, 2016 27999253

Shalev A, Liberzon I, Marmar C: Post-traumatic stress disorder. N Engl J Med 376(25):2459–2469, 2017 28636846

Yasaei R, Saadabadi A: Clonidine [Updated July 17, 2023], in: StatPearls [Internet]. Treasure Island, FL, StatPearls Publishing, 2024. Available at: https://www.ncbi.nlm.nih.gov/books/NBK459124/. Accessed June 21, 2024.

Doxazosin (Nightmares)

I. **Brand Names**: Cardura, Cardura X
II. **Therapeutic Class**: Antihypertensive
III. **Mechanism-Based Class**: Norepinephrine α_1 receptor antagonist
IV. **Mechanism(s) of Action**

A. Doxazosin blocks the effects of norepinephrine mediated through the α_1 receptor.

V. **Indications**

A. FDA adult:

1. Hypertension
2. Benign prostatic hypertrophy

B. Evidence-based[1] off-label uses:

1. Trauma-related nightmares
2. Ureteral calculi
3. Perioperative treatment of pheochromocytoma

C. Other off-label uses (with limited supporting data/evidence):

1. PTSD symptoms

D. FDA pediatric: None

VI. **Major Contraindications and When to Use Caution**

A. **Major contraindications**:

1. Known hypersensitivity to doxazosin.
2. Stop doxazosin before cataract surgery to reduce the incidence of intraoperative floppy iris syndrome (IFIS).

B. **Use caution**: People with low blood pressure or who are taking other antihypertensives in conjunction with doxazosin may require dosage adjustment to avoid hypotension. Older adult patients.

VII. **Dosage Formulations**

A. Brand and generic immediate-release (IR) capsule (1 mg, 2 mg, 4 mg, 8 mg)
B. Brand and generic extended-release (ER) tablet (4 mg, 8 mg)

VIII. **Dosage Ranges and Guidelines**

A. The recommended starting dosage for all disorders is 1 mg/day for at least 2 weeks to reduce the risk of acute hypotension, unless using the ER tablet (do not cut the tablets). Increase in 1- to 2-mg increments every 2 weeks for the IR formulation.
B. Trauma-related nightmares (off-label; adults): Start at 1 mg at bedtime. Increase in 1- to 2-mg increments every 2 weeks, with an initial target dosage of 4 mg/day as tolerated. The dosage can be increased to 8 mg/day as needed, although higher dosages can be used if required.

---

[1]Evidence strength varies; readers are referred to the literature for more detailed information.

C. PTSD (off-label): Doxazosin has been used to treat PTSD symptoms other than nightmares (e.g., daytime hyperarousal). The suggested range is 2–16 mg/day in divided doses, typically with a larger fraction of the dose taken in the evening.
D. Hypertension: Start at 1 mg/day. Advance in 1- to 2-mg increments as required. Maximum dosage is 16 mg/day divided into 2–3 doses.
E. Benign prostatic hypertrophy: Start at 1 mg/day. Increase as needed to 8 mg/day taken in 1 or 2 doses.

IX. **Monitoring**: None

X. **Relevant Pharmacokinetics/Pharmacodynamics**

A. **Metabolism**: Hepatic (cytochrome P450 [CYP] 3A4 [primary pathway], CYP2C19, CYP2D6, and CYP2C19)
B. **Time to peak plasma concentration**:
   1. Immediate-release: 2.4 hours
   2. Extended-release: 8 hours
C. **Half-life**: 22 hours
D. **Effect of food**: There is a slight reduction in blood levels (not considered to be clinically significant) when doxazosin is administered with food.
E. **Hepatic impairment**: Doxazosin is hepatically metabolized, and impairment is likely to lead to increased blood levels and half-life.
F. **Renal impairment**: No effect

XI. **Clinically Relevant Drug Interactions**

A. Metabolized by CYP2C19, CYP2D6, CYP3A4, all to a minor extent
   1. There is no known effect of CYP enzyme inhibitors or inducers.
B. Doxazosin has 98% protein binding and may interact with other highly bound drugs with narrow therapeutic ranges (e.g., warfarin).
C. Use with caution with other antihypertensives.

XII. **Adverse Effects**

A. **Most common**: Orthostatic hypotension, dizziness, edema, fatigue, somnolence. Most side effects improve with continued use and can be reduced by starting at a low dosage and titrating slowly.
B. **Uncommon**: Abdominal discomfort, allergy, anxiety, dry mouth, diaphoresis, dyspnea, edema, increased urinary frequency, insomnia, priapism (very rare), pruritus, rash, syncope, tachycardia.
C. **Risks in pregnancy and lactation**:
   1. Fetal loss was shown in animal studies at extremely high dosages. Fetal malformations were not shown in animal studies at lower or higher dosages. However, risk in pregnancy in humans is unknown.
   2. A relatively high amount of doxazosin is transmitted in breast milk and may result in adverse reactions in infants. Use in breastfeeding is not recommended.

XIII. **Clinical Pearls/Prescribing Tips**

A. Patients taking doxazosin should be warned to get up slowly when rising from a seated or lying position to reduce the risk of dizziness and fainting, especially early in treatment.

B. For older adult patients, use lower dosages and increase in small increments.

C. Even though doxazosin may seem like a more logical choice for the treatment of PTSD than prazosin because of its longer half-life, there has been very little systematic study of its benefits.

D. Given its relatively long half-life, doxazosin can be given once per day unless side effects occur at the time of peak blood concentration (about 3 hours after a dose). Extended-release doxazosin is usually not used/needed.

E. When discontinuing doxazosin, taper dosages to prevent rebound hypertension.

Further Reading

Berger W, Mendlowicz MV, Marques-Portella C, et al: Pharmacologic alternatives to antidepressants in posttraumatic stress disorder: a systematic review. Prog Neuropsychopharmacol Biol Psychiatry 33(2):169–180, 2009 19141307

Doxazosin extended-release prescribing information. U.S. Food and Drug Administration, 2009. Available at: https://www.accessdata.fda.gov/drugsatfda_docs/label/2010/021269s011lbl.pdf. Accessed June 2022.

Doxazosin prescribing information. U.S. Food and Drug Administration, 2009. Available at: https://www.accessdata.fda.gov/drugsatfda_docs/label/2009/019668s021lbl.pdf. Accessed June 2022.

Kim J, Nguyen H: Doxazosin, in StatPearls. Treasure Island, FL, StatPearls Publishing, 2021

Shalev A, Liberzon I, Marmar C: Post-traumatic stress disorder. N Engl J Med 376(25):2459–2469, 2017 28636846

Smith C, Koola MM: Evidence for using doxazosin in the treatment of posttraumatic stress disorder. Psychiatr Ann 46(9):553–555, 2016 27667865

Prazosin (Nightmares)

I. **Brand Names**: Minipress, Minipress XL

II. **Therapeutic Class**: Antihypertensive

III. **Mechanism-Based Class**: Norepinephrine α_1 receptor antagonist

IV. **Mechanism(s) of Action**

A. Prazosin blocks norepinephrine effects mediated via the α_1-adrenergic receptor.

V. **Indications**

A. FDA adult:

1. Hypertension
2. Benign prostatic hypertrophy (prazosin extended release)

B. Evidence-based[1] off-label uses:

1. Trauma-related nightmares
2. PTSD symptoms
3. Raynaud's phenomenon
4. Pheochromocytoma-associated hypertension

C. FDA pediatric: None

VI. **Major Contraindications and When to Use Caution**

A. **Major contraindications**:

1. Known hypersensitivity to prazosin
2. Stop prazosin before cataract surgery to reduce the incidence of intraoperative floppy iris syndrome (IFIS).

B. **Use caution**:

1. People with low blood pressure or those taking other antihypertensives (which may need to be adjusted)
2. Older patients

VII. **Dosage Formulations**

A. Brand and generic immediate-release (IR) capsule (1 mg, 2 mg, 5 mg)

B. Brand and generic extended-release (ER) tablet (2.5 mg, 5 mg)

VIII. **Dosage Ranges and Guidelines**

A. Trauma-related nightmares (off-label) (adults): Start at 1 mg/day. Increase in 1- to 2-mg increments as needed. Maximum dosage is 16 mg/day. Starting at 1 mg/day is generally recommended to ensure that hypotension or other serious adverse effects do not develop.

B. PTSD (off-label): Start at 1–2 mg BID. Dosage can be increased in 2- to 5-mg increments to a maximum of 30 mg/day divided into 2–3 doses.

1. The Veterans Administration minimum recommended dosage (Alexander et al. 2015) is 6 mg/day divided into 2–3 doses.

---

[1]Evidence strength varies; readers are referred to the literature for more detailed information.

C. Hypertension: Start at 1 mg BID. Advance in 1- to 2-mg increments as required. Maximum dosage is 20 mg/day divided into 2–3 doses.
D. Benign prostatic hypertrophy: Start at 0.5–1 mg BID. Increase as needed to 2 mg BID.

IX. **Monitoring**: None

X. **Relevant Pharmacokinetics/Pharmacodynamics**

A. **Metabolism**: Hepatic (cytochrome P450 [CYP] 3A4 and probably other pathways)
B. **Time to peak plasma concentration**:
   1. IR: 3 hours
   2. ER: 12 hours
C. **Half-life**: About 3 hours
D. **Effect of food**: Increases rate of absorption.
E. **Hepatic impairment**: The effects of impairment have not been studied. However, prazosin undergoes extensive/significant first-pass metabolism; therefore, it is likely that impairment will lead to increased blood levels and half-life.
F. **Renal impairment**: Unknown. However, there is only a small amount of direct excretion. Therefore, impairment is unlikely to have significant effects.

XI. **Clinically Relevant Drug Interactions**

A. Although prazosin has high hepatic first-pass metabolism, there is no known effect of CYP enzyme inhibitors or inducers.
B. Prazosin has 97% protein binding and may interact with other highly bound drugs with narrow therapeutic ranges (e.g., warfarin).
C. Use with caution with other antihypertensives.

XII. **Adverse Effects**

A. **Most common**: Orthostatic hypotension, dizziness, fatigue, muscle weakness, nausea, palpitations, somnolence. Most side effects improve with continued use.
B. **Uncommon**: Abdominal discomfort, allergy, alopecia, anxiety, bradycardia, constipation, depression, diaphoresis, diarrhea, dyspnea, edema, elevated transaminases, flushing, hallucinations (extremely rare), impotence, incontinence, increased urinary frequency, lichen planus, paresthesia, priapism, pruritus, rash, syncope, tachycardia, tinnitus, urinary frequency, vertigo, vomiting
C. **Risks in pregnancy and lactation**:
   1. Risk in pregnancy is unknown. Miscarriage and fetal malformations were shown in animal studies at extremely high dosages. Consider consultation with an OB/GYN specialist.
   2. Small amounts of prazosin are transmitted in breast milk and may result in adverse reactions in infants. Use in breastfeeding is not recommended.

XIII. **Clinical Pearls/Prescribing Tips**

A. Warn patients to get up slowly when rising from a seated or lying position to reduce the risk of dizziness and fainting, especially early in treatment. In other words, use caution with position change.

B. Lower dosages with increases in small increments should be used in older adult patients.

C. A single open-label study found that prazosin reduced mortality from scorpion stings in children (Bawaskar and Bawaskar 2011).

Further Reading

Basquez R, Pippin MM: Prazosin, in StatPearls. Treasure Island, FL, StatPearls Publishing, 2022

Berger W, Mendlowicz MV, Marques-Portella C, et al: Pharmacologic alternatives to antidepressants in posttraumatic stress disorder: a systematic review. Prog Neuropsychopharmacol Biol Psychiatry 33(2):169–180, 2009 19141307

Kung S, Espinel Z, Lapid MI: Treatment of nightmares with prazosin: a systematic review. Mayo Clin Proc 87(9):890–900, 2012 22883741

Prazosin extended-release prescribing information. U.S. Food and Drug Administration, 2017. Available at: https://labeling.pfizer.com/ShowLabeling.aspx?id=14828. Accessed June 2022.

Prazosin prescribing information. U.S. Food and Drug Administration, 2009. Available at: https://www.accessdata.fda.gov/drugsatfda_docs/label/2009/017442s033lbl.pdf. Accessed June 2022.

Shalev A, Liberzon I, Marmar C: Post-traumatic stress disorder. N Engl J Med 376(25):2459–2469, 2017 28636846

References

Alexander B, Lund BC, Bernardy NC, et al: Early discontinuation and suboptimal dosing of prazosin: a potential missed opportunity for veterans with posttraumatic stress disorder. J Clin Psychiatry 76(5):e639–e644, 2015 26035198

Bawaskar HS, Bawaskar PH: Efficacy and safety of scorpion antivenom plus prazosin compared with prazosin alone for venomous scorpion (Mesobuthus tamulus) sting: randomised open label clinical trial. BMJ 342:c7136, 2011 21209062

Terazosin (Nightmares)

I. **Brand Name**: Hytrin

II. **Therapeutic Class**: Antihypertensive

III. **Mechanism-Based Class**: Norepinephrine α_1 receptor antagonist

IV. **Mechanism(s) of Action**

A. Terazosin blocks the effects of norepinephrine mediated through the α_1 receptor.

V. **Indications**

A. FDA adult:

1. Hypertension
2. Benign prostatic hypertrophy

B. Evidence-based[1] off-label uses:

1. Trauma-related nightmares
2. PTSD symptoms
3. Ureteral calculi
4. Perioperative treatment of pheochromocytoma

C. FDA pediatric: None

VI. **Major Contraindications and When to Use Caution**

A. **Major contraindications**:

1. Known hypersensitivity to terazosin.
2. Stop terazosin before cataract surgery to reduce the incidence of intraoperative floppy iris syndrome (IFIS).

B. **Use caution**: People with low blood pressure or on other antihypertensives that may need to be adjusted. Older patients.

VII. **Dosage Formulations**: Brand and generic immediate-release (IR) capsule (1 mg, 2 mg, 5 mg)

VIII. **Dosage Ranges and Guidelines**

A. For all disorders, the initial dosage should always be 1 mg/day, continued for at least 2 weeks, to reduce the risk of acute hypotension. Dosage increases should also be made at 2-week intervals.

B. Trauma-related nightmares (adults): Start at 1 mg at bedtime for 2 weeks. The dosage can then be increased in 1- to 2-mg increments as needed and tolerated. There are no clear dosing guidelines, and dosages have varied widely in case reports, most of which used maximum dosages of up to 8 mg/day, although terazosin is approved at 20 mg/day for hypertension.

C. PTSD: Same as for nightmares, with the exception that part of the dosage can be given during the day.

---

[1]Evidence strength varies; readers are referred to the literature for more detailed information.

D. Hypertension: Start at 1 mg/day. Advance in 2- to 5-mg increments as required. Maximum dosage is 20 mg/day divided into 2–3 doses.
E. Benign prostatic hypertrophy: Start at 1 mg/day. Increase to a dosage of 2 mg, 5 mg, or 10 mg/day taken in 1 or 2 doses as needed.

IX. **Monitoring**: None

X. **Relevant Pharmacokinetics/Pharmacodynamics**

A. **Metabolism**: Hepatic (cytochrome P450 [CYP] 3A1 and CYP3A2)
B. **Time to peak plasma concentration**:
   1. Immediate release: 2.4 hours
   2. Extended release: 8 hours
C. **Half-life**: 22 hours
D. **Effect of food**: There is a slight reduction in blood levels (not considered to be clinically significant) when terazosin is administered with food.
E. **Hepatic impairment**: Terazosin is hepatically metabolized, and impairment is likely to lead to increased blood levels and half-life.
F. **Renal impairment**: No effect

XI. **Clinically Relevant Drug Interactions**

A. There is no known effect of CYP enzyme inhibitors or inducers.
B. Terazosin has 90%–94% protein binding and may interact with other highly bound drugs with narrow therapeutic ranges (e.g., warfarin).
C. Use with caution with other antihypertensives.

XII. **Adverse Effects**

A. **Most common**: Orthostatic hypotension, dizziness, edema, fatigue, somnolence. Most side effects improve with continued use and can be reduced by starting at a low dosage and titrating slowly.
B. **Uncommon**: Abdominal discomfort, allergy, anxiety, dry mouth, diaphoresis, dyspnea, increased urinary frequency, insomnia, priapism (very rare), pruritus, rash, syncope, tachycardia.
C. **Risks in pregnancy and lactation**:
   1. Fetal loss was shown in animal studies at extremely high dosages. Fetal malformations were not shown in animal studies at lower or higher dosages. However, risk in pregnancy in humans is unknown. Consider consultation with an OB/GYN specialist.
   2. A relatively high amount of terazosin is transmitted in breast milk and may result in adverse reactions in infants. Use in breastfeeding is not recommended.

XIII. **Clinical Pearls/Prescribing Tips**

A. Warn patients to get up slowly when rising from a seated or reclining position to reduce the risk of dizziness and fainting, especially early in treatment. In other words, patients should be careful with position changes.
B. Lower dosages with increases in small increments should be used in older patients.
C. Even though terazosin may seem to be a more logical choice for treatment of PTSD than prazosin because of its longer half-life, there are only case reports and series supporting its efficacy.

D. Given its relatively long half-life, terazosin can be given once per day unless side effects occur at the time of peak blood concentration (about 2–3 hours after a dose).
E. When discontinuing terazosin, taper dosage to prevent rebound hypertension.

Further Reading

Aphena Pharma Solutions: Terazosin hydrochloride capsule [package insert]. U.S. Food and Drug Administration website. Revised January 2021. Available at: https://www.accessdata.fda.gov/spl/data/b23a32b3-7e6b-4b58-be96-303ac3ef069a/b23a32b3-7e6b-4b58-be96-303ac3ef069a.xml. Accessed June 2022.

Detweiler MB, Pagadala B, Candelario J, et al: Treatment of post-traumatic stress disorder nightmares at a Veterans Affairs Medical Center. J Clin Med 5(12):117, 2016 27999253

Shalev A, Liberzon I, Marmar C: Post-traumatic stress disorder. N Engl J Med 376(25):2459–2469, 2017 28636846

Yang CH, Raja A: Terazosin, in StatPearls. Treasure Island, FL, StatPearls Publishing, 2022

5

Mood Stabilizers

Richard C. Shelton, M.D.

Overview

- Mood stabilizers represent a broad class of drugs with varying mechanisms of action. They are commonly utilized in the treatment of bipolar disorder I and II. Some mood stabilizers are FDA approved to treat specific mood states in bipolar disorder. Mood stabilizers are also sometimes used in the treatment of other mood disorders (e.g., the off-label use of lithium in treatment-resistant major depressive disorder). Some mood-stabilizing agents are clinically used in the treatment of anxiety or psychotic disorders, often as adjunctive agents (off-label). Common off-label and evidence-based uses of mood stabilizers are covered in this Handbook. However, an in-depth review of these off-label uses or a review of less common or less-evidence-based uses goes beyond the scope of this chapter and intent of this book. The evidence-based off-label use of medication blends the art of clinical practice with the clinician's ability to apply the medical literature to individual patients, often harnessing the known clinical effects and mechanisms of action of a specific drug to treat target symptoms

Anticonvulsants and Severe Cutaneous Reactions

- Severe cutaneous adverse reactions, including Stevens-Johnson syndrome (SJS), toxic epidermal necrolysis (TEN), and drug reaction with eosinophilia and systemic symptoms (DRESS) to antiepileptic drugs (AEDs), are rare but result in significant morbidity and mortality. The risk of developing these serious rashes has been found to be higher in populations with an inherited allelic variant of the HLA-B gene (Chung et al. 2021). Accordingly, the FDA recommends screening for the HLA-B*15:02 allele before initiating treatment with AEDs in patients of Asian ancestry, who are known to have high frequencies of this allele.

Anticonvulsant Boxed Warning: Serious Dermatological Reactions

Serious and sometimes fatal dermatological reactions, including **toxic epidermal necrolysis (TEN)** and **Stevens-Johnson syndrome (SJS)**, have been reported during treatment with various anticonvulsant medications, including **carbamazepine, lamotrigine, oxcarbazepine, and valproate**.

Warning signs of SJS/TEN: Severe widespread erythematous rash with tenderness, confluence, or erythema multiforme and exfoliation of skin/mucosa (Lorberg et al. 2009). Systemic symptoms (e.g., fever, malaise, lymphadenopathy) may occur prior to rash. Rash often involves the neck, upper trunk, face, lips, tongue, and/or oral or vaginal mucosa.

Risk factors: Cotherapy of lamotrigine with valproate, rapid dosage escalation, prior rash with an anticonvulsant, young age (age <12 years), genetic factors (see below).

Genetic factors:

- SJS/TEN incidence is much higher among Asian populations in South China, Thailand, Malaysia, parts of the Philippines, and Taiwan than among other population groups.
- Studies in patients of Asian/Chinese ancestry have found a strong association between the risk of developing SJS/TEN and the presence of HLA-B*15:02, an inherited allelic variant of the HLA-B gene. SJS/TEN is associated with HLA-B*44:03 in people of Korean descent and with HLA-B*58:01 in people not of Asian origin (e.g., European, African American, Hispanic, Native American ancestry). HLA-A*31:01 is associated with several types of generalized rashes in European and Asian populations.

References

Chung SJ, Ahn KM, Oh JH, et al: Incidence rates of severe cutaneous adverse reactions due to anti-seizure medication: a nationwide study using health claims data in Korea. Epilepsia 62(1):250–257, 2021 33188522

Lorberg B, Youssef NA, Bhagwagar Z: Lamotrigine-associated rash: to rechallenge or not to rechallenge? Int J Neuropsychopharmacol 12(2):257–265, 2009 18845017

Carbamazepine

I. **Brand Names**: Carbatrol, Carnexiv (discontinued), Epitol, Equetro, Tegretol, Tegretol XR, Teril

II. **Therapeutic Class**: Anticonvulsant

III. **Mechanism-Based Class**: Sodium channel inhibitor

IV. **Mechanism(s) of Action**

A. Carbamazepine's mechanism of action in bipolar disorder is not fully understood.
B. Carbamazepine blocks voltage-gated sodium channels, reducing the high-frequency firing of neurons, thereby decreasing membrane excitability (Macdonald and Kelly 1995).

V. **Indications**

A. FDA adult:

1. Seizures
2. Trigeminal neuralgia
3. Acute bipolar I mania or mixed states (only as Equetro)

B. Evidence-based[1] off-label uses: Bipolar maintenance
C. FDA pediatric: Seizures

VI. **Major Contraindications and When to Use Caution**

A. **Major contraindications**:

1. Known hypersensitivity to carbamazepine or oxcarbazepine
2. Hepatic impairment

B. **Use caution**:

1. History of previous severe medication-induced allergies with other drugs
2. Patients who may become pregnant

VII. **Dosage Formulations**

A. Brand or generic immediate-release (IR) capsule (100 mg, 200 mg, 300 mg)
B. Brand or generic extended-release (ER) capsule (100 mg, 200 mg, 300 mg)
C. Brand or generic chewable tablet (100 mg)
D. Oral suspension (100 mg/5 mL)

VIII. **Dosage Ranges and Guidelines**

A. Adults and children older than 12 years: Start at 200 mg BID. Gradually increase by 200 mg at weekly intervals to achieve appropriate blood levels (see "Monitoring" below), up to a maximum dosage of 1,200 mg/day (age >15 years) or 1,000 mg/day (age 12–15 years).

1. Pediatric (age ≤12 years): Maximum dosage 35 mg/kg/day

B. The dosage can be decreased in 100- to 200-mg increments to manage side effects.

---

[1]Evidence strength varies; readers are referred to the literature for more detailed information.

IX. **Monitoring**

A. **Baseline (before starting carbamazepine)**: Obtain a complete blood count (CBC), a comprehensive metabolic panel (CMP), and a pregnancy test. Check coagulation parameters as clinically indicated.

B. **Consider obtaining human leukocyte antigen (HLA) genotyping**: The FDA recommends screening for the HLA-B*15:02 allele before initiating carbamazepine treatment in patients of Asian ancestry, who are known to have high frequencies of this allele.

C. **Periodic monitoring**: Obtain a CBC and CMP at 3, 6, and 12 months and annually thereafter.

D. **Blood-level monitoring**: The established trough blood level range for seizure disorders is 4–12 µg/mL.

1. Because of carbamazepine's induction of its own metabolism, therapeutic blood levels should be obtained after 3–5 weeks (Tolou-Ghamari et al. 2013)

X. **Relevant Pharmacokinetics/Pharmacodynamics**

A. **Metabolism**: Hepatic (cytochrome P450 [CYP] 3A4 [primary pathway], CYP2C8, CYP3A5, and CYP2B6; uridine 5′-diphospho-glucuronosyltransferase [UGT] 2B7)

B. **Time to peak plasma concentration**:

1. IR: 17 hours
2. ER: 24 hours (with food: 12 hours)

C. **Half-life**: ~20 hours at steady state (16–24 hours; varies according to CYP3A4 genotype). Half-life for a single dose is 36 hours.

1. Carbamazepine undergoes autoinduction, in which clearance increases over time with continued exposure, leading to a reduction in the half-life. As a result, time to reach steady state is approximately 3–5 weeks (Tolou-Ghamari et al. 2013)

D. **Effect of food**: Increases the rate of absorption

E. **Hepatic impairment**: Because of the risk of hepatotoxicity with carbamazepine, use in people with hepatic impairment is not recommended.

F. **Renal impairment**: Effects are unknown, but impairment is unlikely to have major effects on unconjugated blood levels.

XI. **Clinically Relevant Drug Interactions**

A. Carbamazepine is a strong inducer of CYP3A4, so it will *decrease* the blood levels of medications metabolized by that pathway.

1. A large number of medications are metabolized via CYP3A4, including many antidepressants, antipsychotics, benzodiazepines, cardiac medications (e.g., apixaban, rivaroxaban), estrogens, immunological medications, buprenorphine, and others. Use a drug interaction checker before prescribing.
2. Notably, carbamazepine is known to decrease the effectiveness of oral contraceptives (see "Clinical Pearls").

B. Carbamazepine is also metabolized by CYP3A4 (major), CYP2C8, CYPB3A5, CYP2B6, and UGT2B7 (all minor)

1. CYP3A4 inhibitors and inducers significantly affect carbamazepine metabolism. Dosages should be adjusted accordingly.

   a. Commonly used medications that are CYP3A4 strong inhibitors (*increase* carbamazepine levels) include certain protease inhibitors (e.g., indinavir, ritonavir), clarithromycin, and ketoconazole. Moderate inhibitors include ciprofloxacin, diltiazem, erythromycin, fluconazole, fluvoxamine, grapefruit and juice, and verapamil.
   b. Commonly used agents/medications that are CYP3A4 inducers (*decrease* carbamazepine levels) include apalutamide, efavirenz, enzalutamide, phenytoin, rifampin, and St. John's wort.

2. The carbamazepine dosage will need to be adjusted if the dosage of a coadministered inducer or inhibitor is changed or the medication is stopped.

XII. **Adverse Effects**

A. **Most common**:

1. Neuropsychiatric: Ataxia, gait unsteadiness, discoordination, dizziness, drowsiness, concentration (and other cognitive) problems
2. Gastrointestinal: Nausea, vomiting
3. Photosensitivity: Patients should always use sunscreen with any but brief sun exposure.
4. Hyponatremia/syndrome of inappropriate antidiuretic hormone secretion (SIADH): Incidence varies (estimates range from 4%–40% for carbamazepine to 23%–73% for oxcarbazepine [Berghuis et al. 2017]); usually mild/asymptomatic, dosage related; timing of onset varies (Seifert et al. 2021).

B. **Uncommon**:

1. Liver dysfunction:

   a. Asymptomatic transient increases in serum transaminases, γ-glutamyl transferase (GGT), and alkaline phosphatase (ALP) can occur (Carbamazepine 2017).
   b. Signs of hepatotoxicity may include hepatocellular hepatitis, cholestatic hepatitis or mixed hepatitis, intrahepatic cholestasis, or granulomatous hepatitis. Onset is generally between 6 and 12 weeks, but signs can take up to a year to appear. Concomitant use of other antiepileptics, presence of the HLA-A*3101 allele, and longer duration of carbamazepine treatment increase the risk. Hepatotoxicity is usually reversible with discontinuation (Carbamazepine 2017).

2. Cardiac risk: Sinus tachycardia (mostly younger patients in overdose), bradyarrhythmia/atrioventricular conduction delay (mostly older patients), increased risk of cardiac failure, likely related to blockade of sodium channels (Kasarskis et al. 1992).

3. Boxed warning: Delayed hypersensitivity reactions: Ranging from mild to severe rashes (Stevens-Johnson syndrome [SJS]/toxic epidermal necrolysis [TEN]) to drug reaction with eosinophilia and systemic symptoms (DRESS) (Chung et al. 2021).
   a. Obtain HLA genotyping for patients in high-risk groups (see "Anticonvulsant Boxed Warning: Serious Dermatological Reactions" at the beginning of this chapter).
4. Boxed warning: Blood dyscrasias (agranulocytosis, leukopenia, aplastic anemia, pancytopenia, thrombocytopenia): Very rare; timing of onset varies. Monitor CBC.
5. Suicide risk: Noted in drug labeling but not clearly established; likely very low risk (Mula et al. 2013). For a detailed discussion, the reader is referred to comprehensive sources in the literature (e.g., Fergusson et al. 2005).
6. Other uncommon effects: Abnormal vision, alopecia, angioedema, arthralgias, diplopia, edema, irritability/aggression, menstrual disturbance, nystagmus, paresthesias, peripheral edema, pneumonitis, urinary retention, rare anxiety, depression, psychosis (potentially related to hyponatremia)

C. **Risks in pregnancy and lactation:**
   1. Pregnancy: Epidemiological data indicate that carbamazepine is associated with an increased risk of major malformations, including spina bifida. Intrauterine exposure is also associated with developmental delays. Use in pregnancy is not recommended.
   2. Lactation: Significant levels of carbamazepine and its major metabolite are transmitted in breast milk and may result in adverse reactions in infants.

XIII. Clinical Pearls/Prescribing Tips

A. Data support the use of carbamazepine for acute mania and maintenance treatment of bipolar disorder but not for bipolar depression.
B. Carbamazepine may be used in combination with an antipsychotic or another mood stabilizer (monitor for bidirectional effects on blood levels due to interactions).
C. There is some evidence that carbamazepine improves impulsivity in patients with impulse-control disorders.
D. Use caution given the relatively high risk of drug interactions with carbamazepine. More drugs are metabolized by CYP3A4 than by any other CYP enzyme.
E. Carbamazepine significantly decreases the efficacy of hormonal contraceptive methods, and if a pregnancy were to occur, it would pose significant teratogenic risks (Crawford et al. 1990; Davis et al. 2011). Recommend a copper intrauterine device (IUD) as an alternative to hormonal methods of contraception for these patients.
F. Periodically monitor comprehensive metabolic panel (CMP) and complete blood count (CBC) with differential, given the risk of hepatotoxicity, hyponatremia, and blood dyscrasias.
G. Compared with other commonly used mood stabilizers such as lithium or valproate, carbamazepine is less likely to cause significant weight gain.
H. Although a benign rash can occur with carbamazepine, signs of a more serious rash include systemic symptoms, mucosal involvement, and a widespread, confluent painful rash.

I. Because of carbamazepine's induction of its own metabolism, therapeutic blood levels should be obtained after 3–5 weeks.

Further Reading

Al Khalili Y, Sekhon S, Jain S: Carbamazepine toxicity, in StatPearls. Treasure Island, FL, StatPearls Publishing, 2022

Novartis Pharmaceuticals: Tegretol (carbamazepine), Tegretol-EX (carbamazepine extended release) prescribing information. East Hanover, NJ, Novartis Pharmaceuticals Corporation, December 2007. Available at: https://www.accessdata.fda.gov/drugsatfda_docs/label/2007/016608s098lbl.pdf. Accessed June 21, 2024.

Carvalho AF, Firth J, Vieta E: Bipolar disorder. N Engl J Med 383(1):58–66, 2020 32609982

Maan JS: Duong TvH, Saadabadi A: Carbamazepine [Updated July 10, 2023], in StatPearls [Internet]. Treasure Island, FL, StatPearls Publishing, January 2024. Available at: https://www.ncbi.nlm.nih.gov/books/NBK482455/. Accessed March 13, 2024.

Mockenhaupt M, Messenheimer J, Tennis P, et al: Risk of Stevens-Johnson syndrome and toxic epidermal necrolysis in new users of antiepileptics. Neurology 64(7):1134–1138, 2005 15824335

Mullan KA, Anderson A, Illing PT, et al: HLA-associated antiepileptic drug-induced cutaneous adverse reactions. HLA 93(6):417–435, 2019 30895730

References

Berghuis B, van der Palen J, de Haan GJ, et al; EpiPGX Consortium: Carbamazepine- and oxcarbazepine-induced hyponatremia in people with epilepsy. Epilepsia 58(7):1227–1233, 2017 28542738

Carbamazepine [updated January 15, 2017], in LiverTox: Clinical and Research Information on Drug-Induced Liver Injury. Bethesda, MD, National Institute of Diabetes and Digestive and Kidney Diseases, 2012–. Available at: https://www.ncbi.nlm.nih.gov/books/NBK548097/. Accessed March 13, 2024.

Chung SJ, Ahn KM, Oh JH, et al: Incidence rates of severe cutaneous adverse reactions due to antiseizure medication: a nationwide study using health claims data in Korea. Epilepsia 62(1):250–257, 2021 33188522

Crawford P, Chadwick DJ, Martin C, et al: The interaction of phenytoin and carbamazepine with combined oral contraceptive steroids. Br J Clin Pharmacol 30(6):892–896, 1990 2126946

Davis AR, Westhoff CL, Stanczyk FZ: Carbamazepine coadministration with an oral contraceptive: effects on steroid pharmacokinetics, ovulation, and bleeding. Epilepsia 52(2):243–247, 2011 21204827

Fergusson D, Doucette S, Glass KC, et al: Association between suicide attempts and selective serotonin reuptake inhibitors: systematic review of randomised controlled trials. BMJ 330(7488):396, 2005 15718539

Kasarskis EJ, Kuo CS, Berger R, et al: Carbamazepine-induced cardiac dysfunction: characterization of two distinct clinical syndromes. Arch Intern Med 152(1):186–191, 1992 1728915

Lorberg B, Youssef NA, Bhagwagar Z: Lamotrigine-associated rash: to rechallenge or not to rechallenge? Int J Neuropsychopharmacol 12(2):257–265, 2009 18845017

Macdonald RL, Kelly KM: Antiepileptic drug mechanisms of action. Epilepsia 36(Suppl 2):S2–S12, 1995 8784210

Mula M, Kanner AM, Schmitz B, et al: Antiepileptic drugs and suicidality: an expert consensus statement from the Task Force on Therapeutic Strategies of the ILAE Commission on Neuropsychobiology. Epilepsia 54(1):199–203, 2013 22994856

Seifert J, Letmaier M, Greiner T, et al: Psychotropic drug-induced hyponatremia: results from a drug surveillance program-an update. J Neural Transm (Vienna) 128(8):1249–1264, 2021 34196782
Tolou-Ghamari Z, Zare M, Habibabadi JM, et al: A quick review of carbamazepine pharmacokinetics in epilepsy from 1953 to 2012. J Res Med Sci 18(Suppl 1):S81–S85, 2013 23961295

Lamotrigine

I. **Brand Names**: Lamictal, Lamictal extended release

II. **Therapeutic Class**: Mood stabilizer, anticonvulsant

III. **Mechanism-Based Class**: Sodium and calcium channel modulator

IV. **Mechanism(s) of Action**

A. The mechanism of action in bipolar disorder is not fully understood.

B. Lamotrigine blocks both voltage-gated sodium channels and L-type calcium channels.

V. **Indications**

A. FDA adult:

1. Bipolar disorder (maintenance treatment only)
2. Generalized tonic-clonic seizures
3. Partial-onset seizure disorders
4. Generalized seizures of Lennox-Gastaut syndrome

B. Evidence-based[1] off-label uses:

1. Management of impulsivity, including impulsive aggressive behavior.
2. Bipolar depression (based on a meta-analysis of five studies [Geddes et al. 2009])

C. FDA pediatric: Seizure disorders (see "FDA adult" above)

VI. **Major Contraindications and When to Use Caution**

A. **Major contraindications**: Known hypersensitivity to lamotrigine, including skin rash

B. **Use caution**:

1. Patients with a history of prior severe medication-induced skin rash with other drugs
2. Patients with high-risk human leukocyte antigen (HLA) alleles (see "Anticonvulsant Boxed Warning: Serious Dermatological Reactions" at the beginning of this chapter).

VII. **Dosage Formulations**

A. Brand or generic immediate-release (IR) tablet (25 mg, 100 mg, 150 mg, 200 mg)

B. Brand or generic extended-release (ER) tablet (300 mg, 450 mg)

C. Brand or generic chewable (2 mg, 5 mg, 25 mg)

[1]Evidence strength varies; readers are referred to the literature for more detailed information.

D. Brand or generic oral disintegrating tablet (ODT) (25 mg, 50 mg, 100 mg, 200 mg)
E. Brand or generic starter kit (IR or ODT):
   1. Regular dosing: Orange kit
   2. Dosing with inducers: Green kit
   3. Dosing with valproate: Blue kit

VIII. **Dosage Ranges and Guidelines**

A. Follow strict dosing guidelines (Table 5–1 for adults and children age 12 years and older; Table 5–2 for pediatric patients age 2–12 years).
B. Lamotrigine metabolism is induced by carbamazepine, phenytoin, phenobarbital, primidone, estrogens, rifampin, and the protease inhibitors lopinavir/ritonavir and atazanavir/ritonavir. These agents decrease lamotrigine levels.
C. Lamotrigine's metabolism is inhibited by valproate. Concomitant use of valproate will increase lamotrigine levels.
D. Increasing the dosage faster than the recommended schedule can result in a severe rash or Stevens-Johnson syndrome/toxic epidermal necrolysis.
E. In the event of intolerable side effects or lack of benefit, check lamotrigine blood levels (see "Blood-level monitoring" under "Monitoring" below).

Table 5–1. Lamotrigine dosage escalation regimen for adults

Indication	Patients NOT TAKING carbamazepine, phenytoin, phenobarbital, primidone, valproate, or estrogens	Patients TAKING carbamazepine, phenytoin, phenobarbital, primidone, or estrogens, and NOT TAKING valproate	Patients TAKING valproate
Bipolar disorder Seizure disorders Impulsivity	Weeks 1 and 2: 25 mg/day	Weeks 1 and 2: 50 mg/day	Weeks 1 and 2: 25 mg every other day OR 12.5 mg/day
	Weeks 3 and 4: 50 mg/day	Weeks 3 and 4: 100 mg/day	Weeks 3 and 4: 25 mg/day
	Week 5 onward: Increase dosage by 50 mg each week	Week 5 onward: Increase dosage by 100 mg each week	Week 5 onward: Increase dosage by 25 mg each week
	Target dosage range: 200–400 mg/day	Target dosage range: 300–500 mg/day	Target dosage range: 100–200 mg/day
	Maximum approved dosage for bipolar disorder*: 200 mg/day	Maximum approved dosage for bipolar disorder*: 400 mg/day	Maximum approved dosage for bipolar disorder*: 100 mg/day

Note. The dose packs for dosage escalation are color-coded for each of the three scenarios in this table.
*Same maximum dosage also applies to other uses (e.g., impulsivity).

Table 5–2. Lamotrigine dosage escalation regimen for pediatric patients (ages 2–12 years) with seizure disorders

	Patients NOT TAKING carbamazepine, phenytoin, phenobarbital, primidone, or valproate	Patients TAKING carbamazepine, phenytoin, phenobarbital, or primidone,* and NOT TAKING valproate	Patients TAKING valproate
Weeks 1 and 2	0.3 mg/kg/day in 1 or 2 separate doses	0.6 mg/kg/day in 2 divided doses	0.15 mg/kg/day in 1 or 2 separate doses
Weeks 3 and 4	0.6 mg/kg/day in 2 divided doses	1.2 mg/kg/day in 2 divided doses	0.3 mg/kg/day in 1 or 2 separate doses
Week 5 onward to maintenance	Increase dosage every 1–2 weeks: 0.6 mg/kg/day added to previous dosage	Increase dosage every 1–2 weeks: 1.2 mg/kg/day added to previous dosage	Increase dosage every 1–2 weeks: 0.3 mg/kg/day added to previous dosage
Usual maintenance dosage	May need to be increased by as much as 50%, depending on clinical response	May need to be increased by as much as 50%, depending on clinical response	May need to be increased by as much as 50%, depending on clinical response

*For patients taking **carbamazepine**, **phenytoin**, **phenobarbital**, or **primidone**: Round dosage down to nearest whole tablet.

IX. **Monitoring**

A. **Baseline (before starting lamotrigine)**: Obtain a complete blood count (CBC) and liver function tests (LFTs).

B. **Periodic monitoring**: Obtain CBC and LFTs as clinically indicated.

C. **Blood-level monitoring**: The established blood level range for seizure disorders is 3–14 μg/mL.

X. **Relevant Pharmacokinetics/Pharmacodynamics**

A. **Metabolism**: Hepatic (glucuronidation, primarily uridine 5′-diphospho-glucuronosyltransferase [UGT] 1A4)

B. **Time to peak plasma concentration**:

1. Taking no inhibitors or inducers: 2 hours
2. Taking inducers: 2 hours
3. Taking valproate: 5 hours
4. Taking inducer plus valproate: 4 hours

C. **Half-life**:

1. Taking no inducers or valproate: Single dose: 33 hours; multiple doses: 25 hours
2. Taking inducers: Single dose: 14 hours; multiple doses: 13 hours
3. Taking valproate: Single dose: 48 hours, multiple doses: 70 hours
4. Taking inducers plus valproate: 27 hours

D. **Hepatic impairment**: No dosage adjustment is needed in patients with mild liver impairment. Dosages should be reduced by 25% in patients with moderate or severe liver impairment without ascites and by 50% in those with ascites.

E. **Renal impairment**: No dosage adjustment required (100% hepatic clearance), although the half-life is doubled with severe renal impairment.

XI. **Clinically Relevant Drug Interactions**

A. Metabolism induction or inhibition is the result of increased and decreased glucuronidation, respectively.

1. Inducers that *decrease* lamotrigine levels include carbamazepine, phenytoin, phenobarbital, primidone, estrogens, rifampin, and the protease inhibitors lopinavir/ritonavir and atazanavir/ritonavir.
2. Inhibitor that *increases* lamotrigine levels: valproate.
3. The lamotrigine dosage will need to be adjusted if the dosage of a coadministered inducer or inhibitor is changed or the agent is discontinued.

B. Lamotrigine inhibits dihydrofolate reductase, which is involved in the conversion of folic acid to its active form, L-5-methyltetrahydrofolate (also known as L-methylfolate).

XII. **Adverse Effects**

A. **Most common**: Somnolence, benign skin rash (about 10% incidence [Wang et al. 2015]), headache, dizziness, ataxia, blurred vision, diplopia, nausea, vomiting, indigestion, discoordination, dysmenorrhea.

1. Severe photosensitivity: Lamotrigine is associated with severe photosensitivity. Patients should always use sunscreen with any but brief sun exposure.

B. **Uncommon**:

1. Boxed warnings: Delayed hypersensitivity reactions: Ranging from mild to severe rashes (Stevens-Johnson syndrome [SJS]/toxic epidermal necrolysis [TEN]) to drug reaction with eosinophilia and systemic symptoms (DRESS) (Chung et al. 2021).

   a. Benign rash (about 10% incidence [Wang et al. 2015]): Most likely to occur between day 5 and week 8. Usually a simple morbilliform rash, either pruritic or nonpruritic. Rechallenging after rash has been shown to be largely safe in studies (Houser and Graham 2018). Can consider reintroducing at a lower dosage (i.e., as low as 5 mg every other day or daily) (Aiken and Orr 2010).

   b. Rare risk of SJS/TEN (~0.04% incidence [Bloom and Amber 2017]): Most likely to occur between day 5 and week 8. Incidence of SJS/TEN in lamotrigine-treated patients is 4 per 10,000, although the rate may be much lower with slow dosage titration (see "Anticonvulsant Boxed Warning: Serious Dermatological Reactions" at the beginning of this chapter).

2. Hemophagocytic lymphohistiocytosis: Very rare; usually occurs within the first several weeks. Watch out for rash, fever, hepatosplenomegaly, organ system dysfunction, and hematological abnormalities.
3. Aseptic meningitis: Very rare; onset usually within 42 days of initiation. If aseptic meningitis develops, avoid re-exposure.
4. Blood dyscrasias (agranulocytosis, leukopenia, aplastic anemia, pancytopenia, thrombocytopenia): Very rare; onset varies. Monitor CBC as clinically indicated.
5. Suicide risk: Noted in drug labeling, but not clearly established; likely very low risk (Mula et al. 2013).
6. Other uncommon adverse effects: Fatigue, peripheral edema, arthralgias, memory problems, disinhibition, weight loss, angioedema

C. **Risks in pregnancy and lactation**: There is no established relationship between intrauterine exposure to lamotrigine and major malformations. However, teratogenicity was shown in animal studies. Lamotrigine is transmitted in breast milk at significant levels. A thorough risk/benefit discussion with the patient is recommended on continuing versus stopping the medication, including consultation with an OB/GYN specialist and/or lactation expert. See Chapter 15 ("Women: Pregnancy, Postpartum, and Breastfeeding") for more information.

XIII. Clinical Pearls/Prescribing Tips

A. Lamotrigine is FDA approved as monotherapy for bipolar maintenance, although it is more effective in preventing depression than mania (Besag et al. 2021). The opposite is true for lithium, making them a good maintenance combination.
B. There is some evidence that lamotrigine improves mood in acute bipolar depression; however, the data are mixed and largely based on a meta-analysis of five studies (Geddes et al. 2009).
C. Lamotrigine may have some benefit in irritability/anger in borderline personality disorder, although study findings are mixed/limited (Reich et al. 2009; Tritt et al. 2005).
D. SJS/TEN is very rare and is usually caused by increasing the dosage too rapidly. Follow strict dosing guidelines (see Tables 5–1 and 5–2).
E. A benign rash may occur; consider rechallenging with lamotrigine at a lower dosage. Warning signs of a more serious rash include systemic symptoms, mucosal involvement, and a widespread, confluent painful rash.
F. Estrogen-containing oral contraceptive pills (OCPs) can significantly decrease the lamotrigine level, but lamotrigine does not appear to affect OCP effectiveness (Christensen et al. 2007; Reimers et al. 2005).
G. Lamotrigine has no metabolic adverse effects and is safer in pregnancy compared with other mood stabilizers.

Further Reading

Betchel NT, Fariba KA, Saadabadi A: Lamotrigine, in StatPearls. Treasure Island, FL, StatPearls Publishing, 2022

Carvalho AF, Firth J, Vieta E: Bipolar disorder. N Engl J Med 383(1):58–66, 2020 32609982

GlaxoSmithKline: Lamictal XR (lamotrigine) extended-release tablets [package insert]. U.S. Food and Drug Administration website. Revised March 2015. Available at: https://www.accessdata.fda.gov/drugsatfda_docs/label/2015/022115s011s018lbl.pdf. Accessed June 21, 2024.

Mullan KA, Anderson A, Illing PT, et al: HLA-associated antiepileptic drug-induced cutaneous adverse reactions. HLA 93(6):417–435, 2019 30895730

References

Aiken CB, Orr C: Rechallenge with lamotrigine after a rash: a prospective case series and review of the literature. Psychiatry (Edgmont) 7(5):27–32, 2010 20532155

Besag FMC, Vasey MJ, Sharma AN, et al: Efficacy and safety of lamotrigine in the treatment of bipolar disorder across the lifespan: a systematic review. Ther Adv Psychopharmacol 11:20451253211045870, 2021 34646439

Bloom R, Amber KT: Identifying the incidence of rash, Stevens-Johnson syndrome and toxic epidermal necrolysis in patients taking lamotrigine: a systematic review of 122 randomized controlled trials. An Bras Dermatol 92(1):139-141, 2017 28225977

Christensen J, Petrenaite V, Atterman J, et al: Oral contraceptives induce lamotrigine metabolism: evidence from a double-blind, placebo-controlled trial. Epilepsia 48(3):484–489, 2007 17346247

Chung SJ, Ahn KM, Oh JH, et al: Incidence rates of severe cutaneous adverse reactions due to antiseizure medication: a nationwide study using health claims data in Korea. Epilepsia 62(1):250–257, 2021 33188522

Geddes JR, Calabrese JR, Goodwin GM: Lamotrigine for treatment of bipolar depression: independent meta-analysis and meta-regression of individual patient data from five randomised trials. Br J Psychiatry 194(1):4–9, 2009 19118318

Houser J, Graham A. Rechallenge of lamotrigine after development of rash. Ment Health Clin 8(5):247–249, 2018

Lorberg B, Youssef NA, Bhagwagar Z: Lamotrigine-associated rash: to rechallenge or not to rechallenge? Int J Neuropsychopharmacol 12(2):257–265, 2009 18845017

Mula M, Kanner AM, Schmitz B, et al: Antiepileptic drugs and suicidality: an expert consensus statement from the Task Force on Therapeutic Strategies of the ILAE Commission on Neuropsychobiology. Epilepsia 54(1):199–203, 2013 22994856

Reich DB, Zanarini MC, Bieri KA: A preliminary study of lamotrigine in the treatment of affective instability in borderline personality disorder. Int Clin Psychopharmacol 24(5):270–275, 2009 19636254

Reimers A, Helde G, Brodtkorb E: Ethinyl estradiol, not progestogens, reduces lamotrigine serum concentrations. Epilepsia 46(9):1414–1417, 2005 16146436

Tritt K, Nickel C, Lahmann C, et al: Lamotrigine treatment of aggression in female borderline-patients: a randomized, double-blind, placebo-controlled study. J Psychopharmacol 19(3):287–291, 2005 15888514

Wang XQ, Xiong J, Xu WH, et al: Risk of a lamotrigine-related skin rash: current meta-analysis and postmarketing cohort analysis. Seizure 25:52-61, 2015 25645637

Lithium

I. **Brand Names**: Lithane, Eskalith, Eskalith CR, Lithobid, Lithotabs, Lithonate

II. **Therapeutic Class**: Mood stabilizer

III. **Mechanism-Based Class**: Enzyme modulator

IV. **Mechanism(s) of Action**

A. The mechanism of action is not fully understood but lithium works in a variety of ways to exert antimanic effects and mood stabilization.

1. **Lithium has "thymolytic" activity** that reduces affective intensity via multiple mechanisms.
2. **Lithium modulates cellular signaling systems**, including adenylyl cyclase and cyclic adenosine monophosphate (cAMP), inositol monophosphatase (IMPase), inositol polyphosphate 1-phosphatase (IPPase), protein kinase C (PKC), glycogen synthase kinase 3 (GSK-3), brain-derived neurotrophic factor (BDNF), and B-cell lymphoma 2 (Bcl-2) (Malhi et al. 2013):
   a. Inhibits IMPase and IPPase, decreasing myoinositol (i.e., myoinositol depletion hypothesis).
   b. Inhibits PKC and its downstream target myristoylated alanine-rich C-kinase substrates (MARCKS), which is believed to be antimanic.
   c. Inhibits GSK-3, involved in gene transcription and synaptic plasticity, which is believed to be antimanic.
   d. Modulates cell free calcium levels through inhibition of phospholipase C (PLC) and Bcl-2 protein (also known as the mitochondrial permeability transition pore). Modulation of calcium levels has neuroprotective effects, which may impact the progression and cognitive decline associated with bipolar disorder.
   e. Inhibits triphosphoinositol (TPI), a second messenger in limbic neurons, thus decreasing the intensity of neuronal firing rates.
3. **Lithium has neurotransmitter effects**:
   a. Inhibits dopamine (excitatory) via alteration of G protein–coupled receptor (GPCR) subunits involved in the postsynaptic activation of dopamine (antimanic).
   b. Inhibits glutamate (excitatory) via eventual downregulation of *N*-methyl-D-aspartate (NMDA) receptors (Nonaka et al. 1998) (antimanic).
   c. Increases GABA (inhibitory) in the CSF via facilitation of GABA release presynaptically and upregulation of $GABA_B$ receptors postsynaptically. Bipolar patients have been shown to have reduced GABAergic neurotransmission.
   d. Desensitizes serotonergic autoreceptors in the raphe nuclei, increasing serotonin in the frontal/temporal lobes (Wang and Friedman 1988).

4. **Lithium has neuroprotective effects**: Lithium has been shown to preserve gray matter, decrease rates of apoptosis in neurons, and increase the robustness of dendrites (Gerhard et al. 2015; Malhi et al. 2013). It also promotes transcription factors *FOS* (Fos proto-oncogene) and cAMP-responsive element binding protein (CREB), leading to increases in neurotrophic factors such as BDNF and Bcl-2 (Giotakos et al. 2015; Young 2009).

V. **Indications**

A. FDA adult:

1. Bipolar disorder (mania, maintenance)

B. Evidence-based[1] off-label uses:

1. Antidepressant adjunctive therapy for treatment-resistant major depressive disorder
2. Reduce suicidal ideation in patients with mood disorders or schizophrenia
3. Bipolar depression
4. Management of impulsivity, including impulsive aggressive behavior and suicide attempts
5. Adjunct to clozapine to counteract leukopenia (Nykiel et al. 2010).

C. FDA pediatric: Bipolar disorder (age ≥7 years)

VI. **Major Contraindications and When to Use Caution**

A. **Major contraindications**:

1. Severe renal impairment
2. Heart failure
3. Addison's disease
4. Pregnancy (first trimester)

B. **Use caution**:

1. Elderly patients (increased risk of neurotoxicity)
2. Family history of Brugada syndrome or sudden death; sick sinus syndrome
   a. Obtain ECG for patients with a history of cardiac disease or age older than 40 years.

VII. **Dosage Formulations**

A. Brand lithium carbonate immediate-release (IR) capsule (150 mg, 300 mg, 600 mg)—*Eskalith*
B. Generic lithium carbonate IR capsule (150 mg, 300 mg, 600 mg)—*Lithium carbonate*
C. Brand lithium carbonate controlled-release (CR) tablet (450 mg [*scored*])—*Eskalith CR*
D. Brand lithium carbonate extended-release (ER) tablet (300 mg)—*Lithobid*
E. Generic lithium carbonate ER tablet (300 mg, 450 mg)—*Lithium ER*

1. Do not crush, break, or chew the ER tablet.

---

[1]Evidence strength varies; readers are referred to the literature for more detailed information.

VIII. Dosage Ranges and Guidelines

A. IR/ER: Start at 600 mg at bedtime. Increase dosage by 300–600 mg every 1–5 days taken as a single dose or in 2–3 divided doses until the desired serum level is reached. Maximum dosage is 1,800 mg/day.

B. Blood-level target varies depending on indication (see "Monitoring").

C. Less-frequent dosing appears to be more beneficial for kidney function, and lithium's 24-hour half-life makes this feasible (Bowen et al. 1991).

D. Consider lower starting dosages (e.g., 300 mg/day) for elderly adult patients.

E. Dosing for adolescents older than age 12 years is the same as that for adults.

F. Lithium "loading" has been shown to be effective (Keck et al. 2001; Kook et al. 1985).

Table 5–3. Lithium indications and dosage ranges

Indications	Usual dosage range
Bipolar disorder (see "Monitoring" for blood-level guidelines)	900–1,500 mg
Treatment-resistant major depressive disorder* (off-label)	600–900 mg
Impulsivity, suicide risk** (off-label)	600–900 mg

*Lithium has been well studied for treatment-resistant depression (Bschor et al. 2003, 2007; Vázquez et al. 2021), with most studies examining lithium augmentation of tricyclic antidepressants (de Montigny et al. 1983; Januel et al. 2003), although studies also indicate that it can beneficially augment newer antidepressants (Nelson et al. 2014). For TRD, adjust dosage to 600–900 mg/day (Nelson et al. 2014).

**Lithium has a notable antisuicide effect that appears to be independent of its mood benefits (Lewitzka et al. 2015). In contrast to lithium's beneficial effect on other indications, the antisuicide effect may not be dosage dependent (Song et al. 2017). Lithium has been shown to decrease risk of relapse following electroconvulsive therapy (ECT), both alone and with nortriptyline (Lambrichts et al. 2021; Sackeim et al. 2001), although some studies indicate the combination of lithium and ECT increases the risk of cognitive effects and delirium (Patel et al. 2020).

IX. Monitoring

A. **Baseline (before starting lithium)**: Obtain a complete blood count (CBC), electrolytes (including calcium), blood urea nitrogen (BUN), creatinine, estimated glomerular filtration rate (eGFR), and thyroid function tests at baseline; at 3, 6, and 12 months; and every 6–12 months thereafter.

B. **Weight gain**: Check weight prior to treatment and periodically, given the risk of weight gain.

C. **Lithium blood-level monitoring**:

1. Measure the trough blood level after 5 days of continuous dosing.
   a. For divided doses, measure the level 12 hours after the last dose and before the next dose.[1]
   b. For once-daily or nightly dosing, measure the level ~24 hours after the last dose, as 12-hour trough levels would be 1.3 times higher than the true trough. Alternatively, take the 12-hour trough level and divide it by 1.3 (or 18%–25%) to get the true trough (Reddy and Reddy 2014).

2. Target blood levels:
   a. Mania: Adjust dosage to achieve a blood level of **0.8–1.0 mmol/L.**
      i. In some patients, levels of 1.0–1.2 mmol/L may be required for optimal mood stability.
   b. Mood stabilization: Adjust dosage to achieve a blood level range of 0.8–1.0. Some sources recommend lower dosage ranges (i.e., 0.4–0.8), but risk of relapse was higher in patients receiving lower dosages (Gelenberg et al. 1989).
      i. In the face of intolerable side effects, reduce blood levels to 0.6–0.8 mmol/L. In rare cases, patients will not be able to tolerate lithium above a blood level range of 0.4–0.6 mmol/L. Combination with another mood stabilizer will usually be required at lower blood concentrations.
3. Frequency of monitoring:
   a. Five days after starting and after every dosage adjustment
   b. Three weeks after stable dosing
   c. Every 6–12 months thereafter
4. Obtain a lithium level if a new sign of toxicity emerges or a prior toxicity worsens with long-term treatment (e.g., tremor).
5. Lithium level varies inversely with sodium level (lower sodium = higher lithium). (See "Clinically Relevant Drug Interactions.")

X. **Relevant Pharmacokinetics/Pharmacodynamics**

A. **Metabolism**: No hepatic metabolism; renal clearance only.
B. **Time to peak plasma concentration**: 1–3 hours (IR); 2–6 hours (CR/ER) (varies depending on the preparation)
C. **Half-life**: 24 hours
D. **Hepatic impairment**: No adjustment required (no hepatic metabolism).
E. **Renal impairment**: 100% renal clearance:
   1. CrCl ≥ 60 mL/minute: No dosage adjustment required.
   2. CrCl 30–60 mL/minute: Start at lower dosages and check lithium levels more frequently.
   3. CrCl < 30 mL/minute: Avoid lithium use.

---

[1]Historically, reference levels have been based on BID or TID dosing of lithium and 12 hours prior to the last dose. Therefore, there are fewer data on true reference ranges for 24-hour troughs with once-daily ER dosing. Carter et al. (2013) highlighted much of the conjecture in the literature regarding lithium dosing and renal protection and concluded that "because lithium serum levels are [traditionally] based on [twice daily] dosing, patients should be started on [twice daily] dosing to determine an appropriate daily dosage in the therapeutic range, and then switched to [dosing at bedtime]."

If lithium is started as once-daily/nightly ER, it makes sense to obtain 24-hour trough levels (as 12-hour levels are not true "troughs"). However, obtaining 24-hour troughs has not been explicitly studied in the literature. Reddy and Reddy 2014 recommended adjusting 12-hour levels per the guidance above.

XI. Clinically Relevant Drug Interactions

A. **NSAIDs**: Avoid using lithium with nonsteroidal anti-inflammatory drugs (e.g., ibuprofen), which increase lithium blood levels. Sulindac and aspirin may be safer.

B. **Diuretics**: Avoid using lithium with diuretics, which increase lithium blood levels. If a diuretic is required with lithium, start the diuretic first, then start lithium at half the dosage described above (see "Dosage Ranges and Guidelines") and monitor frequently.

C. **ACE inhibitors or ARBs**: Aldosterone-converting enzyme (ACE) inhibitors or angiotensin II receptor blockers (ARBs) may increase lithium levels.

D. **Verapamil/diltiazem**: Lithium neurotoxicity has been reported with verapamil and diltiazem, although the incidence is unknown. It is also not known whether the same toxicity would occur with other calcium channel inhibitors.

E. Lithium prolongs the effects of neuromuscular blocking agents (succinylcholine, pancuronium).

XII. Adverse Effects

A. **Most common**:

1. CNS: Mild ataxia, tremor, memory problems, sedation
   a. Tremor: Symmetric tremor, likely to occur early in treatment or after dosage increases. Lower the dosage or add a centrally active beta-blocker (e.g., propranolol) (Baek et al. 2014).
   b. Subjective cognitive slowing: Mental slowness, dullness, decrease in creativity: Likely dosage related; consider lowering the dosage. These effects may also be secondary to depression or bipolar disorder itself or to comorbid mental disorders (Gitlin 2016).

2. Kidney function: Lithium causes a decrease in urine concentrating capacity as a result of accumulation in the distal renal tubule and desensitization of the receptor for antidiuretic hormone (ADH), leading to nephrogenic diabetes insipidus. This leads to an approximately 20% increase in urine output. Lithium can cause a decrease in eGFR over time, but renal failure is rare (Beunders et al. 2018; Ibbeken et al. 2012). The mechanism for these changes may include interstitial nephritis/fibrosis, nephron atrophy, and/or glomerular damage over long-term treatment. Monitor closely.
   a. Polydipsia/polyuria (incidence up to 70% [Passavanti et al. 1989]): Giving the full daily dose at bedtime may reduce polydipsia/polyuria and allow the kidneys more time to clear lithium (Bowen et al. 1991; Gitlin 2016). Amilioride 5–10 mg/day may also improve urine-concentrating ability (Bedford et al. 2008).

3. Gastrointestinal: Dry mouth, nausea, diarrhea
   a. Diarrhea (~10% incidence): The IR formulation is preferred to avoid diarrhea, due to proximal absorption (although it may increase nausea). Dividing or lowering the dosage may help (Gitlin 2016).
   b. Nausea (10%–20% incidence): The ER formulation is preferred to avoid nausea, due to distal absorption (although it may increase diarrhea). Dividing or lowering the dosage may help (Gitlin 2016).

4. Weight gain: Relatively common; may be up to 10 kg (22 lb) or more (Gitlin 2016). Cause may be multifactorial (e.g., water weight, carbohydrate cravings, increased thirst).
5. Dermatological effects: New onset or exacerbation of existing acne or psoriasis. Moderate/severe psoriasis is a relative (not absolute) contraindication to lithium.
6. Hypothyroidism: May be overt or subclinical (up to 20% incidence [Joseph et al. 2023]). Check thyroid function tests regularly. Can be treated with levothyroxine. Generally resolves with discontinuation of lithium (Gitlin 2016), usually within 3 months (Lieber et al. 2020).

B. **Uncommon**:

1. Cardiac effects (rare): Arrhythmia, bradycardia, sinoatrial node dysfunction (sinoatrial block), abnormal T waves (inversion), ST segment depression, peripheral edema, hypotension, sick sinus syndrome (rare), unmasking of Brugada syndrome (very rare). Cardiac changes are likely related to lithium's effects on sodium-potassium channels and appear to be dosage/blood level dependent.
2. Other uncommon adverse effects: Alopecia, clonus, confusion, delirium, drug reaction with eosinophilia and systemic symptoms (DRESS) (rare), dysarthria, dysgeusia (bad taste), sexual dysfunction, extrapyramidal symptoms, hyperreflexia, increased salivation, hyponatremia, hyperparathyroidism and hypercalcemia (rare), leukocytosis, lithium-induced encephalopathic syndrome (very rare), myoclonus, pseudotumor cerebri (very rare), seizure (very rare), serotonin syndrome (with SSRIs or MAOIs) (very rare)

C. **Risks in pregnancy and lactation**:

1. Gestation period
    a. Cardiac defects (early pregnancy)
        i. Initial data suggested a 400-fold increase in congenital heart disease, but newer data suggest that the risk is much lower, although still significant—cardiac malformations risk ratio OF 1.2–7.7 (ACOG Committee on Practice Bulletins—Obstetrics 2008).
        ii. Fetal gestational exposure increases the risk for Ebstein's anomaly (absolute risk about 1/1,000–1/5,000 live births in exposed infants, which is about three times the incidence in nonexposed infants and approximately double the overall rate of cardiac malformations (2.41% exposed vs. 1.15% nonexposed) (Patorno et al. 2017).
        iii. Cardiac risk appears to be dosage-related; one study demonstrated a risk ratio of 1.1 for dosages of 600 mg/day or lower and >3.2 for dosages of 900 mg/day or higher (Patorno et al. 2017).
    b. Other adverse effects (late pregnancy): Neonatal cardiac arrhythmias, polyhydramnios, hypoglycemia, diabetes insipidus, thyroid changes, premature delivery, floppy infant syndrome, neonatal lithium toxicity. Likely dosage-related (ACOG Committee on Practice Bulletins—Obstetrics 2008).

c. Monitor lithium levels closely and periodically during pregnancy, given the physiological changes occurring in pregnancy (e.g., fluid shifts).

d. Abrupt discontinuation of lithium during pregnancy increases the risk of bipolar relapse—taper slowly, ideally prior to conception (ACOG Committee on Practice Bulletins—Obstetrics 2008).

2. Prior to delivery: Discontinue lithium three or more days prior to the expected delivery date in pregnant women to reduce maternal/infant risk of lithium intoxication due to postpartum fluid volume depletion.
3. Breastfeeding: Lithium is present in large quantities/concentrations in the breast milk; therefore, lithium use during breastfeeding is not recommended.

D. **Signs of lithium toxicity**:

1. Mild (level ≥1.5 mmol/L): Coarse tremor, ataxia, diarrhea, vomiting, drowsiness, muscle weakness and dyscoordination, marked increase in urine output, slurred speech
2. Severe (level ≥2 mmol/L): Confusion, severe ataxia, blurred vision, prolonged QTc interval, severe somnolence, coma, death

E. No allergic reactions have been reported in studies of lithium. However, allergies to the components of tablets, capsules, or solution may occur.

XIII. Clinical Pearls/Prescribing Tips

A. Lithium is the "gold standard" mood stabilizer (Balon 2009; Bauer and Mitchner 2004). Lithium works best when it is started early in the course of illness. It is also unique among the mood stabilizers in that it may be protective against suicide.

B. Lithium appears to be an effective antidepressant augmentation strategy in treatment-resistant depression and prevention of relapse after successful ECT treatment.

C. Lithium is neuroprotective; it was reported to enhance neuroplasticity in a variety of animal and human studies (Dell'Osso et al. 2016).

D. Consider adding lithium to clozapine therapy to counteract leukopenia, which can increase the white blood cell (WBC) count (Nykiel et al. 2010).

E. If lithium is to be used during pregnancy:

1. The dosage will have to be adjusted periodically because of increased fluid volume.
2. Discontinue lithium 3 or more days before the expected delivery date to reduce risk of lithium intoxication in the infant or mother (due to postpartum fluid volume depletion). Restart after immediate postpartum diuresis (about 3 days).
3. Postpartum fluid loss can continue as long as 6 months. Check lithium levels every 1–2 months.

F. Older patients are at greater risk of CNS side effects.

G. Blood levels of lithium are increased by dehydration, NSAIDs, ACE inhibitors/ARBs, and diuretics. Educate patients about these potential interactions and instruct them to remain well hydrated.

H. Although the risk of renal failure is low, monitor the eGFR over time during lithium treatment. Once-daily or nightly dosing appears to be more beneficial for kidney function.

Further Reading

Amdisen A: Serum level monitoring and clinical pharmacokinetics of lithium. Clin Pharmacokinet 2(2):73–92, 1977 324690

Carvalho AF, Firth J, Vieta E: Bipolar disorder. N Engl J Med 383(1):58–66, 2020 32609982

Chokhawala K, Lee S, Saadabadi A: Lithium, in StatPearls. Treasure Island, FL, StatPearls Publishing, 2022. Available at: https://www.ncbi.nlm.nih.gov/books/NBK519062/. Accessed May 2022.

Hedya SA, Avula A, Swoboda HD: Lithium toxicity, in StatPearls. Treasure Island, FL, StatPearls Publishing, 2022. Available at: https://www.ncbi.nlm.nih.gov/books/NBK499992/. Accessed May 2022.

Imaz ML, Torra M, Soy D, et al: Clinical lactation studies of lithium: a systematic review. Front Pharmacol 10:1005, 2019 31551795

Lithium carbonate extended release prescribing information. U.S. Food and Drug Administration, 2020. Available at: https://dailymed.nlm.nih.gov/dailymed/fda/fdaDrugXsl.cfm?setid=1b65d27e-5086-4a87-8387-c49f3d060978&type=display. Accessed May 2022.

Lithium carbonate immediate release prescribing information. U.S. Food and Drug Administration, 2018. Available at: https://www.accessdata.fda.gov/drugsatfda_docs/label/2018/017812s033,018421s032,018558s027lbl.pdf. Accessed May 2022.

Rosen MS: Lithium in child and adolescent bipolar disorder. Am J Psychiatry Resid J 12:3–5, 2017

References

ACOG Committee on Practice Bulletins—Obstetrics: ACOG Practice Bulletin: Clinical management guidelines for obstetrician-gynecologists number 92, April 2008 (replaces practice bulletin number 87, November 2007). Use of psychiatric medications during pregnancy and lactation. Obstet Gynecol 111(4):1001–1020, 2008 18378767

Baek JH, Kinrys G, Nierenberg AA: Lithium tremor revisited: pathophysiology and treatment. Acta Psychiatr Scand 129(1):17–23, 2014 23834617

Balon R: Old but still gold: lithium in stabilizing the mood. Indian J Psychiatry 51(2):157–158, 2009 19823639

Bauer MS, Mitchner L: What is a "mood stabilizer"? An evidence-based response. Am J Psychiatry 161(1):3–18, 2004 14702242

Bedford JJ, Leader JP, Jing R, et al: Amiloride restores renal medullary osmolytes in lithium-induced nephrogenic diabetes insipidus. Am J Physiol Renal Physiol 294(4):F812–F820, 2008 18216143

Beunders AJM, Hillegers MHJ, Regeer EJ, et al: Renal complications of lithium use: to cease or to continue? [in German]. Ned Tijdschr Geneeskd 162:D2683, 2018

Bowen RC, Grof P, Grof E: Less frequent lithium administration and lower urine volume. Am J Psychiatry 148(2):189–192, 1991 1987816

Bschor T, Lewitzka U, Sasse J, et al: Lithium augmentation in treatment-resistant depression: clinical evidence, serotonergic and endocrine mechanisms. Pharmacopsychiatry 36(Suppl 3):S230–S234, 2003 14677084

Bschor T, Lewitzka U, Pfennig A, et al: Twenty-five years of lithium augmentation [in German]. Nervenarzt 78(11):1237–1247, 2007 17458527

Carter L, Zolezzi M, Lewczyk A: An updated review of the optimal lithium dosage regimen for renal protection. Can J Psychiatry 58(10):595–600, 2013 24165107

Dell'Osso L, Del Grande C, Gesi C, et al: A new look at an old drug: neuroprotective effects and therapeutic potentials of lithium salts. Neuropsychiatr Dis Treat 12:1687–1703, 2016 27468233

de Montigny C, Cournoyer G, Morissette R, et al: Lithium carbonate addition in tricyclic antidepressant-resistant unipolar depression: correlations with the neurobiologic actions of tricyclic antidepressant drugs and lithium ion on the serotonin system. Arch Gen Psychiatry 40(12):1327–1334, 1983 6418109

Gelenberg AJ, Kane JM, Keller MB, et al: Comparison of standard and low serum levels of lithium for maintenance treatment of bipolar disorder. N Engl J Med 321(22):1489–1493, 1989 2811970

Gerhard T, Devanand DP, Huang C, et al: Lithium treatment and risk for dementia in adults with bipolar disorder: population-based cohort study. Br J Psychiatry 207(1):46–51, 2015 25614530

Giotakos O, Tsouvelas G, Nisianakis P, et al: A negative association between lithium in drinking water and the incidences of homicides, in Greece. Biol Trace Elem Res 164(2):165–168, 2015 25556933

Gitlin M: Lithium side effects and toxicity: prevalence and management strategies. Int J Bipolar Disord 4(1):27, 2016 27900734

Ibbeken C, Becker JU, Baumgärtel MW: Renal side effects of long-term lithium therapy [in German]. Dtsch Med Wochenschr 137(4):143–148, 2012 22259170

Januel D, Poirier MF, D'alche-Biree F, et al: Multicenter double-blind randomized parallel-group clinical trial of efficacy of the combination clomipramine (150 mg/day) plus lithium carbonate (750 mg/day) versus clomipramine (150 mg/day) plus placebo in the treatment of unipolar major depression. J Affect Disord 76(1–3):191–200, 2003 12943949

Joseph B, Nunez NA, Pazdernik V, et al: Long-term lithium therapy and thyroid disorders in bipolar disorder: a historical cohort study. Brain Sci 13(1):133, 2023 36672114

Keck PE Jr, Strakowski SM, Hawkins JM, et al: A pilot study of rapid lithium administration in the treatment of acute mania. Bipolar Disord 3(2):68–72, 2001 11333065

Kook KA, Stimmel GL, Wilkins JN, et al: Accuracy and safety of a priori lithium loading. J Clin Psychiatry 46(2):49–51, 1985 3918024

Lambrichts S, Detraux J, Vansteelandt K, et al: Does lithium prevent relapse following successful electroconvulsive therapy for major depression? A systematic review and meta-analysis. Acta Psychiatr Scand 143(4):294–306, 2021 33506961

Lewitzka U, Severus E, Bauer R, et al: The suicide prevention effect of lithium: more than 20 years of evidence-a narrative review. Int J Bipolar Disord 3(1):32, 2015 26183461

Lieber I, Ott M, Öhlund L, et al: Lithium-associated hypothyroidism and potential for reversibility after lithium discontinuation: findings from the LiSIE retrospective cohort study. J Psychopharmacol 34(3):293–303, 2020 31670617

Malhi GS, Tanious M, Das P, et al: Potential mechanisms of action of lithium in bipolar disorder: current understanding. CNS Drugs 27(2):135–153, 2013 23371914

Nelson JC, Baumann P, Delucchi K, et al: A systematic review and meta-analysis of lithium augmentation of tricyclic and second generation antidepressants in major depression. J Affect Disord 168:269–275, 2014 25069082

Nonaka S, Hough CJ, Chuang DM: Chronic lithium treatment robustly protects neurons in the central nervous system against excitotoxicity by inhibiting N-methyl-D-aspartate receptor-mediated calcium influx. Proc Natl Acad Sci USA 95(5):2642–2647, 1998 9482940

Nykiel S, Henderson D, Bhide G, et al: Lithium to allow clozapine prescribing in benign ethnic neutropenia. Clin Schizophr Relat Psychoses 4(2):138–140, 2010 20643636

Passavanti G, Buongiorno E, De Fino G, et al: Lithium-induced polyuria and polydipsia, in Drugs, Systemic Diseases, and the Kidney. Edited by Amerio A, Coratelli P, Campese VM, et al. Boston, MA, Springer US, 1989, pp 215–231

Patel RS, Bachu A, Youssef NA: Combination of lithium and electroconvulsive therapy (ECT) is associated with higher odds of delirium and cognitive problems in a large national sample across the United States. Brain Stimul 13(1):15–19, 2020 31492631
Patorno E, Huybrechts KF, Bateman BT, et al: Lithium use in pregnancy and the risk of cardiac malformations. N Engl J Med 376(23):2245–2254, 2017 28591541
Reddy DS, Reddy MS: Serum lithium levels: ideal time for sample collection! Are we doing it right? Indian J Psychol Med 36(3):346–347, 2014 25035570
Sackeim HA, Haskett RF, Mulsant BH, et al: Continuation pharmacotherapy in the prevention of relapse following electroconvulsive therapy: a randomized controlled trial. JAMA 285(10):1299–1307, 2001 11255384
Song J, Sjölander A, Joas E, et al: Suicidal behavior during lithium and valproate treatment: a within-individual 8-year prospective study of 50,000 patients with bipolar disorder. Am J Psychiatry 174(8):795–802, 2017 28595491
Vázquez GH, Bahji A, Undurraga J, et al: Efficacy and tolerability of combination treatments for major depression: antidepressants plus second-generation antipsychotics vs. esketamine vs. lithium. J Psychopharmacol 35(8):890–900, 2021 34238049
Wang HY, Friedman E: Chronic lithium: desensitization of autoreceptors mediating serotonin release. Psychopharmacology (Berl) 94(3):312–314, 1988 3128806
Young W: Review of lithium effects on brain and blood. Cell Transplant 18(9):951–975, 2009 19523343

Oxcarbazepine

I. **Brand Names**: Trileptal, Trileptal extended release, Oxtellar CR

II. **Therapeutic Class**: Anticonvulsant

III. **Mechanism-Based Class**: Sodium channel inhibitor

IV. **Mechanism(s) of Action**

A. Oxcarbazepine's mechanism of action in bipolar disorder is not fully understood.

B. Oxcarbazepine blocks voltage-gated sodium channels, reducing the high-frequency firing of neurons, thereby decreasing membrane excitability (Macdonald and Kelly 1995).

V. **Indications**

A. FDA adult: Seizures, trigeminal neuralgia

B. Evidence-based[1] off-label uses: Bipolar mania and maintenance

C. FDA pediatric: Partial seizure disorders (age 2–6 years)

VI. **Major Contraindications and When to Use Caution**

A. **Major contraindications**: Known hypersensitivity to oxcarbazepine or carbamazepine

B. **Use caution**: History of severe medication-induced allergies with other drugs

---

[1]Evidence strength varies; readers are referred to the literature for more detailed information.

VII. **Dosage Formulations**

A. Brand or generic immediate-release (IR) tablet (150 mg, 300 mg, 600 mg)
B. Brand or generic extended-release (IR) tablet (150 mg, 300 mg, 600 mg)
C. Oral suspension (300 mg/5 mL [60 mg/mL])

VIII. **Dosage Ranges and Guidelines**

A. Adults: Start at 300 mg BID. Gradually increase by 300–600 mg every 2–4 weeks to a maximum dosage of 1,200 mg/day as tolerated.

1. Dosage can be decreased in 150- or 300-mg increments to manage side effects.

B. Pediatric (age 2–16 years): Start at 8–10 mg/kg/day in divided doses. Gradually increase to 30–40 mg/kg twice per day as tolerated, to a maximum of 60 mg/day.

IX. **Monitoring**

A. **Baseline (before starting oxcarbazepine)**: Obtain a complete blood count (CBC), a comprehensive metabolic panel (CMP), and a pregnancy test.
B. **Consider obtaining human leukocyte antigen (HLA) genotyping**: The FDA recommends screening for the HLA-B*15:02 allele before initiating oxcarbazepine treatment in patients of Asian ancestry, who are known to have high frequencies of this allele.
C. **Periodic monitoring**: Obtain a CBC and CMP at 3, 6, and 12 months and annually thereafter.
D. **Blood-level monitoring**: Check trough level after 3–4 days. Blood level range for seizure disorders is 10–35 μg/mL.

X. **Relevant Pharmacokinetics/Pharmacodynamics**

A. **Metabolism**: Hepatic (cytochrome P450 [CYP] 3A4)
B. **Time to peak plasma concentration**:
   1. Immediate release: 4.5 hours
   2. Extended release: 12 hours (9.5–15 hours, depending on preparation)
C. **Half-life**: 10.5 hours
D. **Effect of food**: None
E. **Hepatic impairment**: No dosage adjustment is needed in patients with mild to moderate liver impairment. Although the effects of severe impairment have not been tested, such impairment will likely increase blood levels and side effects.
F. **Renal impairment**: Impairment reduces the clearance of the primary metabolite 10-monohydroxy-oxcarbazepine. In patients with impaired renal function (CrCl <30 mL/minute), start at one-half the usual starting dosage and increase slowly.

XI. **Clinically Relevant Drug Interactions**

A. Metabolized by CYP3A4:

1. CYP3A4 inhibitors and inducers significantly affect carbamazepine metabolism. Dosages should be adjusted accordingly.

   a. Commonly used medications that are CYP3A4 strong inhibitors (*increase* carbamazepine levels) include certain protease inhibitors (e.g., indinavir, ritonavir), clarithromycin, and ketoconazole. Moderate inhibitors include ciprofloxacin, diltiazem, erythromycin, fluconazole, fluvoxamine, grapefruit and juice, and verapamil.

b. Commonly used agents/medications that are CYP3A4 inducers (*decrease* carbamazepine level) include apalutamide, carbamazepine, efavirenz, enzalutamide, phenytoin, rifampin, and St. John's wort.

2. The oxcarbazepine dosage will need to be adjusted if the dosage of a coadministered inducer or inhibitor is changed or the medication is stopped.

B. Weak inducer of CYP3A4

XII. **Adverse Effects**

A. **Most common**:

1. CNS effects: Somnolence, ataxia, discoordination, concentration (and other cognitive) problems, dizziness, speech disturbance, nystagmus, blurred vision, headache (likely dosage related)
2. Hyponatremia: May occur in 46% of patients, with 22% of cases being severe (Berghuis et al. 2017), although most are asymptomatic. Usually appears within the first 3 months of treatment.
3. Photosensitivity: Oxcarbazepine is associated with photosensitivity in some patients. Patients should always use sunscreen with any but the briefest sun exposures.

B. **Uncommon**:

1. Boxed warnings: Delayed hypersensitivity reactions: Ranging from mild to severe rashes (Stevens-Johnson syndrome [SJS]/toxic epidermal necrolysis [TEN]) to drug reaction with eosinophilia and systemic symptoms (DRESS) (Chung et al. 2021).

   a. Consider obtaining HLA genotyping for patients in high-risk groups (see "Anticonvulsant Boxed Warning: Serious Dermatological Reactions" at the beginning of this chapter).

2. Blood dyscrasias (agranulocytosis, leukopenia, aplastic anemia, pancytopenia, thrombocytopenia): Very rare; timing of onset varies; monitor CBC.
3. Suicide risk: Noted in drug labeling but not clearly established; likely very low risk (Mula et al. 2013).
4. Other uncommon adverse effects: Peripheral edema, arthralgias, emotional lability, memory problems, disinhibition, indigestion, irritability/aggression, angioedema, menstrual disturbance

C. **Risks in pregnancy and lactation**:

1. Pregnancy: There is no established relationship between fetal gestational exposure and major malformations. However, teratogenicity was found in animal studies. In addition, pregnancy registries have suggested associations with craniofacial defects (e.g., oral clefts) and cardiac malformations (e.g., ventricular septal defects). Use in pregnancy is not recommended.
2. Lactation: Significant levels of oxcarbazepine and its major metabolite are transmitted in breast milk; therefore, use of oxcarbazepine during breastfeeding is not recommended.

XIII. **Clinical Pearls/Prescribing Tips**

A. Oxcarbazepine is not an established treatment for bipolar disorder.; placebo-controlled trials have been limited. Head-to-head trials comparing oxcarbazepine with established medications such as valproate have shown mixed results, although oxcarbazepine may be more effective in mild to moderate mania (Grunze et al. 2021). Alternative antimanic or mood-stabilizing medications should be considered first.

B. There is some evidence that oxcarbazepine improves impulsivity in patients with bipolar disorder and impulse-control disorders.

C. Oxcarbazepine is a prodrug that is metabolized into its active form, 10-monohydroxy-oxcarbazepine, by CYP3A4. This conversion is affected by gain and loss of functional polymorphisms and by inhibitors and inducers of CYP3A4.

D. Monitor CBC and comprehensive metabolic panel (CMP) periodically, given the risk of blood dyscrasias and hyponatremia.

E. Compared with other commonly used mood stabilizers (e.g., lithium, valproate), oxcarbazepine is less likely to cause significant weight gain.

F. A benign rash can occur with oxcarbazepine, but signs of a more serious rash include systemic symptoms, mucosal involvement, and a widespread, confluent painful rash.

Further Reading

Carvalho AF, Firth J, Vieta E: Bipolar disorder. N Engl J Med 383(1):58–66, 2020 32609982

Mullan KA, Anderson A, Illing PT, et al: HLA-associated antiepileptic drug-induced cutaneous adverse reactions. HLA 93(6):417–435, 2019 30895730

Oxcarbazepine, oxcarbazepine extended release prescribing information. U.S. Food and Drug Administration, 2017. Available at: https://www.accessdata.fda.gov/drugsatfda_docs/label/2017/021014s036lbl.pdf. Accessed June 2022.

Preuss CV, Randhawa G, Wy TJP, et al: Oxcarbazepine, in StatPearls. Treasure Island, FL, StatPearls Publishing, 2022. Available at: https://www.ncbi.nlm.nih.gov/books/NBK482313/, Accessed June 2022.

References

Berghuis B, van der Palen J, de Haan GJ, et al; EpiPGX Consortium: Carbamazepine- and oxcarbazepine-induced hyponatremia in people with epilepsy. Epilepsia 58(7):1227–1233, 2017 28542738

Chung SJ, Ahn KM, Oh JH, et al: Incidence rates of severe cutaneous adverse reactions due to anti-seizure medication: a nationwide study using health claims data in Korea. Epilepsia 62(1):250–257, 2021 33188522

Grunze A, Amann BL, Grunze H. Efficacy of carbamazepine and its derivatives in the treatment of bipolar disorder. Medicina (Kaunas) 57(5):433, 2021

Lorberg B, Youssef NA, Bhagwagar Z: Lamotrigine-associated rash: to rechallenge or not to rechallenge? Int J Neuropsychopharmacol 12(2):257–265, 2009 18845017

Macdonald RL, Kelly KM: Antiepileptic drug mechanisms of action. Epilepsia 36(Suppl 2):S2–S12, 1995 8784210

Mula M, Kanner AM, Schmitz B, et al: Antiepileptic drugs and suicidality: an expert consensus statement from the Task Force on Therapeutic Strategies of the ILAE Commission on Neuropsychobiology. Epilepsia 54(1):199–203, 2013 22994856

Valproate/Divalproex/Valproic Acid

I. **Brand Names**: Depakene, Depakote, Depacon, Epival

II. **Therapeutic Class**: Anticonvulsant

III. **Mechanism-Based Class**: Sodium and potassium channel inhibitor

IV. **Mechanism(s) of Action**

A. The mechanism of action in bipolar disorder is not fully understood, but valproate appears to dampen the excitability of the limbic system, likely giving it antimanic effects.

B. Valproate is an inhibitor of succinic semialdehyde dehydrogenase, which results in GABA transaminase inhibition, reducing the degradation of GABA and increasing GABA levels.

C. Valproate blocks both voltage-gated sodium channels and $K_v7.2$ potassium channels. This activity reduces the high-frequency firing of neurons, thereby decreasing membrane excitability (Macdonald and Kelly 1995; Rahman and Nguyen 2022).

D. Valproate leads to extracellular signal-regulated kinase 1/2 (ERK1/2) cascade phosphorylation, which has a number of downstream effects (e.g., increases in Bcl-2, brain-derived neurotrophic factor [BDNF]). This activation of the ERK pathway provides neuroprotective effects, but also appears to be antimanic (Hao et al. 2004).

E. Valproate also inhibits myoinositol monophosphatase, leading to reduced inositol levels. Effects on Bcl-2 and inositol modulate cytosolic calcium; altered calcium regulation has been demonstrated in bipolar disorder (Harrison et al. 2021).

F. Valproate may also activate *N*-methyl-D-aspartate (NMDA) receptors, reducing neuronal excitation, and may modulate dopaminergic and serotonergic transmission (Perucca 2002).

V. **Indications**

A. FDA adult:

1. Bipolar mania
2. Seizures
3. Migraine prophylaxis
4. Fragile X syndrome
5. Familial adenomatous polyposis

B. Evidence-based[1] off-label uses:

1. Bipolar depression and maintenance
2. Agitation in schizophrenia

C. FDA pediatric: Complex partial seizures (age 10 years and older)

[1]Evidence strength varies; readers are referred to the literature for more detailed information.

VI. Major Contraindications and When to Use Caution

A. **Major contraindications**:

1. Known hypersensitivity to valproate or its components
2. Hepatic impairment
3. Mitochondrial disorders caused by mutations in mitochondrial DNA polymerase γ (e.g., Alpers-Huttenlocher syndrome)
4. Urea cycle disorders
5. Pregnancy

B. **Use caution**:

1. History of prior severe medication-induced allergies or hepatotoxicity with other drugs
2. Women of reproductive potential

VII. Dosage Formulations

A. Valproic acid

1. Brand or generic immediate-release (IR) capsule (250 mg)—*Depakene*

B. Divalproex sodium

1. Brand or generic delayed-release (DR) capsule (125 mg, 250 mg, 500 mg)—*Depakote*
2. Brand or generic extended-release (ER) tablet (250 mg, 500 mg)—*Depakote ER*
   a. Do not break or crush ER tabs.
3. Brand or generic sprinkles capsule (125 mg)—*Depakote sprinkles*
4. Brand valproate sodium crushable tablet (100 mg) (outside the United States)

C. Valproate sodium

1. Brand valproate sodium crushable tablet (100 mg) (outside the United States)
2. Brand or generic IR oral solution (250 mg/5 mL)—*Depakene syrup*
3. Brand or generic IV solution (100 mg/mL)—*Depacon*
   a. *Note*: Sodium valproate is the *sodium salt* of valproic acid and divalproex sodium contains a combination of both sodium valproate and valproic acid.
   b. *Note*: The IR form is more rapidly absorbed but has greater fluctuations in serum levels and a shorter half-life (dosed 2 times daily). The bioavailability of the DR form is higher than that of the ER form. Therefore, if switching from the DR to the ER form, the dosage may need to be increased by about 10%–20% (McGraw 2014).

VIII. Dosage Ranges and Guidelines

A. **Bipolar mania**: Initial dosage is 500–750 mg/day, increasing as rapidly as possible to achieve response or target plasma level.

1. Valproate loading: A loading strategy for divalproex sodium has been tested in multiple studies in acutely manic patients.
   a. A loading dose of 20 mg/kg/day of the immediate-release or 15 mg/kg/day titrated to 30 mg/kg/day of the extended-release formulation has been shown to be effective (Keck et al. 2000).

b. One study used 30 mg/kg/day for 2 days, followed by 20 mg/kg/day of the immediate-release formulation for more rapid loading (Hirschfeld et al. 1999).
c. After initial loading, adjust dosage upward or downward to reach therapeutic blood levels (see "Monitoring").

2. Fixed dosing: Start at 500–750 mg/day (consider nightly dosing, given sedation) taken as a single dose or in 2–4 doses. Increase by 250–500 mg every 1–2 days to a typical dosage of 1,500–2,500 mg/day (Goodwin et al. 2016).

B. Bipolar maintenance and bipolar depression (off-label; see Table 5–4 below).
C. **Seizures**: Start at 10–15 mg/kg/day (for complex partial seizures) or 15 mg/kg/day (for absence seizures), increasing at 1-week intervals by 5–10 mg/kg/day until optimal response and/or therapeutic level is obtained.
D. **Migraine**: The recommended starting dosage is 250 mg twice daily. If needed, the dosage can be increased to 750 or 1,000 mg/day. The maximum recommended dosage is 60 mg/day.

Table 5–4. Valproate/divalproex/valproic acid indications and dosage ranges

Psychiatric indication	Usual dosage range
Bipolar mania	500–750 mg/day → 1,500–2,000 mg/day (BID if delayed release; QD/QHS if extended release) Maximum dosage 60 mg/kg/day Loading (see "Valproate loading" in "Dosage Ranges and Guideline" section
Bipolar maintenance (off-label)	Continue the dosage that stabilized patient
Bipolar depression (off-label)	500–750 mg/day → 1,500–2,500 mg/day (taken as a single dose or in 2–4 doses)
Migraine prophylaxis	500 mg/day → 1,000 mg/day (taken as a single dose or in 2 doses)
Complex partial seizures	10–15 mg/kg/day → 60 mg/kg/day
Absence seizures	15 mg/kg/day → 60 mg/kg/day

Note. BID=twice a day; QD=every day; QHS=every night at bedtime.
Bipolar maintenance: Valproate and lithium have shown similar efficacy for maintenance treatment of bipolar disorder (Bowden et al. 2000; Cipriani et al. 2013; Kang et al. 2020; Yatham et al. 2018), although the combination of valproate and lithium appears to be even more efficacious (Cipriani et al. 2013).
Bipolar depression: Valproate has shown benefit in bipolar depression (Bond et al. 2010). One study showed that depression during mania responded better to valproate than to lithium (Swann et al. 1997). However, the evidence supporting valproate use in bipolar depression is limited.
Other indications: *Schizophrenia*: In a large Cochrane Review, valproate was shown to be beneficial as an augmentation to antipsychotics in schizophrenia and specifically improved overexcitement and agitation (Wang et al. 2016). *Agitation/impulsivity*: Valproate has shown some efficacy in the treatment of agitation and impulsivity across various psychiatric diagnoses, including major depressive disorder, panic disorder, PTSD, and borderline personality disorder (Davis et al. 2000).

IX. **Monitoring**

A. **Baseline (before starting valproate/divalproex/valproic acid)**: Obtain complete blood count (CBC) and liver function tests (LFTs) at baseline; at 1, 3, 6, and 12 months; and every 6–12 months thereafter. For patients with liver dysfunction, consider obtaining baseline albumin and checking periodically.

B. **Weight gain**: Obtain weight at baseline and monitor periodically, given risk of weight gain.

C. **Consider HLA genotyping.**

D. **Blood-level monitoring**:

1. Trough levels: Check 3–4 days after continuous dosing.
   a. Extended-release formulation: Obtain trough level ~24 hours after the once-daily/nightly dose (right before the next dose). If levels must be obtained 12 hours after the dose for convenience, the level may have to be reduced by 18%–25% for accuracy (Damegunta 2014; Reed and Dutta 2006).
   b. Delayed-release formulation: Obtain trough level ~12 hours after the nightly dose (just prior to the morning dose) if given twice daily (McGraw 2014)
2. Target levels:
   a. Mania: 50–125 μg/mL (total level—both bound and free)
      i. At total concentrations less than 50 μg/mL, almost all of valproate is bound to albumin, leaving very little active (unbound) drug to enter the brain.
      ii. Toxicity exists at around 175 μg/mL or more
   b. Seizures: 50–100 μg/mL (total level—both bound and free)
3. *Note*: Valproate is highly protein bound (~90%), and only the free (unbound) portion can enter the brain and exert clinical effects. As the dosage increases, the free fraction increases (for example, at total concentrations less than 50 μg/mL, almost all of the drug is bound by albumin). Serum valproate levels account for both the bound *and* the unbound drug. Therefore, in the presence of hypoalbuminemia, the free drug may be proportionally higher than normal. Other drugs or substances that compete for albumin (e.g., aspirin, NSAIDs, phenytoin) can also lead to a higher proportion of unbound valproate, increasing the risk of toxicity. No specific guidelines exist for adjusting valproate dosing in cases of hypoalbuminemia, so obtaining a free valproate level may be necessary (Tseng et al. 2020; VandenBerg et al. 2018). The therapeutic free valproate level is approximately 10%–15% of the total level: **5–15** μg/mL (Smetana et al. 2015).

X. **Relevant Pharmacokinetics/Pharmacodynamics**

A. **Metabolism**:

1. Hepatic (through both cytochrome P450 [CYP] enzymes and direct glucuronidation via uridine 5′-diphospho-glucuronosyltransferase [UGT] enzymes).
2. Mitochondrial beta oxidation

B. **Time to peak plasma concentration**:
    1. Immediate release (valproate, divalproex): 4 hours (with food: 8 hours)
    2. Extended release: 24 hours
    3. Sprinkles: 3.3 hours (with food: 4 hours)
C. **Half-life**: About 13 hours at steady state (9–16 hours)
D. **Hepatic impairment**: Use not recommended in individuals with hepatic impairment because of the risk of hepatotoxicity.
E. **Renal impairment**: Renal impairment may have a small effect on unconjugated blood levels, but dosage does not require adjustment.

XI. **Clinically Relevant Drug Interactions**

A. Metabolized by CYP2A6, CYP2B6, CYP2C9, and CYP3A5; UGT1A3, UGT1A4, UGT1A6, UGT1A9, UGT1A10, UGT2B7, and UGT2B15; and mitochondrial beta oxidation.
B. Concomitant use of lamotrigine with valproate increases the risk of Stevens-Johnson syndrome/toxic epidermal necrolysis (SJS/TEN). This interaction is posited to involve valproate's inhibition of lamotrigine metabolism, leading to increased lamotrigine blood levels. When lamotrigine is prescribed as an adjunct to valproic acid treatment, dosage titration should be slow.
C. Concomitant use of topiramate may result in hyperammonemia with encephalopathy.
D. Phenytoin, carbamazepine, phenobarbital, and primidone can decrease valproate levels by inducing UGT enzymes. Conversely, valproate can have effects on the metabolism and levels of phenytoin, carbamazepine, phenobarbital, and primidone, potentially leading to increased levels of these medications.

XII. **Adverse Effects**

A. **Most common**:
    1. CNS effects: Usually CNS depression, which involves symptoms such as dizziness (incidence up to 25% [Abbott Laboratories 2011]) and drowsiness (incidence up to 30% [Abbott Laboratories 2011]), but also includes stimulating effects (e.g., nervousness, insomnia, tremor).
    2. Hematological effects: These effects most commonly include thrombocytopenia (incidence up to 24% [Abbott Laboratories 2011]), but can also include aplastic anemia, neutropenia, and/or pure red cell aplasia. Etiology appears to be multifactorial, involving direct bone marrow toxicity, antibody-mediated destruction of thrombocytes, destruction of platelets, and/or inhibition of erythroid differentiation. Onset can occur from 8 days to 16 months after initiation. Effects are likely dosage-related and can usually be reversed with dosage reduction or discontinuation (Acharya and Bussel 2000).
        a. The risk of neutropenia appears to be increased when valproate is combined with clozapine (Malik et al. 2018) or quetiapine (Park and Kim 2016).
    3. Gastrointestinal effects: Nausea (incidence up to 48% [Abbott Laboratories 2011]), vomiting, diarrhea (incidence up to 23%), anorexia, abdominal pain, dyspepsia, constipation

4. Weight gain (incidence about 40% [Biton et al. 2001]): Common; patients treated with valproate may gain 5 kg (11 lb) or more. Weight gain may occur more frequently in women. Etiology unclear but potentially related to dysregulation of the hypothalamic system, hyperinsulinemia, insulin resistance, effect on adipokine levels (i.e., leptin, ghrelin) (Verrotti et al. 2011). Consider adding metformin or topiramate to counteract these effects (White et al. 2013).
5. Other effects: Alopecia (incidence up to 12% [Kakunje et al. 2018]), appetite loss, ataxia, blurred vision, fatigue, headache, nystagmus, orthostatic hypotension, pruritus, rash, weight loss
    a. Valproate is associated with photosensitivity in some patients. Patients should always use sunscreen with any but the very briefest sun exposure.

B. **Uncommon**:

1. Boxed warning: Liver dysfunction:
    a. Hepatocellular injury: Incidence 5%–10% [Valproate 2020]; may develop AST/ALT elevations (usually 1–3 times the upper limit of normal), usually without increases in bilirubin, alkaline phosphatase. Mostly asymptomatic and may self-resolve or improve with dosage decrease or discontinuation (Valproate 2020).
    b. Liver failure: Very rare (1/40,000); more common in children or young adults; usually occurs within the first 3 months of treatment (McKiernan 2014). Risk is higher for patients with developmental delay, metabolic disorders, or certain genetic risks (e.g., mitochondrial diseases), as well as for patients taking multiple antiseizure medications (Bryant and Dreifuss 1996). Multiple potential mechanisms. Monitor for nausea, vomiting, anorexia, impaired consciousness, and ataxia.
2. Boxed warning: Pancreatitis: Rare but life-threatening cases have occurred with hemorrhage and rapid progression to death. Monitor for abdominal pain, anorexia, nausea, and vomiting.
3. Hyperammonemia (and/or hyperammonemic encephalopathy): May be relatively common (~27% in one study [Tseng et al. 2014]) but is usually asymptomatic. Obtain ammonia level if symptomatic (change in mental status including drowsiness, lethargy, cognitive slowing, vomiting, focal neurological signs, change in level of consciousness) or if hypothermia occurs. May occur in the presence or absence of hepatic dysfunction. Onset varies but usually occurs early in treatment. Potentially dosage/concentration related. Typically resolves with discontinuation. If asymptomatic hyperammonemia is discovered incidentally, ammonia levels should be monitored and discontinuation of valproate should be considered if hyperammonemia persists. Risk factors include urea cycle disorders; carnitine deficiency; concurrent use of topiramate, other antiepileptic drugs, or antipsychotic drugs; and overdose (Tseng et al. 2014).
4. CNS: Delirium, hallucinations, parkinsonism, cognitive dysfunction. Likely dosage-related. Risk factors include higher free valproate concentrations (low albumin) and use of multiple antiseizure medications.

5. Other uncommon adverse effects: Agitation, hostility/aggression, hyperammonemia, hyponatremia, SIADH, hypothermia (rare), irritability, pancreatitis, polycystic ovary syndrome, psychosis (rare), reduced bone density, severe hepatotoxicity/hepatic failure, severe thrombocytopenia, SJS/TEN (extremely rare).
6. Boxed warnings: Delayed hypersensitivity reactions: Ranges from mild to severe rashes (Stevens-Johnson syndrome [SJS]/toxic epidermal necrolysis [TEN]) and drug reaction with eosinophilia and systemic symptoms (DRESS) (Chung et al. 2021).
    a. Consider HLA genotyping in high-risk groups (see "Anticonvulsant Boxed Warning: Serious Dermatological Reactions" at the beginning of this chapter).
7. Suicide risk: Noted in drug labeling, but not clearly established, likely very low risk (Mula et al. 2013).

C. **Risks in pregnancy and lactation**:
1. Boxed warning: Pregnancy—Fetal risk: Fetal gestational exposure to valproate is associated with an increased risk of neural tube defects, other malformations (e.g., craniofacial, cardiovascular, and limb malformations; hypospadias), and reduced IQ. Malformation risk is approximately 10% (Andrade 2024). Use in pregnancy is not recommended.
2. Lactation: Significant levels of valproate and its major metabolite are transmitted in breast milk and may result in adverse reactions in infants.

XIII. **Clinical Pearls/Prescribing Tips**

A. Valproate has shown efficacy similar to that of lithium in bipolar maintenance treatment, although it is not FDA approved for this indication. Combined use with other mood stabilizers has been recommended by some (Bowden et al. 2000). Evidence is limited for valproate's efficacy for bipolar depression. In addition, valproate is used to treat impulsivity, agitation, and aggression, although controlled data are lacking.

B. For patients taking valproate, check CBC and liver function periodically, given the risk of hematological and liver dysfunction. Obtain weight at baseline and check periodically, given weight gain risk. Consider use of augmentation agents such as metformin/topiramate to curb weight gain/metabolic effects.

C. Valproate carries a substantial risk of teratogenic effects. Ensure that women of childbearing age who are taking valproate are using contraception.

D. Valproate is highly protein bound, and because no specific guidelines exist for adjusting valproate dosing in cases of hypoalbuminemia, obtaining a free valproate level may be necessary.

E. The DR and ER formulations of divalproex differ in their pharmacokinetic properties (including bioavailability) and their therapeutic blood level monitoring requirements; therefore, dosage adjustment is required when switching between them.

Further Reading

Abbott Laboratories: Depakote (divalproex sodium) tablets for oral use [package insert]. U.S. Food and Drug Administration website. Revised October 2011. Available at: https://www.accessdata.fda.gov/drugsatfda_docs/label/2011/018723s037lbl.pdf. Accessed June 21, 2024.

AbbVie Inc: Depakene (valproic acid), capsules, oral solution [package insert]. U.S. Food and Drug Administration website. Revised November 2016. Available at: https://www.accessdata.fda.gov/drugsatfda_docs/label/2016/018081s065_018082s048lbl.pdf. Accessed June 21, 2024.

AbbVie Inc: Depakote ER (divalproex sodium tablet, extended release) [package insert]. U.S. Food and Drug Administration website. Revised February 2023. Available at: https://www.accessdata.fda.gov/spl/data/c7f33a5e-be13-45a6-8edd-8f6cd7618e1e/c7f33a5e-be13-45a6-8edd-8f6cd7618e1e.xml. Accessed June 21, 2024.

AbbVie Inc: Depakote Sprinkle Capsules (divalproex sodium coated particles in capsules), for oral use [package insert]. U.S. Food and Drug Administration website. Revised July 2013. Available at: https://www.accessdata.fda.gov/drugsatfda_docs/label/2013/019680s035lbl.pdf. Accessed June 21, 2024.

Carvalho AF, Firth J, Vieta E: Bipolar disorder. N Engl J Med 383(1):58–66, 2020 32609982

Jochim J, Rifkin-Zybutz RP, Geddes J, et al: Valproate for acute mania. Cochrane Database Syst Rev 10(10):CD004052, 2019 31621892

Mullan KA, Anderson A, Illing PT, et al: HLA-associated antiepileptic drug-induced cutaneous adverse reactions. HLA 93(6):417–435, 2019 30895730

References

Abbott Laboratories: Depakote (divalproex sodium) tablets for oral use [package insert]. U.S. Food and Drug Administration website. Revised October 2011. Available at: https://www.accessdata.fda.gov/drugsatfda_docs/label/2011/018723s037lbl.pdf. Accessed June 21, 2024.

Acharya S, Bussel JB: Hematologic toxicity of sodium valproate. J Pediatr Hematol Oncol 22(1):62–65, 2000 10695824

Andrade C: Epilepsy, antiepileptic drugs, and adverse pregnancy outcomes, 1: examination and interpretation of recent research. J Clin Psychiatry 85(2):24f15411, 2024 38836866

Biton V, Mirza W, Montouris G, et al: Weight change associated with valproate and lamotrigine monotherapy in patients with epilepsy. Neurology 56(2):172–177, 2001 11160951

Bond DJ, Lam RW, Yatham LN: Divalproex sodium versus placebo in the treatment of acute bipolar depression: a systematic review and meta-analysis. J Affect Disord 124(3):228–234, 2010 20044142

Bowden CL, Calabrese JR, McElroy SL, et al; Divalproex Maintenance Study Group: A randomized, placebo-controlled 12-month trial of divalproex and lithium in treatment of outpatients with bipolar I disorder. Arch Gen Psychiatry 57(5):481–489, 2000 10807488

Bryant AE III, Dreifuss FE: Valproic acid hepatic fatalities, III: U.S. experience since 1986. Neurology 46(2):465–469, 1996 8614514

Chung SJ, Ahn KM, Oh JH, et al: Incidence rates of severe cutaneous adverse reactions due to antiseizure medication: a nationwide study using health claims data in Korea. Epilepsia 62(1):250–257, 2021 33188522

Cipriani A, Reid K, Young AH, et al: Valproic acid, valproate and divalproex in the maintenance treatment of bipolar disorder. Cochrane Database Syst Rev (10):CD003196, 2013 24132760

Damegunta SR: Time matters! When is the right time to estimate serum valproic acid levels? Indian J Psychol Med 36(3):349–350, 2014 25035573

Davis LL, Ryan W, Adinoff B, et al: Comprehensive review of the psychiatric uses of valproate. J Clin Psychopharmacol 20(1)(Suppl 1):1S–17S, 2000 10646685

Goodwin GM, Haddad PM, Ferrier IN, et al: Evidence-based guidelines for treating bipolar disorder: revised third edition recommendations from the British Association for Psychopharmacology. J Psychopharmacol 30(6):495–553, 2016

Hao Y, Creson T, Zhang L, et al: Mood stabilizer valproate promotes ERK pathway-dependent cortical neuronal growth and neurogenesis. J Neurosci 24(29):6590–6599, 2004 15269271

Harrison PJ, Hall N, Mould A, et al: Cellular calcium in bipolar disorder: systematic review and meta-analysis. Mol Psychiatry 26(8):4106–4116, 2021 31801967

Hirschfeld RM, Allen MH, McEvoy JP, et al: Safety and tolerability of oral loading divalproex sodium in acutely manic bipolar patients. J Clin Psychiatry 60(12):815–818, 1999 10665626

Kakunje A, Prabhu A, Sindhu Priya ES, et al: Valproate: its effects on hair. Int J Trichology 10(4):150-153, 2018 30386073

Kang MG, Qian H, Keramatian K, et al: Lithium vs valproate in the maintenance treatment of bipolar I disorder: a post-hoc analysis of a randomized double-blind placebo-controlled trial. Aust N Z J Psychiatry 54(3):298–307, 2020 31845587

Keck PE Jr, McElroy SL, Bennett JA: Pharmacologic loading in the treatment of acute mania. Bipolar Disord 2(1):42–46, 2000 11254019

Lorberg B, Youssef NA, Bhagwagar Z: Lamotrigine-associated rash: to rechallenge or not to rechallenge? Int J Neuropsychopharmacol 12(2):257–265, 2009 18845017

Macdonald RL, Kelly KM: Antiepileptic drug mechanisms of action. Epilepsia 36(Suppl 2):S2–S12, 1995 8784210

Malik S, Lally J, Ajnakina O, et al: Sodium valproate and clozapine induced neutropenia: a case control study using register data. Schizophr Res 195:267–273, 2018 28882687

McGraw D: Therapeutic drug monitoring with valproate—why product selection is an important factor. Ment Health Clin 4(1):31–34, 2014

McKiernan P: Acute liver failure after valproate exposure: liver transplantation may be indicated beyond childhood. Liver Transpl 20(11):1287–1289, 2014 25179873

Mula M, Kanner AM, Schmitz B, et al: Antiepileptic drugs and suicidality: an expert consensus statement from the Task Force on Therapeutic Strategies of the ILAE Commission on Neuropsychobiology. Epilepsia 54(1):199–203, 2013 22994856

Park HJ, Kim JY: Incidence of neutropenia with valproate and quetiapine combination treatment in subjects with acquired brain injuries. Arch Phys Med Rehabil 97(2):183–188, 2016 26427579

Perucca E: Pharmacological and therapeutic properties of valproate: a summary after 35 years of clinical experience. CNS Drugs 16(10):695–714, 2002 12269862

Rahman M, Nguyen H: Valproic acid, in StatPearls. Treasure Island, FL, StatPearls Publishing, 2022. Available at: https://www.ncbi.nlm.nih.gov/books/NBK559112/. Accessed June 2022.

Reed RC, Dutta S: Does it really matter when a blood sample for valproic acid concentration is taken following once-daily administration of divalproex-ER? Ther Drug Monit 28(3):413–418, 2006 16778728

Smetana KS, Cook AM, Bastin ML, et al: Antiepileptic dosing for critically ill adult patients receiving renal replacement therapy. J Crit Care 36:116–124, 2016 27546759

Swann AC, Bowden CL, Morris D, et al: Depression during mania: treatment response to lithium or divalproex. Arch Gen Psychiatry 54(1):37–42, 1997 9006398

Tseng YL, Huang CR, Lin CH, et al: Risk factors of hyperammonemia in patients with epilepsy under valproic acid therapy. Medicine (Baltimore) 93(11):e66, 2014 25192484

Tseng YJ, Huang SY, Kuo CH, et al: Safety range of free valproic acid serum concentration in adult patients. PLoS One 15(9):e0238201, 2020 32877431

Valproate [updated July 31, 2020], in LiverTox: Clinical and Research Information on Drug-Induced Liver Injury [Internet]. Bethesda, MD, National Institute of Diabetes and Digestive and Kidney Diseases, 2012–. Available at: https://www.ncbi.nlm.nih.gov/books/NBK548284/. Accessed March 13, 2024.

VandenBerg A, Broadway J, Lalich C, et al: Valproate serum concentrations in patients with hypoalbuminemia and medical complications. Ment Health Clin 7(1):13–15, 2018 29955492

Verrotti A, D'Egidio C, Mohn A, et al: Weight gain following treatment with valproic acid: pathogenetic mechanisms and clinical implications. Obes Rev 12(5):e32–e43, 2011 20880119

Wang Y, Xia J, Helfer B, et al: Valproate for schizophrenia. Cochrane Database Syst Rev 11(11):CD004028, 2016 27884042

White W, Elmore L, Luthin DR, et al: Psychotropic-induced weight gain: a review of management strategies. Consultant 53(3):153–160, 2013

Yatham LN, Kennedy SH, Parikh SV, et al: Canadian Network for Mood and Anxiety Treatments (CANMAT) and International Society for Bipolar Disorders (ISBD) 2018 guidelines for the management of patients with bipolar disorder. Bipolar Disord 20(2):97–170, 2018 29536616

6

Antipsychotics

Brandon S. Pruett, M.D., Ph.D.
Calley Johnston, M.D.
Bradley G. Burk, Pharm.D., BCPP

Introduction to Antipsychotic Classes

The use of antipsychotics dates back to a serendipitous discovery in the mid-20th century. Prior to antipsychotics, patients with severe mental illness were generally sent to asylums to live out the rest of their lives (Boyd-Kimball et al. 2019; Tandon et al. 2010). In the early 1950s, the French surgeon and neurobiologist Henri Laborit began experimenting with anticholinergic agents as a way of managing surgical shock and found that one such agent in particular, chlorpromazine, when given prior to surgery, produced a calm indifference (Ban 2007; Ramachandraiah et al. 2009; Seeman 2021). This response led Laborit to push for the use of chlorpromazine in managing agitation in psychiatric patients. The first psychiatric patient was treated with chlorpromazine in 1952, and while his agitation did improve, unexpectedly his symptoms of psychosis also largely resolved, so that he was able to be discharged home, an outcome that was exceedingly rare in that day. Further clinical trials by Pierre Deniker and Jean Delay demonstrated the efficacy of chlorpromazine in treating psychosis, and subsequently chlorpromazine became the first antipsychotic drug on the market (Ban 2007; Boyd-Kimball et al. 2019; Ramachandraiah et al. 2009; Seeman 2021).

Although initially slow to gain traction, drugs of both similar (e.g. fluphenazine) and different (e.g. haloperidol) chemical classes but with similar efficacy to chlorpromazine soon became available (Ban 2007; Ramachandraiah et al. 2009; Seeman 2021), and with the advent of medications for treating psychosis came a push, beginning in the 1960s, for the deinstitutionalization of severely mentally ill patients (Boyd-Kimball et al. 2019; Tandon et al. 2010). However, the mechanism of action of these drugs remained unclear until the mid-1970s, when Philip Seeman and Solomon Snyder demonstrated that the efficacy of antipsychotic drugs corresponded directly to their blockade of dopamine D_2 receptors (Seeman 2021; Tandon et al. 2010). The antipsychotic drugs from this time period are often collectively referred to as first-generation (or typical) antipsychotics (FGAs) (Tandon et al. 2010). The D_2 receptors to which the efficacy of these drugs is directly tied are prominent not only in the mesolimbic pathway, which is thought to be the primary target of these drugs, but also in the nigrostriatal and tuberoinfundibular pathways, which mediate some of the most common side effects of the first-generation agents: extrapyramidal symptoms (EPS) (i.e. dystonia, akathisia, parkinsonism) and hyperprolactinemia (Casey and Canal 2017; Seeman 2021).

Around this time, clozapine, a compound synthesized decades earlier, was found to be an even more efficacious antipsychotic than chlorpromazine while also having very low levels of EPS (Ramachandraiah et al. 2009; Weston-Green 2022). However, due to reports linking deaths from agranulocytosis to clozapine, it was removed from the market until 1990, when it was reintroduced for treatment-resistant schizophrenia with a stringent Risk Evaluation and Mitigation Strategy (REMS) program (Leung et al. 2022). Shortly thereafter, a string of new antipsychotic drugs, including risperidone, quetiapine, ziprasidone, and olanzapine, were developed. These drugs are collectively termed second-generation (or atypical) antipsychotics (SGAs), and what distinguishes them is that in addition to antagonism of D_2 receptors, they also antagonize serotonin-2A (5-HT_{2A}) receptors. The addition of 5-HT_{2A} antagonism is thought to allow for similar efficacy to first-generation agents with lower D_2 receptor occupancy (Pani et al. 2007). As a result, this class is less prone to cause EPS (Seeman 2021; Tandon et al. 2010). However, this class is more frequently associated with metabolic side effects, although there is considerable variability among individual agents in this class (Weston-Green 2022).

The next innovation in antipsychotic drugs came with the advent of partial agonists, primarily at the D_2 receptor but also at the 5-HT_{1A} and D_3 receptors, depending on the drug. The first member of this class to hit the market was aripiprazole in 2002, followed by brexpiprazole and cariprazine over the next decade and a half (Casey and Canal 2017; Mohr et al. 2022). Because of their partial agonism at D_2 receptors, partial agonists are thought to predominantly block D_2 receptors in regions where dopamine signaling is elevated (e.g., the mesolimbic pathway) while stimulating D_2 receptors in regions with deficient dopamine signaling (e.g., the mesocortical pathway). They are, therefore, less prone to cause EPS or hyperprolactinemia; in fact, they can actually protect against hyperprolactinemia when used in combination with prolactin-elevating agents (Besag et al. 2021). Furthermore, these agents are thought to be less likely to contribute to cognitive blunting (Casey and Canal 2017).

Although development of newer antipsychotic agents has slowed in recent years, several agents with fairly novel mechanisms have come out in the past few years. First was pimavanserin, which is predominantly an antagonist at 5-HT_{2A} receptors but has minimal activity at D_2 receptors (Tsapakis et al. 2023). Because of its lack of affinity at D_2 receptors, it is primarily used in the treatment of Parkinson's-associated psychotic symptoms. Next was lumateperone, which modulates dopaminergic, serotonergic, and glutamatergic systems through a variety of mechanisms and appears to have a low propensity to cause both EPS and metabolic symptoms. Still, there remains a need for drugs with unique mechanisms of action, and several such agents with mechanisms ranging from the blockade of voltage-gated sodium channels to the stimulation of M_1/M_4 muscarinic acetylcholine receptors, for instance, are currently in clinical trials or under review by the FDA (Tsapakis et al. 2023).

Antipsychotic Class Adverse Effects, Receptor Actions, and FDA-Approved and Off-Label Indications

Table 6–1 provides an overview of antipsychotic class adverse effects. Table 6–2 highlights the known and sometimes theorized effects of specific receptors. Table 6–3A and Table 6–3B present the FDA-labeled and most common off-label uses for the FGAs and SGAs (including partial agonists and newer agents), respectively.

Table 6–1. Antipsychotic class adverse effects

Black box warning: Increased mortality risk in older adults with dementia-related psychosis
• Mortality may be from myriad causes (e.g., cerebrovascular accident, cardiac arrest, pneumonia).
Class side effects associated with receptor activity
• **Sedation:** Due to antihistamine activity; tolerance usually develops with treatment.
• **Anticholinergic effects:** Due to antimuscarinic receptor blockade; can cause tachycardia, dry mouth, constipation, and (rarely) blurred vision, urinary retention, or delirium/confusion.
• **Corrected QT (QTc) prolongation:** Likely related to inhibition of cardiac potassium channel (hERG receptor); QTc prolongation increases the risk of torsades de pointes or lethal arrhythmias and (in rare cases) sudden death. Female sex, older age, and use of multiple QTc-prolonging medications are among the greatest risk factors.
• **Orthostatic hypotension:** Caused by α-adrenergic receptor blockade.
• **Extrapyramidal symptoms (EPS):** Related to a higher ratio of D_2 to 5-HT_{2A} receptor blockade and D_1 receptor activation. May include acute dystonia, akathisia, parkinsonian symptoms (tremor, cogwheel rigidity, bradykinesia) and, with long-term use, tardive dyskinesia (TD). Can also involve esophageal dysfunction. Clinicians should remember that prolonged use of preventive anticholinergics is not hazard-free, given that these agents can increase the risk of TD.
• **Elevated prolactin:** Due to disinhibition of prolactin release via D_2 receptor blockade, leading to gynecomastia, galactorrhea, low libido, menstrual changes, infertility, and bone mass density loss (Grigg et al. 2017).
• **Sexual side effects:** Likely related to antidopaminergic activity, α-adrenergic blockade, and anticholinergic activity (in regard to erectile dysfunction); may include difficulties with libido, arousal, orgasm, erectile dysfunction, or priapism.
Additional adverse effects
• **Neuroleptic malignant syndrome:** Rare but potentially fatal; symptoms may include fever, muscle rigidity, altered mental status, autonomic instability, rhabdomyolysis, creatine kinase elevation. High dosages, FGA use, and dehydration are among the greatest risk factors.
• **Seizure:** Antipsychotics (more commonly SGAs than FGAs) may lower the seizure threshold, although this is rare. Risk factors include preexisting history of seizures and EEG abnormalities.
• **Electrolyte abnormalities:** Hyponatremia (SIADH) may occur.
• **Other effects:** Blood dyscrasias (agranulocytosis, eosinophilia, leukopenia, hemolytic or aplastic anemia, thrombocytopenic purpura, pancytopenia), hepatotoxicity, dermatological reactions, asthma, laryngeal or angioneurotic edema, and anaphylaxis are reported, as well as skin hyperpigmentation, ocular changes (fine particulate deposits in the lens and cornea), cataracts, temperature dysregulation, and catatonia.
Use caution
• **Falls:** Antipsychotics may increase fall risk due to somnolence, postural hypotension, and sensory/motor changes.
• **Beers Criteria:** All antipsychotics are identified as potentially inappropriate for use in adults age 65 years or older, regardless of underlying dementia status (American Geriatrics Society 2023). Caution is especially warranted in persons with baseline hyponatremia.
• **Withdrawal symptoms:** When discontinuing an antipsychotic, a slow taper is recommended to avoid cholinergic rebound, withdrawal dyskinesias, or relapse of symptoms.

Table 6–2. Receptor actions among antipsychotics

Introduction: Receptor Blockade
• Each antipsychotic blocks a specific set of receptors, leading to a specific set of effects, some of which may be intended and some of which may be unintended. For example, olanzapine's effect on psychosis largely comes from its action at the D_2 receptor, whereas its sedative and constipating properties result from its activity at histamine (H_1) receptors and muscarinic cholinergic receptors.
• Prescribers can make rational use of the unintended effects by carefully selecting a medication on the basis of its receptor binding profile (e.g., using an antipsychotic with sedating properties for a patient who has psychosis and insomnia). Such an approach can help reduce the need for use of multiple other medications.
Dopamine-2 Receptor Antagonism
• Blockade of dopamine D_2 receptors affects a variety of pathways in the brain.
• The primary target of D_2 receptor blockade in psychotic disorders has historically been postulated to be in the mesolimbic pathway of the brain, where postsynaptic dopamine receptor blockade can have a therapeutic effect on positive symptoms (i.e., hallucinations, delusions, disorganization) (Lewis and Lieberman 2000).
• Modern literature also links the nigrostriatal pathway to the production of psychotic symptoms (Correll et al. 2022; McCutcheon et al. 2019).
• D_2 receptor blockade also occurs in the nigrostriatal pathway, potentially leading to development of extrapyramidal symptoms (EPS), which can range in severity from nuisance to disabling, or even life-threatening (e.g., airway crisis) (Ali et al. 2021; Loonen and Ivanova 2021).
• Prolonged blockade of the postsynaptic D_2 receptors may lead to dopaminergic supersensitivity, secondary to an upregulation of dopamine receptors, which may be responsible for tardive dyskinesia or developed tolerance to antipsychotics (Chouinard et al. 2017; Rubio et al. 2020).
• Nigrostriatal D_2 receptor blockade may indirectly worsen preexisting negative symptoms or cause new symptoms that seem identical to negative symptoms via EPS (i.e., secondary negative symptoms) (Correll and Schooler 2020; McCutcheon et al. 2020; Mosolov and Yaltonskaya 2022).
• Negative symptoms are the deficit symptoms of schizophrenia and include symptoms such as anhedonia, alogia, and avolition.
• In addition to its effects on the nigrostriatal and mesolimbic pathways, D_2 receptor blockade in the tuberoinfundibular pathway may disinhibit production of prolactin, leading to downregulation of gonadotropins, which can cause sexual dysfunction and calcium loss (Bostwick et al. 2009).
Serotonin-2A Receptor Antagonism/Inverse Agonism
• Antagonism at 5-HT_{2A} receptors increases dopaminergic transmission in nigrostriatal areas and prefrontal cortex and ventromedial prefrontal cortex, potentially improving EPS (Meltzer 1999).
• Conversely, antagonism of the 5-HT_{2A} receptor may decrease dopaminergic transmission in the mesocortical and nigrostriatal areas, leading to improvement of psychosis (Meltzer 1999).
• Whereas SGAs were theorized to improve negative symptoms/cognition, this outcome has never been confirmed in large-scale trials (Meltzer 1999; Romeo et al. 2023).
• Furthermore, these effects could contribute to the antidepressant effects of some SGAs.

Table 6–2. Receptor actions among antipsychotics *(continued)*

Serotonin-2C Receptor Antagonism
• Among other potential mechanisms, 5-HT_{2C} blockade has been linked to the weight gain associated with SGA medications (De Luca et al. 2007; Reynolds et al. 2006).
Alpha-2 Adrenoreceptor (Autoreceptor) Antagonism
• α_2-Adrenergic receptor (autoreceptor) antagonism leads to increased dopamine and norepinephrine release from noradrenergic terminals in the occipital cortex and the medial prefrontal cortex (Devoto et al. 2003). • Antagonism of α_2 receptors was theorized to have therapeutic effects on negative symptoms in schizophrenia, although the effect of SGAs on cognitive and negative symptoms has never been definitively demonstrated • This mechanism may also explain antipsychotic benefits in alcohol/substance use disorders in patients with schizophrenia, but again, evidence is limited (Brosda et al. 2014; Gammon et al. 2021; Proudman et al. 2022).
Serotonin-1A Receptor Partial Agonism
• Partial agonism at the 5-HT_{1A} receptor promotes the release of dopamine in the prefrontal cortex (Meltzer 1999). • The clinical significance of this action is not fully understood but it has been theorized to help with cognitive and negative symptoms (although this effect has never been definitively demonstrated). • Drugs with stronger presynaptic 5-HT_{1A} receptor effects are less likely to demonstrate EPS (Newman-Tancredi 2010). • Additionally, 5-HT_{1A} receptor partial agonism may also be responsible for anxiolytic effects (Mombereau et al. 2017).
Histamine-1 Receptor Antagonism
• H_1 receptor blockade is responsible for sedating effects and, among other mechanisms, can lead to the weight gain that can be a serious side effect of antipsychotics (Kroeze et al. 2003; Sato et al. 2015).
Alpha-1 Adrenergic Receptor Antagonism
• α_1-Adrenergic receptor blockade causing vasodilation is implicated in orthostatic hypotension and priapism as well as sensations of lightheadedness and dizziness (Andersohn et al. 2010; Cohen and Lipinski 1986).
Muscarinic Receptor Antagonism
• Muscarinic cholinergic receptor blockade leads to anticholinergic side effects (dry mouth, constipation, urinary retention, and delirium). • In older adults, anticholinergic effects can lead to confusion (Divac et al. 2014; Ogino et al. 2014). • The propensity for anticholinergic effects is related to the amount of receptor binding by specific antipsychotic drugs (Ozbilen et al. 2012). • Theoretically, agents with higher muscarinic antagonism may protect against acute dystonia or pseudoparkinsonism, because the muscarinic antagonism is a built-in mechanism combating the antidopaminergic action that leads to these side effects (Lieberman 2004).

Note. For additional information on antipsychotic receptor activity profiles, see Olten and Bloch 2018.

Table 6–3A. Labeled (L) and common off-label (OL) indications for first-generation antipsychotics

	BP-Mania	Schz	ASD	OCD	TicDs	Nau/Vm	A/C Agit	Del Inf	Anx (n-Psy)	Hunt Chor
Chlorpromazine	L	L	OL			L	L		L[a]	
Droperidol						L	OL			
Fluphenazine		L			OL		OL	OL		OL
Haloperidol	OL	L	OL	OL	OL	OL	OL	OL		OL
Loxapine		L	OL				L[b]			
Perphenazine		L				L				
Pimozide		OL			L			OL		
Prochlorperazine		L				L			L	
Thiothixene		L								
Trifluoperazine		L						OL	L	

[a]FDA approved for presurgical anxiety.
[b]Inhalation (Adasuve): FDA approved for acute agitation in schizophrenia or bipolar I disorder.

Table 6–3B. Labeled (L) and common off-label (OL) indications for second-generation and other atypical antipsychotics

	BP-Mania	BP-Dprss	MDD	Schz	ASD	PTSD	OCD	TicDs	Park-Psy	A/C Agit	Del Inf	Anx (n-Psy)	Hunt Chor
SGAs													
Asenapine	L	OL		L		OL				OL			
Clozapine	OL			L[a]					OL				
Iloperidone	L			L									
Lurasidone		L	OL	L									
Olanzapine	L	L[b]	L[b]	L	OL	OL	OL	OL	OL	L	OL		OL

Table 6–3B. Labeled (L) and common off-label (OL) indications for second-generation and other atypical antipsychotics *(continued)*

	BP-Mania	BP-Dprss	MDD	Schz	ASD	PTSD	OCD	TicDs	Park-Psy	A/C Agit	Del Inf	Anx (n-Psy)	Hunt Chor
SGAs *(continued)*													
Paliperidone	OL			L	OL		OL	OL			OL		OL
Quetiapine	L	L	L*	L	OL	OL	OL	OL	OL	OL		OL	
Risperidone	L		OL*	L	OL	OL	OL	OL		OL	OL		OL
Ziprasidone	L		OL*	L	OL					L	OL		
Partial agonists													
Aripiprazole	L		L*	L	OL	OL	OL	OL		OL	OL	OL	OL
Brexpiprazole	OL	OL	L*	L		OL				L[c]			
Cariprazine	L	L	L*	L									
Other atypical antipsychotics													
Lumateperone		L		L									
Pimavanserin			OL	OL[d]					L				

Note. A/C Agit=acute/chronic agitation; Anx (n-Psy)=nonpsychotic anxiety; ASD=autism spectrum disorder; BP=bipolar disorder; Del-Inf=delusional infestation; FGA=first-generation antipsychotics; Hunt Chor= Huntington's chorea; MDD=major depressive disorder (unipolar depression); Nau/Vm=nausea/vomiting; Park-Psy=Parkinson's-related psychosis; Schz=schizophrenia; SGAs=second-generation antipsychotics; TicDs=tic disorders.

*Adjunctive therapy with antidepressant.

[a]Including a specific FDA approval for suicidal behavior in schizophrenia or schizoaffective disorder.

[b]Olanzapine-fluoxetine combination is FDA approved for bipolar depression and treatment-resistant unipolar depression.

[c]FDA approved for agitation associated with dementia due to Alzheimer's disease.

[d]Used to target negative symptoms of schizophrenia.

Further Reading

Bird AM, Smith TL, Walton AE: Current treatment strategies for clozapine-induced sialorrhea. Ann Pharmacother 45(5):667–675, 2011 21540404

Camm AJ, Karayal ON, Meltzer H, et al: Ziprasidone and the corrected QT interval: a comprehensive summary of clinical data. CNS Drugs 26(4):351–365, 2012 22452529

Crapanzano C, Damiani S, Guiot C: Quetiapine in the anxiety dimension of mood disorders: a systematic review of the literature to support clinical practice. J Clin Psychopharmacol 41(4):436–449, 2021 34166261

Dahl SG, Strandjord RE: Pharmacokinetics of chlorpromazine after single and chronic dosage. Clin Pharmacol Ther 21(4):437–448, 1977 849674

Delgado A, Velosa J, Zhang J, et al: Clozapine in bipolar disorder: a systematic review and meta-analysis. J Psychiatr Res 125:21–27, 2020 32182485

Huhn M, Nikolakopoulou A, Schneider-Thoma J, et al: Comparative efficacy and tolerability of 32 oral antipsychotics for the acute treatment of adults with multi-episode schizophrenia. Lancet 394(10202):939–951, 2019 31303314

Jiang WL, Cai DB, Yin F, et al: Adjunctive metformin for antipsychotic-induced dyslipidemia: a meta-analysis of randomized, double-blind, placebo-controlled trials. Transl Psychiatry 10(1):117, 2020 32327628

Johnsen E, Kroken RA, Løberg EM, et al: Amisulpride, aripiprazole, and olanzapine in patients with schizophrenia-spectrum disorders (BeSt InTro): a pragmatic, rater-blind, semi-randomised trial. Lancet Psychiatry 7(11):945–954, 2020 33069317

Komossa K, Rummel-Kluge C, Hunger H, et al: Ziprasidone versus other atypical antipsychotics for schizophrenia. Cochrane Database Syst Rev (4):CD006627, 2009 19821380

Lieberman JA, Stroup TS, McEvoy JP, et al: Effectiveness of antipsychotic drugs in patients with chronic schizophrenia. N Engl J Med 353(12):1209–1223, 2005 16172203

Maneeton N, Maneeton B, Woottiluk P, et al: Quetiapine monotherapy in acute treatment of generalized anxiety disorder: a systematic review and meta-analysis of randomized controlled trials. Drug Des Devel Ther 10:259–276, 2016 26834458

Schulte P: What is an adequate trial with clozapine? Therapeutic drug monitoring and time to response in treatment-refractory schizophrenia. Clin Pharmacokinet 42(7):607–618, 2003 12844323

Siskind D, McCartney L, Goldschlager R, et al: Clozapine v. first- and second-generation antipsychotics in treatment-refractory schizophrenia: systematic review and meta-analysis. Br J Psychiatry 209(5):385–392, 2016 27388573

Siskind D, Sharma M, Pawar M, et al: Clozapine levels as a predictor for therapeutic response: a systematic review and meta-analysis. Acta Psychiatr Scand 144(5):422–432, 2021 34374073

Tohen M, Case M, Trivedi MH, et al: Olanzapine/fluoxetine combination in patients with treatment-resistant depression: rapid onset of therapeutic response in a pooled analysis of 5 studies. J Clin Psychiatry 71(4):451–462, 2010 20361905

Villarreal G, Hamner MB, Cañive JM, et al: Efficacy of quetiapine monotherapy in posttraumatic stress disorder. Am J Psychiatry 173(12):1205–1212, 2016 27418378

Wenthur CJ, Lindsley CW: Classics in chemical neuroscience: clozapine. ACS Chem Neurosci 4(7):1018–1025, 2013 24047509

References

American Geriatrics Society Beers Criteria Update Expert Panel: 2023 updated AGS Beers Criteria for potentially inappropriate medication use in older adults. J Am Geriatr Soc 71(7):2052–2081, 2023 37139824

Ali T, Sisay M, Tariku M, et al: Antipsychotic-induced extrapyramidal side effects: a systematic review and meta-analysis of observational studies. PLoS One 16(9):e0257129, 2021 34506552
Andersohn F, Schmedt N, Weinmann S, et al: Priapism associated with antipsychotics: role of alpha1 adrenoceptor affinity. J Clin Psychopharmacol 30(1):68–71, 2010 20075651
Ban TA: Fifty years chlorpromazine: a historical perspective. Neuropsychiatr Dis Treat 3(4):495–500, 2007 19300578
Besag FMC, Vasey MJ, Salim I: Is adjunct aripiprazole effective in treating hyperprolactinemia induced by psychotropic medication? A narrative review. CNS Drugs 35(5):507–526, 2021 33880739
Bostwick JR, Guthrie SK, Ellingrod VL: Antipsychotic-induced hyperprolactinemia. Pharmacotherapy 29(1):64–73, 2009 19113797
Boyd-Kimball D, Gonczy K, Lewis B, et al: Classics in chemical neuroscience: chlorpromazine. ACS Chem Neurosci 10(1):79–88, 2019 29929365
Brosda J, Jantschak F, Pertz HH: A2-Adrenoceptors are targets for antipsychotic drugs. Psychopharmacology (Berl) 231(5):801–812, 2014 24488407
Casey AB, Canal CE: Classics in chemical neuroscience: aripiprazole. ACS Chem Neurosci 8(6):1135–1146, 2017 28368577
Chouinard G, Samaha AN, Chouinard VA, et al: Antipsychotic-induced dopamine supersensitivity psychosis: pharmacology, criteria, and therapy. Psychother Psychosom 86(4):189–219, 2017 28647739
Cohen BM, Lipinski JF: In vivo potencies of antipsychotic drugs in blocking alpha 1 noradrenergic and dopamine D2 receptors: implications for drug mechanisms of action. Life Sci 39(26):2571–2580, 1986 2879204
Correll CU, Schooler NR: Negative symptoms in schizophrenia: a review and clinical guide for recognition, assessment, and treatment. Neuropsychiatr Dis Treat 16:519–534, 2020 32110026
Correll CU, Abi-Dargham A, Howes O: Emerging treatments in schizophrenia. J Clin Psychiatry 83(1):SU21204IP1, 2022
De Luca V, Mueller DJ, de Bartolomeis A, et al: Association of the HTR2C gene and antipsychotic induced weight gain: a meta-analysis. Int J Neuropsychopharmacol 10(5):697–704, 2007 17291373
Devoto P, Flore G, Vacca G, et al: Co-release of noradrenaline and dopamine from noradrenergic neurons in the cerebral cortex induced by clozapine, the prototype atypical antipsychotic. Psychopharmacology (Berl) 167(1):79–84, 2003 12632247
Divac N, Prostran M, Jakovcevski I, et al: Second-generation antipsychotics and extrapyramidal adverse effects. BioMed Res Int 2014:656370, 2014 24995318
Gammon D, Cheng C, Volkovinskaia A, et al: Clozapine: why is it so uniquely effective in the treatment of a range of neuropsychiatric disorders? Biomolecules 11(7):1030, 2021 34356654
Grigg J, Worsley R, Thew C, et al: Antipsychotic-induced hyperprolactinemia: synthesis of worldwide guidelines and integrated recommendations for assessment, management and future research. Psychopharmacology (Berl) 234(22):3279–3297, 2017 28889207
Kroeze WK, Hufeisen SJ, Popadak BA, et al: H1-histamine receptor affinity predicts short-term weight gain for typical and atypical antipsychotic drugs. Neuropsychopharmacology 28(3):519–526, 2003 12629531
Leung JG, de Leon J, Frye MA, et al: The modernization of clozapine: a recapitulation of the past in the United States and the view forward. J Clin Psychopharmacol 42(6):565–580, 2022 36170148
Lewis DA, Lieberman JA: Catching up on schizophrenia: natural history and neurobiology. Neuron 28(2):325–334, 2000 11144342
Lieberman JA III: Managing anticholinergic side effects. Prim Care Companion J Clin Psychiatry 6(Suppl 2):20–23, 2004 16001097
Loonen AJ, Ivanova SA: Neurobiological mechanisms associated with antipsychotic drug-induced dystonia. J Psychopharmacol 35(1):3–14, 2021 32900259
McCutcheon RA, Abi-Dargham A, Howes OD: Schizophrenia, dopamine and the striatum: from biology to symptoms. Trends Neurosci 42(3):205–220, 2019 30621912

McCutcheon RA, Krystal JH, Howes OD: Dopamine and glutamate in schizophrenia: biology, symptoms and treatment. World Psychiatry 19(1):15–33, 2020 31922684
Meltzer HY: The role of serotonin in antipsychotic drug action. Neuropsychopharmacology 21(2)(Suppl):106S–115S, 1999 10432496
Mohr P, Masopust J, Kopecek M: Dopamine receptor partial agonists: do they differ in their clinical efficacy? Front Psychiatry 12:781946, 2022 35145438
Mombereau C, Arnt J, Mørk A: Involvement of presynaptic 5-HT1A receptors in the low propensity of brexpiprazole to induce extrapyramidal side effects in rats. Pharmacol Biochem Behav 153:141–146, 2017 28057524
Mosolov SN, Yaltonskaya PA: Primary and secondary negative symptoms in schizophrenia. Front Psychiatry 12:766692, 2022 35046851
Newman-Tancredi A: The importance of 5-HT1A receptor agonism in antipsychotic drug action: rationale and perspectives. Curr Opin Investig Drugs 11(7):802–812, 2010 20571976
Ogino S, Miyamoto S, Miyake N, et al: Benefits and limits of anticholinergic use in schizophrenia: focusing on its effect on cognitive function. Psychiatry Clin Neurosci 68(1):37–49, 2014 24102938
Olten B, Bloch MH: Meta regression: relationship between antipsychotic receptor binding profiles and side-effects. Prog Neuropsychopharmacol Biol Psychiatry 84(Pt A):272–281, 2018 29410000
Ozbilen M, Adams CE, Marley J: Anticholinergic effects of oral antipsychotic drugs of typicals versus atypicals over medium- and long-term: systematic review and meta-analysis. Curr Med Chem 19(30):5214–5218, 2012 23016549
Pani L, Pira L, Marchese G: Antipsychotic efficacy: relationship to optimal D2-receptor occupancy. Eur Psychiatry 22(5):267–275, 2007 17419008
Proudman RGW, Akinaga J, Baker JG: The affinity and selectivity of ?-adrenoceptor antagonists, antidepressants and antipsychotics for the human ?2A, ?2B, and ?2C-adrenoceptors and comparison with human ?1 and ?-adrenoceptors. Pharmacol Res Perspect 10(2):e00936, 2022 35224877
Ramachandraiah CT, Subramaniam N, Tancer M: The story of antipsychotics: past and present. Indian J Psychiatry 51(4):324-326, 2009 20048463
Reynolds GP, Hill MJ, Kirk SL: The 5-HT2C receptor and antipsychotic-induced weight gain—mechanisms and genetics. J Psychopharmacol 20(4)(Suppl):15–18, 2006 16785265
Romeo B, Willaime L, Rari E, et al: Efficacy of 5-HT2A antagonists on negative symptoms in patients with schizophrenia: a meta-analysis. Psychiatry Res 321:115104, 2023 36774749
Rubio JM, Schoretsanitis G, John M, et al: Psychosis relapse during treatment with long-acting injectable antipsychotics in individuals with schizophrenia-spectrum disorders: an individual participant data meta-analysis. Lancet Psychiatry 7(9):749–761, 2020 32828165
Sato H, Ito C, Hiraoka K, et al: Histamine H1 receptor occupancy by the new-generation antipsychotics olanzapine and quetiapine: a positron emission tomography study in healthy volunteers. Psychopharmacology (Berl) 232(19):3497–3505, 2015 26146015
Seeman MV: History of the dopamine hypothesis of antipsychotic action. World J Psychiatry 11(7):355–364, 2021 34327128
Tandon R, Nasrallah HA, Keshavan MS: Schizophrenia, "just the facts" 5: treatment and prevention—past, present, and future. Schizophr Res 122(1–3):1–23, 2010 20655178
Tsapakis EM, Diakaki K, Miliaras A, et al: Novel compounds in the treatment of schizophrenia—a selective review. Brain Sci 13(8):1193, 2023 37626549
Weston-Green K: Antipsychotic drug development: from historical evidence to fresh perspectives. Front Psychiatry 13:903156, 2022 35782443

First-Generation Antipsychotics

Chlorpromazine

I. **Brand Names**: Thorazine, Aminazine, Chlor-PZ, Klorazine, Promachlor, Promapar, Sonazine, Chlorprom, Chlor-Promanyl, Largactil

II. **Therapeutic Class**: First-generation/typical antipsychotic, antiemetic

III. **Mechanism-Based Class**: Dopamine and serotonin receptor antagonist

IV. **Mechanism(s) of Action**

A. Dopamine D_2 receptor antagonist (Ki=7.244 nM). Some effect on D_1, D_3, D_4 receptors.

B. Serotonin 5-HT_{2A} receptor antagonist (Ki=2.75 nM). Also has effects on other serotonin receptors.

C. Potent α_1- and α_2-adrenergic receptor antagonist (α_{1A} Ki=0.28 nM)

D. M_1/M_2 receptor antagonists (anticholinergic) (M_1 Ki=47 nM)

E. H_1 receptor antagonist (Ki=4.25 nM) (Roth and Driscoll 2023)

V. **Indications**

A. FDA adult:

1. Bipolar disorder (manic episodes)
2. Schizophrenia
3. Agitation/aggression (severe, acute) associated with psychiatric disorders (e.g,, schizophrenia, bipolar disorder)
4. Nausea and vomiting (acute, self-limited)
5. Hiccups (prolonged or intractable)
6. Presurgery anxiety/apprehension
7. Acute intermittent porphyria
8. Adjunct to tetanus treatment

B. Evidence-based[1] off-label uses:

1. Migraine, severe, acute treatment
2. Nausea and vomiting in pregnancy, refractory
3. Acute agitation or delirium, severe behavioral or psychological symptoms of dementia
4. Neonatal abstinence syndrome

C. FDA pediatric:

1. Bipolar disorder (manic episodes)
2. Schizophrenia

---

[1]Evidence strength varies; readers are referred to the literature for more detailed information.

3. Severe behavioral problems (e.g., acute agitation)
4. Nausea and vomiting, including chemotherapy-induced nausea and vomiting (CINV), cyclic vomiting syndrome, and non-CINV nausea and vomiting
5. Presurgery anxiety/apprehension
6. Adjunct to tetanus treatment

VI. Major Contraindications and When to Use Caution

A. **Contraindications**: Hypersensitivity to phenothiazines, comatose state, individuals with significant CNS depression, concomitant use of large quantities of a CNS depressant (e.g., alcohol, benzodiazepines, barbiturates, opioids)

B. **Use caution**: Patients with baseline fall risk, hyponatremia or other electrolyte abnormalities, dysrhythmias (including QTc prolongation), leukopenia/neutropenia, hypotension/syncope (or taking antihypertensive medications), seizures, motor/cognitive impairments (or taking CNS depressants or anticholinergic agents), temperature dysregulation, aspiration, dysphagia, obesity, hyperglycemia, hyperlipidemia, risk factors for neuroleptic malignant syndrome (e.g., dehydration), dementia-related psychosis (boxed warning), pregnancy/lactation, Parkinson's disease.

VII. Dosage Formulations

A. Generic tablet (10 mg, 25 mg, 50 mg, 100 mg, 200 mg)
B. Generic oral concentrate (30 mg/mL [120 mL], 100 mg/mL [240 mL])
C. Generic solution for injection (25 mg/mL [1 mL], 50 mg/2 mL [2 mL])

VIII. Dosage Ranges and Guidelines

A. Refer to Table 6–4 for dosage ranges (initial/maximum) and guidelines. Dosages are for adults unless otherwise specified.

1. Bioavailability is approximately 3 times higher with IM/IV dosing than with PO dosing, so lower IM dosages should be used. For IM/IV administration, the maximum dosage is generally considered to be 200–400 mg/day, although the reader is referred to the package insert for chlorpromazine injection for further information (Eugia US LLC 2024).

B. **Titration** (PO): Increase by 10–50 mg every 3–4 days.

1. Use slower titration in older adults and children.

C. **Discontinuation**: For patients on long-term treatment, taper slowly to avoid rebound psychosis and withdrawal dyskinesias.

Table 6–4. Chlorpromazine indications and dosage guidelines

Schizophrenia or bipolar mania
PO: 10–25 mg BID–TID (for prompt control of severe symptoms, can use 25–50 mg TID). Maximum dosage: 800–1,000 mg/day taken in divided doses (minimal benefit with dosages >1,000 mg/day).
IM/PO: May use IM for first 24–48 hours if necessary, then switch to PO and gradually titrate to effective dosage. See below ("Agitation/aggression") for IM dosing.

Table 6–4. Chlorpromazine indications and dosage guidelines *(continued)*

Agitation/aggression (severe, acute) associated with psychotic disorders (IM)
IM: Give 25 mg IM once. May administer additional 25–50 mg IM after 1 hour if needed. Maximum dosage: 200 mg/day (refer to package insert [Eugia US LLC 2024] for further information).
Nausea and vomiting
Adults/adolescents:
PO: 10–25 mg every 4–6 hours PRN. Maximum dosage: 150 mg/day **IM/IV**: 10–25 mg every 3–4 hours PRN (monitor for hypotension). Maximum dosage: 200 mg/day
Children (age ≥6 months):
PO: 0.55 mg/kg every 4–6 hours PRN. **IM/IV**: 12.5 mg. May repeat initial dose 30 minutes later if no hypotension.
Intractable hiccups
PO: 25–50 mg 3–4 times daily for 2–3 days. Maximum dosage: 200 mg/day. **IM**: 25–50 mg once. **IV**: 25–50 mg once.

IX. **Monitoring**

A. Blood pressure should be monitored at baseline and periodically, given the risk for orthostatic hypotension (higher with parenteral administration).

B. Baseline and periodic:

1. Labs: Complete blood count with differential (rule out hematological changes), liver function tests (LFTs) (rare liver damage risk), renal function, electrolytes
2. Metabolic: Weight, hemoglobin A1c test, lipid panel given chlorpromazine's metabolic risks
3. Extrapyramidal symptoms (EPS): Monitor for abnormal involuntary movements/parkinsonian signs (via Abnormal Involuntary Movement Scale [AIMS]) at baseline and periodically.
4. Consider obtaining an ECG at baseline and periodically if indicated (cardiac risk factors, high-risk medication).
5. Other: Visual changes/ocular exam, sexual changes, mental status changes, falls

C. Consider ordering a drug level if there are concerns regarding compliance or metabolism (proposed reference range for schizophrenia: 30–300 ng/mL)

X. **Relevant Pharmacokinetics/Pharmacodynamics**

A. **Metabolism**: Phase I: cytochrome P450 (CYP) 2D6 (major), CYP1A2 (minor), and CYP3A4 (minor) substrate; Phase II: glucuronidation; numerous metabolites

B. **Time to peak plasma concentration**: 2.8 hours

C. **Onset of action**: Sedation: 30–60 minutes, lasting 4–18 hours; peak antipsychotic effects: 6 weeks to 6 months

D. **Half-life**: Biphasic; initial, 2 hours; terminal, 30 hours

E. **Bioavailability**: 32% (oral)

F. **Volume of distribution**: ~22 L

G. **Hepatic impairment**: No dosage adjustments necessary; use with caution.

H. **Renal impairment**: Less than 1% excreted unchanged in urine. No dosage adjustments necessary; not dialyzable.

XI. **Clinically Relevant Drug Interactions**

A. Metabolized primarily by CYP2D6 and to a lesser extent CYP1A2 and CYP3A4

1. Coadministration with CYP2D6 inhibitors or in known poor CYP2D6 metabolizers can lead to increased plasma levels.
2. Coadministration of chlorpromazine with CYP2D6 substrates can lead to increased levels of these substrates (e.g., propranolol) or decreased production of their active metabolites (e.g., codeine, tamoxifen).

B. Concomitant use with thiazide diuretics may worsen orthostatic hypotension.

C. Concomitant use with anticholinergic drugs and CNS depressants can lead to increased sedative effects.

D. Acute encephalopathy has been reported with concomitant use of lithium.

E. Concomitant use with other QTc-prolonging medications may enhance the risk for torsades de pointes.

F. Use of chlorpromazine may diminish benefits from acetylcholinesterase inhibitors (e.g., donepezil).

XII. **Adverse Effects**

A. **See Table 6–1 ("Antipsychotic Class Adverse Effects") at beginning of chapter.**

B. Chlorpromazine's adverse effects include metabolic syndrome, anticholinergic effects, QTc prolongation, orthostatic hypotension, EPS, prolactin elevation, sexual dysfunction, NMS, temperature dysregulation, hyponatremia/syndrome of inappropriate antidiuretic hormone secretion (SIADH), seizures

1. For the full scope of potential adverse effects, see the chlorpromazine prescribing information (Sun Pharmaceutical Industries 2022).

C. **Boxed warning**: Increased mortality in older patients with dementia-related psychosis

D. Chlorpromazine has significant antihistamine effects, leading to sedation and a relatively higher risk of weight gain.

E. Chlorpromazine has significant α_1-adrenergic receptor blockade, leading to hypotension risk and priapism.

F. Chlorpromazine's built-in anticholinergic activity leads to anticholinergic side effects such as tachycardia, dry mouth, constipation, and blurred vision, but likely decreases the relative risk of EPS (acute dystonia and parkinsonism) compared with other FGAs.

G. Cholestatic jaundice is rare but may occur with chlorpromazine, usually early in treatment. Consider LFTs.

H. Chlorpromazine is known to carry a risk of ocular effects (pigmentary retinopathy, lenticular/corneal deposits) and potentially photosensitivity and skin depigmentation (slate gray), especially at higher dosages.

I. Chlorpromazine may have the highest risk of seizures among the FGAs.

XIII. **Clinical Pearls/Prescribing Tips**

A. Oral bioavailability is around one-third of an equivalent IM dose, so lower IM doses should be used. Maximum PO dosage is 800–1,000 mg.
B. IM/IV administration requires the use of a filter needle because the medication is extracted from a glass ampule.
C. For IV administration, dilute 1:1 with normal saline. IV solution should be administered no faster than 1 mg/minute (0.5 mg/minute in children) to avoid hypotension. Patients should remain supine for at least 30 minutes after injection.
D. Chlorpromazine has relatively strong anticholinergic, alpha-blocking, antihistaminergic, and QTc-prolonging effects, leading to a higher risk of delirium, orthostatic hypotension, sedation/weight gain, and torsades de pointes, respectively. Use with caution in older individuals or patients with cardiac risk factors.
E. Chlorpromazine's built-in anticholinergic effects make its risk for acute dystonia and parkinsonism relatively lower compared with other FGAs.
F. Monitor blood pressure with chlorpromazine, especially with IM/IV administration.
G. Chlorpromazine has benefits for hiccups, nausea, and vomiting.

Further Reading

Adams CE, Rathbone J, Thornley B, et al: Chlorpromazine for schizophrenia: a Cochrane Systematic Review of 50 years of randomised controlled trials. BMC Med 3:15, 2005 16229742

Boyd-Kimball D, Gonczy K, Lewis B, et al: Classics in chemical neuroscience: chlorpromazine. ACS Chem Neurosci 10(1):79–88, 2019 29929365

References

Eugia US LLC: Chlorpromazine hydrochloride injection (package insert). Revised July 2024. Available at: https://dailymed.nlm.nih.gov/dailymed/drugInfo.cfm?setid=07e6144a-b460-4887-b8e2-dd371c14a55c&audience=professional. Accessed July 30, 2024.

Roth BL, Driscoll J: PDSP Ki Database. Psychoactive Drug Screening Program (PDSP). University of North Carolina at Chapel Hill and the United States National Institute of Mental Health, 2023

Sun Pharmaceutical Industries: Chlorpromazine hydrochloride tablet (package insert). Revised January 2022. Available at: https://dailymed.nlm.nih.gov/dailymed/drugInfo.cfm?setid=432cd4ca-c728-48ff-beec-2485f5e02512. Accessed July 6, 2024.

Droperidol

I. **Brand Names**: Inapsine, Droleptan, Dridol, Xomolix, Innovar

II. **Therapeutic Class**: First-generation/typical antipsychotic, antiemetic

III. **Mechanism-Based Class**: Dopamine receptor antagonist

IV. **Mechanism(s) of Action**

A. D_2 receptor blockade (Ki = 0.25 nM)

V. **Indications**

A. FDA adult:

1. Postoperative nausea/vomiting

B. Evidence-based[1] off-label uses:

1. May be used for agitation in hospital settings

C. FDA pediatric:

1. Postoperative nausea/vomiting

VI. **Major Contraindications and When to Use Caution**

A. **Contraindications**: Known or suspected QT prolongation (QTc >440 ms in men and >450 ms in women); known hypersensitivity

B. **Use caution**: Patients with baseline fall risk, hyponatremia or other electrolyte abnormalities, dysrhythmias (including QTc prolongation), leukopenia/neutropenia, hypotension/syncope or on antihypertensive medications, seizures, motor/cognitive impairments or on CNS depressants or anticholinergic agents, temperature dysregulation, aspiration, dysphagia, obesity, hyperglycemia, hyperlipidemia, risk factors for NMS (e.g., dehydration), or dementia-related psychosis (boxed warning), pregnancy/lactation, or Parkinson's disease.

C. Severe hypertension and tachycardia have been seen in individuals diagnosed with pheochromocytoma following droperidol administration.

VII. **Dosage Formulations**

A. Generic solution for injection (2.5 mg/mL [2 mL vial])

VIII. **Dosage Ranges and Guidelines**

A. Refer to Table 6–5 for dosage ranges (initial/maximum) and guidelines. Dosages are for adults unless otherwise specified.

1. Older adults: Lower dosages are typically used and are titrated more slowly.

IX. **Monitoring**:

A. Obtain 12-lead ECG prior to use to determine baseline QTc, and continue for 2–3 hours after treatment to monitor for arrhythmias.

B. Electrolytes, including magnesium and potassium

[1]Evidence strength varies; readers are referred to the literature for more detailed information.

Table 6–5. Droperidol dosage guidelines

Postoperative nausea/vomiting
Adults/adolescents:
IM/IV: Initial dose 0.625–1.25 mg (no more than 2.5 mg). May give an additional 1.25 mg if necessary, but only if benefits outweigh risks.
Children (age 2–12 years):
IM/IV: Initial dose 0.05–0.075 mg (no more than 0.1 mg/kg). Safety/efficacy have not been established for children younger than 2 years.
Acute agitation (off-label)
IM/IV: 2.5–10 mg alone or in combination with a benzodiazepine (Taylor et al. 2017).

C. Other vitals, including blood pressure and temperature, should also be monitored routinely, and fluids/countermeasures available to manage hypotension should it develop.

X. **Relevant Pharmacokinetics/Pharmacodynamics**

A. **Metabolism**: Metabolized and conjugated in liver

B. **Time to peak plasma concentration**: 30 minutes

C. **Onset of action**: 3–10 minutes, with peak response up to 30 minutes; sedation from a single dose can last for 2–4 hours, while altered consciousness can last up to 12 hours.

D. **Half-life**: 2 hours

E. **Bioavailability**: Extensive

F. **Distribution**: 85%–90% plasma protein bound

G. **Hepatic impairment**: Extensive liver metabolism; caution should be used, but no specific dosage adjustments are provided.

H. **Renal impairment**: Less than 1% excreted unchanged in urine; caution should be used, but no specific dosage adjustments are provided.

XI. **Clinically Relevant Drug Interactions**:

A. No known cytochrome P450 (CYP) interactions.

B. Droperidol should not be used in combination with other drugs that can prolong the QTc interval (e.g., class I/III antiarrhythmics, antihistamines, antimalarials, calcium channel blockers, antipsychotics, antidepressants [including monoamine oxidase inhibitors]) or that can induce hypokalemia or hypomagnesemia (e.g., diuretics, laxatives, mineralocorticoid-active agents).

C. CNS depressants (e.g,. barbiturates, benzodiazepines, opioids, general anesthetics) can have additive/potentiating effects in combination with droperidol.

D. Combinations with fentanyl or other IV analgesics have been reported to cause hypertension; concomitant use of epidural or spinal anesthesia increases the likelihood of hypotension.

XII. **Adverse Effects:**

A. **See Table 6–1 ("Antipsychotic Class Adverse Effects") at beginning of chapter.**

B. Droperidol's adverse effects include anticholinergic effects, QTc prolongation, orthostatic hypotension, extrapyramidal symptoms (EPS), prolactin elevation, sexual side effects, NMS, and seizures.

1. Cardiac conduction: QT interval prolongation, torsades de pointes, cardiac arrest, and ventricular tachycardia have been reported.
2. For the full scope of potential adverse effects, see drug labeling (Droperidol package insert).

C. **Boxed warning**: Arrhythmia risk due to QTc prolongation

D. **Common**: Mild to moderate hypotension and tachycardia that are usually self-limited; dysphoria, drowsiness, restlessness, hyperactivity, anxiety, extrapyramidal symptoms, postoperative hallucinatory episodes

E. **Less common**: Anaphylaxis, dizziness, chills, laryngospasm, bronchospasm

XIII. **Clinical Pearls/Prescribing Tips**

A. Droperidol is mainly used for nausea/vomiting in hospital settings; available only in IM/IV forms.

B. Slow IV push administration over at least 2–5 minutes is required to prevent hypotension and cardiac events.

C. Dopamine blockade in the chemoreceptor trigger zone is responsible for droperidol's antiemetic effect.

D. Droperidol has notable D_2 receptor blockade, alpha blockade, and QTc prolongation risk.

Further Reading

deSouza IS, Thode HC Jr, Shrestha P, et al: Rapid tranquilization of the agitated patient in the emergency department: a systematic review and network meta-analysis. Am J Emerg Med 51:363–373, 2022 34823192

Droperidol injection package insert. Daily Med. Available at: https://dailymed.nlm.nih.gov/dailymed/fda/fdaDrugXsl.cfm?setid=147e033d-d997-4ef6-8bb5-a9ba372590b2andtype=display. Accessed March 13, 2024.

Khokhar MA, Rathbone J: Droperidol for psychosis-induced aggression or agitation. Cochrane Database Syst Rev (12):CD002830, 2016 27976370

Roth BL, Driscoll J: PDSP Ki Database. Psychoactive Drug Screening Program (PDSP). University of North Carolina at Chapel Hill and the United States National Institute of Mental Health, 2023

References

Taylor DM, Yap J, Knott JC, et al: Midazolam-droperidol, droperidol, or olanzapine for acute agitation: a randomized clinical trial. Ann Emerg Med 69(3):318–326.e1, 2017 27745766

Fluphenazine

I. **Brand Names**: Prolixin, Prolixin decanoate, Permitil, Modecate, Moditen

II. **Therapeutic Class**: First-generation/typical antipsychotic

III. **Mechanism-Based Class**: Dopamine receptor antagonist

IV. **Mechanism(s) of Action**

A. Potent dopamine D_2 receptor antagonist (Ki=0.89 nM). Some action at other dopamine receptors.

B. Serotonin 5-HT_{2A} receptor antagonist (Ki=3.8–98 nM). Some action at other serotonin receptors.

C. Alpha-1 (α_1) greater than alpha-2 (α_2) receptor antagonist (α_{1A} Ki=6.4–9 nM)

D. H_1 receptor antagonist (Ki=7.3–70 nM) (Roth and Driscoll 2023)

V. **Indications**

A. FDA adult:

1. Psychotic disorders/schizophrenia

B. Evidence-based[1] off-label uses:

1. Severe behavioral or psychological symptoms of dementia
2. Tourette's disorder, management of tics
3. Huntington's chorea
4. Acute psychosis-related aggression/agitation

C. FDA pediatric: None; off-label for tic disorders

VI. **Major Contraindications and When to Use Caution**

A. **Contraindications**:

1. Suspected or known subcortical brain damage; patients on large dosages of hypnotics; comatose or severely cognitively depressed states; presence of blood dyscrasias or liver disease
2. Hypersensitivity to fluphenazine or other phenothiazine derivatives
3. Sesame seed allergies (fluphenazine decanoate only)

B. **Use caution**: Patients with baseline fall risk, hyponatremia or other electrolyte abnormalities, dysrhythmias (including QTc prolongation), leukopenia/neutropenia, hypotension/syncope or on antihypertensive medications, seizures, motor/cognitive impairments or on CNS depressants or anticholinergic agents, temperature dysregulation, aspiration, dysphagia, obesity, hyperglycemia, hyperlipidemia, risk factors for NMS (e.g., dehydration), or dementia-related psychosis (boxed warning), pregnancy/lactation, or Parkinson's disease.

VII. **Dosage Formulations**

A. Generic tablet (1 mg, 2.5 mg, 5 mg, 10 mg)

B. Generic oral concentrate (5 mg/mL [120 mL])

---

[1]Evidence strength varies; readers are referred to the literature for more detailed information.

C. Generic oral elixir (2.5 mg/5 mL [60 mL, 473 mL])
D. Generic solution for injection (hydrochloride, short-acting) (2.5 mg/mL [10 mL])
E. Generic solution for injection (decanoate, long-acting) (25 mg/mL [5 mL])

VIII. **Dosage Ranges and Guidelines**

A. Refer to Table 6–6 for dosage ranges (initial/maximum) and guidelines. Dosages are for adults unless otherwise specified.

1. Older adults: Use lower initial dosages (1–2.5 mg/day).

B. **Titration**: Not specified in labeling, but in general can increase by 2.5–5 mg every 5–7 days if tolerated; can increase by smaller increments (0.5–1 mg) for Tourette's disorder or in older patients.

C. **Conversion of IM/IV formulations to PO**:

1. The short-acting fluphenazine hydrochloride IM/IV dosage is about one-third to one-half of the PO dosage because of differences in bioavailability.
2. Conversion to PO should be made as soon as possible/feasible.
3. Consider concomitant IM/IV anticholinergic or benzodiazepine medications to prevent acute dystonic reactions.

D. **Discontinuation**: For patients on long-term treatment, taper slowly to avoid rebound psychosis and withdrawal dyskinesias.

Table 6–6. Fluphenazine indications and dosage guidelines

Psychotic disorders
Psychotic disorders (PO)
Initial: 2.5–10 mg/day (divided into 3–4 doses). Maximum dosage: 12–20 mg/day (divided). Some recommendations allow for dosages up to 40 mg/day.
Psychotic disorders (acute psychosis-related aggression/agitation) (short-acting IM)
Initial: 2.5–10 mg/day in divided doses (e.g., every 6–8 hours). Usual maximum is 10 mg/day.
Psychotic disorders (long-acting injectable [LAI] IM/subcutaneous)
Note: Tolerance/efficacy of PO fluphenazine should be established prior to initiation of LAI. **Dosing**: • LAI IM/subcutaneous dose (every 3 weeks) = PO dose multiplied by 1.25. • LAI IM/subcutaneous dosage range: 6.25–25.0 mg every 3–4 weeks. Maximum dosage: 100 mg (This dosage range is given in the package insert, although anecdotally a frequency of 2–4 weeks is often also used.) • **PO taper**: PO dose should be decreased by half after the initial injection. Consider discontinuation of PO dosing after the second injection.

Table 6–6. Fluphenazine indications and dosage guidelines *(continued)*

Severe behavioral or psychological symptoms of dementia (off-label) (PO)
1–2.5 mg/day (given as a single dose or in 2 divided doses)
Tourette's disorder, management of tics (off-label) (PO)
Initial: 0.5–1 mg/day. Usual range: 2.5–10 mg/day (given as a single dose or in 2–3 divided doses). Maximum dosages up to 24 mg/day have been studied.
Huntington's chorea (off-label) (PO)
Initial: 0.5–1 mg/day. Usual range: 6–8 mg/day (given as a single dose or in 2–3 divided doses).

IX. **Monitoring**:

A. Baseline and periodic:

1. Labs: CBC with differential (rule out hematological changes), LFTs (rare liver damage risk), renal function, electrolytes (given label instructions to stop the medication if BUN is abnormal)
2. Metabolic: Weight, hemoglobin A1c test, lipid panel given metabolic risk (although lower with fluphenazine)
3. Extrapyramidal symptoms (EPS): Monitor for abnormal involuntary movements/parkinsonian signs (via Abnormal Involuntary Movement Scale [AIMS]) at baseline and periodically.
4. Consider obtaining an ECG at baseline and periodically if indicated (cardiac risk factors, high-risk medication).
5. Other: Visual changes/ocular exam, sexual changes, mental status changes, blood pressure changes, falls

B. Consider ordering a drug level if there are concerns regarding compliance or metabolism (proposed reference range for schizophrenia: 1–10 ng/mL).

X. **Relevant Pharmacokinetics/Pharmacodynamics**

A. **Metabolism**: Phase I: CYP2D6 (minor) substrate; Phase II: glucuronidation
B. **Time to peak plasma concentration**: PO: 2 hours; short-acting injectable (SAI): 1.5–2 hours; long-acting injectable (LAI): 8–10 hours
C. **Onset of action**: Tranquilizing effect (IM): within 1 hour; schizophrenia (PO): within 4–6 weeks
D. **Half-life**: PO: 14.4–16.4 hours; LAI: 6–9 days following single injection and 14–26 days following multiple doses
E. **Bioavailability**: 35% (oral)
F. **Volume of distribution**: 398 L
G. **Hepatic impairment**: Use is contraindicated with hepatic impairment given risk of cholestatic jaundice.
H. **Renal impairment**: Use with caution; no dosage adjustments necessary. Per package labeling, if blood urea nitrogen (BUN) is abnormal, discontinue treatment.

XI. **Clinically Relevant Drug Interactions**:

A. Metabolized to a minor extent by CYP2D6:

1. Coadministration with CYP2D6 inhibitors (e.g., fluoxetine, paroxetine) or in known CYP2D6 poor metabolizers can lead to increased plasma levels.

B. Hypotension can occur in combination with anesthetics and CNS depressants.

C. Anticholinergic effects of atropine and other similar agents may be potentiated in combination with fluphenazine.

D. Acute encephalopathy has been reported with concomitant use of lithium.

XII. **Adverse Effects**

A. **See Table 6–1 ("Antipsychotic Class Adverse Effects") at beginning of chapter.**

B. Fluphenazine's adverse effects include metabolic syndrome, anticholinergic effects, QTc prolongation, orthostatic hypotension, EPS, prolactin elevation, sexual dysfunction, NMS, temperature dysregulation, hyponatremia/SIADH, seizures

1. For the full scope of potential adverse effects, see drug labeling (Fluphenazine package insert).

C. **Boxed warning**: Increased mortality in older patients with dementia-related psychosis

D. **Other**: Dystonia, hypertension/fluctuations in blood pressure, tachycardia, peripheral edema, lactation, gynecomastia, menstrual irregularities, sexual dysfunction, allergic reactions (skin reactions ranging from urticarial to exfoliative dermatitis as well as anaphylaxis), blood dyscrasias (leukopenia, agranulocytosis, thrombocytopenic/nonthrombocytopenic purpura, eosinophilia, pancytopenia), liver damage (cholestatic jaundice)

E. **Uncommon/rare**: Neuroleptic malignant syndrome (NMS), systemic lupus erythematosus (SLE)–like syndrome, hypotension, altered ECG/ECG tracings, cerebral edema, asthma, laryngeal edema, angioneurotic edema, sudden death

F. Fluphenazine's potent D_2 blockade leads to a higher risk of EPS and hyperprolactinemia.

G. If fluphenazine is given as a short-acting injection, consider adding an IM anticholinergic medication (e.g., benztropine, diphenhydramine) or a benzodiazepine (e.g., lorazepam) to protect against acute dystonia risk.

H. Liver test abnormalities are relatively common, although usually mild and transient. There have been reports of acute liver damage and cholestatic jaundice with fluphenazine, (similar to damage caused other phenothiazines such as chlorpromazine). Per labeling, fluphenazine use is contraindicated with hepatic impairment.

XIII. **Clinical Pearls/Prescribing Tips**

A. Fluphenazine is a potent D_2 receptor antagonist and has less effect on serotonin and histamine receptors compared with SGAs; thus, it has a higher risk of EPS and a lower risk of metabolic syndrome.

B. LAI formulations of FGAs (e.g., fluphenazine, haloperidol) are generally less expensive than the LAI formulations of SGAs.

C. For fluphenazine decanoate, decrease the oral dose by half when administering the first injection, and consider stopping the PO formulation completely after the second injection.

D. Fluphenazine decanoate administration should be performed via the Z-track technique to avoid spillage of dose.
E. Short-acting injectable/IM doses should be approximately one-third to one-half of PO doses.

Further Reading

Fluphenazine hydrochloride package insert. Daily Med. Available at: https://dailymed.nlm.nih.gov/dailymed/search.cfm?labeltype=all&query=Fluphenazine+hydrochloride&audience=professional. Accessed March 13, 2024.

Matar HE, Almerie MQ, Sampson SJ: Fluphenazine (oral) versus placebo for schizophrenia. Cochrane Database Syst Rev (6):CD006352, 2018 29893410

References

Roth BL, Driscoll J: PDSP Ki Database. Psychoactive Drug Screening Program (PDSP). University of North Carolina at Chapel Hill and the United States National Institute of Mental Health, 2023

Haloperidol

I. **Brand Names**: Haldol, Haldol Decanoate
II. **Therapeutic Class**: First-generation/typical antipsychotic
III. **Mechanism-Based Class**: Dopamine receptor antagonist
IV. **Mechanism(s) of Action**

A. Potent dopamine D_2 receptor antagonist (Ki=0.7 nM); Some action at other dopamine receptors.
B. Relatively potent α_1 receptor antagonist (Ki=3 nM for the metabolite HPP+ {(4-(4-chlorophenyl)-1-[4-(4-fluorophenyl)-4-oxobutyl]-pyridinium)}
C. Weak 5-HT_{2A} antagonism (Ki=53 nM) (Roth and Driscoll 2023); greater at higher doses; some action at other serotonin receptors.
D. Low potency at H_1 and M_1 receptors

V. **Indications**

A. FDA adult and pediatric:

1. Psychosis (adults; patients age 3–17 years)
2. Tics associated with Tourette's disorder (adults; patients age 3–17 years)
3. Severe behavioral disorders (patients age 3–17 years)

B. Evidence-based[1] off-label uses:

1. Acute mania
2. Agitation/aggression associated with psychiatric disorders

---

[1]Evidence strength varies; readers are referred to the literature for more detailed information.

3. Nausea and vomiting (chemotherapy-induced, palliative, postoperative)
4. Intractable hiccups
5. Severe behavioral or psychological symptoms of dementia
6. Hyperactive delirium

VI. Major Contraindications and When to Use Caution

A. **Contraindications**:

1. Comatose or severely cognitively depressed states
2. Hypersensitivity to haloperidol
3. Parkinson's disease/dementia with Lewy bodies
4. Sesame seed allergies (haloperidol decanoate only)

B. **Use caution**: Patients with baseline fall risk, hyponatremia or other electrolyte abnormalities, dysrhythmias (including QTc prolongation), leukopenia/neutropenia, hypotension/syncope or on antihypertensive medications, seizures, motor/cognitive impairments or on CNS depressants or anticholinergic agents, temperature dysregulation, aspiration, dysphagia, obesity, hyperglycemia, hyperlipidemia, risk factors for neuroleptic malignant syndrome (NMS) (e.g., dehydration), or dementia-related psychosis (boxed warning), pregnancy/lactation, or Parkinson's disease.

VII. Dosage Formulations

A. Generic tablet (0.5 mg, 1 mg, 5 mg, 10 mg, 20 mg [*mostly scored*])
B. Generic oral concentrate (2 mg/mL [5 mL, 15 mL, 120 mL])
C. Generic solution for injection (short acting) (5 mg/mL [1 mL, 10 mL])
D. Generic and brand (Haldol decanoate) solution for injection (long acting) (50 mg/mL [1 mL, 5 mL]), for generic only; 100 mg/mL [1 mL, 5 mL], for generic only)

VIII. Dosage Ranges and Guidelines

A. Refer to Table 6–7 and Table 6–8 for dosage ranges (initial/maximum) and guidelines. Dosages are for adults unless otherwise specified.

B. **Titration**: Increase dosages in increments of <5 mg/day every few days for psychosis and by 0.5–2 mg/day for tics. For children, increase by 0.5 mg/day every 5–7 days.

1. For first-episode psychosis and in children and older adults, use lower dosages and slower titrations.

C. **Conversion of IM/IV formulations to PO**:

1. Conversion to PO should be made as soon as possible/feasible.
2. Consider combining with benzodiazepines and/or anticholinergic medications to protect against acute dystonic reactions. However, clinicians should bear in mind that use of preventive anticholinergics is not risk-free, given that these agents can prolong the risk of tardive dyskinesia.
3. When treating an acutely ill individual, estimate the initial daily dosage by totaling the short-acting injectable (SAI) doses given over the previous 24 hours; dosing for PO and SAI are roughly similar.

D. **Discontinuation**: For patients on long-term treatment, taper slowly to avoid rebound psychosis and withdrawal dyskinesias.

Table 6–7. Haloperidol PO/short-acting IM/IV indications and dosages

Schizophrenia/psychosis (PO)/Acute mania (off-label) (PO)
Adults:
Initial: 1.5–10 mg/day (taken as a single dose or in 2–3 divided doses). Dosage range: 6–20 mg/day. Maximum dosage: 100 mg/day. *Note*: Dosages >30 mg/day are not likely to confer benefit and may increase side-effect risk.
Adolescents:
Initial: 0.5–5 mg/day (taken as a single dose or in 2–3 divided doses).
Children:
Initial: 0.5 mg/day (taken as a single dose or in 2–3 divided doses). Dosage range: 0.05–0.15 mg/kg/day.
Agitation/aggression associated with psychotic disorders (off-label) (PO/short-acting IM/IV)
PO: Initial: 2–10 mg every 6 hours. Maximum dosage: 30 mg/day. **IM/IV**: Initial: 2–5 mg every 15 minutes to 1 hour, then every 4–8 hours. Maximum dosage: 20 mg/day. The IM formulation can be given up to 10 mg every 1–4 hours PRN if necessary.
Agitation in children/adolescents (PO/IM)
Weight based: 0.023–0.075 mg/kg/dose every 1–2 hours. Maximum dosage: 6 mg/day if ≤40 kg, 15 mg/day if >40 kg. **Fixed dosage**: 0.5–2 mg (children), 2–5 mg (adolescents) every 1–2 hours. Maximum dosage: 6 mg/day if ≤40 kg, 15 mg/day if >40 kg **Usual dosing (children age 3–12 years)**: 0.5 mg/day divided and given by mouth 2 or 3 times daily. Daily dosage may be increased in increments of 0.5 mg once every 5–7 days until the desired effect is achieved. **Usual dosage range/strategy (children older than 12 years)**: 0.5–2.0 mg/day for moderate symptoms, 3–5 mg/day for severe symptoms, with dosage divided and given in 2 or 3 separate doses. *Note*: Use in agitation in children/adolescents is off-label. However, there are package labeling dosing instructions for severe behavioral disorders.
Tics associated with Tourette's disorder (PO)
Adults: Initial: 1–2 mg/day (taken as a single dose or in 2–3 divided doses). Maximum dosage: 12 mg/day. **Children**: Refer to the medical literature regarding pediatric dosing. There is established guidance on dosing in Tourette's disorder.
Nausea and vomiting (off-label) (PO/IV/subcutaneous)
Chemotherapy/palliative (PO/IV/subcutaneous): Initial: 0.5–2.0 mg every 6 hours PRN. Maximum dosage: ~20 mg/day. **Postoperative (IV)**: Initial: 0.5–2.0 mg once.

Table 6–7. Haloperidol PO/short-acting IM/IV indications and dosages *(continued)*

Delirium (off-label) (PO/IM/IV)
Agitation: Mild: 0.5–2.0 mg once. Moderate: 5–10 mg once. Severe: 10 mg once. Repeat every 15–30 minutes until calm, then every 6 hours PRN. Maximum dosage: 20–30 mg/day.
Severe behavioral or psychological symptoms of dementia (off-label) (PO)
Initial: 0.25–0.5 mg 1–2 times daily. Titrate upward gradually by 0.5 mg every 4–7 days if needed. DO NOT USE in Parkinson's disease or Lewy body dementia.
Intractable hiccups (off-label) (IM)
2–5 mg once.

IX. **Monitoring**

A. Baseline and periodic:

1. Labs: CBC with differential (rule out hematological changes)
2. Metabolic: Weight, hemoglobin A1c test, lipid panel for metabolic risk (although lower with haloperidol)
3. Extrapyramidal symptoms (EPS): Monitor for abnormal involuntary movements/parkinsonian signs (via Abnormal Involuntary Movement Scale [AIMS]) at baseline and periodically.
4. Consider obtaining an ECG at baseline and periodically if indicated (cardiac risk factors, high-risk medication).
5. Other: Visual changes/ocular exam, sexual changes, mental status changes, blood pressure changes, falls

B. Consider ordering a drug level if there are concerns regarding compliance or metabolism (proposed reference range for schizophrenia: 1–10 ng/mL).

X. **Relevant Pharmacokinetics/Pharmacodynamics**

A. **Metabolism**: Phase I: cytochrome P450 (CYP) 2D6 (major), CYP3A4 (major), and CYP1A2 (minor) substrate. Phase II: glucuronidation

B. **Time to peak plasma concentration**: PO: 4–6 hours; SAI: 20–40 minutes; LAI: ~6 days

C. **Onset of action**: Tranquilizing effect (IM/IV): within 15 minutes. Mania (PO): Within 1–2 weeks. Schizophrenia: Within 4–6 weeks.

D. **Half-life**: Immediate-release: ~16 hours (range: 12–37 hours); LAI: ~3 weeks

E. **Bioavailability**: Oral: 40%–70%

F. **Volume of distribution**: ~9.5–21.7 L

G. **Time to steady state**: LAI: by third to fourth dose

H. **Hepatic impairment**: Given extensive hepatic metabolism, caution should be used, but no specific dosage adjustments are provided by manufacturer.

I. **Renal impairment**: 1% excreted unchanged in urine; does not appear that dosage adjustments are needed; likely not dialyzable.

Table 6–8. Haloperidol administration guidelines for long-acting IM dosing

Standard strategy (PO overlap required)

Initial loading dose(s):

1. If 10 mg/day PO, LAI IM dose is 10–15 times PO dose (e.g., if taking 10 mg/day PO, initial loading dose(s) should total 100–150 mg IM).
2. If > 10 mg/day PO, LAI IM dose is 20 times PO dose (e.g., if taking 20 mg/day PO, initial loading dose(s) should total 400 mg IM).

The first injection should never exceed 100 mg. If an initial dose of more than 100 mg is needed, give 100 mg initially, followed by the remaining amount in 3–7 days (e.g., if initial loading dose is 400 mg, give 100 mg LAI IM followed by 300 mg LAI IM in 3–7 days). Maximum total initial dosage should not exceed 450 mg.

Maintenance dosing/PO taper:

1. Maintenance IM dose =10–15 times the PO dose every 4 weeks (usually 50–200 mg IM). Maximum is 450 mg every 4 weeks. Dosages higher than 200 mg (3 mL) may require separate injections.
2. The PO dose should be tapered and discontinued after the loading doses. Usual procedure is to taper by ~25% weekly during the second and third months of LAI treatment.

Alternative strategy (no PO overlap required) (Ereshefsky et al. 1993):

Initial loading dose(s):

1. LAI IM dose = 20 times the PO dose (e.g., if taking 10 mg/day PO, initial loading dose(s) should total 200 mg LAI IM).
2. **Stop** PO dosing immediately before giving the loading dose (injection is close to C_{max} by day 5–8).

The first injection should never exceed 100 mg. If an initial dose of more than 100 mg is needed, give 100 mg initially, followed by the remaining amount in 3–7 days (e.g., if initial loading dose is 400 mg, give 100 mg LAI IM, followed by 300 mg LAI IM in 3–7 days).

Maintenance dosing:

1. Maintenance dosing should start 4 weeks after the INITIAL loading dose.
2. Reduce the decanoate dose by ~25% (of the initial loading dose) monthly for the second shot (i.e., the first maintenance dose), and then adjust further based on response/tolerability. (For example, if the initial loading dose is 400 mg, the first maintenance dose is 300 mg, and the second maintenance dose begins as 200 mg every 4 weeks.)

Usual maintenance dose is 10–15 times the PO dose. Maximum is 450 mg every 4 weeks.

Note. Tolerance/efficacy of PO haloperidol should be established prior to initiation of LAI.

XI. Clinically Relevant Drug Interactions

A. Metabolized primarily by CYP2D6 and CYP3A4, and CYP1A2 to a minor extent

1. Coadministration with CYP2D6 inhibitors (e.g., fluoxetine, paroxetine, bupropion) or in known poor metabolizers of CYP2D6 can lead to increased plasma levels.
2. Coadministration with CYP3A4 inhibitors (clarithromycin, some antifungals/antivirals, nefazodone, grapefruit juice) can lead to increased plasma levels.
3. Polycyclic aromatic hydrocarbons in tobacco smoke can induce the CYP1A2-mediated metabolism of haloperidol and decrease its plasma concentrations (although likely only to a minor extent).
4. Coadministration of haloperidol with CYP3A4 inducers (e.g., rifampin, carbamazepine) can lead to decreased plasma levels.

B. Concomitant use with anticholinergic drugs (e.g., benztropine) can lead to increased intraocular pressure.

C. Possible dementia has been reported with concomitant use of methyldopa.

D. Acute encephalopathy has been reported with concomitant use of lithium.

E. May potentiate effects of other CNS depressants (e.g., anesthetics, opioids, alcohol).

XII. Adverse Effects

A. **See Table 6–1 ("Antipsychotic Class Adverse Effects") at beginning of chapter.**

B. Haloperidol's adverse effects include metabolic syndrome, anticholinergic effects, QTc prolongation, orthostatic hypotension, EPS, prolactin elevation, sexual dysfunction, NMS, temperature dysregulation, hyponatremia/syndrome of inappropriate antidiuretic hormone secretion (SIADH), and seizures.

C. **Boxed warning**: Increased mortality in older patients with dementia-related psychosis

D. EPS (dystonia, akathisia, parkinsonism) and eventual tardive dyskinesia are more prevalent with haloperidol than with many SGAs, given haloperidol's potent D_2 blockade and lack of significant anticholinergic effect.

E. Hematological abnormalities have occurred with haloperidol (e.g., leukopenia, neutropenia, thrombocytopenia, agranulocytosis [in rare cases], pancytopenia). These effects usually emerge early in treatment; risk factors include baseline low absolute neutrophil count (ANC) or white blood cell (WBC) count, history of drug-induced hematological changes, and older age. Consider obtaining a complete blood count (CBC) with differential at baseline and periodically after the first month of treatment.

F. Hyperprolactinemia can occur with haloperidol and is likely dosage dependent; monitor for sexual dysfunction, amenorrhea in women, and gynecomastia/galactorrhea.

G. QTc prolongation risk is higher with IV administration; use caution.

H. Given its receptor profile, haloperidol is relatively less likely than SGAs to cause weight gain, metabolic changes, and anticholinergic effects.

I. Use in mania may lead to a rapid swing into depression.

XIII. **Clinical Pearls/Prescribing Tips**

A. Haloperidol's use is contraindicated in Parkinson's disease or dementia with Lewy bodies

B. Haloperidol's receptor profile confers a higher risk of EPS, a moderate risk of hyperprolactinemia and hematological abnormalities, and a lower risk of metabolic syndrome, sedation, and anticholinergic effects.

C. Continuous telemetry monitoring is recommended for patients receiving IV haloperidol because of the risk of arrhythmias. IV haloperidol administration is not FDA approved and should be performed only when a patient is being monitored via continuous telemetry. Slowing the administration rate may improve tolerability.

D. When treating an acutely ill individual, estimate the initial daily dosage by totaling the short-acting injectable (SAI) doses given over the previous 24 hours; dosing for PO and SAI are roughly similar.

E. Haloperidol decanoate administration should be performed via the Z-track technique to avoid spillage of the dose.

F. The standard switch from haloperidol PO to a long-acting injectable (LAI) requires tapering the PO haloperidol after the second IM injection. However, an alternative strategy would be to use a higher loading dose, which would obviate the need for PO overlap.

Further Reading

Adams CE, Bergman H, Irving CB, et al: Haloperidol versus placebo for schizophrenia. Cochrane Database Syst Rev (11):CD003082, 2013 24242360

Haloperidol package insert. Daily Med. Available at: https://dailymed.nlm.nih.gov/dailymed/fda/fdaDrugXsl.cfm?setid=9a9e20dd-646a-4fe9-a345-1b5bda8e7775&type=display. Accessed March 13, 2024.

Tyler MW, Zaldivar-Diez J, Haggarty SJ: Classics in chemical neuroscience: haloperidol. ACS Chem Neurosci 8(3):444–453, 2017 28170220

References

Ereshefsky L, Toney G, Saklad SR, et al: A loading-dose strategy for converting from oral to depot haloperidol. Hosp Community Psychiatry 44(12):1155–1161, 1993 7907570

Roth BL, Driscoll J: PDSP Ki Database. Psychoactive Drug Screening Program (PDSP). University of North Carolina at Chapel Hill and the United States National Institute of Mental Health, 2023

Loxapine

I. **Brand Names**: Adasuve, Loxitane

II. **Therapeutic Class**: First-generation/typical antipsychotic

III. **Mechanism-Based Class**: Dopamine and serotonin receptor antagonist

IV. **Mechanism(s) of Action**

A. Potent 5-HT_{2A} antagonist (loxapine Ki=6.6 nM, metabolite amoxapine Ki=2.5); some action at other serotonin receptors.

B. Dopamine D_2 receptor antagonist (Ki=11 nM); some action at other dopamine receptors.

C. Histamine-1 antagonist (Ki=2.2–4.9)

D. Alpha-1 (α_1)-adrenergic receptor antagonist (α_{1A} Ki=31)

E. M_1 receptor antagonist (Ki=120) (Roth and Driscoll 2023)

F. Loxapine is metabolized to multiple active metabolites, including amoxapine, which is a tricyclic antidepressant.

V. **Indications**

A. FDA adult:

1. Schizophrenia
2. Acute agitation associated with schizophrenia or bipolar disorder

B. Evidence-based[1] off-label uses:

1. Severe behavioral or psychological symptoms of dementia
2. Add-on therapy for irritability associated with autism spectrum disorder (ASD)

C. FDA pediatric: None

VI. **Major Contraindications and When to Use Caution**

A. **Contraindications**:

1. Comatose or severely cognitively depressed states
2. Hypersensitivity to loxapine, amoxapine, or other dibenzoxazepines; hypersensitivity to clozapine.
3. Specific to inhalational formulation: Current diagnosis or history of pulmonary diseases associated with bronchospasm (e.g., asthma, chronic obstructive pulmonary disease [COPD]) or taking medications for these diseases, acute respiratory signs/symptoms (e.g., wheezing, dyspnea), individuals with a history of inhalational loxapine-induced bronchospasm.

B. **Use caution**: Patients with baseline fall risk, hyponatremia or other electrolyte abnormalities, dysrhythmias (including QTc prolongation), leukopenia/neutropenia, hypotension/syncope or on antihypertensive medications, seizures, motor/cognitive impairments or on CNS depressants or anticholinergic agents, temperature dysregulation, aspiration, dysphagia, obesity, hyperglycemia, hyperlipidemia, risk factors for neuroleptic malignant syndrome (NMS) (e.g., dehydration), or dementia-related psychosis (boxed warning), pregnancy/lactation, or Parkinson's disease.

---

[1]Evidence strength varies; readers are referred to the literature for more detailed information.

VII. **Dosage Formulations**

A. Generic capsule (5 mg, 10 mg, 25 mg, 50 mg)
B. Brand (Adasuve) aerosol powder for inhalation (10 mg)

VIII. **Dosage Ranges and Guidelines**

A. Refer to Table 6–9 for dosage ranges (initial/maximum) and guidelines. Dosages are for adults unless otherwise specified.
   1. Older adults: Same as in younger adults, although lower dosages are typically used and are titrated more slowly.
   2. Children/adolescents: Safety/efficacy have not been established for this age group.

B. **Titration**: Increase by 5–10 mg every 4–7 days.
   1. In severe cases, may titrate quickly over the first 7–10 days until an effective dosage is achieved.

C. **Discontinuation**: For patients on long-term treatment, taper slowly to avoid rebound psychosis and withdrawal dyskinesias.

Table 6–9. Loxapine indications and dosage guidelines

Schizophrenia (PO)
Initial: 10 mg BID (up to 50 mg if severe). Dosage range: 60–100 mg/day (taken at bedtime or in 2–4 divided doses). Maximum dosage: 250 mg/day.
Acute agitation associated with schizophrenia or bipolar disorder (inhalation—Adasuve)
Initial: 10 mg once. Maximum dosage: 10 mg/day.

IX. **Monitoring**

A. Baseline and periodic:
   1. Labs: CBC with differential (rule out hematological changes), LFTs (rare liver damage risk)
   2. Metabolic: Weight, hemoglobin A1c test, lipid panel for metabolic risk
   3. Extrapyramidal symptoms (EPS): Monitor for abnormal involuntary movements/parkinsonian signs (via Abnormal Involuntary Movement Scale [AIMS]) at baseline and periodically.
   4. Consider obtaining an ECG at baseline and periodically if indicated (cardiac risk factors, high-risk medication).
   5. Other: Visual changes/ocular exam, sexual changes, mental status changes, blood pressure changes, falls

B. Because of the requirement to monitor the patient for bronchospasm, inhaled loxapine must only be administered at a health care facility enrolled in this program. Enrollment in the Adasuve Risk Evaluation and Mitigation Strategy (REMS) program is required for administration.

C. Consider ordering a drug level if there are concerns regarding compliance or metabolism (proposed reference range for schizophrenia: 5–10 ng/mL).

X. **Relevant Pharmacokinetics/Pharmacodynamics**

A. **Metabolism**: Phase I: cytochrome P450 (CYP) 1A2, CYP2D6, and CYP3A4, P-glycoprotein substrate. Phase II: glucuronidation, sulfation. Several active metabolites, namely amoxapine, a tricyclic antidepressant.

B. **Time to peak plasma concentration**: PO: 1–3 hours. Oral inhalation: 2 minutes

C. **Onset of action**: PO: sedation in 20–30 minutes, peaking at 1.5–3 hours and lasting 12 hours; antipsychotic effects within 2–4 weeks

D. **Half-life**: PO: 4 hours (loxapine), 12 hours (active metabolites). Oral inhalation: 7.6 hours

E. **Bioavailability**: Inhalation: 91%; Oral: ~70%

F. **Volume of distribution**: Unclear

G. **Hepatic impairment**: No dosage adjustments per labeling.

H. **Renal impairment**: No dosage adjustments per labeling.

XI. **Clinically Relevant Drug Interactions**

A. Metabolized to a minor extent by CYP1A2, CYP2D6, CP3A4

B. Concomitant use with lorazepam has in rare cases been reported to cause significant respiratory depression, stupor, and/or hypotension.

C. Loxapine may have additive effects with other CNS depressants (e.g., anesthetics, opioids, alcohol).

D. Loxapine may potentiate the effects of anticholinergic drugs.

E. Anticonvulsants (e.g., carbamazepine, phenobarbital, phenytoin) may decrease plasma loxapine levels.

F. Loxapine may lower phenytoin levels.

G. Acute encephalopathy can occur when loxapine is used concomitantly with lithium.

H. Concomitant use with beta-blockers may further lower the blood pressure.

XII. **Adverse Effects**

A. **See Table 6–1 ("Antipsychotic Class Adverse Effects") at beginning of chapter.**

B. Loxapine's adverse effects include metabolic syndrome, anticholinergic effects, QTc prolongation, orthostatic hypotension, extrapyramidal symptoms, prolactin elevation, sexual dysfunction, NMS, temperature dysregulation, hyponatremia/syndrome of inappropriate antidiuretic hormone secretion (SIADH), seizure

C. **Boxed warnings**:

1. Increased mortality in older patients with dementia-related psychosis.
2. Adasuve inhalation: Risk of bronchospasm, which can cause respiratory distress/arrest; higher risk in patients with lung disease.

D. **Somewhat common**: Sedation, dizziness

E. Loxapine has a relatively potent D_2 blockade, making EPS (dystonia, akathisia, parkinsonism, tardive dyskinesia) fairly common, but not as common as with other FGAs such as haloperidol.

F. Loxapine is structurally similar to clozapine, but with a lower risk of agranulocytosis, slightly more potent D_2 blockade compared with clozapine, and less risk of metabolic effects/weight gain.

G. **Specific to inhalation formulation**: Respiratory distress (i.e., bronchospasm, cough, chest pain, dyspnea, wheezing); dysgeusia, sedation, hypotension, syncope

XIII. **Clinical Pearls/Prescribing Tips**

A. Loxapine is known as a typical antipsychotic, but is felt to behave in some ways like an SGA (i.e., it has both dopamine and serotonin receptor blockade). Loxapine and clozapine are very similar in structure. However, loxapine has D_2 blockade that is somewhat more potent and has a lower risk of agranulocytosis and metabolic effects/weight gain. Given these factors, loxapine is an attractive alternative for patients who are unable to tolerate clozapine (Shrestha et al. 2021).

B. Loxapine is unique given its inhaled formulation, although this requires enrolling in a REMS program and patients must be observed for potential bronchospasm. No IM formulation is available in the United States.

C. Loxapine inhaler indicator light notifies the provider as to complete/incomplete dose administration.

D. Loxapine has a short half life (4 hours) but has several active metabolites, namely amoxapine (a tricyclic antidepressant).

Further Reading

Chakrabarti A, Bagnall A, Chue P, et al: Loxapine for schizophrenia. Cochrane Database Syst Rev (4):CD001943, 2007 17943763

Faden J, Citrome L: Examining the safety, efficacy, and patient acceptability of inhaled loxapine for the acute treatment of agitation associated with schizophrenia or bipolar I disorder in adults. Neuropsychiatr Dis Treat 15:2273–2283, 2019 31496709

Loxapine [package insert]. Daily Med. Available at: https://dailymed.nlm.nih.gov/dailymed/fda/fdaDrugXsl.cfm?setid=a6107bb1-3e23-4c5d-bbf4-5e29deff6728&type=display. Accessed March 13, 2024.

References

Roth BL, Driscoll J: PDSP Ki Database. Psychoactive Drug Screening Program (PDSP). University of North Carolina at Chapel Hill and the United States National Institute of Mental Health, 2023

Shrestha S, Agha RS, Khan Z, et al: Considering loxapine instead of clozapine: a case series and literature review. Cureus 13(1):e12919, 2021 33654602

Perphenazine

I. **Brand Names**: Trilafon, Etrafon, Triavil (in combination with amitriptyline [Elavil]), Phenazine, Etaperazin

II. **Therapeutic Class**: First-generation/typical antipsychotic

III. **Mechanism-Based Class**: Dopamine receptor antagonist

IV. **Mechanism(s) of Action**

A. Potent dopamine D_2 receptor antagonist (Ki=0.765 nM); some action at other dopamine receptors.

B. 5-HT_{2A} receptor antagonist (Ki=5.6 nM); some action at other serotonin receptors.
C. Histamine-1 (H_1) receptor antagonist (Ki=8 nM)
D. Alpha-1 (α_1)-adrenergic receptor antagonist (α_{1A} Ki=10 nM) (Roth and Driscoll 2023)

V. **Indications**

A. FDA adult:

1. Schizophrenia
2. Severe nausea/vomiting
3. Depression with anxiety (as Triavil)
4. Psychosis with depression (as Triavil)

B. Evidence-based[1] off-label uses:

1. Severe behavioral or psychological symptoms of dementia
2. Intractable hiccups

C. FDA pediatric: None

VI. **Major Contraindications and When to Use Caution**

A. **Contraindications**:

1. Comatose or severely cognitively depressed states
2. Hypersensitivity to perphenazine, other phenothiazines (chlorpromazine, thioridazine), or sulfites
3. Hepatic impairment
4. Existing blood dyscrasias or bone marrow depression
5. Known or suspected subcortical brain damage, with or without hypothalamic damage, as hyperthermic reactions with temperatures >104°F can occur, patients receiving large dosages of CNS depressants (e.g., during surgery)

B. **Use caution**: Patients with baseline fall risk, hyponatremia or other electrolyte abnormalities, dysrhythmias (including QTc prolongation), leukopenia/neutropenia, hypotension/syncope or on antihypertensive medications, seizures, motor/cognitive impairments or on CNS depressants or anticholinergic agents, temperature dysregulation, aspiration, dysphagia, obesity, hyperglycemia, hyperlipidemia, risk factors for NMS (e.g., dehydration), or dementia-related psychosis (boxed warning), pregnancy/lactation, or Parkinson's disease.

VII. **Dosage Formulations**

A. Generic tablet (2 mg, 4 mg, 8 mg, 16 mg)
B. As Triavil (generic perphenazine-amitriptyline) (2 mg/10 mg, 2 mg/25 mg, 4 mg/10 mg, 4 mg/25 mg, 4 mg/50 mg)

VIII. **Dosage Ranges and Guidelines**

A. Refer to Table 6–10 for dosage ranges (initial/maximum) and guidelines. Dosages are for adults unless otherwise specified.

1. Children: Safety/efficacy have not been established for this age group.

---

[1]Evidence strength varies; readers are referred to the literature for more detailed information.

B. **Titration**: Increase gradually (frequency not defined).

   1. Older adults: Same as in younger adults, although lower dosages are typically used and are titrated more slowly (titrate by 2–4 mg every 4–7 days).

C. **Discontinuation**: For patients on long-term treatment, taper slowly to avoid rebound psychosis and withdrawal dyskinesias.

Table 6–10. Perphenazine indications and dosage guidelines

Schizophrenia (PO)
Initial: 4–8 mg (in 2–3 divided doses) for moderate symptoms or 8–16 mg (in 2–4 divided doses) for hospitalized patients. Usual maximum: 24 mg/day. Do not exceed 64 mg/day. Can switch to nightly or twice-daily dosing (one-third every morning and two-thirds at bedtime) once stable.
Nausea and vomiting (PO)
Initial: 8–16 mg/day (in 2–4 divided doses). Maximum dosage: 24 mg/day.
Severe behavioral or psychological symptoms of dementia (off-label) (PO)
Initial: 2–4 mg/day (taken as a single dose or in 2–3 divided doses). Maximum dosage: 24 mg/day.
Intractable hiccups (off-label) (PO)
Initial: 8–16 mg/ day (in 2–3 divided doses). Maximum dosage: 24 mg/day.
Depression with anxiety (Triavil)
Start at 2 mg/10 mg BID–QID and titrate slowly. Maximum dosage: 32 mg/200 mg/day.
Psychosis with depression (Triavil)
Start at 2 mg/10 mg BID–QID and titrate upward slowly. Maximum dosage: 32 mg/200 mg/day.

IX. Monitoring

A. Baseline and periodic:

   1. Labs: CBC with differential (rule out hematological changes), LFTs (liver damage risk [rare]; contraindicated in hepatic impairment), renal function, electrolytes
   2. Metabolic: Weight, hemoglobin A1c test, lipid panel for metabolic risk
   3. Extrapyramidal symptoms (EPS): Monitor for abnormal involuntary movements/parkinsonian signs (via Abnormal Involuntary Movement Scale [AIMS]) at baseline and periodically.
   4. Consider obtaining an ECG at baseline and periodically if indicated (cardiac risk factors, high-risk medication).
   5. Other: Visual changes/ocular exam, sexual changes, mental status changes, blood pressure changes, falls

B. Consider ordering a drug level if there are concerns regarding compliance or metabolism (proposed reference range for schizophrenia: 0.6–2.4 ng/mL)

C. Can also order a blood level for amitriptyline for patients taking perphenazine/amitriptyline. See the 'Tricyclic Antidepressants" section in Chapter 2, "Antidepressants," for more details on monitoring, side effects, and pharmacokinetics/pharmacodynamics of amitriptyline. See also the established literature, including the work of Sheldon Preskorn, M.D., and David Flockhart, M.D., on therapeutic drug monitoring and drug-drug interactions.

X. **Relevant Pharmacokinetics/Pharmacodynamics**

A. **Metabolism**: Cytochrome P450 (CYP) 2D6 (major), and multiple minor pathways (including CYP1A2, CYP2C9, CYP2C19, and CYP3A4) substrate. Phase II: glucuronidation. Metabolite (7-hydroxy perphenazine) is ~70% as active as parent drug.

B. **Time to peak plasma concentration**: 1–3 hours

C. **Onset of action**: Schizophrenia: 4–6 weeks

D. **Half-life**: 9–12 hours (perphenazine), 10–19 hours (active metabolite)

E. **Bioavailability**: 20%–40%

F. **Volume of distribution**: 10–34 L

G. **Time to steady state**: Reached within 72 hours when given 4 mg every 8 hours.

H. **Hepatic impairment**: Use contraindicated in individuals with significant hepatic impairment.

I. **Renal impairment**: Use caution, but no specific dosage adjustments provided per labeling.

1. Due to low plasma concentrations and extensive tissue distribution, hemodialysis is not effective in removing perphenazine.

XI. **Clinically Relevant Drug Interactions**

A. Metabolized primarily by CYP2D6, but also by CYP1A2, CYP2C19, CYP2C9, CYP3A4 to a more minor extent

1. Coadministration with CYP2D6 inhibitors (e.g., fluoxetine, paroxetine, bupropion) or in known CYP2D6 poor metabolizers can lead to increased plasma levels.
2. Polycyclic aromatic hydrocarbons in tobacco smoke can induce the CYP1A2-mediated metabolism of perphenazine and decrease its plasma concentrations (although likely only to a minor extent).

B. May potentiate effects with other CNS depressants (e.g., analgesics, antihistamines, barbiturates, opioids, alcohol)

C. May have additive effects with atropine or other anticholinergic drugs

D. Acute encephalopathy has been reported with concomitant use of lithium.

E. Concomitant use of epinephrine or dopamine can lead to hypotension

XII. **Adverse Effects**

A. **See Table 6–1 ("Antipsychotic Class Adverse Effects") at beginning of chapter.**

B. Perphenazine's adverse effects include metabolic syndrome, anticholinergic effects, QTc prolongation, orthostatic hypotension, EPS, prolactin elevation, sexual dysfunction, NMS, temperature dysregulation, hyponatremia/SIADH, seizure

C. **Boxed warning**: Increased mortality in older patients with dementia-related psychosis.

D. Side-effect profile is similar to that of chlorpromazine but is less anticholinergic.
E. Potent D_2 receptor blockade leads to a higher risk of EPS (dystonia, akathisia, parkinsonism, tardive dyskinesia) and hyperprolactinemia (changes in libido, sexual function, menstruation)
F. May be sedating and could cause weight gain, dizziness, orthostasis, photosensitivity, temperature dysregulation risk.
G. **Other**: Photosensitivity; can predispose to hyperthermia; prolactin elevation.

XIII. **Clinical Pearls/Prescribing Tips**

A. Considered a "medium potency" FGA based on D_2 receptor affinity.
B. Perphenazine has a low to moderate risk of sedation, orthostasis, and anticholinergic side effects.
C. Perphenazine's ue is contraindicated in hepatic impairment.
D. Lower dosages may be required in CYP2D6 poor metabolizers.

Further Reading

Hartung B, Sampson S, Leucht S: Perphenazine for schizophrenia. Cochrane Database Syst Rev (3):CD003443, 2015 25749632

Perphenazine package insert. Daily Med. Available at: https://dailymed.nlm.nih.gov/dailymed/fda/fdaDrugXsl.cfm?setid=003fe32c-a55d-4191-99fa-1013522b1b2e&type=display. Accessed March 13, 2024.

Rosenheck R, Lin H: Noninferiority of perphenazine vs. three second-generation antipsychotics in chronic schizophrenia. J Nerv Ment Dis 202(1):18–24, 2014 24375207

Schnabel A, Eberhart LH, Muellenbach R, et al: Efficacy of perphenazine to prevent postoperative nausea and vomiting: a quantitative systematic review. Eur J Anaesthesiol 27(12):1044–1051, 2010 20739894

References

Roth BL, Driscoll J: PDSP Ki Database. Psychoactive Drug Screening Program (PDSP). University of North Carolina at Chapel Hill and the United States National Institute of Mental Health, 2023

Pimozide

I. **Brand Names**: Orap
II. **Therapeutic Class**: First-generation/typical antipsychotic
III. **Mechanism-Based Class**: Dopamine receptor antagonist
IV. **Mechanism(s) of Action**

A. Potent dopamine D_2 antagonist (Ki = 0.33 nM); some action at other dopamine receptors.
B. Potent serotonin 5-HT_7 blockade (Ki = 0.5 nM); may have antidepressant effects.
C. Serotonin 5-HT_{2A} blockade (Ki = 48.4 nM); some action at other 5-HT receptors.

D. Potent hERG receptor (cardiac potassium channel) antagonist (Ki = 18 nM) (Roth and Driscoll 2023)
E. Weak alpha, histamine, and muscarinic receptor blockade

V. **Indications**

A. FDA adult:

1. Tics in individuals with Tourette's disorder who have failed to respond to standard treatment

B. Evidence-based[1] off-label uses:

1. Delusional parasitosis not responsive to standard therapy
2. Schizophrenia not responsive to standard therapy

C. FDA pediatric:

1. Tics in Tourette's disorder (not a first-line choice)

VI. **Major Contraindications and When to Use Caution**

A. **Contraindications**:

1. Hypersensitivity to pimozide
2. Tics not associated with Tourette's disorder; use with drugs known to be associated with tics (e.g., pemoline, methylphenidate, amphetamines) unless they have been ruled out as a cause for the tics.
3. Individuals with long QT syndrome, history of cardiac arrhythmias, taking drugs that prolong QT interval (e.g., sertraline, escitalopram, citalopram), or with hypokalemia/hypomagnesemia.
4. Comatose or severely cognitively depressed states
5. Individuals taking cytochrome P450 (CYP) 3A4 or CYP2D6 inhibitors (see "Clinically Relevant Drug Interactions" below)

B. **Use caution**: Patients with baseline fall risk, hyponatremia or other electrolyte abnormalities, dysrhythmias (including QTc prolongation), leukopenia/neutropenia, hypotension/syncope or on antihypertensive medications, seizures, motor/cognitive impairments or on CNS depressants or anticholinergic agents, temperature dysregulation, aspiration, dysphagia, obesity, hyperglycemia, hyperlipidemia, risk factors for NMS (e.g., dehydration), or dementia-related psychosis (boxed warning), pregnancy/lactation, or Parkinson's disease.

VII. **Dosage Formulations**

A. Generic tablet (1 mg, 2 mg [*both scored*])

VIII. **Dosage Ranges and Guidelines**

A. Refer to Table 6–11 for dosage ranges (initial/maximum) and guidelines. Dosages are for adults unless otherwise specified.

1. Older adults: Same as in younger adults, although lower dosages are typically used and are titrated more slowly.
2. Children (age 8–12 years): Safety/efficacy not well established for this age group.

---

[1]Evidence strength varies; readers are referred to the literature for more detailed information.

B. **Titration**:

1. Tourette's disorder: Increase by 0.5–2 mg every other day for adults and every third day for children.
2. Delusional parasitosis: Increase in 1- to 2-mg increments every 3–7 days.

C. For patients with CYP2D6 poor metabolism, a maximum dosage of 4 mg/day is recommended, and doses should not be increase more frequently than every 14 days.

D. Dosage reduction is recommended if QTc increases to >520 ms (or >25% above baseline).

E. **Discontinuation**: For patients on long-term treatment, taper slowly to avoid rebound psychosis and withdrawal dyskinesias.

1. Delusional parasitosis: Taper in increments of 1 mg/day or more weekly after symptoms have been relieved for 1 month. Long-term treatment may be indicated in some cases.

Table 6–11. Pimozide indications and dosage guidelines

Tourette's disorder (second-line choice) (PO)
Adults:
Initial: 1–2 mg per day (taken as a single dose or in 2 divided doses). Maximum dosage: 10 mg/day or 0.2 mg/kg (whichever is less); 4 mg/day maximum for CYP2D6 poor metabolizers.
Children (age 8–12 years) and adolescents:
Initial: 0.05 mg/kg/day or 0.5–1 mg/day (usually dosed nightly). Dosage range: 1–6 mg/day. Maximum dosage: 10 mg/day or 0.2 mg/kg/day (or 0.05 mg/kg/day for CYP2D6 poor metabolizers). Not studied thoroughly in children younger than 12 years.
Delusional parasitosis (second line; off-label) (PO)
Initial: 0.5–2 mg/day (taken as a single dose or in 2 divided doses). Dosage range: 2–4 mg/day. Maximum dosage: 10 mg/day (or 4 mg/day for CYP2D6 poor metabolizers).

Note. CYP=cytochrome P450.

IX. Monitoring

A. Due to potential for toxicity, CYP2D6 genotyping is required, especially at dosages >4 mg/day.

B. Baseline and periodic:

1. Labs: CBC with differential (rule out hematological changes), LFTs, renal function, electrolytes
2. Metabolic: Weight, hemoglobin A1c test, lipid panel for metabolic risk
3. Extrapyramidal symptoms (EPS): Monitor for abnormal involuntary movements/parkinsonian signs (via Abnormal Involuntary Movement Scale [AIMS]) at baseline and periodically.

4. Consider obtaining an ECG at baseline and periodically (given pimozide's high risk of ECG changes).
5. Other: Visual changes/ocular exam, sexual changes, mental status changes, blood pressure changes, falls

C. Consider ordering a drug level if there are concerns regarding compliance or metabolism (proposed reference range for schizophrenia: 15–20 ng/mL).

X. **Relevant Pharmacokinetics/Pharmacodynamics**

A. **Metabolism**: CYP3A4 (major), CYP2D6 (major), and CYP1A2 (minor) substrate
B. **Time to peak plasma concentration**: 6–8 hours
C. **Onset of action**: Schizophrenia—4–6 weeks
D. **Half-life**: 55–66 hours
E. **Bioavailability**: 50%
F. **Volume of distribution**: ~28 L
G. **Hepatic impairment**: Use caution, but no specific dosage adjustments provided.
H. **Renal impairment**: Use caution. but no specific dosage adjustments provided.

XI. **Clinically Relevant Drug Interactions**

A. Metabolized primarily by CYP2D6 and CYP3A4, and to a lesser extent CYP1A2
1. Coadministration with CYP2D6 inhibitors (e.g., fluoxetine, paroxetine, bupropion) or in known CYP2D6 poor metabolizers can lead to increased plasma levels.
   a. Do not exceed 4 mg/day in patients who are poor CYP2D6 metabolizers (per manufacturer, genotyping should be conducted if dosage >4 mg/day is required).
2. Coadministration with CYP3A4 inhibitors (clarithromycin, some antifungals/antivirals, nefazodone, grapefruit juice) can lead to increased plasma levels.
3. Coadministration with CYP3A4 inducers (e.g., rifampin, carbamazepine) can lead to decreased plasma levels.
4. Polycyclic aromatic hydrocarbons in tobacco smoke can induce the CYP1A2-mediated metabolism of pimozide and decrease its plasma concentrations (although likely only to a minor extent).

B. Additive prolongation of QT interval can be seen with phenothiazines, tricyclic antidepressants, antiarrhythmic agents, and other drugs that also prolong QT interval.
C. Pimozide may potentiate the effects of other CNS depressants (e.g., analgesics, antihistamines, barbiturates, opioids, alcohol).

XII. **Adverse Effects**

A. **See Table 6–1 ("Antipsychotic Class Adverse Effects") at beginning of chapter.**
B. Pimozide's adverse effects include metabolic syndrome, anticholinergic effects, QTc prolongation, orthostatic hypotension, EPS, prolactin elevation, sexual dysfunction, NMS, temperature dysregulation, hyponatremia/syndrome of inappropriate antidiuretic hormone secretion (SIADH), and seizures.
C. **Boxed warning**: Increased mortality in older patients with dementia-related psychosis

D. Potent D_2 blockade leads to a higher risk of EPS (dystonia, akathisia, parkinsonism, tardive dyskinesia); also oculogyric crises and opisthotonos have occurred; higher risk of hyperprolactinemia given potent D_2 blockade
E. Potent hERG blockade leads to higher risk of ECG changes, including prolonged QTc interval, flattening/notching/inversion of the T wave, and appearance of U waves.
F. Sedation may occur, but it less common with pimozide than with other antipsychotics because of pimozide's lower affinity for the H_1 receptor.
G. **Gastrointestinal**: Dry mouth, constipation
H. **Other**: Sexual side effects; ocular changes (visual disturbance, decreased accommodation)

XIII. **Clinical Pearls/Prescribing Tips**

A. Pimozide is not recommended as a first-line treatment for any of its indications.
B. Potent D_2 blockade leads to a higher risk of EPS (dystonia, akathisia, parkinsonism, tardive dyskinesia) and hyperprolactinemia (changes in libido, sexual function, menstruation).
C. Because of pimozide's potential for toxicity, CYP2D6 genotyping is required, especially at dosages higher than 4 mg/day.
D. Pimozide is contraindicated with concomitant use of CYP3A4 and CYP2D6 inhibitors.
E. Potent hERG (cardiac potassium channel) blockade means a higher risk of delaying cardiac repolarization and inducing ECG changes such as prolonged QTc (Kang et al. 2000).

Further Reading

Mothi M, Sampson S: Pimozide for schizophrenia or related psychoses. Cochrane Database Syst Rev (11):CD001949, 2013 24194433

Pimozide [package insert]. Daily Med. Available at: https://dailymed.nlm.nih.gov/dailymed/fda/fdaDrugXsl.cfm?setid=70b079e2-a1f7-4a93-8685-d60a4d7c1280&type=display. Accessed March 13, 2024.

Pringsheim T, Marras C: Pimozide for tics in Tourette's syndrome. Cochrane Database Syst Rev (2):CD006996, 2009 19370666

References

Kang J, Wang L, Cai F, et al: High affinity blockade of the HERG cardiac K(+) channel by the neuroleptic pimozide. Eur J Pharmacol 392(3):137–140, 2000 10762666

Roth BL, Driscoll J: PDSP Ki Database. Psychoactive Drug Screening Program (PDSP). University of North Carolina at Chapel Hill and the United States National Institute of Mental Health, 2023

Prochlorperazine

I. **Brand Names**: Compazine, Compro
II. **Therapeutic Class**: First-generation/typical antipsychotic, antiemetic
III. **Mechanism-Based Class**: Dopamine receptor antagonist
IV. **Mechanism(s) of Action**

A. Dopamine D_2 receptor antagonist (Ki=2.24 nM); some action at other dopamine receptors.
B. Serotonin 5-HT_{2A} receptor antagonist (Ki=7.24 nM); some action at other serotonin receptors.
C. Histamine H_1 receptor antagonist (Ki=6.03 nM)
D. Alpha-1 (α_1)-receptor antagonist (Ki=24 nM)
E. Weak muscarinic receptor antagonist (M_1 Ki=776 nM) (Roth and Driscoll 2023)

V. **Indications**

A. FDA adult:
1. Schizophrenia (not often used for this indication)
2. Severe nausea/vomiting
3. Short-term treatment of generalized nonpsychotic anxiety (not considered a first-line treatment)

B. Evidence-based[1] off-label uses:
1. Intractable severe migraine (adults: 10 mg IM/IV)

C. FDA pediatric:
1. Chemotherapy-induced nausea and vomiting, refractory
2. Migraine, intractable
3. Nausea and vomiting, severe

VI. **Major Contraindications and When to Use Caution**

A. **Contraindications**:
1. Comatose or severely cognitively depressed states
2. Hypersensitivity to phenothiazines
3. Pediatric surgery; patients younger than 2 years or weighing less than 20 lbs (9 kg); do not use off-label in children

B. **Use caution**: Patients with baseline fall risk, hyponatremia or other electrolyte abnormalities, dysrhythmias (including QTc prolongation), leukopenia/neutropenia, hypotension/syncope or on antihypertensive medications, seizures, motor/cognitive impairments or on CNS depressants or anticholinergic agents, temperature dysregulation, aspiration, dysphagia, obesity, hyperglycemia, hyperlipidemia, risk factors for neuroleptic malignant syndrome (NMS) (e.g., dehydration), or dementia-related psychosis (boxed warning), pregnancy/lactation, or Parkinson's disease.

[1]Evidence strength varies; readers are referred to the literature for more detailed information.

VII. **Dosage Formulations**

A. Generic tablet (5 mg, 10 mg [*some scored*])
B. Generic and brand (Compro) rectal suppository (25 mg)
C. Generic solution for injection (10 mg/2 mL)

VIII. **Dosage Ranges and Guidelines**

A. Refer to Table 6–12 for dosage ranges (initial/maximum) and guidelines. Dosages are for adults unless otherwise specified.
   1. Older adults: Same as in younger adults, although lower dosages are typically used and are titrated more slowly.

B. **Titration**: Increase in small increments (~10 mg) every 2–3 days.

C. **Discontinuation**: For patients on long-term treatment, taper slowly to avoid rebound psychosis and withdrawal dyskinesias.

Table 6–12. Prochlorperazine indications and dosage guidelines

Severe nausea and vomiting (PO/IM/IV)
Adults:
PO: 5–10 mg (in 3–4 divided doses). Maximum dosage: 40 mg/day.
Rectal: 25 mg BID. Maximum dosage: 50 mg/day.
IM/IV: 2.5–10 mg every 3–4 hours PRN. Maximum dosage: 10 mg as a single dose; daily maximum: 40 mg. Can start lower, at 2.5 mg, for IV.
IM/IV (preoperative): 5–10 mg taken 1–2 hours prior to anesthesia induction. May repeat one time after 30 minutes if needed.
Children (age 2–12 years):
PO/rectal: If 9–13 kg, 2.5 mg daily BID. If 14–17 kg, 2.5 mg BID–TID. Maximum dosage: up to 15 mg/day (depending on weight).
IM/IV: 0.132 mg/kg (in 3–4 divided doses). Maximum dosage 10 mg/day on the first day of treatment.
Schizophrenia (PO/IM)
Adults:
PO: 5–10 mg 3–4 times daily. Dosage range: 50–150 mg/day. Maximum dosage: 150 mg/day.
IM (for acute management of schizophrenia symptoms): 10–20 mg IM every 1–4 hours PRN. Convert to PO as soon as possible. Maximum dosage: 150 mg/day.
Children (age 2–12 years):
PO: 2.5 mg 2–3 times daily.
IM: 0.132 mg/kg IM once. Convert to PO as soon as possible. Maximum dosage: 10 mg/day on first day of treatment.
Short-term treatment of nonpsychotic anxiety (not a first-line choice) (PO)
PO: 5–10 mg 3–4 times daily or 25 mg every 12 hours. Maximum dosage: 20 mg/day.

IX. **Monitoring**

A. Baseline and periodic:

1. Labs: CBC with differential (rule out hematological changes), LFTs, renal function, electrolytes
2. Metabolic: Weight, hemoglobin A1c test, lipid panel for metabolic risk
3. Extrapyramidal symptoms (EPS): Monitor for abnormal involuntary movements/parkinsonian signs (via Abnormal Involuntary Movement Scale [AIMS]) at baseline and periodically.
4. Consider obtaining an ECG at baseline and periodically if indicated (cardiac risk factors, high-risk medication).
5. Other: Visual changes/ocular exam, sexual changes, mental status changes, blood pressure changes, falls.

X. **Relevant Pharmacokinetics/Pharmacodynamics**

A. **Metabolism**: Extensively metabolized with some glucuronidation; primary active metabolite: *N*-desmethyl prochlorperazine
B. **Onset of action**: 30–60 minutes
C. **Duration of action**: 4–6 hours
D. **Half-life**: PO: 6–10 hours (single dose), 14–22 hours (repeated); IV: 6–10 hours
E. **Hepatic impairment**: Use caution but no specific dosage adjustments provided.
F. **Renal impairment**: Does not appear that dosage adjustments are needed.

XI. **Clinically Relevant Drug Interactions**

A. No major cytochrome P450 (CYP)450 interactions
B. Prochlorperazine may potentiate the effects of other CNS depressants (e.g., analgesics, antihistamines, barbiturates, opioids, alcohol).
C. Acute encephalopathy has been reported with concomitant use of lithium.
D. Prochlorperazine can reduce the effectiveness of oral anticoagulants.
E. Worsening of orthostatic hypotension can be seen with concomitant use of thiazide diuretics.
F. Antihypertensive effects of guanethidine and related compounds may be counteracted by phenothiazines.
G. Phenothiazines may interfere with phenytoin metabolism and lead to toxicity.
H. Concomitant use with anticholinergic drugs (e.g., atropine) may potentiate anticholinergic effects
I. Concomitant use with propranolol may lead to increased plasma concentrations of both

XII. **Adverse Effects**

A. **See Table 6–1 ("Antipsychotic Class Adverse Effects") at beginning of chapter.**
B. Prochlorperazine's adverse effects include metabolic syndrome, anticholinergic effects, QTc prolongation, orthostatic hypotension, EPS, prolactin elevation, sexual dysfunction, NMS, temperature dysregulation, hyponatremia/syndrome of inappropriate antidiuretic hormone secretion (SIADH), and seizure.
C. **Boxed warning**: Increased mortality in older patients with dementia-related psychosis.

D. Potent D_2 blockade leads to a higher risk of EPS (dystonia, akathisia, parkinsonism, tardive dyskinesia) and hyperprolactinemia (changes in libido, sexual function, menstruation)
E. Given prochlorperazine's potent antihistamine effects, sedation, dizziness, motor dysfunction may occur. Use caution in older adults.
F. Anticholinergic effects, orthostatic hypotension may occur (Beers Criteria [American Geriatrics Society 2023]).

XIII. **Clinical Pearls/Prescribing Tips**

A. Prochlorperazine is mostly used in nausea and vomiting rather than for psychiatric indications and is usually indicated for short-term treatment. Use caution in older adults given high risk of sedation, dizziness and potential anticholinergic effects. Potent D_2 blockade can lead to EPS and hyperprolactinemia.
B. Prochlorperazine is very similar in structure to chlorpromazine and perphenazine
C. Prochlorperazine has multiple forms including PO, IM, IV and rectal suppository.
D. Administration via IV should be done slowly (no more than 5 mg/minute) to avoid hypotension. Do not administer via subcutaneous route to avoid local irritation.
E. May cause false-positive phenylketonuria test

Further Reading

Furyk JS, Meek RA, Egerton-Warburton D: Drugs for the treatment of nausea and vomiting in adults in the emergency department setting. Cochrane Database Syst Rev (9):CD010106, 2015 26411330

Golikhatir I, Cheraghmakani H, Bozorgi F, et al: The efficacy and safety of prochlorperazine in patients with acute migraine: a systematic review and meta-analysis. Headache 59(5):682–700, 2019 30990883

Prochlorperazine maleate package insert. Daily Med. Available at: https://dailymed.nlm.nih.gov/dailymed/fda/fdaDrugXsl.cfm?setid=50ce4381-94ef-49ff-8794-cfde0ee803b4&type=display. Accessed March 13, 2024.

References

American Geriatrics Society Beers Criteria Update Expert Panel: 2023 updated AGS Beers Criteria for potentially inappropriate medication use in older adults. J Am Geriatr Soc 71(7):2052–2081, 2023 37139824

Roth BL, Driscoll J: PDSP Ki Database. Psychoactive Drug Screening Program (PDSP). University of North Carolina at Chapel Hill and the United States National Institute of Mental Health, 2023

Thioridazine

I. **Brand Names**: Mellaril (discontinued)

II. **Therapeutic Class**: First-generation/typical antipsychotic

III. **Mechanism-Based Class**: Dopamine receptor antagonist

IV. **Mechanism(s) of Action**

A. Dopamine D_2 receptor antagonist (Ki=0.4–4.3 nM); some action at other dopamine receptors.
B. Histamine-1 (H_1) receptor antagonist (Ki=1.8–16.5 nM)
C. Alpha-1 (α_1)-receptor antagonist (Ki=2–3.2 nM)
D. M_1 receptor antagonist (anticholinergic) (Ki=10–12.8 nM)
E. hERG (potassium ion channel) antagonist (Ki=191 nM)

V. **Indications**

A. FDA adult: Schizophrenia, refractory
B. Evidence-based off-label uses: None reported
C. FDA pediatric: None

VI. **Major Contraindications and When to Use Caution**

A. **Contraindications**:

1. Use with other QTc-prolonging medications, in patients with congenital long QT syndrome, or in patients with a known history of cardiac arrhythmias
2. Use with strong cytochrome P450 (CYP) 2D6 inhibitors (e.g., fluoxetine, bupropion) or in patients who are CYP2D6 poor metabolizers
3. Patients in comatose or severely cognitively depressed states

B. **Use caution**: Patients with baseline fall risk, hyponatremia or other electrolyte abnormalities, dysrhythmias (including QTc prolongation), leukopenia/neutropenia, hypotension/syncope or on antihypertensive medications, seizures, motor/cognitive impairments or on CNS depressants or anticholinergic agents, temperature dysregulation, aspiration, dysphagia, obesity, hyperglycemia, hyperlipidemia, risk factors for NMS (e.g., dehydration), or dementia-related psychosis (boxed warning), pregnancy/lactation, or Parkinson's disease.

VII. **Dosage Formulations**

I. Generic capsule (10 mg, 25 mg, 50 mg, 100 mg)

II. **Dosage Ranges and Guidelines**

A. Refer to Table 6–13 for dosage ranges (initial/maximum) and guidelines. Dosages are for adults unless otherwise specified.

1. Older adults: Same as in younger adults, although lower dosages are typically used and are titrated more slowly.
2. Children (age 1–11 years)/infants: Safety/efficacy have not been established for this age group.

B. **Titration**: Increase gradually (frequency not defined).
C. **Discontinuation**: For patients on long-term treatment, taper slowly to avoid rebound psychosis and withdrawal dyskinesias.

Table 6–13. Thioridazine indications and dosage guidelines

Schizophrenia (PO), refractory*
Adults:
Initial: 50–100 mg 3 times/day. Maximum dosage: 800 mg/day in 2–4 divided doses.
Children and adolescents:
Refer to the medical literature for guidance and the best evidence on dosing (Mylan Pharmaceuticals 2019).

*Reserved for refractory schizophrenia (defined as failure to respond to two or more antipsychotics).

III. **Monitoring**

A. Baseline and periodic:

1. Labs: CBC with differential (rule out hematological changes), renal function, liver function, electrolytes
2. Metabolic: Weight, hemoglobin A1c test, lipid panel for metabolic risk
3. Extrapyramidal symptoms (EPS): Monitor for abnormal involuntary movements/parkinsonian signs (via Abnormal Involuntary Movement Scale [AIMS]) at baseline and periodically.
4. Obtain an ECG at baseline (do not initiate treatment if QTc >450 ms) and periodically if indicated (cardiac risk factors, high-risk medication).
5. Other: Visual changes/ocular exam (routine exam every year for individuals age ≥40 years; every other year for individuals age <40 years), sexual changes, mental status changes, blood pressure changes, falls

B. Consider ordering a drug level if there are concerns regarding compliance or metabolism (proposed reference range for schizophrenia: 100–200 ng/mL).

IV. **Relevant Pharmacokinetics/Pharmacodynamics**

A. **Metabolism**: CYP2D6 (major) and CYP2C19 (minor) substrate; inhibits CYP2D6 (moderate); induces CYP3A4 (weak); active metabolites: mesoridazine and sulphordiazine
B. **Time to peak plasma concentration**: 1–4 hours
C. **Onset of action**: Schizophrenia: 4–6 weeks
D. **Half-life**: ~22 hours
E. **Bioavailability**: 25%–33%
F. **Volume of distribution**: 1.8–17.8 L
G. **Hepatic impairment**: Use caution due to hepatic metabolism, but no specific dosage adjustments provided.
H. **Renal impairment**: Use caution, but no specific dosage adjustments provided.

V. **Clinically Relevant Drug Interactions**

A. Metabolized primarily by CYP2D6:

1. Coadministration with strong CYP2D6 inhibitors (e.g., fluoxetine, paroxetine, bupropion) may increase thioridazine serum concentrations (considered a contraindication)

B. Moderate inhibitor of CYP2D6 activity:
   1. Coadministration with CYP2D6 substrates (e.g., aripiprazole or tamoxifen) may increase serum concentrations of substrate (consider therapy modification)
C. May potentiate effects of other CNS depressants (e.g., analgesics, antihistamines, barbiturates, opioids, alcohol).
D. May potentiate effects of atropine or other anticholinergic drugs.
E. Coadministration with antihypertensive agents may result in additive hypotensive effects.

VI. **Adverse Effects**

A. **See Table 6–1 ("Antipsychotic Class Adverse Effects") at beginning of chapter.**
B. Thioridazine's adverse effects include metabolic syndrome, anticholinergic effects, QTc prolongation, orthostatic hypotension, EPS, prolactin elevation, sexual dysfunction, NMS, temperature dysregulation, hyponatremia/SIADH, seizures
C. **Boxed warnings**:
   1. Proarrhythmic effects (including torsades de pointes and sudden cardiac death)
   2. Increased mortality in older patients with dementia-related psychosis
D. Potent D_2 blockade leads to a higher risk of EPS (dystonia, akathisia, parkinsonism, tardive dyskinesia) and hyperprolactinemia (changes in libido, sexual function, menstruation).
E. Given thioridazine's potent antihistamine effects, sedation, dizziness, and motor dysfunction may occur; use caution in older adults.
F. QTc prolongation and torsades de pointes (dosage-related risk; discontinue in patients with QTc >500 ms)
G. In rare cases, retinitis pigmentosa (diminished visual acuity, brownish coloring of vision, with deposits in fundus on exam) has been seen during long-term use.
H. Photosensitivity, dermatitis, and hyperpigmentation of the skin may occur (rare).

VII. **Clinical Pearls/Prescribing Tips**

A. Considered a "low potency" FGA similar to chlorpromazine, based on D_2 receptor affinity.
B. H_1 and α_1 receptor antagonism are relatively potent; watch for sedation and orthostasis, respectively.
C. Thioridazine is reserved for treatment-refractory cases because of the high risk of QTc prolongation (a dosage-related side effect secondary to hERG [potassium ion channel] inhibition). Do not initiate in patients with baseline QTc >450 ms; discontinue in patients with QTc >500 ms.
D. Retinitis pigmentosa has been associated with prolonged use of thioridazine and with dosages >800 mg/day. A baseline eye exam and an exam every 1–2 years (based on age) are recommended during use.
E. Strongly metabolized by CYP2D6; moderate inhibitor of CYP2D6.
F. May cause false-positive results on urine pregnancy tests.

Further Reading

Roth BL, Driscoll J: PDSP Ki Database. Psychoactive Drug Screening Program (PDSP). University of North Carolina at Chapel Hill and the United States National Institute of Mental Health, 2023

References

Mylan Pharmaceuticals: Thioridazine hydrochloride [package insert]. Revised September 2019. Available at: https://dailymed.nlm.nih.gov/dailymed/fda/fdaDrugXsl.cfm?setid=56b3f4c2-52af-4947-b225-6808ae9f26f5&type=display. Accessed March 13, 2024.

Thiothixene

I. **Brand Names**: Navane (discontinued)
II. **Therapeutic Class**: First-generation/typical antipsychotic
III. **Mechanism-Based Class**: Dopamine receptor antagonist
IV. **Mechanism(s) of Action**

A. Potent dopamine D_2 receptor antagonist (Ki=0.03–1.4 nM); some action at other dopamine receptors.
B. Histamine-1 (H_1) receptor antagonist (Ki=4.0–12 nM)
C. Alpha-1 (α_1)-receptor antagonist (Ki=19 nM)
D. Muscarinic M_1 receptor antagonism (Ki>2,000 nM)

V. **Indications**

A. FDA adult: Schizophrenia
B. Evidence-based[1] off-label uses:

1. Severe behavioral or psychological symptoms of dementia

C. FDA pediatric: None

VI. **Major Contraindications and When to Use Caution**

A. **Contraindications**: Comatose or severely cognitively depressed states; circulatory collapse; blood dyscrasias; hypersensitivity to thiothixene or other phenothiazines derivatives
B. **Use caution**: Patients with baseline fall risk, hyponatremia or other electrolyte abnormalities, dysrhythmias (including QTc prolongation), leukopenia/neutropenia, hypotension/syncope or on antihypertensive medications, seizures, motor/cognitive impairments or on CNS depressants or anticholinergic agents, temperature dysregulation, aspiration, dysphagia, obesity, hyperglycemia, hyperlipidemia, risk factors for NMS (e.g., dehydration), or dementia-related psychosis (boxed warning), pregnancy/lactation, or Parkinson's disease.

[1]Evidence strength varies; readers are referred to the literature for more detailed information.

VII. **Dosage Formulations**

A. Generic capsule (1 mg, 2 mg, 5 mg, 10 mg)

VIII. **Dosage Ranges and Guidelines**

A. Refer to Table 6–14 for dosage ranges (initial/maximum) and guidelines. Dosages are for adults unless otherwise specified.

1. Older adults: Same as in younger adults, although lower dosages are typically used and are titrated more slowly.
2. Children (age 1–11 years)/infants: Safety/efficacy have not been established for this age group.

B. **Titration**: Increase gradually (frequency not defined)

C. **Discontinuation**: For patients on long-term treatment, taper slowly to avoid rebound psychosis and withdrawal dyskinesias.

Table 6–14. Thiothixene indications and dosage guidelines

Schizophrenia (PO)
Adults, children, and adolescents (age ≥ 12 years*):
2–5 mg 2–3 times/day up to 60 mg/day in 2–3 divided doses. Maximum dosage: 60 mg/day.
Severe behavioral or psychological symptoms of dementia (off-label) (PO)
1–2 mg BID up to 30 mg/day (in divided doses).

*Package insert states that use in children younger than 12 years is not recommended.

IX. **Monitoring**

A. Baseline and periodic:

1. Labs: CBC with differential (rule out hematological changes), renal function, electrolytes
2. Metabolic: Weight, hemoglobin A1c test, lipid panel for metabolic risk
3. Extrapyramidal symptoms (EPS): Monitor for abnormal involuntary movements/parkinsonian signs (via Abnormal Involuntary Movement Scale [AIMS]) at baseline and periodically.
4. Consider obtaining an ECG at baseline and periodically if indicated (cardiac risk factors, high-risk medication).
5. Other: Visual changes/ocular exam (baseline and every 1–2 years, depending on age), sexual changes, mental status changes, blood pressure changes, falls

X. **Relevant Pharmacokinetics/Pharmacodynamics**

A. **Metabolism**: Cytochrome P450 (CYP) 1A2 (moderate) substrate
B. **Time to peak plasma concentration**: 1–2 hours
C. **Onset of action**: Schizophrenia: within 4–6 weeks
D. **Half-life**: biphasic; initial: 3.4 hours; terminal: 34 hours
E. **Bioavailability**: ~50%
F. **Volume of distribution**: Unclear

G. **Hepatic impairment**: Use caution but no specific dosage adjustments provided.
H. **Renal impairment**: Use caution but no specific dosage adjustments provided.

XI. **Clinically Relevant Drug Interactions**

A. Metabolized by CYP1A2 (moderate)

1. Concomitant use of CYP1A2 inducers (e.g., carbamazepine, phenytoin, phenobarbital) may lead to decreased plasma levels of thiothixene. In addition, the polycyclic aromatic hydrocarbons present in cigarette smoke (as well as in emissions from other tobacco products, charred meats, and wood-burning stoves) are also inducers of CYP1A2, and exposure to any of these sources may lead to CYP enzyme induction.

B. May potentiate effects of other CNS depressants (e.g., analgesics, antihistamines, barbiturates, opioids, alcohol).
C. May potentiate the effects of atropine or other anticholinergic drugs.
D. Tricyclic antidepressants may increase plasma thiothixene concentrations.
E. Beta-blockers (e.g., propranolol), cimetidine, and isoniazid may decrease thiothixene clearance.
F. Concurrent use of antihypertensive agents may lead to additive hypotensive effects.
G. Acute encephalopathy has been reported with concomitant use of lithium.

XII. **Adverse Effects**

A. **See Table 6–1 ("Antipsychotic Class Adverse Effects") at beginning of chapter.**
B. Thiothixene's adverse effects include metabolic syndrome, anticholinergic effects, QTc prolongation, orthostatic hypotension, EPS, prolactin elevation, sexual dysfunction, NMS, temperature dysregulation, hyponatremia/SIADH, seizure
C. **Boxed warning**: Increased mortality in older adults with dementia-related psychosis
D. Potent D_2 blockade leads to a higher risk of EPS (dystonia, akathisia, parkinsonism, tardive dyskinesia) and hyperprolactinemia (changes in libido, sexual function, menstruation)
E. Corneal pigmentation can in rare case occur with prolonged use.
F. Photosensitivity, dermatitis, and hyperpigmentation of the skin may occur (rare).

XIII. **Clinical Pearls/Prescribing Tips**

A. Thiothixene is a "high potency" FGA. Potent D_2 blockade can lead to EPS and hyperprolactinemia.
B. Thiothixene has a relatively low risk of anticholinergic side effects, sedation, and orthostasis.
C. Thiothixene can cause false-positive results on urine pregnancy tests.

Further Reading

Roth BL, Driscoll J: PDSP Ki Database. Psychoactive Drug Screening Program (PDSP). University of North Carolina at Chapel Hill and the United States National Institute of Mental Health, 2023

Thiothixene package insert. Daily Med. Available at: https://dailymed.nlm.nih.gov/dailymed/fda/fdaDrugXsl.cfm?setid=81c40311-7dc4-4332-8920-a39a8466aea6&type=display. Accessed March 13, 2024.

Trifluoperazine

I. **Brand Names**: Stelazine (discontinued)

II. **Therapeutic Class**: First-generation/typical antipsychotic

III. **Mechanism-Based Class**: Dopamine and serotonin receptor antagonist

IV. **Mechanism(s) of Action**

A. Dopamine D_2 receptor antagonist (Ki = 0.96–2.6 nM)

B. Serotonin 5-HT_{2A} receptor antagonist (Ki = 13–135 nM)

C. Histamine (H_1) receptor antagonist (Ki = 62 nM)

D. Low affinity for α_1-adrenergic and M_1 receptor antagonism

V. **Indications**

A. FDA adult:

1. Schizophrenia
2. Short-term treatment of generalized nonpsychotic anxiety (not first line)

B. Evidence-based[1] off-label uses: Agitation

C. FDA pediatric: None

VI. **Major Contraindications and When to Use Caution**

A. **Contraindications**: Comatose or severely cognitively depressed states; hypersensitivity to trifluoperazine, other phenothiazines, or sulfites; existing blood dyscrasias or bone marrow depression; preexisting hepatic impairment

B. **Use caution**: Patients with baseline fall risk, hyponatremia or other electrolyte abnormalities, dysrhythmias (including QTc prolongation), leukopenia/neutropenia, hypotension/syncope or on antihypertensive medications, seizures, motor/cognitive impairments or on CNS depressants or anticholinergic agents, temperature dysregulation, aspiration, dysphagia, obesity, hyperglycemia, hyperlipidemia, risk factors for NMS (e.g., dehydration), or dementia-related psychosis (boxed warning), pregnancy/lactation, or Parkinson's disease.

VII. **Dosage Formulations**

A. Generic tablet (1 mg, 2 mg, 5 mg, 10 mg)

VIII. **Dosage Ranges and Guidelines**

A. Refer to Table 6–15 for dosage ranges (initial/maximum) and guidelines. Dosages are for adults unless otherwise specified.

1. Older adults: Same as in younger adults, although lower dosages are typically used and are titrated more slowly.
2. Children (age <6 years): Safety/efficacy have not been established for this age group.

B. **Titration**: Increase gradually (frequency not defined)

C. **Discontinuation**: For patients on long-term treatment, taper slowly to avoid rebound psychosis and withdrawal dyskinesias.

---

[1]Evidence strength varies; readers are referred to the literature for more detailed information.

Table 6–15. Trifluoperazine indications and dosage guidelines

Schizophrenia (PO)
Adults/adolescents:
Initial: 2–5 mg 1–2 times daily. Usual dosage: 15–20 mg/day (divided). Maximum dosage: 40 mg/day.
Children (age 6–12 years):
Initial: 1 mg 2–3 times daily. Maximum dosage: 15 mg/day.
Short-term treatment of generalized nonpsychotic anxiety (not first line) (PO)
Initial: 1–2 mg 1–2 times daily; limit treatment to ≤12 weeks. Maximum dosage 6 mg/day.

IX. **Monitoring**

A. Baseline and periodic:

1. Labs: CBC with differential (rule out hematological changes), LFTs (rare liver damage risk, contraindicated in hepatic impairment), renal function, electrolytes
2. Metabolic: Weight, hemoglobin A1c test, lipid panel for metabolic risk
3. Extrapyramidal symptoms (EPS): Monitor for abnormal involuntary movements/parkinsonian signs (via Abnormal Involuntary Movement Scale [AIMS]) at baseline and periodically.
4. Consider obtaining an ECG at baseline and periodically if indicated (cardiac risk factors, high-risk medication).
5. Other: Visual changes/ocular exam, sexual changes, mental status changes, blood pressure changes, falls

X. **Relevant Pharmacokinetics/Pharmacodynamics**

A. **Metabolism**: Phase I: cytochrome P450 (CYP) 1A2 (moderate). Phase II: human uridine 5′-diphospho-glucuronosyltransferase (UGT) 1A4.
B. **Time to peak plasma concentration**: 1.5–6 hours
C. **Onset of action**: Schizophrenia: within 4–6 weeks
D. **Half-life**: 3–19 hours
E. **Bioavailability**: Unclear
F. **Volume of distribution**: Unclear
G. **Hepatic impairment**: Contraindicated in patients with preexisting hepatic impairment.
H. **Renal impairment**: Use caution, but no specific dosage adjustments provided.

XI. **Clinically Relevant Drug Interactions**:

A. Metabolized by CYP1A2 (moderate):

1. Concomitant use of CYP1A2 inducers (e.g., carbamazepine, phenytoin, phenobarbital) may lead to decreased plasma levels of trifluoperazine. In addition, the polycyclic aromatic hydrocarbons present in cigarette smoke (as well as in emissions from other tobacco products, charred meats, and wood-burning stoves) are also inducers of CYP1A2, and exposure to any of these sources may lead to CYP enzyme induction.

B. Trifluoperazine may potentiate effects with other CNS depressants (e.g., analgesics, antihistamines, barbiturates, opioids, alcohol).
C. Acute encephalopathy has been reported with concomitant use of lithium.
D. Trifluoperazine can reduce the effectiveness of oral anticoagulants.
E. Concomitant use with propranolol may lead to increased plasma concentrations of both.
F. Worsening of orthostatic hypotension can be seen with concomitant use of thiazide diuretics.

XII. **Adverse Effects**:

A. **See Table 6–1 ("Antipsychotic Class Adverse Effects") at beginning of chapter.**
B. Trifluoperazine's adverse effects include metabolic syndrome, anticholinergic effects, QTc prolongation, orthostatic hypotension, EPS, prolactin elevation, sexual dysfunction, NMS, temperature dysregulation, hyponatremia/syndrome of inappropriate antidiuretic hormone secretion (SIADH), and seizure.
C. **Boxed warning**: Increased mortality in older patients with dementia-related psychosis
D. Hepatic dysfunction and cholestatic jaundice may occur (rare).
E. Corneal pigmentation is a rare effects that occurs with prolonged use.
F. Photosensitivity, dermatitis, and hyperpigmentation of the skin may occur (rare).

XIII. **Clinical Pearls/Prescribing Tips**

A. Trifluoperazine is a "high potency" FGA; potent D_2 blockade can lead to EPS and hyperprolactinemia.
B. Trifluoperazine has a relatively low risk of anticholinergic side effects, sedation, and orthostasis.
C. Trifluoperazine may cause a false-positive phenylketonuria test.
D. Trifluoperazine is contraindicated in preexisting hepatic disease.

Further Reading

Koch K, Mansi K, Haynes E, et al: Trifluoperazine versus placebo for schizophrenia. Cochrane Database Syst Rev (1):CD010226, 2014 24414883

Roth BL, Driscoll J: PDSP Ki Database. Psychoactive Drug Screening Program (PDSP). University of North Carolina at Chapel Hill and the United States National Institute of Mental Health, 2023

Trifluoperazine hydrochloride package insert. Daily Med. Available at: https://dailymed.nlm.nih.gov/dailymed/fda/fdaDrugXsl.cfm?setid=c2575a86-19e5-44df-8603-ff066bb9c9c5&type=display. Accessed March 13, 2024.

Second-Generation Antipsychotics

Asenapine

I. **Brand Names**: Saphris (sublingual), Secuado (transdermal system [patch])

II. **Therapeutic Class**: Atypical antipsychotic

III. **Mechanism-Based Class**: Dopamine, serotonin, and norepinephrine receptor antagonist

IV. **Mechanism(s) of Action**

A. Potent dopamine D_2 receptor antagonist (Ki=0.765 nM); some action at other dopamine receptors.

B. 5-HT_{2A} receptor antagonist (Ki=5.6 nM); 5-HT_{1A} partial agonist (Ki=2.5); some action at other serotonin receptors.

C. Histamine-1 (H_1) receptor antagonist (Ki=8 nM)

D. Alpha-1 (α_1)-adrenergic receptor antagonist (α_{1A} Ki=10 nM) (Roth and Driscoll 2023)

E. Norepinephrine α_1-adrenergic receptor antagonist (α_{2A} Ki=8.9 nM, α_{2B} Ki=9.5 nM, α_{2C} Ki=8.9 nM)

V. **Indications**

A. FDA adult and pediatric:

1. Schizophrenia
2. Acute monotherapy treatment of manic or mixed episodes in adults and pediatric patients age 10–17 years
3. Adjunct to lithium or valproate treatment in adults with bipolar disorder
4. Maintenance monotherapy treatment of bipolar disorder in adults

B. Evidence-based[1] off-label uses:

1. Severe behavioral or psychological symptoms of dementia (dosage not established)
2. Agitation/aggression (severe, acute) associated with psychiatric disorders (e.g., bipolar disorder, schizophrenia), substance intoxication, or other organic causes (alternative agent) (off-label use)

VI. **Major Contraindications and When to Use Caution**

A. **Contraindications**: Severe hepatic impairment (Child-Pugh Class C), hypersensitivity to asenapine

B. **Use caution**: Patients with baseline fall risk, hyponatremia or other electrolyte abnormalities, dysrhythmias (including QTc prolongation), leukopenia/neutrope-

[1]Evidence strength varies; readers are referred to the literature for more detailed information.

nia, hypotension/syncope or on antihypertensive medications, seizures, motor/cognitive impairments or on CNS depressants or anticholinergic agents, temperature dysregulation, aspiration, dysphagia, obesity, hyperglycemia, hyperlipidemia, risk factors for NMS (e.g., dehydration), or dementia-related psychosis (boxed warning), pregnancy/lactation, or Parkinson's disease.

C. Patch formulation: Use caution with excessive exposure to external heat.

D. Use caution in individuals with phenylketonuria (tablets may contain aspartame).

VII. **Dosage Formulations**

A. Brand and generic sublingual (SL) tablet (2.5 mg, 5 mg, 10 mg)

B. Brand (Secuado) 24-hour transdermal patch (3.8 mg/24 hours, 5.7 mg/24 hours, 7.6 mg/24 hours)

VIII. **Dosage Ranges and Guidelines**

A. Refer to Table 6–16 for dosage ranges (initial/maximum) and guidelines. Dosages are for adults unless otherwise specified.

1. Older adults: Same as in younger adults, although lower dosages are typically used and are titrated more slowly.
2. Children (age <10 years) and children/adolescents (age ≥10–17 years): The safety/efficacy of the transdermal/patch formulation have not been established in these age groups.
3. See "Clinically Relevant Drug Interactions" below and adjust dosages accordingly.

B. **Titration**:

1. Adults: SL tablet: Increase by 10 mg per day (divided) every week. Transdermal patch: Increase by 1.9 mg/24 hours every week.
2. Children (SL): Increase by 2.5–5 mg BID every 3–7 days.

C. **Conversion**: 5 mg SL BID is equivalent to 3.8 mg patch/24 hours, and 10 mg SL BID is equivalent to 7.6 mg patch/24 hours.

D. **Discontinuation**: For patients on long-term treatment, taper slowly to avoid rebound psychosis and withdrawal dyskinesias.

Table 6–16. Asenapine indications and dosage guidelines

Schizophrenia (SL tablet/transdermal patch)
SL tablet: Initial: 5 mg BID. Maximum dosage: 10 mg BID.
Transdermal patch: Initial: 3.8 mg/24 hours. Maximum dosage: 7.6 mg/24 hours.
Bipolar I disorder, mania/mixed episodes (SL tablet)
Adults:
Initial: 5–10 mg BID. Maximum dosage: 10 mg BID.
Children/adolescents (age ≥10 years):
Initial: 2.5 mg BID. Maximum dosage: 10 mg BID.

Table 6–16. Asenapine indications and dosage guidelines *(continued)*

Bipolar I disorder, maintenance treatment (SL tablet)
Adults: Initial: 5–10 mg BID. Maximum dosage: 10 mg BID.
Agitation (off-label) (SL tablet)
Adults: 5–10 mg once. Maximum dosage: 20 mg/day in divided doses.

IX. **Monitoring**

A. Baseline and periodic:

1. Labs: CBC with differential (rule out hematological changes), LFTs (liver damage risk [rare]; contraindicated in hepatic impairment), renal function, electrolytes
2. Metabolic: Weight, hemoglobin A1c test, lipid panel for metabolic risk
3. Extrapyramidal symptoms (EPS): Monitor for abnormal involuntary movements/parkinsonian signs (via Abnormal Involuntary Movement Scale [AIMS]) at baseline and periodically.
4. Consider obtaining an ECG at baseline and periodically if indicated (cardiac risk factors, concomitant use of high-risk medication).
5. Other: Visual changes/ocular exam, sexual changes, mental status changes, blood pressure changes, falls

X. **Relevant Pharmacokinetics/Pharmacodynamics**

A. **Metabolism**: Phase I: cytochrome P450 (CYP) 1A2 (major), CYP3A4/CYP2D6 (minor); Phase II: glucuronidation by human uridine 5′-diphospho-glucuronosyltransferase (UGT) 1A4

B. **Time to peak plasma concentration**: SL: 0.5–1.5 hours; transdermal: 12–24 hours

C. **Excretion**: 50% renally, 40% biliary

D. **Bioavailability**: 35% (SL and transdermal patch)

E. **Distribution**: 95% plasma protein bound

F. **Half-life**: SL: 13–39 hours; transdermal: 30 hours

G. **Time to steady state**: ~5 days (SL and transdermal patch)

H. **Absorption**: External heat sources may increase rate/extent of patch absorption.

I. **Hepatic impairment**: No dosage adjustment required for mild to moderate impairment (Child-Pugh Class A/B); contraindicated with severe impairment.

J. **Renal impairment**: No dosage adjustment required.

XI. **Clinically Relevant Drug Interactions**

A. Metabolized by CYP1A2 (minor), but also by CYP2D6, CYP3A4 (minor)

1. Use caution/decrease dose when coadministered with strong CYP1A2 inhibitors (e.g., fluvoxamine, ciprofloxacin).
2. Polycyclic aromatic hydrocarbons in tobacco smoke can induce the CYP1A2-mediated metabolism of asenapine and decrease its plasma concentrations (although likely only to a minor extent).
3. Use caution when coadministered with CYP3A4 inducers (e.g., carbamazepine).

B. **Weak inhibitor of CYP2D6**

1. May see increased levels of CYP2D6 substrates/inhibitors (e.g., paroxetine) when given with asenapine.

C. Use caution with other drugs known to prolong the QTc, antihypertensive drugs, other CNS depressants, and anticholinergic agents.

D. Valproic acid can slightly increase asenapine levels.

XII. **Adverse Effects**

A. **See Table 6–1 ("Antipsychotic Class Adverse Effects") at beginning of chapter.**

B. Asenapine's adverse effects include metabolic syndrome, anticholinergic effects, QTc prolongation, orthostatic hypotension, EPS, prolactin elevation, sexual dysfunction, NMS, temperature dysregulation, hyponatremia/syndrome of inappropriate antidiuretic hormone secretion (SIADH), seizure. Dysgeusia (bad taste) is often reported anecdotally by patients, including with the flavored SL formulation.

1. Because of asenapine's potent D_2 blockade, EPS (including akathisia, dystonia, parkinsonism, tardive dyskinesia) is relatively common.
2. For the full scope of potential adverse effects, see drug labeling (Asenapine package insert).

C. **Boxed warning**: Increased mortality in older patients with dementia-related psychosis.

D. Application site reactions (patch)

E. **Most common**: Akathisia, sedation, dizziness, weight gain, oral hypoesthesia

F. **Rare**: Allergic reactions including anaphylaxis, swollen tongue, angioedema, rash, orthostatic hypotension, syncope

XIII. **Clinical Pearls/Prescribing Tips**

A. The sublingual tablet is a good option for patients who have difficulty swallowing pills or those who have undergone a gastric bypass (resulting in intestinal absorption that cannot be relied on). Avoid eating or drinking for 10 minutes following SL administration, as food or drink can decrease asenapine exposure by 10%–20%. Oral bioavailability when swallowed is less than 2%.

B. External heat may increase rate/extent of asenapine patch absorption.

C. Compared with other SGAs, asenapine carries a lower risk of weight gain, sedation, and EPS but a higher risk of QTc prolongation.

D. Asenapine is contraindicated in severe hepatic impairment.

E. Asenapine SL 5 mg BID is roughly equivalent to 3.8 mg/24 hour patch.

Further Reading

Asenapine package insert. U.S Food and Drug Administration, 2023. Available at: https://www.accessdata.fda.gov/spl/data/f1f1f3b2-6b49-a523-e053-2995a90ad0c9/f1f1f3b2-6b49-a523-e053-2995a90ad0c9.xml. Accessed March 13, 2024.

Citrome L: Asenapine review, part I: chemistry, receptor affinity profile, pharmacokinetics and metabolism. Expert Opin Drug Metab Toxicol 10(6):893–903, 2014 24793403

Citrome L: Asenapine review, part II: clinical efficacy, safety and tolerability. Expert Opin Drug Saf 13(6):803–830, 2014 24793161

Hay A, Byers A, Sereno M, et al: Asenapine versus placebo for schizophrenia. Cochrane Database Syst Rev (11):CD011458, 2015 26599405
Marazziti D, Mucci F, Falaschi V, et al: Asenapine for the treatment of bipolar disorder. Expert Opin Pharmacother 20(11):1321–1330, 2019 31132287
Zhou M, Derakhshanian S, Rath A, et al: Asenapine transdermal patch for the management of schizophrenia. Psychopharmacol Bull 50(4):60–82, 2020 33012873

References

Roth BL, Driscoll J: PDSP Ki Database. Psychoactive Drug Screening Program (PDSP). University of North Carolina at Chapel Hill and the United States National Institute of Mental Health, 2023

Clozapine

I. **Brand Names**: Clozaril, Versacloz, FazaClo
II. **Therapeutic Class**: Atypical antipsychotic
III. **Mechanism-Based Class**: Dopamine, serotonin, and norepinephrine receptor antagonist
IV. **Mechanism(s) of Action**

A. 5-HT_{2A} antagonism/inverse agonism (Ki=5.35 nM)

1. At doses of 300–600 mg of clozapine, approx. 96% of the serotonin 5-HT_{2A} receptors are occupied (compared with risperidone, which blocks 100% of the receptors at doses of 6 mg) (Seeman 2014).

B. 5-HT_{2C} antagonism (Ki=9.44 nM).
C. Norepinephrine α_1-adrenergic receptor (autoreceptor) antagonism (α_{2A} Ki=37 nM, α_{2B} Ki=26.5 nM, α_{2C} Ki=6 nM)
D. Weak dopamine D_2 receptor antagonism (Ki=157 nM)

1. Clozapine binds "loosely" to the D_2 receptor, meaning it dissociates quickly from the receptor after a dose is given, allowing endogenous dopamine to bind thereafter, notably in the motor-controlling brain regions, likely leading to decreased risk of motor side effects. For example, an oral dose of 350 mg of clozapine decreases D_2 occupancy from 72% down to less than 30% at 24 hours, compared with haloperidol, which strongly occupies D_2 receptors for 27 hours after a dose (Seeman 2014). Quetiapine also has loose binding similar to that of clozapine.

E. D_1 activity in clozapine (Ki=290–540 nM) is similar to D_2 activity, which is unique for clozapine, although it is still unclear whether clozapine acts as an agonist or an antagonist of D_1 (Tauscher et al. 2004).
F. D_4 activity in clozapine (Ki=26.4 nM) may affect frontotemporal function such as cognition, negative symptoms (Semba 2004).
G. Histamine-1 (H_1) receptor antagonism (Ki=1.13 nM)
H. α_1-Adrenergic receptor antagonism (α_{1A} Ki=1.62 nM) (Roth and Driscoll 2023)

I. Muscarinic receptor antagonism (M_1 Ki=6.17); exception—agonistic activity on M_4 receptor (Ki=15.33 nM)

J. Reductions in glutamate in the caudate nucleus could also contribute to clozapine's effectiveness as an antipsychotic (McQueen et al. 2021).

V. **Indications**

A. FDA adult:

1. Treatment-resistant schizophrenia
2. Reduce risk of suicidal behavior in schizophrenia or schizoaffective disorder

B. Evidence-based[1] off-label uses:

1. Bipolar disorder
2. Parkinson's disease psychosis
3. Schizoaffective disorder
4. Schizophrenia with comorbid depression
5. Tardive dyskinesia in individuals with schizophrenia or schizoaffective disorder

C. FDA pediatric: None; off-label use for treatment-resistant schizophrenia (children age ≥6 years)

VI. **Major Contraindications and When to Use Caution**

A. **Contraindications**: Hypersensitivity to clozapine

B. **Use caution**: Patients with baseline fall risk, hyponatremia or other electrolyte abnormalities, dysrhythmias (including QTc prolongation), leukopenia/neutropenia, hypotension/syncope or on antihypertensive medications, seizures, motor/cognitive impairments or on CNS depressants or anticholinergic agents, temperature dysregulation, aspiration, dysphagia, obesity, hyperglycemia, hyperlipidemia, risk factors for neuroleptic malignant syndrome (NMS) (e.g., dehydration), or dementia-related psychosis (boxed warning), pregnancy/lactation, or Parkinson's disease; also patients with acute infections or inflammatory processes, or with severe constipation or bowel impaction.

VII. **Dosage Formulations**

A. Brand and generic oral tablet (25 mg, 50 mg, 100 mg, 200 mg)

B. Generic oral disintegrating tablet (12.5 mg, 25 mg, 100 mg, 150 mg, 200 mg)

C. Brand (Versacloz) suspension (50 mg/mL [100 mL])

VIII. **Dosage Ranges and Guidelines**

A. Refer to Table 6–17 for dosage ranges (initial/maximum) and guidelines. Dosages are for adults unless otherwise specified.

1. Older adults: Same as in younger adults, although lower dosages are typically used and are titrated more slowly.
2. Children/adolescents: Start with 6.25–12.5 mg once daily, increase by 12.5–25 mg every 3–5 days to a targeted dosage of 200–400 mg/day taken in divided doses.
3. See "Clinically Relevant Drug Interactions" below and adjust dosages accordingly.

---

[1]Evidence strength varies; readers are referred to the literature for more detailed information.

B. **Titration**: Increase by 25–50 mg every 1–3 days to achieve a target dosage of 300–450 mg after 2 weeks. Some patients may require dosages up to the maximum of 900 mg/day.

   1. Increased risk of seizures, hypotension, myocarditis, and other adverse effects with rapid titration and dosages >600 mg/day. Strict adherence to slow titration is highly recommended. If patient has been off clozapine for ≥48 hours, re-titration is required.

C. **Clozapine Risk Evaluation Mitigation Strategy (REMS) program**:

   1. Because of the risk of severe neutropenia, clozapine is available only through a REMS program.
   2. To prescribe clozapine, providers must first enroll in—and then complete training to be certified by—the REMS program (www.newclozapinerems.com/home).
   3. Patients must be enrolled in the REMS program and adhere to absolute neutrophil count (ANC) testing, as detailed below (see "Monitoring").
   4. Pharmacies must be certified with the REMS program and must verify the eligibility of patients in order to dispense clozapine.

D. **Discontinuation**: For patients on long-term treatment, taper slowly to avoid rebound psychosis, withdrawal dyskinesias, and cholinergic rebound.

Table 6–17. Clozapine indications and dosage guidelines

Treatment-resistant schizophrenia **Suicidality related to schizophrenia or schizoaffective disorder** **Schizoaffective disorder (off-label)**
Adults:
12.5 mg BID or 25 mg QHS for 2–3 days
25 mg BID or 50 mg QHS for 2–3 days
50 mg BID or 100 mg QHS for 2–3 days
75 mg BID or 150 mg QHS for 2–3 days
100 mg BID or 200 mg QHS for 2–3 days
125 mg BID or 250 mg QHS for 2–3 days
150 mg BID or 300 mg QHS for 2–3 days
After 300–450 mg, dosage can be increased by 100 mg once or twice weekly.
175 mg BID or 350 mg QHS
200 mg BID or 400 mg QHS, and so on
Maximum dosage: 900 mg/day
Note: If the patient is actively smoking, can start at a higher dosage.
Parkinson's disease psychosis (off-label)
Initial: 6.25 mg QHS. Increase by 6.25 mg every 2–3 days. Maximum dosage: ~50 mg/day.

Note. BID=twice a day; QHS=every night at bedtime.

IX. Monitoring

A. ANC monitoring is mandatory per REMS program:

1. Routine ANC monitoring:
   a. Baseline (within 7 days of initiation) ANC must be ≥1,500 /μL for general population and ≥1,000/μL for individuals with benign ethnic neutropenia (BEN) before initiation of clozapine.
   b. After initiation of clozapine, ANC must be checked **weekly for 6 months.**
   c. If after 6 months the ANC remains within normal range (i.e., ≥1,500/μL for general population and ≥1,000/μL for BEN), ANC can be checked **every 2 weeks for 6 months.**
   d. If after an additional 6 months ANC remains within normal range, ANC can be checked **every 4 weeks thereafter for remainder of time on clozapine.**
   e. If a patient is off clozapine for **30 days or more,** monitoring must be restarted from baseline as if they were a new patient.
   f. If a patient develops fever with neutropenia, necessitating clozapine discontinuation, continuation of ANC monitoring is required for 2 more weeks based on general population versus BEN population and degree of neutropenia.
2. If patient develops neutropenia:
   a. General population:
      i. Mild neutropenia (ANC=1,000–1,499/μL):
         (a) Repeat ANC within 24 hours for confirmation of low level.
         (b) Can continue clozapine treatment.
         (c) Increase ANC monitoring to 3 times per week until ANC ≥1,500/μL.
         (d) Once ANC is within the normal range, can resume prior ANC monitoring interval.
      ii. Moderate neutropenia (ANC=500–999/μL):
         (a) Repeat ANC within 24 hours for confirmation of low level.
         (b) Hematology consultation is recommended.
         (c) May weigh risks and benefits of interrupting clozapine treatment.
         (d) Increase frequency of ANC checks to daily until ANC ≥1,000/μL, then 3 times/week until ANC ≥1,500/μL, and then weekly for 4 weeks.
         (e) If ANC returns to and remains within normal range, can resume prior ANC monitoring interval.
         (f) Can resume clozapine treatment once ANC ≥1,000/μL.
      iii. Severe neutropenia (ANC <500/μL):
         (a) Repeat ANC within 24 hours for confirmation of low level.
         (b) Interrupt clozapine treatment.
         (c) Same monitoring as for moderate neutropenia, except that patient should not be rechallenged with clozapine unless the benefits clearly outweigh the risks.
         (d) If patient is rechallenged, they should resume treatment as if they were a "new" patient.

b. Benign ethnic neutropenia (BEN):

i. BEN moderate (ANC 500–999/μL):

(a) Repeat ANC within 24 hours for confirmation of low level.
(b) Hematology consultation is recommended.
(c) Can continue clozapine treatment.
(d) Increase frequency of ANC checks to **3 times per week until ANC ≥1,000/μL, then check weekly for 4 weeks**.
(e) If ANC returns to and remains within normal range, can resume prior ANC monitoring interval.

ii. BEN severe (ANC <500/μL):

(a) Repeat ANC within 24 hours for confirmation of low level.
(b) Hematology consultation is recommended.
(c) Interrupt clozapine treatment.
(d) Do not rechallenge with clozapine unless benefits clearly outweigh risks.
(e) Increase frequency of ANC checks to daily until ANC ≥500/μL, then 3 times per week until ANC ≥1,000/μL
(f) If patient is rechallenged, they should resume treatment as if they were a "new" patient.

B. Monitor ECG (see "Adverse Effects").
C. Monitor for constipation and urinary retention (see "Adverse Effects").
D. Monitor for metabolic changes (see "Adverse Effects").
E. Monitor for hypothermia and hyperthermia (see "Adverse Effects").
F. Periodically monitor hepatic function and signs/symptoms of hepatotoxicity (e.g., fatigue, malaise, anorexia, nausea, jaundice, bilirubinemia, coagulopathy, hepatic encephalopathy); if such signs are present, obtain liver function tests (LFTs). If hepatitis or elevated transaminases occur, and systemic symptoms are also present, consider permanent discontinuation of clozapine.
G. If eosinophilia or elevated C-reactive protein (CRP) occurs, evaluate for signs/symptoms of systemic reactions and inflammation (e.g., rash/allergic symptoms, myocarditis, pancreatitis, hepatitis, colitis, nephritis, venous thromboembolism), and if these are present, consider stopping clozapine.
H. Monitor for sialorrhea and aspiration pneumonia, especially in patients with excessive sedation or dysphagia.
I. If patient develops fever (temperature >101.3°F), evaluate for severe neutropenia, infection, or NMS and consider discontinuing clozapine.
J. In the event that a patient develops an acute infection, it may be prudent to decrease the clozapine dosage by as much as 50%, because inflammatory processes have been shown to decrease activity of cytochrome P450 (CYP) 1A2, leading to clozapine toxicity (Leung et al. 2014).
K. **Clozapine/norclozapine serum concentrations**:

1. Check a trough level once at steady state for a given dosage (~3–5 days), with any dosage adjustments, or as clinically indicated if toxicity or nonadherence is suspected.

2. Conventionally, normal lab values are largely based on **12-hour trough levels**, so if BID dosing, draw prior to either the morning or the night dose. If clozapine is given nightly at bedtime, draw 12 hours after the last dose (in the morning).
3. The therapeutic range is **350–600 ng/mL** (clozapine), although adverse effects increase at higher levels. Below 350 ng/mL, response is limited. Levels above 600–700 ng/mL increase the risk of adverse effects, although such levels may be required in certain patients (Remington et al. 2013; Stark and Scott 2012).
4. Evidence indicates that high C reactive protein levels and obesity correlate with poor metabolism of clozapine, requiring lower dosages for therapeutic effect, and that DNA ancestry group may also dictate metabolism of clozapine (de Leon et al. 2022; Shelton et al. 2022).
5. Some fluctuation can occur with repeated levels at the same dosage, but marked fluctuations may indicate nonadherence.
6. The **clozapine:norclozapine ratio** is helpful in determining metabolic status or drug interaction significance.
   a. The normal clozapine:norclozapine ratio is approximately **1.32**. This ratio is obtained by dividing the clozapine level by the norclozapine level.
   b. If the clozapine:norclozapine ratio is greater than 1.32 (meaning that the clozapine level is greater than the norclozapine level), this may indicate that a CYP1A2 or CYP2D6 inhibitor is present, that the patient is a CYP1A2 or CYP2D6 poor metabolizer, or that the metabolism has been saturated (zero-order kinetics), which could mean that the level was drawn at a peak (i.e., clozapine has not had time to metabolize to norclozapine).
   c. If the clozapine:norclozapine ratio is greater than 3.0 (marked), consider whether severe bacterial/viral infections may be present, as these can lead to an inhibition of CYP1A2 activity.
   d. If the clozapine:norclozapine ratio is less than 1.32 (meaning that the norclozapine level is greater than the clozapine level), this may indicate that a CYP1A2 inducer is present or that the patient is a CYP1A2 or CYP2D6 ultrarapid metabolizer.

X. **Relevant Pharmacokinetics/Pharmacodynamics**

A. **Metabolism**: Phase I: CYP1A2 (major), CYP3A4 (major), CYP2C19 (minor), CYP2C9 (minor), and CYP2D6 (minor):
   1. Metabolized to the active metabolite *N*-desmethylclozapine (NMDC; also known as norclozapine)

B. **Time to peak plasma concentration**: ~2.5 hours

C. **Half-life**: For clozapine, 8 hours following a single dose; 12 hours once steady state achieved. For NDMC, 20 hours.

D. **Time to steady state**: Within 1 week

E. **Hepatic impairment**: May be necessary to reduce clozapine dosage.

F. **Renal impairment**: May be necessary to reduce clozapine dosage.

XI. Clinically Relevant Drug Interactions

A. Metabolized by CYP1A2 (major), CYP3A4 (major), CYP2C19 (minor), CYP2C9 (minor), and CYP2D6 (minor)

1. Use caution/decrease dosage when coadministered with strong CYP1A2 inhibitors (e.g., fluvoxamine, ciprofloxacin, enoxacin), strong CYP2D6 inhibitors (e.g., fluoxetine, paroxetine, bupropion), or CYP3A4 inhibitors (e.g., erythromycin, terbinafine, nefazodone).
2. Concomitant use of clozapine with a strong CYP3A4 inducer (e.g., phenytoin, carbamazepine, St. John's wort, rifampin) or a CYP1A2 inducer (e.g., **tobacco smoke**) can significantly decrease the clozapine concentration.
3. Use caution/adjust dosage when clozapine is coadministered with other CYP2D6, CYP3A4, or CYP1A2 substrates, because concomitant use can lead to increased levels of these substrates, and lower dosages of both drugs may be necessary.
4. Valproic acid and related products have mixed data regarding their effects on increasing or decreasing clozapine levels.

B. Studies are inconsistent with respect to correlation between the number of cigarettes smoked per day and clozapine levels, but 7 cigarettes per day may be enough to induce CYP1A2 activity significantly (Mayerova et al. 2018). When a patient stops smoking, steadily decreasing the dosage of clozapine by up to 30% is recommended (Wagner et al. 2020).

C. Avoid use of carbamazepine with clozapine, which can increase the risk of neutropenia.

D. Avoid use of systemic anticholinergics (e.g., glycopyrrolate, benztropine), which may increase risk of constipation or urinary retention.

E. Use of valproic acid or related products may increase the risk of myocarditis or neutropenia,

F. Minimize use of clozapine with benzodiazepines to avoid additive sedation, respiratory depression, and delirium.

G. Minimize use of clozapine with other drugs known to cause orthostatic hypotension.

H. Minimize use of clozapine with other drugs known to prolong the QT interval.

XII. Adverse Effects

A. **See Table 6–1 ("Antipsychotic Class Adverse Effects") at beginning of chapter.**

B. Clozapine's adverse effects include metabolic syndrome, anticholinergic effects, QTc prolongation, orthostatic hypotension, EPS, prolactin elevation, sexual dysfunction, NMS, temperature dysregulation, hyponatremia/syndrome of inappropriate antidiuretic hormone secretion (SIADH), seizures

1. For the full scope of potential adverse effects, see drug labeling (Clozapine package insert).

C. **Boxed warnings**:

1. Agranulocytosis (see "Monitoring" section above)
2. Seizure risk: Use caution in patients with a history of seizures or predisposing risk factors for seizures (e.g., alcohol abuse, CNS pathology, other medications that lower the seizure threshold)
   a. Seizure risk increases at dosages >600 mg/day. If benefits of clozapine outweigh risks and if seizures occur, can consider adding an antiepileptic medication such as valproic acid (although these medications may have additive hematological or other adverse effects).
3. Myocarditis, cardiomyopathy, mitral valve incompetence (see "Monitoring" section above)
4. Other severe cardiovascular and respiratory effects (orthostatic hypotension, syncope, bradycardia, cardiac arrest); use caution in patients with cardiovascular/cerebrovascular disease or with predisposing factors for hypotension.
5. Increased mortality in older patients with dementia-related psychosis

D. **Most common**:

1. Sedation: Largely due to H_1 antagonism; may switch to all nightly dosing until dosages >600 mg are reached.
2. Weight gain/metabolic: Obtain baseline and periodic weight, hemoglobin A1c test, lipids; monitor weight regularly.
   a. Consider lifestyle/behavioral interventions (nutrition, exercise) or the addition of metformin, topiramate, or aripiprazole (Dayabandara et al. 2017).
3. Sialorrhea:
   a. Sialorrhea may be treated with oral systemic antimuscarinic agents (e.g., glycopyrrolate 1 mg BID, benztropine 1 mg BID, trihexyphenidyl 5–15 mg nightly at bedtime) or with clonidine; however, these agents may be less preferred compared with locally administered antimuscarinic agents (atropine sulfate solution, 1%, 1 drop SL nightly at bedtime; ipratropium bromide spray, 0.06%, 1 spray SL nightly at bedtime), which have the advantage of limited systemic adverse effects.
4. Constipation/gastrointestinal hypomotility: Largely dosage dependent. Screen for constipation prior to clozapine initiation and treat as indicated. Monitor bowel function closely, looking for changes in frequency/character of bowel movements and any signs/symptoms of hypomotility-related complications such as nausea, vomiting, abdominal distension, or abdominal pain. Consider abdominal films if needed.
   a. To mitigate risk, consider use of prophylactic laxatives (e.g., polyethylene glycol, bisacodyl, sennosides).

5. Orthostatic hypotension (defined as decrease in systolic blood pressure (SBP) of ≥20 mmHg or diastolic blood pressure (DBP) of ≥10 mmHg within 3 minutes of standing; dosage dependent):
   a. If inpatient, consider measuring periodic orthostatic vitals during titration. If orthostatic hypotension is identified, consider lowering the dose and slowing titration. Assess for any dizziness of lightheadedness, especially when standing; If these occur, slow the titration and replete fluids if needed.
   b. Minimize coadministration with other orthostasis-causing medications (particularly agents with α_1 antagonist activity). Consider slower titration if unable to taper these other medications prior to starting clozapine.
6. Tachycardia:
   a. Largely secondary to anticholinergic effects
   b. Ensure that tachycardia is not simply related to orthostatic hypotension.
   c. Can treat with a beta-blocker.
7. Temperature dysregulation (hypothermia/hyperthermia) and drug-induced fever:
   a. Idiosyncratic; possibly more common during titration
   b. Hyperthermia is possibly secondary to anticholinergic or antidopaminergic effects, whereas hypothermia is possibly secondary to alpha antagonism or 5-HT_{2A} antagonism.
8. QT interval prolongation: Obtain baseline medical history, medication history, physical exam, ECG, and basic metabolic panel (BNP) and correct any electrolyte abnormalities prior to initiation. Stop medication if QTc >500 ms. If a patient develops symptoms suggestive of torsades de pointes/other arrhythmias (e.g., syncope, presyncope, dizziness, palpitations), stop the medication and obtain cardiac evaluation.

E. **Rare adverse effects**:

1. Myocarditis/cardiomyopathy: Monitor for signs/symptoms of myocarditis/cardiomyopathy (e.g., chest pain, dyspnea, persistent tachycardia at rest, palpitations, fever, flu-like symptoms, hypotension, other signs/symptoms of heart failure, ECG changes [low voltages, ST-T abnormalities, arrhythmias, right-axis deviation, poor R wave progression])
   a. Most common within the first 2 months of therapy.
   b. Titration related; increased risk with use of valproic acid or related agents.
   c. If myocarditis/cardiomyopathy is suspected, clozapine should be stopped and a cardiac evaluation obtained, including troponin, C-reactive protein (CRP), and ECG.
   d. Patients with clozapine-induced myocarditis/cardiomyopathy should generally not be rechallenged with clozapine unless the benefits clearly outweigh the risks.

2. Severe neutropenia or agranulocytosis:
   a. Neutropenia is most common within the first 18 weeks of therapy
   b. Idiosyncratic, not dose, titration, or level related; mechanism largely unknown
   c. See "Monitoring" section above.
3. Seizures
   a. Likely dosage related (>600 mg/day conferring higher risk), possibly titration related
   b. Mechanism not well elucidated.
   c. May not necessitate clozapine discontinuation (weigh risks and benefits); dosage reduction should be considered along with adequate treatment of seizures; consider splitting the dosage if >500 mg/day.

XIII. Clinical Pearls/Prescribing Tips

A. If clozapine initiation is desired, ensure that a thorough baseline workup is performed, including labs and physical examination/history.

B. Minimize concomitant use of benzodiazepines, anticholinergic medications, and medications that are prone to causing orthostatic hypotension.

C. Consider prophylactic laxatives when starting clozapine, given the risk of hypomotility/constipation. See "Adverse Effects" for strategies to mitigate/treat adverse effects.

D. NDMC (norclozapine metabolite) has a different binding profile than clozapine and may be responsible for varying side effects and efficacy than the parent compound.

E. Tobacco/cannabis smoking can significantly decrease clozapine levels and should be evaluated at baseline and monitored (see "Clinically Relevant Drug Interactions").

F. Clozapine levels have become a standard of care and should be considered for all patients after initial titration or dosage adjustments.

G. Clozapine has been shown to be beneficial for patients with suicidality secondary to schizophrenia or schizoaffective disorder, regardless of their treatment-resistant status (FDA-approved indication).

H. Because clozapine has low antidopaminergic activity, it is an ideal agent for Parkinson's disease–related psychosis. Often, clozapine dosages required to treat this indication are lower than those needed to treat other indications.

I. Although many of clozapine's side effects (e.g., sialorrhea, seizures, orthostasis, hypotension) are dosage/blood level dependent, the risk of neutropenia appears to be very idiosyncratic and unrelated to these parameters.

J. If the patient is off clozapine for more than 48 hours, re-titration is necessary to prevent orthostatic hypotension and myocarditis.

K. In individuals with moderate or severe tardive dyskinesia, clozapine has been shown to reduce symptoms. In those with mild tardive dyskinesia, clozapine does not appear to worsen symptoms.

Further Reading

Clozaril [package insert]. U.S Food and Drug Administration website. Revised December 2022. Available at: https://www.accessdata.fda.gov/spl/data/c9536339-ee33-4a5f-95fc-80cbb5e048a3/c9536339-ee33-4a5f-95fc-80cbb5e048a3.xml. Accessed March 13, 2024.

Devoto P, Flore G, Vacca G, et al: Co-release of noradrenaline and dopamine from noradrenergic neurons in the cerebral cortex induced by clozapine, the prototype atypical antipsychotic. Psychopharmacology (Berl) 167(1):79–84, 2003 12632247

Gammon D, Cheng C, Volkovinskaia A, et al: Clozapine: why is it so uniquely effective in the treatment of a range of neuropsychiatric disorders? Biomolecules 11(7):1030, 2021 34356654

References

Dayabandara M, Hanwella R, Ratnatunga S, et al: Antipsychotic-associated weight gain: management strategies and impact on treatment adherence. Neuropsychiatr Dis Treat 13:2231–2241, 2017 28883731

de Leon J, Schoretsanitis G, Smith RL, et al: An international adult guideline for making clozapine titration safer by using six ancestry-based personalized dosing titrations, CRP, and clozapine levels. Pharmacopsychiatry 55(2):73–86, 2022 34911124

Leung JG, Nelson S, Takala CR, et al: Infection and inflammation leading to clozapine toxicity and intensive care: a case series. Ann Pharmacother 48(6):801–805, 2014 24619948

Mayerova M, Ustohal L, Jarkovsky J, et al: Influence of dose, gender, and cigarette smoking on clozapine plasma concentrations. Neuropsychiatr Dis Treat 14:1535–1543, 2018 29950838

McQueen G, Sendt KV, Gillespie A, et al: Changes in brain glutamate on switching to clozapine in treatment-resistant schizophrenia. Schizophr Bull 47(3):662–671, 2021 33398325

Remington G, Agid O, Foussias G, et al: Clozapine and therapeutic drug monitoring: is there sufficient evidence for an upper threshold? Psychopharmacology (Berl) 225(3):505–518, 2013 23179967

Roth BL, Driscoll J: PDSP Ki Database. Psychoactive Drug Screening Program (PDSP). University of North Carolina at Chapel Hill and the United States National Institute of Mental Health, 2023

Semba J: Functional role of dopamine D4 receptor in schizophrenia [in Japanese]. Nihon Shinkei Seishin Yakurigaku Zasshi 24(1):13–20, 2004 15027326

Seeman P: Clozapine, a fast-off-D2 antipsychotic. ACS Chem Neurosci 5(1):24–29, 2014 24219174

Shelton C, Ruan CJ, Ertu?rul A, et al: Should we routinely add CRP to clozapine titrations? Learning from three cases. Neuropsychopharmacol Hung 24(4):153–161, 2022 36775960

Stark A, Scott J: A review of the use of clozapine levels to guide treatment and determine cause of death. Aust N Z J Psychiatry 46(9):816–825, 2012 22327098

Tauscher J, Hussain T, Agid O, et al: Equivalent occupancy of dopamine D1 and D2 receptors with clozapine: differentiation from other atypical antipsychotics. Am J Psychiatry 161(9):1620–1625, 2004 15337652

Wagner E, McMahon L, Falkai P, et al: Impact of smoking behavior on clozapine blood levels—a systematic review and meta-analysis. Acta Psychiatr Scand 142(6):456–466, 2020 32869278

Iloperidone

I. **Brand Names**: Fanapt

II. **Therapeutic Class**: Atypical antipsychotic

III. **Mechanism-Based Class**: Dopamine and serotonin receptor antagonist

IV. **Mechanism(s) of Action**

A. D_2 receptor antagonist (Ki=6.3 nM); D_3 receptor antagonist (Ki=7.1 nM).

B. 5-HT_{2A} receptor antagonist (Ki=5.6 nM); some action at other serotonin receptors.

C. Potent norepinephrine a1/a2 receptor antagonist (a1 Ki=0.36 nM)

D. Weak histamine-1 (H_1) receptor antagonist (Ki=437 nM)

E. Negligible activity at muscarinic receptors (Ki >1,000 nM)

V. **Indications**

A. FDA adult:

1. Schizophrenia
2. Acute treatment of manic or mixed episodes associated with bipolar I disorder

B. Evidence-based off-label uses: None at this time

C. FDA pediatric: None

VI. **Major Contraindications and When to Use Caution**

A. **Contraindications**: Hypersensitivity to iloperidone

B. **Use caution**: Patients with baseline fall risk, hyponatremia or other electrolyte abnormalities, dysrhythmias (including QTc prolongation), leukopenia/neutropenia, hypotension/syncope or on antihypertensive medications, seizures, motor/cognitive impairments or on CNS depressants or anticholinergic agents, temperature dysregulation, aspiration, dysphagia, obesity, hyperglycemia, hyperlipidemia, risk factors for NMS (e.g., dehydration), or dementia-related psychosis (boxed warning), pregnancy/lactation, or Parkinson's disease.

VII. **Dosage Formulations**

A. Brand tablet (1 mg, 2 mg, 4 mg, 6 mg, 8 mg, 10 mg, 12 mg)

1. Some formularies offer a titration pack to help prescribers and patients to manage titration and use the dosing in the package insert.

VIII. **Dosage Ranges and Guidelines**

A. Initial: 1 mg BID. Maximum dosage: 12 mg BID (24 mg/day).

B. **Titration**: For schizophrenia, gradually increase by 4 mg/day (divided). For bipolar disorder, increase by no more than 3 mg BID (6 mg/day).

1. Titrate slowly to avoid hypotension. Must restart titration if doses are missed for more than 3 days.
2. Older adults: Same as in younger adults, although lower dosages are typically used and are titrated more slowly.
3. Children/adolescents: Safety/efficacy is not established in this population.
4. See "Clinically Relevant Drug Interactions" below and adjust dosages accordingly.

C. **Discontinuation**: For patients on long-term treatment, taper slowly to avoid rebound psychosis and withdrawal dyskinesias.

IX. Monitoring

A. Baseline and periodic:

1. Labs: CBC with differential (rule out hematological changes), LFTs (rare liver damage risk, contraindicated in hepatic impairment), renal function, electrolytes
2. Metabolic: Weight, hemoglobin A1c test, lipid panel for metabolic risk
3. Extrapyramidal symptoms (EPS): Monitor for abnormal involuntary movements/parkinsonian signs (via Abnormal Involuntary Movement Scale [AIMS]) at baseline and periodically.
4. Consider obtaining an ECG at baseline and periodically if indicated (cardiac risk factors, concomitant high-risk medication).

   1. Iloperidone should be stopped if QTc is found to be persistently >500 ms.

2. Other: Visual changes/ocular exam, sexual changes, mental status changes, blood pressure changes, falls

B. Consider ordering a drug level if there are concerns regarding compliance or metabolism (proposed reference range for schizophrenia: 5–10 ng/mL).

X. Relevant Pharmacokinetics/Pharmacodynamics

A. **Metabolism**: Phase I: cytochrome P450 (CYP) 2D6 (major) and CYP3A4 (major)
B. **Time to peak plasma concentration**: 2–4 hours
C. **Half-life**: 18 hours (CYP2D6 extensive metabolizers) to 33 hours (CYP2D6 poor metabolizers)
D. **Time to steady state**: 3–4 days
E. **Bioavailability**: 96%
F. **Hepatic impairment**: Mild: no dosage adjustment necessary. Moderate: caution recommended; may need dosage reduction. Severe: avoid use.
G. **Renal impairment**: No adjustment should be required

XI. Clinically Relevant Drug Interactions

A. Metabolized primarily by CYP2D6 and CYP3A4:

1. The manufacturer recommends specific reduction of one-half the dose in patients who are poor CYP2D6 metabolizers or who are taking strong inhibitors of CYP2D6 (e.g., fluoxetine, paroxetine, bupropion) or CYP3A4 (e.g., ketoconazole, clarithromycin).
2. Use caution with other drugs known to prolong the QT interval.
3. Potential additive effects can occur with other CNS depressants (e.g., analgesics, antihistamines, barbiturates, opioids, alcohol).
4. As a result of its α_1-adrenergic receptor antagonism, iloperidone may enhance the effects of certain antihypertensives.

B. Weak inhibitor of CYP1A2:
C. Use caution with other drugs known to prolong the QTc, antihypertensive drugs, other CNS depressants, and anticholinergic agents.

XII. **Adverse Effects**

A. **See Table 6–1 ("Antipsychotic Class Adverse Effects") at beginning of chapter.**

B. Iloperidone's adverse effects include metabolic syndrome, anticholinergic effects, QTc prolongation, orthostatic hypotension, EPS, prolactin elevation, sexual dysfunction, NMS, temperature dysregulation, hyponatremia/syndrome of inappropriate antidiuretic hormone secretion (SIADH), seizures

1. For the full scope of potential adverse effects, see drug labeling (Iloperidone package insert).

C. **Boxed warning**: Increased mortality in older patients with dementia-related psychosis

D. **Notable adverse effects**: Hypotension and priapism (both due to potent alpha blockade), weight gain, and QTc prolongation

E. **Other**: Tachycardia, nausea, diarrhea, dizziness, nasal congestion

XIII. **Clinical Pearls/Prescribing Tips**

A. Iloperidone can be administered without regard to meals.

B. Because of iloperidone's high rates of α_1 receptor antagonism, it is recommended that dosages be increased slowly while monitoring for orthostatic hypotension. In addition, monitoring for priapism may be prudent, given iloperidone's binding affinity for this receptor.

C. Iloperidone has a higher risk of QTc prolongation than most other antipsychotics.

D. Iloperidone has two active metabolites (P88 and P95) with varying receptor affinities.

E. While iloperidone may have a lower incidence of EPS, the incidence of weight gain with iloperidone is higher than that with most other SGAs (on par with quetiapine [Huhn et al. 2019]).

Further Reading

Citrome L: Iloperidone: chemistry, pharmacodynamics, pharmacokinetics and metabolism, clinical efficacy, safety and tolerability, regulatory affairs, and an opinion. Expert Opin Drug Metab Toxicol 6(12):1551–1564, 2010 21034370

Iloperidone package insert. U.S Food and Drug Administration, 2022. Available at: https://www.accessdata.fda.gov/spl/data/dcf849c7-acfc-4b32-ab2e-2e3d30c636f2/dcf849c7-acfc-4b32-ab2e-2e3d30c636f2.xml. Accessed March 13, 2024.

Nair A, Salem A, Asamoah AL, et al: An update on the efficacy and safety of iloperidone as a schizophrenia therapy. Expert Opin Pharmacother 21(15):1793–1798, 2020 32735148

Roth BL, Driscoll J: PDSP Ki Database. Psychoactive Drug Screening Program (PDSP). University of North Carolina at Chapel Hill and the United States National Institute of Mental Health, 2023

References

Huhn M, Nikolakopoulou A, Schneider-Thoma J, et al: Comparative efficacy and tolerability of 32 oral antipsychotics for the acute treatment of adults with multi-episode schizophrenia: a systematic review and network meta-analysis. Lancet 394(10202):939-951, 2019 31303314

Lurasidone

I. **Brand Names**: Latuda
II. **Therapeutic Class**: Atypical antipsychotic
III. **Mechanism-Based Class**: Dopamine and serotonin receptor antagonist
IV. **Mechanism(s) of Action**

A. D_2 receptor antagonist (Ki=1.68 nM)
B. 5-HT_{2A} receptor antagonist (Ki=2.03 nM); 5-HT_{1A} receptor partial agonist (Ki=6.75 nM) and 5-HT_7 antagonist (Ki=0.5 nM) (Roth and Driscoll 2023)
C. No significant α_1 receptor antagonism (K=47.9 nM), antihistamine or anticholinergic activity

V. **Indications**

A. FDA adult and pediatric:

1. Schizophrenia (adults and adolescents age 13–17 years)
2. Bipolar I disorder depressive episodes as monotherapy or as adjunct to lithium or valproate treatment (adults and pediatric patients age 10–17 years)

B. Evidence-based[1] off-label uses:

1. Major depressive disorder with mixed features
2. Bipolar major depressive episode with mixed features
3. Impulse-control disorders

VI. **Major Contraindications and When to Use Caution**

A. **Contraindications**: Hypersensitivity to lurasidone; concomitant use with strong cytochrome P450 (CYP) 3A4 inhibitors, including grapefruit/grapefruit juice, or strong CYP3A4 inducers
B. **Use caution**: Patients with baseline fall risk, hyponatremia or other electrolyte abnormalities, dysrhythmias (including QTc prolongation), leukopenia/neutropenia, hypotension/syncope or on antihypertensive medications, seizures, motor/cognitive impairments or on CNS depressants or anticholinergic agents, temperature dysregulation, aspiration, dysphagia, obesity, hyperglycemia, hyperlipidemia, risk factors for NMS (e.g., dehydration), or dementia-related psychosis (boxed warning), pregnancy/lactation, or Parkinson's disease.

VII. **Dosage Formulations**

A. Brand tablet (20 mg, 40 mg, 60 mg, 80 mg, 120 mg)

VIII. **Dosage Ranges and Guidelines**

A. Refer to Table 6–18 for dosage ranges (initial/maximum) and guidelines. Dosages are for adults unless otherwise specified.

1. **Lurasidone must be taken with at least 350 calories of food for adequate absorption.**

---

[1]Evidence strength varies; readers are referred to the literature for more detailed information.

2. Older adults: Same as in younger adults, although lower dosages are typically used and are titrated more slowly.
3. Children (age <10 years): Safety/efficacy is not established in this age group.
4. See "Clinically Relevant Drug Interactions" below and adjust dosages accordingly.

B. **Titration**: Increase in increments of 20 mg every 2 or more days.

C. **Discontinuation**: For patients on long-term treatment, taper slowly to avoid rebound psychosis and withdrawal dyskinesias.

Table 6–18. Lurasidone indications and dosage guidelines

Schizophrenia (PO)
Adults:
Initial: 40 mg/day with meals. Usual dosage: 40–160 mg/day. Maximum dosage: 160 mg/day.
Adolescents (age 13–17 years):
Initial: 40 mg/day with meals. Usual dosage: 40–80 mg/day. Maximum dosage: 80 mg/day.
Bipolar I disorder, depression (PO)
Adults:
Initial: 20 mg/day with meals. Usual dosage: 20–120 mg/day. Maximum dosage: 120 mg/day. *Note*: Dosages >80 mg/day are usually not more effective, in the experience of the authors.
Children/adolescents (age 10–17 years):
Initial: 20 mg/day with meals. Usual dosage: 20–80 mg/day. Maximum dosage: 80 mg/day.

IX. Monitoring

A. Baseline and periodic:

1. Labs: CBC with differential (rule out hematological changes), LFTs (rare liver damage risk, contraindicated in hepatic impairment), renal function, electrolytes
2. Metabolic: Weight, hemoglobin A1c test, lipid panel for metabolic risk
3. Extrapyramidal symptoms (EPS): Monitor for abnormal involuntary movements/parkinsonian signs (via Abnormal Involuntary Movement Scale [AIMS]) at baseline and periodically.
4. Consider obtaining an ECG at baseline and periodically if indicated (cardiac risk factors, concomitant high-risk medication).
5. Other: Visual changes/ocular exam, sexual changes, mental status changes, blood pressure changes, falls

B. Although low risk, monitor for treatment-emergent manic or hypomanic episodes.

C. Consider ordering a drug level if there are concerns regarding compliance or metabolism (proposed reference range for schizophrenia: 15–40 ng/mL).

X. Relevant Pharmacokinetics/Pharmacodynamics

A. **Metabolism**: Phase I: CYP3A4 (major); 2 active metabolites (ID-14283 and ID-14326)
B. **Time to peak plasma concentration**: 1–3 hours
C. **Half-life**: 18 hours
D. **Bioavailability**: 9%–19%
E. **Distribution**: 99% protein bound
F. **Time to steady state**: ~7 days
G. **Use with food**: Must be taken with at least 350 calories for adequate absorption.
H. **Hepatic impairment**:
   1. Mild: No dosage adjustment needed.
   2. Moderate (Child-Pugh B): Initial: 20 mg/day PO; do not exceed 80 mg/day.
   3. Severe (Child-Pugh C): Initial: 20 mg/day PO; do not exceed 40 mg/day.
I. **Renal impairment**:
   1. CrCl≥50 mL/minute: no dosage adjustment needed.
   2. CrCl<50 mL/minute: Initial: 20 mg/day PO, do not exceed 80 mg/day.

XI. Clinically Relevant Drug Interactions

A. Metabolized by CYP3A4 (major):
   1. Use of lurasidone is contraindicated with strong CYP3A4 inhibitors (e.g., ketoconazole, clarithromycin, ritonavir, grapefruit/grapefruit juice).
   2. Use caution/decrease dose when using lurasidone with moderate CYP3A4 inhibitors (e.g., diltiazem). The following is recommended by the manufacturer:
      a. With concomitant moderate CYP3A4 inhibitors, administer half of usual dose, initiate at 20 mg/day and use maximum dosage of 80 mg/day.
   3. Use of lurasidone is contraindicated with strong CYP3A4 inducers (e.g., carbamazepine, St. John's wort, rifampin, phenytoin).
B. Weak inhibitor of CYP3A4
C. Use caution with other drugs known to prolong the QTc, antihypertensive drugs, other CNS depressants, and anticholinergic agents.

XII. Adverse Effects

A. **See Table 6–1 ("Antipsychotic Class Adverse Effects") at beginning of chapter.**
B. Lurasidone's adverse effects include metabolic syndrome, anticholinergic effects, QTc prolongation, orthostatic hypotension, EPS, prolactin elevation, sexual dysfunction, NMS, temperature dysregulation, hyponatremia/SIADH, seizures
   1. For the full scope of potential adverse effects, see drug labeling (Aurobindo Pharma LTD 2023).
C. **Boxed warnings**:
   1. Increased mortality in older patients with dementia-related psychosis
   2. Potential increased risk of suicidal thoughts/behaviors in pediatric/young adult patients. Monitor closely for emergence of suicidal thoughts. For detailed information, the reader is referred to comprehensive sources in the literature (e.g., Fergusson et al. 2005).

D. **Most common**: Sedation, gastrointestinal effects (nausea, vomiting, diarrhea), akathisia and parkinsonism (both dosage-related), agitation

E. **Rare**: Blurry vision, orthostatic hypotension, dizziness, lightheadedness

XIII. **Clinical Pearls/Prescribing Tips**

A. Consider timing dose with meals as in order to achieve adequate absorption; must be taken with food (≥350 cal)

B. Lurasidone's evidence (as monotherapy) for bipolar disorder is primarily with bipolar depression, rather than maintenance treatment or mania.

C. Lurasidone is FDA approved for bipolar I depression in children age 10 years and older and for schizophrenia in adolescents age 13 years and older.

D. Lurasidone has demonstrated a lower risk of metabolic effects/weight gain compared with other SGAs.

E. Lurasidone appears to be relatively weight-neutral, although may cause more weight gain in children.

F. Potent $5\text{-}HT_7$ blockade theoretically portends some cognitive benefit, although this has not been clearly demonstrated in studies.

Further Reading

Greenberg WM, Citrome L: Pharmacokinetics and pharmacodynamics of lurasidone hydrochloride, a second-generation antipsychotic: a systematic review of the published literature. Clin Pharmacokinet 56(5):493–503, 2017 27722855

Ostacher M, Ng-Mak D, Patel P, et al: Lurasidone compared to other atypical antipsychotic monotherapies for bipolar depression: a systematic review and network meta-analysis. World J Biol Psychiatry 19(8):586–601, 2018 28264635

Srisurapanont M, Suttajit S, Likhitsathian S, et al: A network meta-analysis of the dose-response effects of lurasidone on acute schizophrenia. Sci Rep 11(1):5571, 2021 33692392

Wang H, Xiao L, Wang HL, et al: Efficacy and safety of lurasidone versus placebo as adjunctive to mood stabilizers in bipolar I depression: a meta-analysis. J Affect Disord 264:227–233, 2020 32056755

Zheng W, Cai DB, Yang XH, et al: Short-term efficacy and tolerability of lurasidone in the treatment of acute schizophrenia: a meta-analysis of randomized controlled trials. J Psychiatr Res 103:244–251, 2018 29906709

References

Aurobindo Pharma LTD: Lurasidone hydrochloride tablet [package insert]. Revised March 2023. Available at: https://www.accessdata.fda.gov/spl/data/6ab7b492-d568-4fae-a993-f52921691c6a/6ab7b492-d568-4fae-a993-f52921691c6a.xml. Accessed March 13, 2024.

Fergusson D, Doucette S, Glass KC, et al: Association between suicide attempts and selective serotonin reuptake inhibitors: systematic review of randomised controlled trials. BMJ 330(7488):396, 2005 15718539

Roth BL, Driscoll J: PDSP Ki Database. Psychoactive Drug Screening Program (PDSP). University of North Carolina at Chapel Hill and the United States National Institute of Mental Health, 2023

Olanzapine

I. **Brand Names**: Zyprexa, Zyprexa Zydis (orally disintegrating tablets [ODT]), Symbyax (with fluoxetine), Lybalvi (with samidorphan), Zyprexa Relprevv (long-acting injectable)

II. **Therapeutic Class**: Atypical antipsychotic

III. **Mechanism-Based Class**: Dopamine and serotonin receptor antagonist

IV. **Mechanism(s) of Action**

A. D_2 receptor agonist (Ki = 3–106 nM)

B. 5-HT_{2A} inverse agonist (Ki = 1.32–24.2 nM), 5-HT_{2C} inverse agonist (Ki = 6.4–29 nM), 5-HT_{1A} antagonist (Ki = 2,400 nM). Some action at other serotonin receptors.

C. Potent H_1 inverse agonist (Ki = 0.65–4.9 nM)

D. Relatively potent M_1 receptor antagonist (Ki = 2.5–73 nM)

E. Alpha-1a (α_1) receptor (Ki = 109–115 nM)

V. **Indications**

A. FDA adult (and pediatric where indicated):

1. Schizophrenia (adults; adolescents age 13 years and older).
2. Bipolar I disorder, acute treatment of manic/mixed episodes (adults; adolescents age 13 years and older); as monotherapy or as adjunct to lithium or valproate treatment
3. Bipolar I disorder maintenance treatment, as monotherapy or as adjunct to lithium or valproate treatment
4. Bipolar I disorder, major depressive episodes (olanzapine with fluoxetine [Symbyax]) (adults; children age 10 years and older)
5. Acute agitation associated with schizophrenia or bipolar mania (IM)
6. Treatment-resistant depression (TRD; *treatment resistant* is defined as nonresponse to 2 antidepressants of adequate dosage/duration during current episode]) (with fluoxetine [Symbyax])
7. Reduction in weight gain in patients taking olanzapine (Lybalvi)

B. Evidence-based[1] off-label uses:

1. Schizophrenia in children age 6–12 years
2. Agitation associated with schizophrenia or bipolar mania in children age 12 years and older
3. Severe behavioral or psychological symptoms of dementia
4. Anorexia nervosa
5. Chemotherapy-induced nausea/vomiting prophylaxis
6. Delusional infestation
7. Huntington's disease chorea
8. Hyperactive delirium
9. Impulse-control disorders

---

[1]Evidence strength varies; readers are referred to the literature for more detailed information.

VI. Major Contraindications and When to Use Caution

A. **Contraindications**: Hypersensitivity to olanzapine; concomitant use with opioids or in patients undergoing acute opioid withdrawals (Lybalvi); concomitant use of an MAOI (including methylene blue or linezolid) or within 2 weeks of stopping an MAOI (Symbyax); concomitant use of pimozide or thioridazine (Symbyax)

B. **Use caution**: Patients with baseline fall risk, hyponatremia or other electrolyte abnormalities, dysrhythmias (including QTc prolongation), leukopenia/neutropenia, hypotension/syncope or on antihypertensive medications, seizures, motor/cognitive impairments or on CNS depressants or anticholinergic agents, temperature dysregulation, aspiration, dysphagia, obesity, hyperglycemia, hyperlipidemia, risk factors for NMS (e.g., dehydration), or dementia-related psychosis (boxed warning), pregnancy/lactation, or Parkinson's disease.

VII. Dosage Formulations

A. Brand and generic tablet (2.5 mg, 5 mg, 7.5 mg, 10 mg, 15 mg, 20 mg)

B. Brand and generic disintegrating tablet (5 mg, 10 mg, 15 mg, 20 mg)

C. Brand and generic short-acting IM solution (10 mg/2 mL)

D. Brand long-acting IM suspension (210 mg, 300 mg, 405 mg)

E. Brand (Lybalvi) tablet (olanzapine 10 mg/samidorphan 10 mg, 15 mg/10 mg, 20 mg/10 mg)

F. Brand (Symbyax) and generic capsule (olanzapine 3 mg/fluoxetine 25 mg, 6 mg/25 mg, 6 mg/50 mg, 12 mg/50 mg)

VIII. Dosage Ranges and Guidelines

A. Refer to Table 6–19 for dosage ranges (initial/maximum) and guidelines. Dosages are for adults unless otherwise specified.

1. Older adults: Same as in younger adults, although lower dosages are typically used and are titrated more slowly.
2. Children:
   a. Age 13 years and older: Approved for schizophrenia, bipolar manic/mixed episodes, and bipolar depression (in combination with fluoxetine [Symbyax]), although used off-label for other indications. Generally use lower dosages and slower titration in this age group.
   b. Age 10 years and older: Approved for bipolar depression (in combination with fluoxetine [Symbyax]); In general, use lower dosages and slower titration.
   c. Age younger than 10 years: All uses are off-label; if used, use lower doses and slower titration.
3. See "Clinically Relevant Drug Interactions" below and adjust dosages accordingly.

B. **Titration**: In general, increase by 5 mg no more frequently than daily.

C. **Notes on long-acting injectable olanzapine (Zyprexa Relprevv)**:

1. Tolerability/efficacy of PO olanzapine should be established before initiating LAI.
2. Dosage/frequency of LAI is determined by effective/tolerated dosage of oral olanzapine (see Table 6–19, "Schizophrenia [long-acting injection (LAI)]").
3. For individuals not at risk of hypotension, efficacy has been established for 150–300 mg IM every 2 weeks or 405 mg IM every 4 weeks.

4. Because of the risk of severe hypotension, sedation (including coma), and delirium, this LAI must be given in a registered health care facility with easy access to emergency response services, and each patient must be monitored at this facility for at least 3 hours following each injection and be accompanied by someone after this period of time.
5. Because of the risk of hypotension, sedation (including coma), and delirium, Zyprexa Relprevv is available only through the Zyprexa Relprevv Patient Care Program, which requires enrollment of the health care provider, the health care facility, the patient, and the pharmacy.
6. Doses of Zyprexa Relprevv should be administered in the gluteal muscle.

D. **Discontinuation**: For patients on long-term treatment, taper slowly to avoid rebound psychosis, withdrawal dyskinesias, and cholinergic rebound.

Table 6–19. Olanzapine indications and dosage guidelines

Schizophrenia (PO)
Adults:
Initial: 10–15 mg/day. Usual dosage: 5–20 mg/day. Maximum dosage: 20 mg/day (may require lower dosages if used as an adjunct to lithium/valproate)
Adults (Lybalvi):
Initial: olanzapine 10 mg/samidorphan 10 mg. Usual dosage: olanzapine 10 mg/samidorphan 10 mg → olanzapine 20 mg/samidorphan 10 mg. Maximum dosage: olanzapine 20 mg/samidorphan 10 mg/day. *Note*: Off-label olanzapine dosages of up to 30 mg/day have been reported anecdotally in clinical practice as well as in published literature. However, clinicians should bear in mind that fluoxetine can increase the AUC of olanzapine by ~17%. Readers are referred to the medical literature for more detailed information (Gannon et al. 2023).
Adolescents:
Initial: 2.5–5 mg/day. Usual dosage: 2.5–20 mg/day. Maximum dosage: 20 mg/day.
Schizophrenia (long-acting injection [LAI])
See "Notes on long-acting injectable olanzapine (Zyprexa Reprevv)" (Item C under "Dosage Ranges and Guidelines" section above).
Conversion from PO maintenance dosage to IM maintenance dosage
Adults:
Starting IM dosage during first 8 weeks: • 10 mg/day PO ≈ 210 mg IM every 2 weeks or 405 mg IM every 4 weeks • 15–20 mg/day PO ≈ 300 mg IM every 2 weeks
Recommended maintenance IM dosage following 8 weeks of treatment: • 10 mg/day PO ≈ 150 mg IM every 2 weeks or 300 mg IM every 4 weeks • 15 mg/day PO ≈ 210 mg IM every 2 weeks or 405 mg IM every 4 weeks • 20 mg/day PO ≈ 300 mg IM every 2 weeks

Table 6–19. Olanzapine indications and dosage guidelines *(continued)*

Older adults (age ≥65 years):
Initial: 150 mg IM every 4 weeks. Titrations should be done cautiously.
Bipolar I disorder, manic/mixed episodes
Adults (olanzapine tablets or orally disintegrating tablets [ODTs]):
Initial: 10–15 mg/day. Usual dosage: 5–20 mg/day. Maximum dosage: 20 mg/day (may require lower dosages if used as an adjunct to lithium/valproate).
Adults (Lybalvi):
Initial: olanzapine 10 mg/samidorphan 10 mg. Usual dosage: olanzapine 10 mg/samidorphan 10 mg → olanzapine 20 mg/samidorphan 10 mg. Maximum dosage: olanzapine 20 mg/samidorphan 10 mg/day.
Adolescents:
Initial: 2.5–5 mg/day. Usual dosage: 2.5–20 mg/day. Maximum dosage: 20 mg/day.
Acute agitation associated with schizophrenia or bipolar mania (short-acting IM)
Note: IM olanzapine formulation may be given via the IV route for off-label use, but should only be administered in settings where patients can be closely monitored for respiratory depression.
Adults:
Initial: 5–10 mg once; can repeat dose every 4–6 hours Maximum dosage: 30 mg/day in divided doses Lower dosages (2.5 mg) are recommended for older adults. Conversion to PO therapy should be made as soon as possible/feasible. Dose equivalence for olanzapine PO-to-SAI conversion is 1:1.
Bipolar I disorder, depressed episodes, in combination with fluoxetine (Symbyax)
Adults:
Initial: Olanzapine 5 mg + fluoxetine 20 mg/day. Usual dosage: Olanzapine 3–12 mg/day + fluoxetine 25–50 mg/day. Maximum dosage: Olanzapine 12 mg/day, fluoxetine 50 mg/day.
Children/adolescents (age ≥10 years):
Initial: Olanzapine 2.5 mg/day + fluoxetine 20 mg/day. Maximum: Olanzapine 12 mg/day + fluoxetine 50 mg/day.
Treatment-resistant depression (TRD) in combination with fluoxetine (Symbyax)
Adults:
Initial: Olanzapine 5 mg + fluoxetine 20 mg/day. Usual dosage: Olanzapine 3–12 mg/day + fluoxetine 25–50 mg/day. Maximum dosage: Olanzapine 12 mg/day + fluoxetine 50 mg/day.

IX. **Monitoring**

A. Baseline and periodic:

1. Labs: CBC with differential (rule out hematological changes), LFTs (rare liver damage risk; contraindicated in hepatic impairment), renal function, electrolytes
2. Metabolic: Weight, hemoglobin A1c test, lipid panel for metabolic risk
3. Extrapyramidal symptoms (EPS): Monitor for abnormal involuntary movements/parkinsonian signs (via Abnormal Involuntary Movement Scale [AIMS]) at baseline and periodically.
4. Consider obtaining an ECG at baseline and periodically if indicated (cardiac risk factors, concomitant high-risk medication).
5. Other: Visual changes/ocular exam, sexual changes, mental status changes, blood pressure changes, falls

B. Consider ordering a drug level if there are concerns regarding compliance or metabolism (proposed reference range for schizophrenia: 20–80 ng/mL).

X. **Relevant Pharmacokinetics/Pharmacodynamics**

A. **Metabolism**: Phase I: cytochrome P450 (CYP) 1A2 (major), CYP2D6 (minor), Flavin-containing monooxygenase; Phase II: glucuronidation
B. **Time to peak plasma concentration**: PO: 6 hours; SAI: 15–45 minutes; peak concentration ~5 times greater with SAI than with PO
C. **Half-life**: PO: 30 hours; LAI: 30 days
D. **Time to steady state**: PO: 1 week; LAI: 3 months
E. **Bioavailability**: 60%
F. **Distribution**: 93% plasma protein bound
G. **Excretion**: 57% renally, 30% biliary
H. **Hepatic impairment**: Dosages may need modification; the recommended starting dosage is 2.5–5 mg PO, with careful titration, when used as an adjunct for treatment-resistant depression/bipolar depression; for other indications, there are no specific recommendations, although cautious use and careful titration are recommended.
I. **Renal impairment**: No dosage adjustment is needed for olanzapine tablets, ODT, or olanzapine-fluoxetine combination; olanzapine-samidorphan use is not recommended in individuals with an estimated glomerular filtration rate (eGFR) <15 mL/minute.
J. **Special populations**: The mean elimination half-life of olanzapine is 1.5 times greater in older adults (age ≥65 years) than in younger adults. In addition, clearance is ~30% lower in women than in men and ~40% higher in smokers than in nonsmokers; clearance in young smoking males may be 3 times higher than that in older nonsmoking females.

XI. **Clinically Relevant Drug Interactions**

A. Metabolized by CYP1A2 (major) and CYP2D6 (minor):

1. Use caution/decrease dosage with CYP1A2 inhibitors (namely fluvoxamine).
2. Concomitant use with CYP1A2 inducers (e.g., carbamazepine, ritonavir, and notably tobacco smoking) can significantly decrease olanzapine concentrations. Adjust dosages accordingly.

3. Use caution/decrease dosage when coadministered with CYP2D6 inhibitors (e.g., fluoxetine, bupropion, paroxetine), although the effect on plasma concentrations is more minor than with CYP1A2 interactions.

B. CYP2D6 strong inhibition (Symbyax only):

1. Use caution with CYP2D6 substrates (e.g., tamoxifen, aripiprazole).

C. Use caution with other drugs known to prolong the QTc interval, antihypertensive drugs, other CNS depressants, and anticholinergic agents.

D. Olanzapine may antagonize the effects of levodopa and dopamine agonists.

E. Concomitant use of parenteral olanzapine and benzodiazepines can lead to excessive sedation and cardiorespiratory depression (see "Adverse Effects" below).

F. Concomitant use of opioids (e.g., fentanyl, morphine) is contraindicated with Lybalvi due to the antagonistic effects of samidorphan on opioid receptors.

G. Concomitant use of a monoamine oxidase inhibitor (MAOI) (e.g., phenelzine, linezolid) is contraindicated with Symbyax because of the risk of serotonin syndrome with fluoxetine. Concomitant use of other serotonergic medications should likewise be avoided.

XII. **Adverse Effects**

A. **See Table 6–1 ("Antipsychotic Class Adverse Effects") at beginning of chapter.**

B. Olanzapine's adverse effects include metabolic syndrome, anticholinergic effects, QTc prolongation, orthostatic hypotension, EPS, prolactin elevation, sexual dysfunction, NMS, temperature dysregulation, hyponatremia/syndrome of inappropriate antidiuretic hormone secretion (SIADH), seizures

1. For the full scope of potential adverse effects, see drug labeling (Olanzapine package insert).

C. **Boxed warnings**:

1. Increased mortality in older patients with dementia-related psychosis
2. Zyprexa Relprevv: Postinjection delirium/sedation syndrome

D. **Eli Lilly Warning**: Eli Lilly provided a warning of potentially fatal respiratory depression with concomitant IM olanzapine and parenteral benzodiazepines after reports of fatalities related to IM olanzapine/benzodiazepine combinations in 2004–2005 (Marder et al. 2010). However, it is unclear whether the fatalities were directly related to the medication combination, and subsequent controlled studies indicated that the combination is likely safe (Williams 2018; Wilson et al. 2012). Given this controversy, it may be prudent to separate the administration of IM/IV olanzapine and the administration of parenteral benzodiazepines by at least 1 hour (per guidelines from the European Medicines Agency) or to avoid the combination altogether.

E. Olanzapine is notable for its sedating properties and potential for weight gain (at times significant; can be up to 30 lbs or more)/metabolic effects. Olanzapine has moderate anticholinergic activity as well. Taking the entire daily dosage at night can ameliorate daytime sedation.

F. Given their similarities in structure to clozapine, olanzapine and quetiapine may both have a higher incidence of hematological adverse effects (e.g., leucopenia, neutropenia, thrombocytopenia, agranulocytosis, pancytopenia) compared with other SGAs (Arslan et al. 2016; Lander and Bastiampillai 2011; Pang et al. 2017). Monitor CBC with differential routinely.

XIII. **Clinical Pearls/Prescribing Tips**

A. Olanzapine has been shown to be one of the more effective and well-tolerated antipsychotics (Huhn et al. 2019; Lieberman et al. 2005), although its use is often limited by its metabolic side effects; concomitant use with agents such as metformin can reduce these metabolic side effects and weight gain (de Silva et al. 2016; Jiang et al. 2020). A more recently approved combination drug, Lybalvi, which contains olanzapine and samidorphan (an opioid receptor antagonist), has also been shown to reduce the risk of weight gain and metabolic side effects.

B. The daily dosage should be taken at night to reduce the likelihood of daytime sedation.

C. Olanzapine is not removed by hemodialysis.

D. It is notable that for oral or disintegrating olanzapine, time to peak plasma concentration is 5–6 hours, so if rapid effects are desired, consider an alternative option or the short-acting IM formulation of olanzapine.

E. Concentrations of olanzapine are affected by age (increased half-life in older persons), sex (lower clearance in females), and smoking status (higher clearance in smokers), as well as by other drug interactions (mainly CYP1A2).

F. While very rare (0.07%), a postinjection hypotension/delirium syndrome has been documented after administration of the olanzapine long-acting IM injection (Zyprexa Relprevv). This adverse effect may be the result of "dose dumping" (i.e., rapid release of a medication designed for extended release) or accidental IV administration of the medication.

G. To avoid the risks of excessive sedation, respiratory depression, and hypotension, parenteral olanzapine (IM/IV) should not be administered earlier than 1 hour after administration of parenteral benzodiazepine.

H. Dose equivalence for olanzapine PO-to-SAI conversion is 1:1.

Further Reading

Cipriani A, Rendell J, Geddes JR: Olanzapine in the long-term treatment of bipolar disorder: a systematic review and meta-analysis. J Psychopharmacol 24(12):1729–1738, 2010 19828571

Detke HC, McDonnell DP, Brunner E, et al: Postinjection delirium/sedation syndrome in patients with schizophrenia treated with olanzapine long-acting injection, I: analysis of cases. BMC Psychiatry 10:43, 2010 20537128

Kishi T, Matsunaga S, Iwata N: Intramuscular olanzapine for agitated patients: a systematic review and meta-analysis of randomized controlled trials. J Psychiatr Res 68:198–209, 2015 26228420

Komossa K, Rummel-Kluge C, Hunger H, et al: Olanzapine versus other atypical antipsychotics for schizophrenia. Cochrane Database Syst Rev (3):CD006654, 2010 20238348

McDonnell DP, Detke HC, Bergstrom RF, et al: Postinjection delirium/sedation syndrome in patients with schizophrenia treated with olanzapine long-acting injection, II: investigations of mechanism. BMC Psychiatry 10:45, 2010

Olanzapine [package insert]. U.S Food and Drug Administration, 2022. Available at: https://www.accessdata.fda.gov/spl/data/07ce1a1f-b10a-4dfc-a96e-15d1d7db3678/07ce1a1f-b10a-4dfc-a96e-15d1d7db3678.xml. Accessed March 13, 2024.

Roth BL, Driscoll J: PDSP Ki Database. Psychoactive Drug Screening Program (PDSP). University of North Carolina at Chapel Hill and the United States National Institute of Mental Health, 2023

Silva MT, Zimmermann IR, Galvao TF, et al: Olanzapine plus fluoxetine for bipolar disorder: a systematic review and meta-analysis. J Affect Disord 146(3):310–318, 2013 23218251

Tohen M, Calabrese JR, Sachs GS, et al: Randomized, placebo-controlled trial of olanzapine as maintenance therapy in patients with bipolar I disorder responding to acute treatment with olanzapine. Am J Psychiatry 163(2):247–256, 2006 16449478

References

Arslan FC, Aykut DS, Ince C, et al: Neutropenia and thrombocytopenia induced by quetiapine monotherapy: a case report and review of literature. Klinik Psikofarmakol BBülteni 26(3):319–323, 2016

de Silva VA, Suraweera C, Ratnatunga SS, et al: Metformin in prevention and treatment of antipsychotic induced weight gain: a systematic review and meta-analysis. BMC Psychiatry 16(1):341, 2016 27716110

Gannon L, Reynolds J, Mahon M, et al: High-dose olanzapine in treatment-resistant schizophrenia: a systematic review. Ther Adv Psychopharmacol 13:20451253231168788, 2023 37187727

Huhn M, Nikolakopoulou A, Schneider-Thoma J, et al: Comparative efficacy and tolerability of 32 oral antipsychotics for the acute treatment of adults with multi-episode schizophrenia: a systematic review and network meta-analysis. Lancet 394(10202):939–951, 2019 31303314

Jiang WL, Cai DB, Yin F, et al: Adjunctive metformin for antipsychotic-induced dyslipidemia: a meta-analysis of randomized, double-blind, placebo-controlled trials. Transl Psychiatry 10(1):117, 2020 32327628

Lander M, Bastiampillai T: Neutropenia associated with quetiapine, olanzapine, and aripiprazole. Aust N Z J Psychiatry 45(1):89, 2011 21058927

Lieberman JA, Stroup TS, McEvoy JP, et al: Effectiveness of antipsychotic drugs in patients with chronic schizophrenia. N Engl J Med 353(12):1209–1223, 2005 16172203

Marder SR, Sorsaburu S, Dunayevich E, et al: Case reports of postmarketing adverse event experiences with olanzapine intramuscular treatment in patients with agitation. J Clin Psychiatry 71(4):433–441, 2010 20156413

Pang N, Thrichelvam N, Naing KO: Olanzapine-induced pancytopenia: a rare but worrying complication. East Asian Arch Psychiatry 27(1):35–37, 2017 28387211

Williams AM: Coadministration of intramuscular olanzapine and benzodiazepines in agitated patients with mental illness. Ment Health Clin 8(5):208–213, 2018

Wilson MP, MacDonald K, Vilke GM, et al: A comparison of the safety of olanzapine and haloperidol in combination with benzodiazepines in emergency department patients with acute agitation. J Emerg Med 43(5):790–797, 2012 21601409

Paliperidone

I. **Brand Names**: Invega, Invega Sustenna, Invega Trinza, Invega Hafyera

II. **Therapeutic Class**: Atypical antipsychotic

III. **Mechanism-Based Class**: Dopamine, serotonin, and norepinephrine receptor antagonist

IV. **Mechanism(s) of Action**

A. Dopamine D_2, serotonin 5-HT_{2A}, and norepinephrine α_2 receptor antagonist
B. D_2 receptor antagonist (Ki = 1.6 nM)
C. 5-HT_{2A} receptor antagonist (Ki = 1.1 nM), 5-HT7 receptor antagonist (Ki = 2.7); 5-HT_{1A} receptor antagonist (Ki = 617). Some action at other serotonin receptors.
D. H_1 receptor antagonist (Ki = 19 nM)
E. Alpha 1a receptor antagonist (Ki = 2.5 nM)
F. Alpha 2a receptor antagonist (Ki = 3.9 nM)
G. No significant anticholinergic activity

V. **Indications**

A. FDA adult and pediatric:

1. Schizophrenia (adults; adolescents age 12–17 years)
2. Schizoaffective disorder (monotherapy or as adjunct to mood stabilizers and/or antidepressants)

B. Evidence-based[1] off-label uses:

1. Mania associated with bipolar disorder
2. Severe behavioral or psychological symptoms of dementia
3. Impulse-control disorders

VI. **Major Contraindications and When to Use Caution**

A. **Contraindications**: Hypersensitivity to paliperidone or its parent compound, risperidone
B. **Use caution**: Patients with baseline fall risk, hyponatremia or other electrolyte abnormalities, dysrhythmias (including QTc prolongation), leukopenia/neutropenia, hypotension/syncope or on antihypertensive medications, seizures, motor/cognitive impairments or on CNS depressants or anticholinergic agents, temperature dysregulation, aspiration, dysphagia, obesity, hyperglycemia, hyperlipidemia, risk factors for NMS (e.g., dehydration), or dementia-related psychosis (boxed warning), pregnancy/lactation, or Parkinson's disease.
C. Paliperidone extended-release (ER) tablets should not be given to patients with preexisting severe gastrointestinal narrowing or who cannot swallow the tablets whole.

VII. **Dosage Formulations**

A. Brand and generic 24-hour ER tablet (1.5 mg, 3 mg, 6 mg, 9 mg)

1. Do not crush, chew, or divide ER tablet.

---

[1]Evidence strength varies; readers are referred to the literature for more detailed information.

B. Invega Sustenna IM suspension prefilled syringe (39 mg/0.25 mL [0.25 mL]; 78 mg/0.5 mL [0.5 mL]; 117 mg/0.75 mL [0.75 mL]; 156 mg/mL [1 mL]; 234 mg/1.5 mL [1.5 mL])
C. Invega Trinza IM suspension prefilled syringe (410 mg/1.315 mL [1.315 mL]; 273 mg/0.875 mL [0.875 mL]; 546 mg/1.75 mL [1.75 mL]; 819 mg/2.625 mL [2.625 mL])
D. Invega Hafyera IM suspension prefilled syringe (1,092 mg/3.5 mL [3.5 mL]; 1,560 mg/5 mL [5 mL])

VIII. **Dosage Ranges and Guidelines**

A. Refer to Table 6–20 for dosage ranges (initial/maximum) and guidelines. Dosages are for adults unless otherwise specified.
   1. Older adults: Same as in younger adults, although lower dosages are typically used and are titrated more slowly.
   2. See "Clinically Relevant Drug Interactions" below and adjust dosages accordingly.
B. **Titration**: For schizophrenia or schizoaffective disorder, increase by 3-mg increments every 5 or more days. For bipolar mania (off-label), increase in increments of 3 mg/day at intervals of at least 2 days.
C. **Discontinuation**: For patients on long-term treatment, taper slowly to avoid rebound psychosis and withdrawal dyskinesias.

Table 6–20. Paliperidone indications and dosage guidelines

Schizophrenia or schizoaffective disorder (PO) **Mania associated with bipolar disorder (off-label) (PO)**
Adults:
Initial: 6 mg/day. Maximum dosage: 12 mg/day.
Children age ≥12 years:
Initial: 3 mg/day. Maximum dosage: 12 mg if weight ≥51 kg; 6 mg/day if weight <51 kg.
Schizophrenia or schizoaffective disorder (LAI)
Note: Tolerability/efficacy of PO paliperidone or risperidone should be established prior to initiation of LAI.
Invega Sustenna (every 4 weeks)
Loading dose (regardless of PO dose):
Day 0: 234 mg IM injection in the deltoid muscle
Day 7 (±4): 156 mg IM injection in the deltoid muscle
Maintenance dose:
First maintenance dose is typically given 5 weeks after first initiation dose; can be delivered to deltoid or gluteal muscle; can be given up to 7 days before or after monthly due date.

Table 6–20. Paliperidone indications and dosage guidelines *(continued)*

Conversion from PO paliperidone to Invega Sustenna
3 mg/day PO ≈ 39–78 mg IM/month
6 mg/day PO ≈ 117 mg IM/month
9 mg/day PO ≈ 156 mg IM/month
12 mg/day PO ≈ 234 mg IM/month
Conversion from PO risperidone to Invega Sustenna:
1–2 mg PO ~ 39–78 mg IM/month
3 mg PO ~ 117 mg IM/month
4–5 mg PO ~ 156 mg IM/month
6 mg or more PO ~ 234 mg IM/month*
*Because of the higher bioavailability of PO risperidone, 234 mg of Invega Sustenna may not provide comparable levels of paliperidone.
Invega Trinza (every 3 months)
Must be stable on once-monthly LAI (Invega Sustenna) for at least 4 months prior to initiation. Can give initial Invega Trinza injection within 7 days of when next once monthly LAI (Invega Sustenna) would be due. Can be given up to 2 weeks before or after every 3-month due date.
Conversion from Invega Sustenna to Invega Trinza:
78 mg IM/month (Invega Sustenna) ≈ 273 mg IM every 3 months (Invega Trinza)
117 mg IM/month (Invega Sustenna) ≈ 410 mg IM every 3 months (Invega Trinza)
156 mg IM/month (Invega Sustenna) ≈ 546 mg IM every 3 months (Invega Trinza)
234 mg IM/month (Invega Sustenna) ≈ 819 mg IM every 3 months (Invega Trinza)
Invega Hafyera (every 6 months)
Must be stable on Invega Sustenna for at least 4 months or Invega Trinza for at least one 3-month cycle before transitioning to Invega Hafyera. Can give initial Invega Hafyera gluteal injection within 7 days of when next Invega Sustenna injection would be due, or within 2 weeks of when next Invega Trinza injection would be due. Can be given up to 2 weeks before or 3 weeks after every 6-month due date.
Conversion from Invega Sustenna or Invega Trinza to Invega Hafyera
156 mg IM/month (Invega Sustenna) ≈ 546 mg IM every 3 months (Invega Trinza) ≈ 1,092 mg IM every 6 months (Invega Hafyera)
234 mg IM/month (Invega Sustenna) ≈ 819 mg IM every 3 months (Invega Trinza) ≈ 1,560 mg IM every 6 months (Invega Hafyera)

IX. **Monitoring**

A. Baseline and periodic:

1. Labs: CBC with differential (rule out hematological changes), LFTs (rare liver damage risk), renal function, electrolytes
2. Metabolic: Weight, hemoglobin A1c test, lipid panel for metabolic risk
3. Extrapyramidal symptoms (EPS): Monitor for abnormal involuntary movements/parkinsonian signs (via Abnormal Involuntary Movement Scale [AIMS]) at baseline and periodically.

4. Consider obtaining an ECG at baseline and periodically if indicated (cardiac risk factors, concomitant high-risk medication).
5. Other: Visual changes/ocular exam, sexual changes, mental status changes, blood pressure changes, falls

B. Consider ordering a prolactin level if patients exhibit signs of hyperprolactinemia such as sexual dysfunction or gynecomastia/galactorrhea.
C. Consider modifying the paliperidone dosage if starting/titrating carbamazepine or divalproex (see "Clinically Relevant Drug Interactions").
D. Taking paliperidone ER tablets with food may increase paliperidone exposure.
E. Consider ordering a drug level if there are concerns regarding compliance or metabolism (proposed reference range for schizophrenia: 20–60 ng/mL)

X. **Relevant Pharmacokinetics/Pharmacodynamics**

A. **Metabolism**: Phase I: cytochrome P450 (CYP) 2D6 (minor), CYP3A4 (minor); drug transporters: P-glycoprotein
B. **Time to peak plasma concentration**: PO: 24 hours; LAI: Invega Sustenna: 13 days; Invega Trinza: 30–33 days; Invega Hafyera: 29–32 days
C. **Half-life**: PO: 23 hours; LAI (prolonged with gluteal administration): Invega Sustenna: 25–49 days; Invega Trinza: 84–139 days; Invega Hafyera: 148–159 days
D. **Time to steady state**: PO: 4–5 days; LAI: after 4–5 doses
E. **Excretion**: 80% renally (with 59% excreted unchanged); 11% biliary
F. **Bioavailability**: 28%; increased with food
G. **Distribution**: 74% plasma protein bound
H. **Use with food**: Taking paliperidone ER tablets with food may increase paliperidone bioavailability.
I. **Hepatic impairment**: No dosage adjustment needed for PO or LAI with mild to moderate impairment; has not been studied in patients with severe impairment.
J. **Renal impairment**:

1. CrCl <90 mL/minute:
   a. Invega Hafyera: Use not recommended.
2. CrCl ≥80 mL/minute:
   a. PO/Invega Sustenna/Invega Trinza: No dosage adjustment needed.
3. CrCl = 50–79 mL/minute:
   a. PO: Initial: 3 mg/day. Maximum: 6 mg/day.
   b. Invega Sustenna: Loading: 156 mg IM on day 1 and 117 mg IM on day 8. Maintenance: 78 mg IM/month.
   c. Invega Trinza: 273 mg IM every 3 months
4. CrCl = 10–49 mL/minute:
   a. PO: Initial: 1.5 mg/day. Maximum: 3 mg/day.
   b. Invega Sustenna/Invega Trinza: Use not recommended.
5. CrCl < 10 mL/minute:
   a. PO/LAI: Use not recommended.

XI. Clinically Relevant Drug Interactions

A. Metabolized by CYP3A4 (minor), CYP2D6 (minor), P-glycoprotein /ABCB1 (minor):

1. Concomitant use with carbamazepine, a potent inducer of P-glycoprotein, decreases the mean steady-state C_{max} and AUC of paliperidone by 37%.
2. Concomitant use with divalproex increases the C_{max} and AUC of paliperidone by 50%.
3. Concomitant use with paroxetine may lead to increased paliperidone AUC in CYP2D6 extensive metabolizers.

B. Use caution with other drugs known to prolong the QTc, antihypertensive drugs, other CNS depressants, and anticholinergic agents.

C. May antagonize the effects of levodopa and dopamine agonists; may have additive effects in combination with antihypertensive agents.

XII. Adverse Effects

A. **See Table 6–1 ("Antipsychotic Class Adverse Effects") at beginning of chapter.**

B. Paliperidone's adverse effects include metabolic syndrome, anticholinergic effects, QTc prolongation, orthostatic hypotension, EPS, prolactin elevation, sexual dysfunction, NMS, temperature dysregulation, hyponatremia/SIADH, seizures

1. For the full scope of potential adverse effects, see drug labeling (Paliperidone package insert).

C. **Boxed warning**: Increased mortality in older patients with dementia-related psychosis

D. Compared with other SGAs, risperidone and paliperidone are known to have a higher risk of prolactin elevation, with subsequent sexual dysfunction, gynecomastia, and potential galactorrhea.

E. The high D_2 potency of risperidone and paliperidone compared with other SGAs also means a higher risk of EPS.

F. Paliperidone may cause both insomnia or somnolence.

G. The controlled-release formulation could potentially lodge in the gastrointestinal tract, so avoid prescribing for patients with preexisting gastrointestinal tract narrowing or strictures.

XIII. Clinical Pearls/Prescribing Tips

A. Paliperidone (9-hydroxyrisperidone) is the active metabolite of risperidone, so converting between these formulations—including going from an oral formulation of risperidone to an LAI formulation of paliperidone—is fairly straightforward (see Table 6–20). Nonetheless, clinicians should be aware of pharmacogenomic differences between risperidone and paliperidone that can lead to differing concentrations of these medications.

B. Paliperidone utilizes an osmotic controlled-release oral delivery system (OROS) to provide a prolonged release of paliperidone in the gastrointestinal tract. Patients may see a tablet shell in their stool.

C. The first two doses of Invega Sustenna should be given in the deltoid muscle to attain therapeutic concentrations rapidly.

D. Because of the high amounts of paliperidone excreted unchanged in the urine, caution/dosage adjustments are warranted for patients with renal impairment.
E. Except as discussed in the "Clinically Relevant Drug Interactions" section above, paliperidone has minimal drug-drug interactions, and levels are generally not affected by the activity of CYP enzymes, making paliperidone an ideal choice for patients on complex pharmacological regimens or patients who are extensive/poor metabolizers of CYP enzymes that commonly metabolize other antipsychotic agents (e.g., CYP1A2, CYP3A4, CYP2D6).
F. Paliperidone and risperidone are some of the worst offenders when it comes to prolactin elevation, so clinical monitoring is strongly encouraged. Consider augmenting with—or switching to—a partial D_2 receptor agonist, such as aripiprazole, in this case.
G. Invega may be less sedating in comparison with its parent molecule risperidone.

Further Reading

Nussbaum AM, Stroup TS: Paliperidone for treatment of schizophrenia. Schizophr Bull 34(3):419–422, 2008 18375569

Nussbaum AM, Stroup TS: Paliperidone palmitate for schizophrenia. Cochrane Database Syst Rev (6):CD008296, 2012 22696377

Paliperidone [package insert]. U.S Food and Drug Administration, 2022. Available at: https://www.accessdata.fda.gov/spl/data/ea0d63fc-69e1-4447-b98f-62197f385aaa/ea0d63fc-69e1-4447-b98f-62197f385aaa.xml. Accessed March 13, 2024.

Roth BL, Driscoll J: PDSP Ki Database. Psychoactive Drug Screening Program (PDSP). University of North Carolina at Chapel Hill and the United States National Institute of Mental Health, 2023

Quetiapine

I. **Brand Names**: Seroquel, Seroquel XR
II. **Therapeutic Class**: Atypical antipsychotic
III. **Mechanism-Based Class**: Dopamine, serotonin, and norepinephrine receptor antagonist
IV. **Mechanism(s) of Action**

A. Weak D_2 receptor antagonist (Ki=245 nM). Some action at other dopamine receptors.

1. Quetiapine, like clozapine, binds "loosely" to the D_2 receptor, meaning that it dissociates quickly from the receptor after a dose is given, allowing endogenous dopamine to bind thereafter, notably in motor-controlling brain regions, likely leading to decreased risk of motor side effects. However, these frequent "off" periods may require multiple daily dosing to sustain antipsychotic effects throughout the day.

2. Higher dosages correlate with increased D_2 receptor occupancy, with one study indicating that the dosage of quetiapine ER required to occupy 50% of the D_2 receptor is 638 mg/day (Nord et al. 2011).

B. 5-HT_{2A} receptor antagonist (Ki=96–101). 5-HT_{1A} receptor partial agonist (Ki=320–432). Some action at other serotonin receptors.

C. Potent H_1 receptor antagonist (Ki=2.2–11 nM)

D. Weak α_1 receptor antagonist (Ki=220–3,651 nM)

E. Weak M_1 receptor antagonist (Ki=858 nM)

F. The primary active metabolite of quetiapine is norquetiapine, which acts as an inhibitor at the norepinephrine transporter (NET Ki ~7.54 nM) and as a partial agonist at 5-HT_{1A} receptors (Ki ~6.24 nM), likely contributing to quetiapine's antidepressant and antianxiety activity (Cross et al. 2016).

V. **Indications**

A. FDA adult and pediatric:

1. Bipolar disorder, manic or mixed episodes (adults; children age 10 years and older) as monotherapy or as adjunct to lithium or valproate
2. Bipolar disorder, maintenance as adjunct to lithium or valproate
3. Bipolar I or II disorder, depression
4. Major depressive disorder (MDD), as adjunct to antidepressants
5. Schizophrenia (adults; adolescents age 13 years and older)

B. Evidence-based[1] off-label uses:

1. Monotherapy for MDD
2. Rapid-cycling bipolar disorder
3. Adjunctive treatment of refractory OCD
4. Neurocognitive symptoms (e.g., impulsivity) in borderline personality disorder
5. Severe behavioral or psychological symptoms of dementia
6. Neuropsychiatric symptoms of dementia with Lewy bodies not responsive to other treatments
7. Insomnia
8. Impulse-control disorders
9. PTSD
10. Anxiety disorders

VI. **Major Contraindications and When to Use Caution**

A. **Contraindications**: Hypersensitivity to quetiapine

B. **Use caution**: Patients with baseline fall risk, hyponatremia or other electrolyte abnormalities, dysrhythmias (including QTc prolongation), leukopenia/neutropenia, hypotension/syncope or on antihypertensive medications, seizures, motor/cognitive impairments or on CNS depressants or anticholinergic agents, temperature dysregulation, aspiration, dysphagia, obesity, hyperglycemia, hyperlipidemia, risk factors for neuroleptic malignant syndrome (NMS) (e.g., dehydration), or dementia-related psychosis (boxed warning), pregnancy/lactation, or Parkinson's disease.

---

[1]Evidence strength varies; readers are referred to the literature for more detailed information.

VII. **Dosage Formulations**

A. Brand and generic tablet (25 mg, 50 mg, 100 mg, 200 mg, 300 mg, 400 mg)
B. Brand and generic extended-release (ER) 24-hour tablet (50 mg, 150 mg, 200 mg, 300 mg, 400 mg)

VIII. **Dosage Ranges and Guidelines**

A. Refer to Table 6–21 for dosage ranges (initial/maximum) and guidelines. Dosages are for adults unless otherwise specified.
B. **Titration**:
   1. MDD: Increase by 50 mg every 2 or more days.
   2. Bipolar manic/mixed/depressive/maintenance, schizophrenia: Increase by 50–100 mg immediate-release (IR) increments (or up to 300 mg ER increments) every 1–4 days.
   3. See "Clinically Relevant Drug Interactions" below and adjust dosages accordingly.
C. A maximum dosage of 800–1,200 mg/day PO is suggested although not definitive. The FDA-defined maximum is 800 mg/day, although anecdotally dosages up to 1,200 mg/day have been used, including in the authors' practice.
D. Older adults: Maximum dosage: 200–800 mg/day PO is suggested, although not definitive; Lower dosages are typically used in older adults and are titrated more slowly, especially in patients with Lewy body dementia or Parkinson's disease.
E. Patients who are debilitated or at risk for hypotension may require lower dosages and slower titrations.
F. Quetiapine can generally be restarted at the previous maintenance dosage if the interruption of treatment has lasted less than 7 days, but if more than 7 days, should re-titrate based on the initial dosing schedule to avoid orthostatic hypotension risks.
G. **Discontinuation**: For patients on long-term treatment, taper slowly to avoid rebound psychosis, withdrawal dyskinesias, and cholinergic rebound.

Table 6–21. Quetiapine indications and dosage guidelines

Major depressive disorder, adjunctive (PO, ER)
Adults:
Initial: 50 mg QHS. Usual dosage: 150–300 mg/day. Maximum dosage: 300 mg/day.
Bipolar disorder (PO, IR, ER), manic/mixed episodes or maintenance
Adults:
IR: Initial: 50 mg BID. Usual dosage: 400–800 mg/day. Maximum dosage: 800 mg/day.
ER: Initial: 300 mg QHS. Usual dosage 400–800 mg/day. Maximum dosage: 800 mg/day.
Children/adolescents (age ≥10 years):
IR: Initial: 25 mg BID. Usual dosage: 400–600 mg/day. Maximum dosage: 600 mg/day.
ER: Initial: 50 mg QHS. Usual dosage: 400–600 mg/day. Maximum dosage: 600 mg/day.

Table 6–21. Quetiapine indications and dosage guidelines *(continued)*

Bipolar I and II disorder (PO, IR, ER), depressive episodes
Adults:
IR/ER: Initial: 50 mg QHS. Usual dosage: 300 mg/day. Maximum dosage: 600 mg/day (IR), 300 mg/day (ER).
Schizophrenia (PO, IR, ER)
Adults:
IR: Initial: 25 mg BID. Usual dosage: 400–800 mg/day. Maximum dosage: 800 mg/day.
ER: Initial: 300 mg QHS. Usual dosage: 400–800 mg/day. Maximum dosage: 800 mg/day.
Adolescents:
IR: Initial: 25 mg BID. Usual dosage: 400–800 mg/day. Maximum dosage: 800 mg/day.
ER: Initial: 50 mg QHS. Usual dosage 400–800 mg/day. Maximum dosage: 800 mg/day.

Note. BID=twice a day; QHS=every night at bedtime.

IX. **Monitoring**

A. Baseline and periodic:

1. Labs: CBC with differential (rule out hematological changes), LFTs (rare liver damage risk), renal function, electrolytes
2. Metabolic: Weight, hemoglobin A1c test, lipid panel for metabolic risk
3. Extrapyramidal symptoms (EPS): Monitor for abnormal involuntary movements/parkinsonian signs (via Abnormal Involuntary Movement Scale [AIMS]) at baseline and periodically.
4. Consider obtaining an ECG at baseline and periodically if indicated (cardiac risk factors, concomitant high-risk medication).
5. Other: Visual changes/ocular exam, sexual changes, mental status changes, blood pressure changes, falls

B. As when starting any new antidepressant, monitor closely for clinical worsening, suicidality, and behavioral changes, especially during the first few months of treatment and when making dosage adjustments. Families and caregivers of patients should be warned to monitor for agitation, irritability, behavioral changes, and suicidality and to report these to health care providers if they are observed. This topic continues to generate controversy. For a detailed discussion, the reader is referred to comprehensive sources in the literature (e.g., Fergusson et al. 2005).

C. Consider ordering a drug level if there are concerns regarding compliance or metabolism (proposed reference range for schizophrenia: 100–500 ng/mL).

X. **Relevant Pharmacokinetics/Pharmacodynamics**

A. **Metabolism**: Phase I: cytochrome P450 (CYP) 3A4 (major), CYP2D6 (minor); the major active metabolite is norquetiapine, which is an norepinephrine reuptake inhibitor and partial 5-HT_{1A} agonist.

B. **Excretion**: 73% renally (less than 1% excreted unchanged), 20% biliary

C. **Bioavailability**: 9%

D. **Distribution**: 83% plasma protein bound

E. **Time to peak plasma concentration**: 1.5 hours (IR); 6 hours (ER)

1. Pharmacokinetic studies show that quetiapine ER/XR provides a lower peak and a more stable plasma concentration than the IR formulation.

F. **Half-life**: 6 hours

G. **Time to steady state**: 2 days

H. **Hepatic impairment**: 30% lower mean quetiapine clearance

1. Immediate-release: Start with 25 mg/day PO and increase in increments of 25–50 mg/day based on response/tolerability and give in twice daily divided doses.
2. Extended-release: Start with 50 mg/day PO and increase in increments of 50 mg/day based on response/tolerability.

I. **Renal impairment**: For CrCl ≥10 mL/minute, no dosage adjustment necessary; no dosing guidelines available for CrCl <10 mL/minute.

J. **Special populations**: AUC and C_{max} are 41% and 39% lower, respectively, in children/adolescents compared with adults; mean plasma clearance is reduced by 30%–50% in older adults relative to younger adults.

XI. **Clinically Relevant Drug Interactions**

A. Metabolized primarily by CYP3A4 and CYP2D6 to a lesser extent.

1. Use caution/decrease dosage with strong CYP3A4 inhibitors (e.g., ketoconazole, itraconazole, indinavir, ritonavir, nefazodone).
   a. When coadministering quetiapine with a potent CYP3A4 inhibitor, reduce the quetiapine dosage to one-sixth of the original dosage.
2. Concomitant use with CYP3A4 inducers (e.g., phenytoin, carbamazepine, rifampin, St. John's wort) decreases quetiapine concentrations.
   a. When coadministering quetiapine with potent CYP3A4 inducers, increase the quetiapine dosage to as much as 5 times the original dose. When the CYP3A4 inducer is discontinued, the quetiapine dosage should be reduced to the original level over 7–14 days.

B. Use caution with other drugs known to prolong the QTc, antihypertensive drugs, other CNS depressants, and anticholinergic agents.

XII. **Adverse Effects**

A. **See Table 6–1 ("Antipsychotic Class Adverse Effects") at beginning of chapter.**

B. Quetiapine's adverse effects include metabolic syndrome, anticholinergic effects, QTc prolongation, orthostatic hypotension, EPS, prolactin elevation, sexual dysfunction, NMS, temperature dysregulation, hyponatremia/syndrome of inappropriate antidiuretic hormone secretion (SIADH), seizures

1. For the full scope of potential adverse effects, see drug labeling (Quetiapine package insert).

C. **Boxed warnings**:

   1. Increased mortality in older patients with dementia-related psychosis
   2. Potential increased risk of suicidal thoughts/behaviors in pediatric/young adult patients. Monitor closely for emergence of suicidal thoughts. For detailed information, the reader is referred to comprehensive sources in the literature (e.g., Fergusson et al. 2005).

D. Given their similarities in structure to clozapine, olanzapine and quetiapine may both have a higher incidence of hematological adverse effects (leucopenia, neutropenia, thrombocytopenia, agranulocytosis, pancytopenia) compared with other SGAs (Arslan et al. 2016; Lander and Bastiampillai 2011; Pang et al. 2017). Monitor CBC with differential routinely.

E. Weight gain and sedation are relatively common adverse effects with quetiapine.

XIII. **Clinical Pearls/Prescribing Tips**

A. Target dosages vary based on indication: 150–300 mg/day for adjunctive treatment in MDD, 300–600 mg/day for bipolar depression, and 400–800 mg/day for both bipolar mania/maintenance treatment and schizophrenia.

B. Whereas IR and ER quetiapine are considered bioequivalent, IR dosing should generally be split into 2–3 doses per day. ER/XR dosing is beneficial for maintaining D_2 receptor blockade above the therapeutic threshold (>60%) for optimal antipsychotic effects throughout the day.

C. May potentially result in false-positive results for methadone and tricyclic antidepressants.

D. Quetiapine may be a good choice for patients who have experienced hyperprolactinemia or parkinsonism with other antipsychotic agents due to its low propensity for both; however, quetiapine has high rates of anticholinergic effects, leading to more constipation, urinary retention, and confusion.

E. Quetiapine has evidence of efficacy in PTSD (Villarreal et al. 2016) and generalized anxiety disorder (Maneeton et al. 2016), as well as improving anxiety in the context of mood disorders (Crapanzano et al. 2021); thus, quetiapine may be a reasonable choice for minimizing polypharmacy in patients with co-occurring psychiatric disorders responsive to quetiapine (e.g., a patient with bipolar disorder and PTSD). There is also evidence to support quetiapine's use in treatment-resistant generalized anxiety disorder.

F. Although quetiapine can be quite sedating, this effect can usually be minimized by giving the majority or all of the daily dosage at bedtime. Patients may actually benefit from this effect, particularly if they are experiencing insomnia as part of their clinical picture (although not recommended for insomnia alone). The majority of H_1 receptors are occupied at a quetiapine dosage of ~50 mg, which is far from the maximum recommended dosage for this medication.

G. Norquetiapine, the primary active metabolite of quetiapine, has effects at the NET and $5\text{-}HT_{1A}$ receptors that likely explain the unique antidepressant and antianxiety properties of quetiapine.

Further Reading

Hutton P, Taylor PJ, Mulligan L, et al: Quetiapine immediate release v. placebo for schizophrenia: systematic review, meta-analysis and reappraisal. Br J Psychiatry 206(5):360–370, 2015 25934300

Kishi T, Ikuta T, Sakuma K, et al: Comparison of quetiapine immediate- and extended-release formulations for bipolar depression: a systematic review and network meta-analysis of double-blind, randomized placebo-controlled trials. J Psychiatr Res 115:121–128, 2019 31128502

Quetiapine package insert. U.S Food and Drug Administration, 2022. Available at: https://www.accessdata.fda.gov/spl/data/1b417ed8-bf67–42e5–9e56–53397d40fd5d/1b417ed8-bf67–42e5–9e56–53397d40fd5d.xml. Accessed March 13, 2024.

Roth BL, Driscoll J: PDSP Ki Database. Psychoactive Drug Screening Program (PDSP). University of North Carolina at Chapel Hill and the United States National Institute of Mental Health, 2023

References

Arslan FC, Aykut DS, Ince C, et al: Neutropenia and thrombocytopenia induced by quetiapine monotherapy: a case report and review of literature. Klinik Psikofarmakol BBülteni 26(3):319–323, 2016

Crapanzano C, Damiani S, Guiot C: Quetiapine in the anxiety dimension of mood disorders: a systematic review of the literature to support clinical practice. J Clin Psychopharmacol 41(4):436–449, 2021 34166261

Cross AJ, Widzowski D, Maciag C, et al: Quetiapine and its metabolite norquetiapine: translation from in vitro pharmacology to in vivo efficacy in rodent models. Br J Pharmacol 173(1):155–166, 2016 26436896

Fergusson D, Doucette S, Glass KC, et al: Association between suicide attempts and selective serotonin reuptake inhibitors: systematic review of randomised controlled trials. BMJ 330(7488):396, 2005 15718539

Lander M, Bastiampillai T: Neutropenia associated with quetiapine, olanzapine, and aripiprazole. Aust N Z J Psychiatry 45(1):89, 2011 21058927

Maneeton N, Maneeton B, Woottiluk P, et al: Quetiapine monotherapy in acute treatment of generalized anxiety disorder: a systematic review and meta-analysis of randomized controlled trials. Drug Des Devel Ther 10:259–276, 2016 26834458

Nord M, Nyberg S, Brogren J, et al: Comparison of D2 dopamine receptor occupancy after oral administration of quetiapine fumarate immediate-release and extended-release formulations in healthy subjects. Int J Neuropsychopharmacol 14(10):1357–1366, 2011 21477416

Pang N, Thrichelvam N, Naing KO: Olanzapine-induced pancytopenia: a rare but worrying complication. East Asian Arch Psychiatry 27(1):35–37, 2017 28387211

Villarreal G, Hamner MB, Cañive JM, et al: Efficacy of quetiapine monotherapy in posttraumatic stress disorder: a randomized, placebo-controlled trial. Am J Psychiatry 173(12):1205–1212, 2016 27418378

Risperidone

I. **Brand Names**: Risperdal, Risperdal M-Tab (ODT), Risperdal Consta, Perseris, Rykindo, Uzedy

II. **Therapeutic Class**: Atypical antipsychotic

III. **Mechanism-Based Class**: Dopamine, serotonin, and norepinephrine receptor antagonist

IV. **Mechanism(s) of Action**

A. D_2 receptor antagonist (Ki=3.57 nM); Some action at other dopamine receptors.

B. Potent 5-HT_{2A} receptor antagonist/inverse agonist (Ki=0.17 nM); 5-HT_{2C} receptor inverse agonist (Ki=12.0 nM); 5-HT_{1A} receptor antagonist (Ki=423). Some action at other serotonin receptors.

C. Histamine-1 (H_1) receptor antagonist/inverse agonist (Ki=20.1 nM)

D. Alpha-1 (α_1)-adrenergic receptor antagonist (α_{1A} Ki=5.0 nM) (Roth and Driscoll 2023)

E. Alpha-2 (α_2)-adrenergic receptor antagonist (α_{2A} Ki=16.5 nM)

F. Negligible anticholinergic activity

V. **Indications**

A. FDA adult and pediatric:

1. Schizophrenia (adults; children age 13 years and older)
2. Bipolar I disorder manic/mixed episodes (adults; children age 10 years and older) as monotherapy or adjunct to lithium or valproate
3. Irritability associated with autism spectrum disorder (ASD) (children age 5 years and older)

B. Evidence-based[1] off-label uses:

1. Moderate to severe tics associated with Tourette's disorder
2. Severe disruptive behaviors associated with oppositional defiant disorder or other disruptive behavioral disorders
3. Delirium in the pediatric intensive care unit
4. Severe behavioral or psychological symptoms of dementia
5. OCD

VI. **Major Contraindications and When to Use Caution**

A. **Contraindications**: Hypersensitivity to risperidone or paliperidone

B. **Use caution**: Patients with baseline fall risk, hyponatremia or other electrolyte abnormalities, dysrhythmias (including QTc prolongation), leukopenia/neutropenia, hypotension/syncope or on antihypertensive medications, seizures, motor/cognitive impairments or on CNS depressants or anticholinergic agents, temperature dysregulation, aspiration, dysphagia, obesity, hyperglycemia, hyperlipidemia, risk factors for NMS (e.g., dehydration), or dementia-related psychosis (boxed warning), pregnancy/lactation, or Parkinson's disease.

[1]Evidence strength varies; readers are referred to the literature for more detailed information.

VII. **Dosage Formulations**

A. Brand and generic tablet (0.25 mg [generic only], 0.5 mg, 1 mg, 2 mg, 3 mg, 4 mg)
B. Generic disintegrating tablet (0.25 mg, 0.5 mg, 1 mg, 2 mg, 3 mg, 4 mg)
C. Brand and generic oral solution (1 mg/mL [30 mL])
D. Brand (Risperdal Consta) intramuscular extended-release (ER) suspension (12.5 mg, 25 mg, 37.5 mg, 50 mg)
E. Brand (Perseris) subcutaneous prefilled syringe (90 mg, 120 mg)
F. Brand (Rykindo) reconstituted ER suspension (12.5 mg, 25 mg, 37.5 mg, 50 mg)
G. Brand (Uzedy) subcutaneous prefilled syringe (50 mg, 75 mg, 100 mg, 125 mg, 150 mg, 200 mg, 250 mg)

VIII. **Dosage Ranges and Guidelines**

A. Refer to Table 6–22 for dosage ranges (initial/maximum) and guidelines. Dosages are for adults unless otherwise specified.
   1. Older adults: Same as in younger adults, although lower dosages are typically used and are titrated more slowly.
   2. Children age <5 years: Safety/efficacy not established; safety/efficacy of LAI has not been established in this population.
   3. See "Clinically Relevant Drug Interactions" section below and adjust dosages accordingly.

B. **Titration**: Increase dosage in increments of 1–2 mg every 24 hours for adults, and in increments of 0.5–1 mg/day for adolescents:
   1. Irritability associated with ASD: Can increase from 0.25 mg (if 15–19 kg [33–42 lb]) or 0.5 mg (if ≥20 kg [44 lb]) to 0.5 mg and 1 mg, respectively, after 4 days. Then, after 14 days, increase in increments of 0.25 and 0.5 mg, respectively, every 2 weeks or more.

C. **Discontinuation**: For patients on long-term treatment, taper slowly to avoid rebound psychosis and withdrawal dyskinesias.

Table 6–22. Risperidone **indications and dosage guidelines**

Schizophrenia (PO)
Adults:
Initial: 1–2 mg/day (1–2 times daily). Usual dosage: 4–8 mg/day. Maximum dosage: 16 mg/day. *Note:* Dosages >8 mg/day are associated with increased side effects and minimal benefit and are thus not generally recommended.
Adolescents:
Initial: 0.5 mg/day (1–2 times daily). Usual dosage: 1–6 mg/day. Maximum dosage: 6 mg/day.
Schizophrenia (long-acting IM/subcutaneous)
Note: Tolerability/efficacy of PO paliperidone or risperidone should be established prior to initiation of LAI.

Table 6–22. Risperidone indications and dosage guidelines *(continued)*

Risperdal Consta (every 2 weeks)
Intramuscular in deltoid or gluteal muscle only
No loading doses
Usual dosage: 25 mg every 2 weeks. Maximum dosage: 50 mg every 2 weeks.
Supplement with PO dosing for 3 weeks following initial injection.
Can increase dosage at intervals of 4 weeks or greater.
Consider initial dose of 12.5 mg IM every 2 weeks in patients with renal/hepatic dysfunction, those on medications that increase plasma risperidone levels, and those with a history of poor tolerability.
Conversion from PO risperidone:
1 mg/day PO ≈ 12.5 mg IM/2 weeks
2–3 mg/day PO ≈ 25 mg IM/2 weeks
3–5 mg/day PO ≈ 37.5 mg IM/2 weeks
4–5 mg/day PO ≈ 50 mg IM/2 weeks*
*Manufacturer recommends maximum dosage of 50 mg/2 weeks. *Note:* Other sources may recommend a different conversion approach. Readers are referred to the manufacturer's full prescribing information for guidance (Janssen Pharmaceuticals 2021).
Perseris (once monthly)
Subcutaneous in abdomen or back of upper arm only
No loading doses
No oral supplementation required per manufacturer.
Initial: 90 or 120 mg subcutaneous once monthly
Maximum: 120 mg subcutaneous monthly
Conversion from PO risperidone:
3 mg/day PO ≈ 90 mg subcutaneous/month
4 mg/day PO ≈ 120 mg subcutaneous/month
Note: Patients on dosages < 3 mg/day or > 4 mg/day may not be candidates for Perseris.
Bipolar mania/maintenance (PO) as monotherapy or adjunct to lithium/valproate
Adults:
Initial: 2–3 mg/day taken as a single dose or in 2 divided doses. Usual dosage: 1–6 mg/day. Maximum dosage: 6 mg/day.
Note: Risperidone is FDA approved for the maintenance treatment of bipolar disorder in the Risperdal Consta formulation.
Children/adolescents (age 10–17 years):
Initial: 0.5mg/day. Usual dosage 1–2.5 mg/day. Maximum dosage: 6 mg/day.

Table 6–22. Risperidone indications and dosage guidelines *(continued)*

Irritability associated with autism spectrum disorder (PO)
Children/adolescents:
Weight 15–19 kg: Initial: 0.25 mg/day. Usual dosage: 0.5–3 mg/day. Maximum dosage: 3 mg/day.
Weight ≥20 kg: Initial: 0.5 mg/day. Usual dosage: 0.5–3 mg/day. Maximum dosage: 3 mg/day.
Moderate to severe tics associated with Tourette's disorder (off-label) (PO)
Adults:
Initial: 0.5 mg/day. Usual dosage: 1–4 mg/day. Maximum dosage: 6 mg/day.
Children/adolescents:
Initial: 0.125–0.5 mg/day. Usual dosage: 1–4 mg/day. Maximum dosage: 6 mg/day.
Obsessive-compulsive disorder, refractory (off-label) (PO)
Initial: 0.25–0.5 mg/day. Usual dosage: 0.5–2 mg/day. Maximum dosage: 3 mg/day.

IX. Monitoring

A. Baseline and periodic:

1. Labs: CBC with differential (rule out hematological changes), LFTs (rare liver damage risk, contraindicated in hepatic impairment), renal function, electrolytes
2. Metabolic: Weight, hemoglobin A1c test, lipid panel for metabolic risk
3. Extrapyramidal symptoms (EPS): Monitor for abnormal involuntary movements/parkinsonian signs (via Abnormal Involuntary Movement Scale [AIMS]) at baseline and periodically.
4. Consider obtaining an ECG at baseline and periodically if indicated (cardiac risk factors, concomitant high-risk medication).
5. Other: Visual changes/ocular exam, sexual changes, mental status changes, blood pressure changes, falls

B. Consider ordering a prolactin level if patients exhibit signs of hyperprolactinemia such as sexual dysfunction or gynecomastia/galactorrhea.

C. Consider ordering a drug level if there are concerns regarding compliance or metabolism (proposed therapeutic range for schizophrenia: 20–60 ng/mL); levels for risperidone are calculated as the total of the parent compound plus paliperidone (9-hydroxyrisperidone).

X. Relevant Pharmacokinetics/Pharmacodynamics

A. **Metabolism**: Phase I: cytochrome P450 (CYP) 2D6 (major), CYP3A4 (minor); drug transporters: P-glycoprotein (major); active metabolite is 9-hydroxyrisperidone (paliperidone)

B. **Bioavailability**: 70%

C. **Distribution**: 90% plasma protein bound
D. **Time to peak plasma concentration**: PO: 1–2 hours (prolonged to 17 hours in poor metabolizers); LAI: subcutaneous (Perseris): first peak 4–6 hours, second peak 10–14 days
E. **Half-life**: PO: 3–20 hours; LAI–IM (Risperdal Consta): 3–6 days; subcutaneous (Perseris): 9–11 days
F. **Time to steady state**: PO: 1–5 days (extensive vs. poor metabolizers); LAI–IM (Risperdal Consta): achieved after 4 injections; subcutaneous (Perseris): by the end of second injection
G. **Excretion**: 70% renally (as paliperidone), 14% biliary
H. **Hepatic impairment**:
   1. Child-Pugh A or B: Reduced dosages may be needed.
   2. Child-Pugh C: PO: Start with 0.5 mg BID and titrate in increments of 0.5 mg or less. For dosages above 1.5 mg BID, titrations should be at intervals of 1 week or greater. IM: Start at 12.5–25 mg every 2 weeks. Subcutaneous: May use 90 mg/month if patient tolerates 3 mg PO risperidone.
I. **Renal impairment**:
   1. CrCl>60 mL/minute:
      a. PO/IM/subcutaneous: No adjustments needed.
   2. CrCl=30–60 mL/minute:
      a. PO: Initiate at 50%–75% of usual dose for specific indication; titrate cautiously; maximum dosage 75% of usual indication dosage.
   3. CrCl 10–<30 mL/minute PO or 10–60 mL/minute LAI IM/subcutaneous:
      a. PO: Initiate at 50% of usual dose for specific indication; titrate cautiously; maximum dose 50% of usual indication dose.
      b. IM: Caution recommended (consider therapeutic drug monitoring). Start at 12.5–25 mg every 2 weeks with incremental titrations of 12.5 mg not more often than every 4 weeks.
      c. Subcutaneous: Caution recommended (consider therapeutic drug monitoring); in general, one 90 mg/month dose recommended (if patient is able to tolerate 3 mg/day PO risperidone)
   4. CrCl<10 mL/minute:
      a. PO: Alternative agents recommended; maximum dosage 25% of usual indication dosage.
      b. IM: Alternative agents recommended (consider therapeutic drug monitoring); do not exceed 12.5–25 mg every 2 weeks.
      c. Subcutaneous: Avoid use.
J. **Special populations**: In older individuals, renal clearance is decreased and elimination half-lives are increased.

XI. Clinically Relevant Drug Interactions

A. Metabolized by CYP2D6 (major), CYP3A4 (major), and substrate of P-glycoprotein/ABCB1

1. Use caution/decrease dosage with strong CYP3A4 inhibitors (e.g., ketoconazole, itraconazole, indinavir, ritonavir, nefazodone).
2. Concomitant use with CYP3A4 inducers (e.g., carbamazepine, phenytoin, St. John's wort, rifampin, phenobarbital) may significantly decrease serum concentrations of risperidone. The following recommendations are provided from the manufacturer:
    a. For Perseris: Increase 90 mg to 120 mg and consider starting supplemental PO risperidone. In patients on 120 mg already, consider starting supplemental PO risperidone.
3. Use caution/decrease dosage with strong CYP2D6 inhibitors (e.g., fluoxetine, bupropion, paroxetine). The following recommendations are provided from the manufacturer:
    a. For Perseris: In patients on 120 mg, it is recommended to decrease to 90 mg.

B. Use caution with other drugs known to prolong the QTc, antihypertensive drugs, other CNS depressants and anticholinergic agents

C. May antagonize the effects of levodopa and dopamine agonists.

XII. Adverse Effects

A. **See Table 6–1 ("Antipsychotic Class Adverse Effects") at beginning of chapter.**

B. Risperidone's adverse effects include metabolic syndrome, anticholinergic effects, QTc prolongation, orthostatic hypotension, EPS, prolactin elevation, sexual dysfunction, NMS, temperature dysregulation, hyponatremia/SIADH, seizures

1. For the full scope of potential adverse effects, see drug labeling (Risperidone package insert).

C. **Boxed warning**: Increased mortality in older patients with dementia-related psychosis

D. Compared with other SGAs, risperidone and paliperidone are known to carry a higher risk of prolactin elevation, with subsequent sexual dysfunction, gynecomastia, and potential galactorrhea.

E. The high D_2 potency of risperidone and paliperidone compared with other SGAs also means a higher risk of EPS.

F. Compared with paliperidone, risperidone is somewhat less sedating, and in general is moderately sedating compared with other atypical antipsychotics. However, insomnia is also possible.

G. Weight gain risk is moderate with risperidone and paliperidone, although likely not as significant as with olanzapine and clozapine.

XIII. Clinical Pearls/Prescribing Tips

A. Risperidone is generally well tolerated, effective, and inexpensive, so it is often a good first-choice agent when starting an antipsychotic in an individual who has never used these medications.

B. Because the active metabolite of risperidone is paliperidone, oral risperidone can also be easily converted to an LAI formulation of paliperidone (see Table 6–20).
C. Paliperidone and risperidone are some of the worst offenders when it comes to prolactin elevation, so clinical monitoring is strongly encouraged. Consider augmenting with, or switching to, a partial D_2 agonist such as aripiprazole in this case.
D. Because the active metabolite of risperidone (paliperidone) is largely eliminated unchanged in the urine, dosage adjustments for risperidone are required for those with renal dysfunction.

Further Reading

Chopko TC, Lindsley CW: Classics in chemical neuroscience: risperidone. ACS Chem Neurosci 9(7):1520–1529, 2018 29695153

Rattehalli RD, Zhao S, Li BG, et al: Risperidone versus placebo for schizophrenia. Cochrane Database Syst Rev 12(12):CD006918, 2016 27977041

Risperidone package insert. U.S Food and Drug Administration, 2022. Available at: https://www.accessdata.fda.gov/spl/data/d5dfbee0-a196-0c56-e053-2995a90a3547/d5dfbee0-a196-0c56-e053-2995a90a3547.xml. Accessed March 13, 2024.

References

Janssen Pharmaceuticals: Risperdal Consta (risperidone) long-acting injection (package insert). Revised February 2021. Available at: https://www.janssenlabels.com/package-insert/product-monograph/prescribing-information/RISPERDAL+CONSTA-pi.pdf. Accessed July 30, 2024.

Roth BL, Driscoll J: PDSP Ki Database. Psychoactive Drug Screening Program (PDSP). University of North Carolina at Chapel Hill and the United States National Institute of Mental Health, 2023

Ziprasidone

I. **Brand Names**: Geodon
II. **Therapeutic Class**: Atypical antipsychotic
III. **Mechanism-Based Class**: Dopamine and serotonin receptor antagonist
IV. **Mechanism(s) of Action**

A. D_2 receptor antagonist (Ki=4.8 nM); some action at other dopamine receptors.
B. Potent 5-HT_{2A} receptor antagonist (Ki=0.08–1.4 nM); 5-HT_{1A} partial agonist (Ki 2.5–76 nM). Some action at other serotonin receptors.
C. Weak histamine-1 (H_1) receptor antagonist (Ki=15–130 nM)
D. Alpha-1 (α_1)-adrenergic receptor antagonist (α_{1A} Ki=18 nM) (Roth and Driscol 2023)
E. Negligible anticholinergic activity
F. hERG (potassium ion channel) antagonist (Ki=169)

V. **Indications**

A. FDA adult:

1. Schizophrenia
2. Bipolar I disorder manic/mixed episodes (monotherapy)
3. Bipolar I disorder maintenance treatment (as adjunct to lithium or valproate)
4. Acute agitation associated with schizophrenia

B. Evidence-based[1] off-label uses:

1. Acute agitation associated with schizophrenia in geriatric or child/adolescent patients or acute agitation associated with other psychiatric illnesses
2. Bipolar I manic/mixed episodes in children age 10–17 years
3. Tourette's disorder
4. Severe behavioral or psychological symptoms of dementia

C. FDA pediatric: None

VI. **Major Contraindications and When to Use Caution**

A. **Contraindications**: Hypersensitivity to ziprasidone; those with known history of QT prolongation, recent acute myocardial infarction, uncompensated heart failure, or cardiac arrhythmias; concomitant use with other drugs known to prolong QT interval

B. **Use caution**: Patients with baseline fall risk, hyponatremia or other electrolyte abnormalities, dysrhythmias (including QTc prolongation), leukopenia/neutropenia, hypotension/syncope or on antihypertensive medications, seizures, motor/cognitive impairments or on CNS depressants or anticholinergic agents, temperature dysregulation, aspiration, dysphagia, obesity, hyperglycemia, hyperlipidemia, risk factors for NMS (e.g., dehydration), or dementia-related psychosis (boxed warning), pregnancy/lactation, or Parkinson's disease.

VII. **Dosage Formulations**

A. Brand or generic oral capsule (20 mg, 40 mg, 60 mg, 80 mg)
B. Brand or generic short-acting IM solution (20 mg)

VIII. **Dosage Ranges and Guidelines**

A. Refer to Table 6–23 for dosage ranges (initial/maximum) and guidelines. Dosages are for adults unless otherwise specified.

B. **Titration**: Increase in increments of 40 mg (or 20 mg BID) every 2 days to 1–2 weeks.

1. Older adults: Same as in younger adults, although lower dosages are typically used and are titrated more slowly.
2. Children/adolescents: All uses in this age group are off-label.
3. See "Clinically Relevant Drug Interactions" below and adjust dosages accordingly.

C. **Absorption of ziprasidone is 2 times greater in the presence of food (requires 500 calories for adequate absorption).**

D. **Discontinuation**: For patients on long-term treatment, taper slowly to avoid rebound psychosis and withdrawal dyskinesias.

---

[1]Evidence strength varies; readers are referred to the literature for more detailed information.

Table 6–23. Ziprasidone indications and dosage guidelines

Schizophrenia (PO)
Adults:
Initial: 20 mg BID with food. Usual dosage 60–80 mg BID. Maximum dosage 80 mg BID.
Bipolar I disorder— manic/mixed episodes (monotherapy) (PO) maintenance treatment (as adjunct to lithium/valproate therapy) (PO)
Adults:
Initial: 40 mg BID with food. Usual dosage: 60–80 mg BID. Maximum dosage: 80 mg BID.
Acute agitation associated with schizophrenia (short-acting IM)
Adults:
Only give 10–20 mg per dose. Give as 10 mg every 2 hours or 20 mg every 4 hours. Maximum dosage: 40 mg/day. Do not use IM for more than 3 consecutive days. Convert to PO as soon as able.
Bipolar I disorder— manic/mixed episodes (age 10–17 years) (off-label use)
Children age 10–17 years, weight <45 kg (99 lb):
Start 20 mg QPM for 1 day, then increase by 20 mg/day every 2 days. Usual dosage: 30–40 mg BID. Maximum dosage: 80 mg BID.
Children age 10–17 years, weight >45 kg (99 lb):
Start 20 mg QPM for 1 day, then increase by 20 mg/day every 2 days. Usual dosage: 40–80 mg BID. Maximum dosage: 80 mg BID
Tourette's disorder (age 7–16 years) (off-label use)
Usual dosage: 20 mg BID. Maximum dosage: 40 mg/day.

Note. BID=twice daily; QPM=once a day after noon.

IX. Monitoring

A. Baseline and periodic:

1. Labs: CBC with differential (rule out hematological changes), LFTs (rare liver damage risk), renal function, electrolytes
2. Metabolic: Weight, hemoglobin A1c test, lipid panel for metabolic risk
3. Extrapyramidal symptoms (EPS): Monitor for abnormal involuntary movements/parkinsonian signs (via Abnormal Involuntary Movement Scale [AIMS]) at baseline and periodically.

4. Consider obtaining an ECG at baseline and periodically if indicated (cardiac risk factors, concomitant high-risk medication).
5. Other: Visual changes/ocular exam, sexual changes, mental status changes, blood pressure changes, falls

B. Consider ordering a drug level if there are concerns regarding compliance or metabolism (proposed reference range for schizophrenia: 50–200 ng/mL).

X. Relevant Pharmacokinetics/Pharmacodynamics

A. **Metabolism**: Phase I: reduction (66%) by glutathione and aldehyde oxidase, oxidation (33%) by cytochrome P450 (CYP) 3A4 and CYP1A2 (minor); Phase II: thiol methyltransferase
B. **Time to peak plasma concentration**: PO: 6–8 hours; SAI: 1 hour
C. **Half-life**: PO: 7 hours; SAI: 2–5 hours
D. **Time to steady state**: 1–3 days
E. **Excretion**: 20% renally (less than 1% unchanged in urine), 66% biliary.
F. **Bioavailability**: PO: 60% (with food; decreased substantially without food); IM: 100%
G. **Distribution**: 99% plasma protein bound
H. **Use with food**: Absorption of ziprasidone is 2 times greater with food (requires 500 calories for adequate absorption).
I. **Hepatic impairment**: Although AUC and half-life of PO ziprasidone are increased in individuals with cirrhosis, there are no guidelines for dosage adjustments in persons with hepatic impairment.
J. **Renal impairment**: Dosage adjustments are not required; IM formulation contains cyclodextrin excipient; use with caution
K. **Special populations**: No significant age- or gender-related differences in metabolism.

XI. Clinically Relevant Drug Interactions

A. Metabolized by CYP1A2 (minor) and CYP3A4 (minor):
   1. CYP3A4 inducers (e.g., carbamazepine) can decrease ziprasidone levels.
   2. CYP3A4 inhibitors (e.g., ketoconazole) can increase ziprasidone levels.

B. Use caution with other drugs known to prolong the QTc, antihypertensive drugs, other CNS depressants and anticholinergic agents.
C. May antagonize effects of levodopa and dopamine agonists.

XII. Adverse Effects

A. **See Table 6–1 ("Antipsychotic Class Adverse Effects") at beginning of chapter.**
B. Ziprasidone's adverse effects include metabolic syndrome, anticholinergic effects, QTc prolongation, orthostatic hypotension, EPS, prolactin elevation, sexual dysfunction, NMS, temperature dysregulation, hyponatremia/syndrome of inappropriate antidiuretic hormone secretion (SIADH), seizures
C. **Boxed warning**: Increased mortality in older patients with dementia-related psychosis
D. QTc prolongation: Higher risk of QTc prolongation compared with most other antipsychotics; dosage dependent (see "Monitoring").

XIII. **Clinical Pearls/Prescribing Tips**

A. Pros of ziprasidone: Less weight gain and sedation, minimal CYP450 drug interactions; Cons of ziprasidone: It must be taken twice daily with food (500 calories or more); increased QTc prolongation risk.

B. Because of ziprasidone's inhibition of the human-Ether-a-go-go-Related Gene (*hERG*) encoding a subunit of potassium ion channels, caution is warranted in patients with QTc prolongation risk. Monitor ECG and electrolytes at baseline and periodically, and correct abnormalities if indicated.

C. Secondary to ziprasidone's poor PO bioavailability, the dose equivalence for ziprasidone PO-to-short-acting IM conversion is 4:1.

Further Reading

Komossa K, Rummel-Kluge C, Hunger H, et al: Ziprasidone versus other atypical antipsychotics for schizophrenia. Cochrane Database Syst Rev (4):CD006627, 2009 19821380

Camm AJ, Karayal ON, Meltzer H, et al: Ziprasidone and the corrected QT interval: a comprehensive summary of clinical data. CNS Drugs 26(4):351–365, 2012 22452529

Ziprasidone hydrochloride [package insert]. U.S Food and Drug Administration website. Revised December 2022. Available at: https://www.accessdata.fda.gov/spl/data/f0d2ddca-ee8f-7a31-e053-2995a90a5faa/f0d2ddca-ee8f-7a31-e053-2995a90a5faa.xml. Accessed March 13, 2024.

References

Roth BL, Driscol J: PDSP Ki Database. Psychoactive Drug Screening Program (PDSP). University of North Carolina at Chapel Hill and the United States National Institute of Mental Health, 2023

Partial Agonist Atypical Antipsychotics

Aripiprazole

I. **Brand Names**: Abilify, Abilify DiscMelt (ODT) Abilify Maintena (aripiprazole monohydrate), Abilify Asimtufii, Aristada (aripiprazole lauroxil), Aristada Initio (aripiprazole lauroxil), Abilify MyCite

II. **Therapeutic Class**: Atypical antipsychotic

III. **Mechanism-Based Class**: Dopamine and serotonin partial agonist and serotonin antagonist

IV. **Mechanism(s) of Action**

A. D_2 receptor partial agonist (Ki=3.3 nM); some action at other dopamine receptors.
B. 5-HT_{2A} receptor antagonist (Ki=3.4–35 nM); 5-HT_{1A} partial agonist (Ki=1.7–5.6 nM). Some action at other serotonin receptors.
C. Weak H_1 receptor antagonist (Ki=27.9–61 nM)
D. Weak α_1-adrenergic receptor antagonist (α_{1A} Ki=25.9 nM) (Roth and Driscoll 2023)
E. Negligible anticholinergic activity

V. **Indications**

A. FDA adult:
1. Schizophrenia
2. Bipolar I disorder (acute mania/mixed episodes) as monotherapy or adjunct to lithium or valproate
3. Bipolar I disorder (maintenance treatment) as monotherapy or adjunct to lithium or valproate
4. Adjunct to antidepressant treatment of major depressive disorder
5. Short-term treatment of irritability associated with autism spectrum disorder (ASD)
6. Tourette's disorder, tic disorders

B. Evidence-based[1] off-label uses:
1. Acute agitation associated with schizophrenia or bipolar mania
2. Severe behavioral or psychological symptoms of dementia
3. Conduct disorder; aggression

C. FDA pediatric:
1. Bipolar disorder manic/mixed episodes (age 10–17 years), schizophrenia (age 13–17 years), irritability in ASD (age 6–17 years), Tourette's disorder (age 6–18 years)

---

[1]Evidence strength varies; readers are referred to the literature for more detailed information.

VI. **Major Contraindications and When to Use Caution**

A. **Contraindications**: Hypersensitivity to aripiprazole

B. **Use caution**: Patients with baseline fall risk, hyponatremia or other electrolyte abnormalities, dysrhythmias (including QTc prolongation), leukopenia/neutropenia, hypotension/syncope or on antihypertensive medications, seizures, motor/cognitive impairments or on CNS depressants or anticholinergic agents, temperature dysregulation, aspiration, dysphagia, obesity, hyperglycemia, hyperlipidemia, risk factors for NMS (e.g., dehydration), or dementia-related psychosis (boxed warning), pregnancy/lactation, or Parkinson's disease.

VII. **Dosage Formulations**

A. Brand and generic tablet (2 mg, 5 mg, 10 mg, 15 mg, 20 mg, 30 mg)

B. Generic disintegrating tablet (10 mg, 15 mg, 20 mg, 30 mg)

C. Oral solution (1 mg/mL [150 mL])

D. **Long-acting IM injection**:

1. Abilify Maintena:

   a. Prefilled syringes or suspension for reconstitution (300 mg, 400 mg)

2. Aristada:

   a. Prefilled syringes (441 mg, 662 mg, 882 mg, 1,064 mg)

3. Aristada Initio:

   a. Prefilled syringe (675 mg)

VIII. **Dosage Ranges and Guidelines**

A. Refer to Table 6–24 for dosage ranges (initial/maximum) and guidelines. Dosages are for adults unless otherwise specified.

B. **Titration**: Increase in increments of 5 mg every 1–2 weeks. Because of prolonged half-life, tolerability may take 14 days to fully assess.

1. Older adults: Same as in younger adults, although lower dosages are typically used and are titrated more slowly.
2. See "Clinically Relevant Drug Interactions" below and adjust dosages accordingly.

C. **Discontinuation**: For patients on long-term treatment, taper slowly to avoid rebound psychosis and withdrawal dyskinesias.

Table 6–24. Aripiprazole indications and dosage guidelines

Schizophrenia (PO)
Adults:
Initial: 5–15 mg/day. Usual dosage: 10–30 mg/day. Maximum dosage: 30 mg/day (PO) or 25 mg/day (oral solution).
Adolescents (age 3–13 years):
Initial: 2 mg/day. Usual dosage: 10 mg/day. Maximum dosage: 30 mg/day (PO) or 25 mg/day (oral solution).

Table 6–24. Aripiprazole indications and dosage guidelines *(continued)*

Schizophrenia (long-acting injectable [LAI])

Note: Tolerability/efficacy of PO aripiprazole should be established prior to initiation of LAI.

Abilify Maintena (every month)

Initial: 400 mg IM once.

Once stable, can reduce dosage to 300 mg IM once monthly based on tolerability.

Maintenance dosage: The authors commonly use 300 mg IM monthly for patients on < 15 mg/day and 400 mg IM monthly for patients on ≥15 mg/day or more of aripiprazole (Mallikaarjun et al. 2013).

PO overlap: Continue PO aripiprazole for 14 days after initial injection.

Abilify Lauroxil (Aristada) (every 1–2 months based on dosage)

Initiation: Aristada initiation dosage is same as maintenance dosage.

Option 1: Administer Aristada Initio 675 mg IM + 1 dose of aripiprazole 30 mg PO + first dose of Aristada IM; no further oral overlap is required

Option 2: Following first Aristada IM injection, continue oral overlap with PO aripiprazole for 21 days

Conversion from PO aripiprazole:

10 mg/day PO ≈ 441 mg IM/month

15 mg/day PO ≈ 662 mg IM/month or 882 mg IM every 6 weeks or 1,064 mg IM every 2 months

20 mg/day PO or higher ≈ 882 mg IM/month

Bipolar I disorder—
maintenance treatment
treatment of acute mixed/manic episodes

Adults:

Initial: 10–15 mg/day. Usual dosage: 15 mg/day. Maximum dosage: 30 mg/day.

Children/adolescents (age ≥10 years):

Initial: 2 mg/day. Usual dosage: 10 mg/day. Maximum dosage: 30 mg/day.

Note: Aripiprazole monohydrate (Abilify Maintena) is approved only for maintenance treatment. Use the same dosing used for schizophrenia.

Acute agitation associated with schizophrenia or bipolar mania (short-acting IM)

Adults:

Initial: 9.75 mg IM as a single dose (5.25 mg if clinically indicated [i.e., CYP2D6 poor metabolizer]). Repeat dose after 2 hours. Maximum dosage: 30 mg/day.

Note: Immediate-release aripiprazole IM is no longer commercially available in the U.S.

Table 6–24. Aripiprazole indications and dosage guidelines *(continued)*

Adjunct to antidepressant treatment of major depressive disorder (PO)
Adults:
Initial: 2–5 mg/day. Usual dosage: 2–15 mg/day. Maximum dosage: 15 mg/day.
Short-term treatment of irritability associated with autism spectrum disorder (PO)
Children/adolescents (age ≥6 years):
Initial: 2 mg/day. Usual dosage: 5–10 mg/day. Maximum dosage: 15 mg/day.
Tourette's disorder (age 6–18 years)
<50 kg: Start 2 mg/day for 2 days, then 5 mg/day. Can increase dosage gradually every week. Maximum dosage: 10 mg/day.
≥50 kg: Start 2 mg/day for 2 days, then 5 mg/day for 5 days, then 10 mg/day. May increase by 5 mg/day every week. Maximum dosage: 20 mg/day.

Note. Additional PO-to-LAI dosage adjustments for drug-drug interactions and genetic polymorphisms are provided below (see "Clinically Relevant Drug Interactions" section).

IX. **Monitoring**

A. Baseline and periodic:

1. Labs: CBC with differential (rule out hematological changes), LFTs (rare liver damage risk, contraindicated in hepatic impairment), renal function, electrolytes
2. Metabolic: Weight, hemoglobin A1c test, lipid panel for metabolic risk
3. Extrapyramidal symptoms (EPS): Monitor for abnormal involuntary movements/parkinsonian signs (via Abnormal Involuntary Movement Scale [AIMS]) at baseline and periodically;
4. Consider obtaining an ECG at baseline and periodically if indicated (cardiac risk factors, concomitant high-risk medications).
5. Other: Visual changes/ocular exam, sexual changes, mental status changes, blood pressure changes, falls

B. As when starting any new antidepressant, monitor closely for clinical worsening, suicidality, and behavioral changes, especially during first few months of treatment and when making dosage adjustments; families and caregivers of patients should be warned to monitor for agitation, irritability, behavioral changes, and suicidality and to report these symptoms to health care providers if they occur.

C. Consider ordering a drug level if there are concerns regarding compliance or metabolism (proposed reference range for schizophrenia: 100–350 ng/mL).

D. Although risk is low, monitor for treatment-emergent manic/hypomanic episodes.

X. **Relevant Pharmacokinetics/Pharmacodynamics**

A. **Metabolism**: Phase I: CYP2D6 and CYP3A4:

B. **Time to peak plasma concentration**: PO: 3–5 hours; LAI: Abilify Maintena: 5–7 days; Aristada Initio: 16–35 days

C. **Half-life**: PO: 75 hours (CYP2D6 extensive metabolizers); 146 hours (CYP2D6 poor metabolizers); LAI: Abilify Maintena: 30–47 days; Aristada: 54–57 days; Aristada Initio: 15–18 days
D. **Bioavailability**: 87%
E. **Distribution**: 99% plasma protein bound
F. **Time to steady state**: PO: 14 days (for extensive CPY2D6 metabolizers; longer for others); LAI: by the 4th dose
G. **Excretion**: 25% renally, 55% biliary
H. **Hepatic impairment**: No dosage adjustment required.
I. **Renal impairment**: No dosage adjustment required.
J. **Special populations**: No significant age- or gender-related differences in metabolism.

XI. **Clinically Relevant Drug Interactions**

A. Metabolized by CYP2D6 (major) and CYP3A4 (major):

1. Use caution/decrease dose when combined with strong CYP2D6 inhibitors (e.g., fluoxetine, paroxetine, bupropion) or strong CYP3A4 inhibitors (e.g., erythromycin, terbinafine, nefazodone). The following recommendations are provided by the manufacturer:

a. Use of PO aripiprazole:

i. With concomitant use of strong CYP2D6 ***or*** CYP3A4 inhibitors: Administer half of usual dose.
ii. With use in known CYP2D6 poor metabolizers: Administer half of usual dose
iii. With concomitant use of strong CYP2D6 ***and*** CYP3A4 inhibitors: Administer one-quarter of usual dose.
iv. With use in known CYP2D6 poor metabolizers taking CYP3A4 inhibitors: Administer one-quarter of usual dose.

b. Use of Abilify Maintena:

i. With concomitant use of strong CYP2D6 ***or*** CYP3A4 inhibitors: 200–300 mg (based on current LAI dose)
ii. With concomitant use of strong CYP2D6 ***and*** CYP3A4 inhibitors: 160–200 mg (based on current LAI dose)
iii. With use in known CYP2D6 poor metabolizers taking CYP3A4 inhibitors: 200 mg

c. Use of Aristada:

i. With concomitant use of strong CYP2D6 ***or*** CYP3A4 inhibitors: Reduce dose of Aristada to next lower strength (no adjustments required for 441 mg Aristada, if tolerated).
ii. With use in known CYP2D6 poor metabolizers taking CYP3A4 inhibitors: Maximum dose 441 mg
iii. With concomitant use of strong CYP2D6 ***and*** CYP3A4 inhibitors: Maximum dose 441 mg

2. Concomitant use with strong CYP3A4 inducers (e.g., carbamazepine, rifampin) can decrease aripiprazole concentrations. The following recommendations are provided by the manufacturer:
   a. Use of PO aripiprazole:
      i. With strong CYP3A4 inducers: Double usual dosage over 1–2 weeks.
   b. Use of Abilify Maintena:
      i. With strong CYP3A4 inducers: Avoid use.
   c. Use of Aristada:
      i. With strong CYP3A4 inducers: Patients taking 441 mg should have dosage increased to 662 mg (no adjustments necessary for higher dosages).

XII. **Adverse Effects**

A. **See Table 6–1 ("Antipsychotic Class Adverse Effects") at beginning of chapter.**

B. Aripiprazole's adverse effects include metabolic syndrome, anticholinergic effects, QTc prolongation, orthostatic hypotension, EPS, prolactin elevation, sexual dysfunction, NMS, temperature dysregulation, hyponatremia/SIADH, seizures
   1. For the full scope of potential adverse effects, see the drug labeling (Aripiprazole package insert).

C. **Boxed warnings**:
   1. Increased mortality in older patients with dementia-related psychosis
   2. Potential increased risk of suicidal thoughts/behaviors in pediatric/young adult patients. Monitor closely for emergence of suicidal thoughts. For detailed information, the reader is referred to comprehensive sources in the literature (e.g., Fergusson et al. 2005).

D. Akathisia, insomnia, anxiety, tremors are relatively common, although sedation can occur as well.

E. There have been rare reports of pathological gambling or other impulse-control disorders with aripiprazole (potentially related to D_2 receptor partial agonist activity).

F. Aripiprazole tends to be more weight-neutral compared with other antipsychotics, although it may cause more weight gain in children than in adults.

G. Aripiprazole carries low risk for hyperprolactinemia, and in fact can be used to treat hyperprolactinemia (off-label).

H. Aripiprazole carries low risk of QTc prolongation and may possibly decrease the QTc interval.

XIII. **Clinical Pearls/Prescribing Tips**

A. Aripiprazole, brexpiprazole, and cariprazine (think "ABC") are all very similar in their receptor binding activity (all are partial dopamine agonists) and thus have similar downstream effects. (Partial agonists have intrinsic activity, but to a lesser extent than the endogenous ligand.)

B. Aripiprazole is generally well tolerated and tends to have lower metabolic symptoms as well as little to no prolactin elevation, so it is a good option if trying to avoid these common side effects of other antipsychotic agents (Preda and Shapiro

2020). Aripiprazole may also be favored in patients with QTc prolongation or risks thereof, as it can actually decrease the QTc interval.

C. Aripiprazole may reduce and potentially normalize hyperprolactinemia when added as an adjunct to other antipsychotic agents (Besag et al. 2021).

D. When used as an adjunct to antidepressant treatment of major depressive disorder, lower dosages are typically prescribed.

E. Aripiprazole has multiple LAI formulations which can be very useful for improving treatment adherence.

F. As with cariprazine and brexpiprazole, impulse-control and related disorders may be seen with aripiprazole.

G. Secondary to the higher bioavailability of the oral solution versus the tablet, the aripiprazole 25 mg oral solution is equivalent to the 30 mg tablet.

H. Abilify MyCite is a tablet formulated as a drug-device combination product with an Ingestible Event Marker intended to be used in conjunction with a nonmedicated patch. This patch contains a pod that digitally logs (through a smartphone application) the time at which the patient ingests the pill.

Further Reading

Aripiprazole package insert. U.S Food and Drug Administration, 2018. Available at: https://www.accessdata.fda.gov/spl/data/ae9e2824–8741–4973-b349-a18ce05cb334/ae9e2824–8741–4973-b349-a18ce05cb334.xml. Accessed March 13, 2024.

Casey AB, Canal CE: Classics in chemical neuroscience: aripiprazole. ACS Chem Neurosci 8(6):1135–1146, 2017 28368577

Li DJ, Tseng PT, Stubbs B, et al: Efficacy, safety and tolerability of aripiprazole in bipolar disorder: an updated systematic review and meta-analysis of randomized controlled trials. Prog Neuropsychopharmacol Biol Psychiatry 79(Pt B):289–301, 2017

References

Besag FMC, Vasey MJ, Salim I: Is adjunct aripiprazole effective in treating hyperprolactinemia induced by psychotropic medication? A narrative review. CNS Drugs 35(5):507–526, 2021 33880739

Fergusson D, Doucette S, Glass KC, et al: Association between suicide attempts and selective serotonin reuptake inhibitors: systematic review of randomised controlled trials. BMJ 330(7488):396, 2005 15718539

Mallikaarjun S, Kane JM, Bricmont P, et al: Pharmacokinetics, tolerability and safety of aripiprazole once-monthly in adult schizophrenia: an open-label, parallel-arm, multiple-dose study. Schizophr Res 150(1):281–288, 2013 23890595

Preda A, Shapiro BB: A safety evaluation of aripiprazole in the treatment of schizophrenia. Expert Opin Drug Saf 19(12):1529–1538, 2020 33064050

Roth BL, Driscoll J: PDSP Ki Database. Psychoactive Drug Screening Program (PDSP). University of North Carolina at Chapel Hill and the United States National Institute of Mental Health 2023

Brexpiprazole

I. **Brand Names**: Rexulti

II. **Therapeutic Class**: Atypical antipsychotic

III. **Mechanism-Based Class**: Dopamine and serotonin partial agonist and serotonin antagonist

IV. **Mechanism(s) of Action**

A. Potent D_2 receptor partial agonist (Ki=0.30 nM); some action at other dopamine receptors.

B. Potent 5-HT_{2A} receptor antagonist (Ki=0.47 nM); potent 5-HT_{1A} receptor partial agonist (Ki=0.12); 5-HT_{2C} receptor partial agonist (Ki=12–34); some action at other serotonin receptors.

C. Histamine-1 (H_1) receptor antagonist (Ki=19 nM)

D. Alpha-1 (α_1)-adrenergic receptor antagonist (α_{1A} Ki=3.8 nM) (Roth and Driscoll 2023)

E. Negligible anticholinergic activity

V. **Indications**

A. FDA adult:

1. Schizophrenia
2. Adjunct to antidepressant treatment of major depressive disorder

B. Evidence-based[1] off-label uses:

1. Severe behavioral or psychological symptoms of dementia (dosage not established).

C. FDA pediatric: Schizophrenia (age 13–17 years)

VI. **Major Contraindications and When to Use Caution**

A. **Contraindications**: Hypersensitivity to brexpiprazole

B. **Use caution**: Patients with baseline fall risk, hyponatremia or other electrolyte abnormalities, dysrhythmias (including QTc prolongation), leukopenia/neutropenia, hypotension/syncope or on antihypertensive medications, seizures, motor/cognitive impairments or on CNS depressants or anticholinergic agents, temperature dysregulation, aspiration, dysphagia, obesity, hyperglycemia, hyperlipidemia, risk factors for NMS (e.g., dehydration) or dementia-related psychosis (boxed warning), pregnancy/lactation, or Parkinson's disease.

VII. **Dosage Formulations**

A. Brand tablet: (0.25 mg, 0.5 mg, 1 mg, 2 mg, 3 mg, 4 mg)

VIII. **Dosage Ranges and Guidelines**

A. Refer to Table 6–25 for dosage ranges (initial/maximum) and guidelines. Dosages are for adults unless otherwise specified.

---

[1]Evidence strength varies; readers are referred to the literature for more detailed information.

B. **Titration**: Start at 0.5 mg/day (MDD) or 1 mg/day (schizophrenia); double dose on day 5–7, then increase by 1 mg/day in weekly intervals to the maximum dose for a given indication.

1. Older adults: Same as in younger adults, although lower dosages are typically used and are titrated more slowly.
2. Adolescents: Same as in adults
3. Children: Safety/efficacy not established.
4. See "Clinically Relevant Drug Interactions" below and adjust dosages accordingly.

C. **Discontinuation**: For patients on long-term treatment, taper slowly to avoid rebound psychosis and withdrawal dyskinesias.

Table 6–25. Brexpiprazole indications and dosage guidelines

Schizophrenia (PO)
Adults:
Initial: 1 mg/day. Usual dosage: 2–4 mg/day. Maximum 4 mg/day.
Adolescents (age 13–17 years):
Initial: 0.5 mg/day. Usual dosage 2–4 mg/day. Maximum dosage: 4 mg/day.
Adjunct to antidepressant treatment of major depressive disorder (PO)
Adults:
Initial: 0.5–1 mg/day. Usual dosage: 2 mg/day. Maximum dosage: 3 mg/day.

Note. Additional dosage adjustments for drug-drug interactions and genetic polymorphisms are provided below (see "Clinically Relevant Drug Interactions").

IX. Monitoring

A. Baseline and periodic:

1. Labs: CBC with differential (rule out hematological changes), LFTs (rare liver damage risk), renal function, electrolytes
2. Metabolic: Weight, hemoglobin A1c test, lipid panel for metabolic risk
3. Extrapyramidal symptoms (EPS): Monitor for abnormal involuntary movements/parkinsonian signs (via Abnormal Involuntary Movement Scale [AIMS]) at baseline and periodically.
4. Consider obtaining an ECG at baseline and periodically if indicated (cardiac risk factors, concomitant high-risk medications).
5. Other: Visual changes/ocular exam, sexual changes, mental status changes, blood pressure changes, falls

B. As when starting any new antidepressant, monitor closely for clinical worsening, suicidality, and behavioral changes, especially during first few months of treatment and when making dosage adjustments. Families and caregivers of patients should be warned to monitor for agitation, irritability, behavioral changes, and suicidality and to report these to health care providers if they are observed. This topic continues to generate controversy. For a detailed discussion, the reader is referred to comprehensive sources in the literature (e.g., Fergusson et al. 2005).

C. Consider ordering a drug level if there are concerns regarding compliance or metabolism (proposed reference range for schizophrenia: 40–140 ng/mL).

D. Although risk is low, monitor for treatment-emergent manic or hypomanic episodes.

X. Relevant Pharmacokinetics/Pharmacodynamics

A. **Metabolism**: Phase I: cytochrome P450 (CYP) 2D6 (major) and CYP3A4 (major)

B. **Time to peak plasma concentration**: 4 hours

C. **Half-life**: 91 hours

D. **Time to steady state**: Within 10–12 days

E. **Excretion**: 25% renally, 46% biliary

F. **Bioavailability**: 95%

G. **Distribution**: >99% plasma protein bound

H. **Hepatic impairment**: Mild: No dosage adjustment required. Moderate to severe (Child-Pugh ≥7): Maximum recommended dosage is 2 mg/day for major depressive disorder and 3 mg/day for schizophrenia.

I. **Renal impairment**: CrCl<60 mL/minute: Maximum recommended dosage is 2 mg/day for major depressive disorder and 3 mg/day for schizophrenia.

J. **Special populations**: No significant age- or gender-related differences in metabolism.

XI. Clinically Relevant Drug Interactions

A. Metabolized primarily by CYP2D6 (major) and CYP3A4 (major):

1. Use caution/decrease dosage when combined with CYP2D6 inhibitors (e.g., fluoxetine, paroxetine, bupropion) or CYP3A4 inhibitors (e.g., erythromycin, terbinafine, nefazodone). The following recommendations are provided by the manufacturer:

    a. With concomitant use of strong CYP2D6 ***or*** CYP3A4 inhibitors: Administer half of usual dose.

    b. With use in known CYP2D6 poor metabolizers: Administer half of usual dose.

    c. With concomitant use of strong/moderate CYP2D6 ***and*** CYP3A4 inhibitors: Administer one-quarter of usual dose.

    d. With use in known CYP2D6 poor metabolizers taking CYP3A4 inhibitors: Administer one-quarter of usual dose.

2. Concomitant use with strong CYP3A4 inducers (e.g., carbamazepine, rifampin) can decrease brexpiprazole concentrations. The following recommendation is provided from the manufacturer:

    a. With concomitant use of strong CYP3A4 inducers: Administer double the usual dose and monitor closely for response (Brexpiprazole package insert 2022).

XII. Adverse Effects

A. **See Table 6–1 ("Antipsychotic Class Adverse Effects") at beginning of chapter.**

B. Brexpiprazole's adverse effects include metabolic syndrome, anticholinergic effects, QTc prolongation, orthostatic hypotension, EPS, prolactin elevation, sexual dysfunction, NMS, temperature dysregulation, hyponatremia/syndrome of inappropriate antidiuretic hormone secretion (SIADH), seizures

   1. For full scope of potential adverse effects, see drug labeling (Brexpiprazole package insert).

C. **Boxed warnings**:

   1. Increased mortality in older patients with dementia-related psychosis
   2. Potential increased risk of suicidal thoughts/behaviors in pediatric/young adult patients. Monitor closely for emergence of suicidal thoughts. For detailed information, the reader is referred to comprehensive sources in the literature (e.g., Fergusson et al. 2005).

D. Akathisia may occur, but it appears to be less common with brexpiprazole than with aripiprazole.

E. Brexpiprazole has a low risk of weight gain, similar to that of aripiprazole,

F. Like aripiprazole, brexpiprazole can cause both insomnia and somnolence/sedation.

G. Rare instances of aripiprazole-induced pathological gambling or other impulse-control disorders have been reported (potentially related to aripiprazole's partial agonist D_2 activity).

H. Brexpiprazole is associated with a low risk of QTc prolongation and can perhaps decrease the QTc interval.

XIII. Clinical Pearls/Prescribing Tips

A. Aripiprazole, brexpiprazole, and cariprazine (think "ABC") are all very similar in receptor binding activity (all are partial dopamine agonists) and thus have similar downstream effects.

B. Brexpiprazole is similar to aripiprazole in terms of its receptor-binding profile, although it has less intrinsic activity at D_2 receptors. Brexpiprazole's safety/tolerability/efficacy profile is similar to that of aripiprazole, although it tends to have less EPS, particularly akathisia (Citrome et al. 2016); thus, it may be a good choice if a patient had a good clinical response to aripiprazole but experienced intolerable akathisia.

C. Unlike aripiprazole, brexpiprazole may not be beneficial for bipolar mania (McIntyre et al. 2011; Vieta et al. 2021).

D. As with aripiprazole, lower dosages of brexpiprazole are typically used adjunctively with antidepressants to treat major depressive disorder (Furukawa et al. 2022).

E. As with aripiprazole and cariprazine, impulse-control and related disorders may be seen with brexpiprazole.

F. Brexpiprazole is unlikely to increase prolactin or the QTc interval.

G. Specific dosage adjustments are provided by the manufacturer for strong/moderate CYP3A4 inhibitors/inducers and CYP2D6 inhibitors/polymorphisms (Brexpiprazole package insert 2022).

Further Reading

Antoun Reyad A, Girgis E, Mishriky R: Efficacy and safety of brexpiprazole in acute management of psychiatric disorders: a meta-analysis of randomized controlled trials. Int Clin Psychopharmacol 35(3):119–128, 2020 32141908

Brexpiprazole [package insert]. U.S Food and Drug Administration website. Revised December 2022. Available at: https://www.accessdata.fda.gov/spl/data/10d2049f-580a-4add-abab-77e458ccb246/10d2049f-580a-4add-abab-77e458ccb246.xml. Accessed March 13, 2024.

Kane JM, Skuban A, Hobart M, et al: Overview of short- and long-term tolerability and safety of brexpiprazole in patients with schizophrenia. Schizophr Res 174(1–3):93–98, 2016 27188270

References

Citrome L, Ota A, Nagamizu K, et al: The effect of brexpiprazole (OPC-34712) and aripiprazole in adult patients with acute schizophrenia: results from a randomized, exploratory study. Int Clin Psychopharmacol 31(4):192–201, 2016 26963842

Fergusson D, Doucette S, Glass KC, et al: Association between suicide attempts and selective serotonin reuptake inhibitors: systematic review of randomised controlled trials. BMJ 330(7488):396, 2005 15718539

Furukawa Y, Oguro S, Obata S, et al: Optimal dose of brexpiprazole for augmentation therapy of antidepressant-refractory depression: a systematic review and dose-effect meta-analysis. Psychiatry Clin Neurosci 76(9):416–422, 2022 35716011

McIntyre RS, Yoon J, Jerrell JM, et al: Aripiprazole for the maintenance treatment of bipolar disorder: a review of available evidence. Neuropsychiatr Dis Treat 7:319–323, 2011 21655345

Roth BL, Driscoll J: PDSP Ki Database. Psychoactive Drug Screening Program (PDSP). University of North Carolina at Chapel Hill and the United States National Institute of Mental Health, 2023

Vieta E, Sachs G, Chang D, et al: Two randomized, double-blind, placebo-controlled trials and one open-label, long-term trial of brexpiprazole for the acute treatment of bipolar mania. J Psychopharmacol 35(8):971–982, 2021 33691517

Cariprazine

I. **Brand Names**: Vraylar

II. **Therapeutic Class**: Atypical antipsychotic

III. **Mechanism-Based Class**: Dopamine and serotonin partial agonist and serotonin antagonist

IV. **Mechanism(s) of Action**

A. Dopamine D_2 and serotonin 5-HT_{1A} receptor partial agonist; serotonin 5-HT_{2A} receptor antagonist

B. Potent dopamine D_2 receptor partial agonist (Ki=0.49 nM); potent dopamine D_3 receptor partial agonist (Ki=0.085); some action at other dopamine receptors.

C. 5-HT_{2A} receptor partial agonist (Ki=18.8 nM); some action at other serotonin receptors.

D. Histamine-1 receptor antagonist (Ki=23.2 nM)
E. Weak α_1-adrenergic receptor antagonist (α_{1A} Ki=155 nM) (Roth and Driscoll 2023)
F. Negligible anticholinergic activity

V. **Indications**

A. FDA adult:

1. Schizophrenia
2. Bipolar disorder (manic/mixed episodes)
3. Bipolar depression
4. Adjunct to antidepressant treatment of major depressive disorder

B. Evidence-based[1] off-label uses:

1. Negative symptoms of schizophrenia

C. FDA pediatric: None

VI. **Major Contraindications and When to Use Caution**

A. **Contraindications**: Hypersensitivity to brexpiprazole
B. **Use caution**: Patients with baseline fall risk, hyponatremia or other electrolyte abnormalities, dysrhythmias (including QTc prolongation), leukopenia/neutropenia, hypotension/syncope or on antihypertensive medications, seizures, motor/cognitive impairments or on CNS depressants or anticholinergic agents, temperature dysregulation, aspiration, dysphagia, obesity, hyperglycemia, hyperlipidemia, risk factors for neuroleptic malignant syndrome (NMS) (e.g., dehydration) or dementia-related psychosis (boxed warning), pregnancy/lactation, or Parkinson's disease.

VII. **Dosage Formulations**

A. Brand capsule (1.5 mg, 3 mg, 4.5 mg, 6 mg)

VIII. **Dosage Ranges and Guidelines**

A. Refer to Table 6–26 for dosage ranges (initial/maximum) and guidelines. Dosages are for adults unless otherwise specified.

1. Older adults: Same as in younger adults, although lower dosages are typically used and are titrated more slowly.
2. Adolescents: Same as in adults
3. Children: Safety/efficacy not established.
4. See "Clinically Relevant Drug Interactions" below and adjust dosages accordingly.

B. **Titration**: Can increase from 1.5 to 3 mg/day on day 2, then adjust by 1.5–3 mg/day, generally on a weekly or every-2-week basis. Because of the prolonged half-life, tolerability may take 14–21 days to fully assess.
C. **Discontinuation**: For patients on long-term treatment, taper slowly to avoid rebound psychosis and withdrawal dyskinesias.

---

[1]Evidence strength varies; readers are referred to the literature for more detailed information.

Table 6–26. Cariprazine indications and dosage guidelines

Schizophrenia (PO)
Adults:
Initial: 1 mg/day. Usual dosage: 2–4 mg/day. Maximum 4 mg/day.
Bipolar disorder (manic/mixed) (PO)
Adults:
Initial: 0.5 mg/day. Usual dosage: 2–4 mg/day. Maximum dosage: 4 mg/day.
Bipolar depression (PO)
Adults:
Initial: 1.5 mg/day. Usual dosage: 1.5–3 mg/day. Maximum dosage: 3 mg/day
Adjunct to antidepressant treatment of major depressive disorder (PO)
Adults:
Initial: 1.5 mg/day. Usual dosage: 1.5–3 mg. Maximum dosage: 3 mg/day

IX. **Monitoring**

A. Baseline and periodic:

1. Labs: CBC with differential (rule out hematological changes), LFTs (rare liver damage risk, contraindicated in hepatic impairment), renal function, electrolytes
2. Metabolic: Weight, hemoglobin A1c test, lipid panel for metabolic risk
3. Extrapyramidal symptoms (EPS): Monitor for abnormal involuntary movements/parkinsonian signs (via Abnormal Involuntary Movement Scale [AIMS]) at baseline and periodically.
4. Consider obtaining an ECG at baseline and periodically if indicated (cardiac risk factors, concomitant high-risk medications).
5. Other: Visual changes/ocular exam, sexual changes, mental status changes, blood pressure changes, falls

B. As when starting any new antidepressant, monitor closely for clinical worsening, suicidality, and behavioral changes, especially during first few months of treatment and when making dosage adjustments; families and caregivers of patients should be warned to monitor for agitation, irritability, behavioral changes, and suicidality and to report these to health care providers. This topic continues to generate controversy. For a detailed discussion, the reader is referred to comprehensive sources in the literature (e.g., Fergusson et al. 2005).

C. Consider ordering a drug level if there are concerns regarding compliance or metabolism (proposed reference range for schizophrenia: 10–20 ng/mL).

D. Although low risk, monitor for treatment-emergent manic or hypomanic episodes.

X. **Relevant Pharmacokinetics/Pharmacodynamics**

A. **Metabolism**: Phase I: cytochrome P450 (CYP) 2D6 (minor) and CYP3A4 (major)

B. **Time to peak plasma concentration**: 3–6 hours

C. **Half-life**: 48–120 hours (cariprazine); 1–3 weeks (didesmethyl cariprazine)

D. **Time to steady state**: Within 1–2 weeks or longer, depending on the individual's genetic metabolic capabilities (cariprazine); 4–8 weeks (didesmethyl cariprazine)
E. **Excretion**: 21% renally
F. **Bioavailability**: High
G. **Distribution**: 91%–97% plasma protein bound
H. **Hepatic impairment**: Use not recommended for individuals with severe hepatic impairment (Child-Pugh ≥10).
I. **Renal impairment**: Use not recommended for individuals with severe renal impairment (CrCl<30 mL/minute).
J. **Special populations**: No significant age- or gender-related differences in metabolism.

XI. **Clinically Relevant Drug Interactions**

A. Metabolized by CYP2D6 (minor) and CYP3A4 (major)

1. Use caution/decrease dose when combined with strong CYP2D6 inhibitors (e.g., fluoxetine, paroxetine, bupropion) or strong CYP3A4 inhibitors (e.g., erythromycin, terbinafine, nefazodone). The following recommendation is provided by the manufacturer:
   a. With concomitant strong CYP3A4 inhibitors: Administer half of usual dose.
2. Concomitant use with strong CYP3A4 inducers (e.g., carbamazepine, rifampin) can decrease brexpiprazole concentrations. The following recommendation is provided by the manufacturer:
   a. With concomitant strong CYP3A4 inducers: Use not recommended.

XII. **Adverse Effects**

A. **See Table 6–1 ("Antipsychotic Class Adverse Effects") at beginning of chapter.**
B. Cariprazine's adverse effects include metabolic syndrome, anticholinergic effects, QTc prolongation, orthostatic hypotension, EPS, prolactin elevation, sexual dysfunction, NMS, temperature dysregulation, hyponatremia/syndrome of inappropriate antidiuretic hormone secretion (SIADH), seizures
   1. For the full scope of potential adverse effects, see drug labeling (Cariprazine package insert).
C. **Boxed warnings**:
   1. Increased mortality in older patients with dementia-related psychosis
   2. Potential increased risk of suicidal thoughts/behaviors in pediatric/young adult patients. Monitor closely for emergence of suicidal thoughts. For detailed information, the reader is referred to comprehensive sources in the literature (e.g., Fergusson et al. 2005).
D. As with aripiprazole, akathisia is relatively common with cariprazine.
E. Cariprazine's effects on weight are similar to those of aripiprazole.
F. Cariprazine can cause either insomnia or somnolence/sedation.
G. As with aripiprazole and brexpiprazole, impulse-control and related disorders may be seen with cariprazine.
H. Cariprazine carries a low risk of QTc prolongation and can perhaps decrease the QTc interval.

XIII. **Clinical Pearls/Prescribing Tips**

A. Aripiprazole, brexpiprazole, and cariprazine (think "ABC") are all very similar in receptor binding activity (all are partial dopamine agonists) and thus have similar downstream effects.

B. Cariprazine has two active metabolites, desmethyl cariprazine (DCAR) and didesmethyl cariprazine (DDCAR), which are considered to be pharmacologically equipotent to cariprazine.

C. Because of the long half-life of cariprazine and its metabolites, dosage adjustments may take several weeks to be reflected in plasma level changes.

D. Although cariprazine is associated with parkinsonism and akathisia, it has a very favorable metabolic profile, particularly in regard to lipids.

E. Cariprazine is unique among the partial dopamine agonists in that it has an FDA indication for bipolar depression, whereas aripiprazole and brexpiprazole have an FDA indication for adjunctive use with antidepressants in the treatment of major depressive disorder (however, aripiprazole is used off-label for bipolar depression).

F. Cariprazine is unlikely to increase prolactin or the QTc interval.

Further Reading

Cooper H, Mishriky R, Reyad AA: Efficacy and safety of cariprazine in acute management of psychiatric disorders: a meta-analysis of randomized controlled trials. Psychiatr Danub 32(1):36–45, 2020 32303028

Pinto JV, Saraf G, Vigo D, et al: Cariprazine in the treatment of bipolar disorder: a systematic review and meta-analysis. Bipolar Disord 22(4):360–371, 2020 31618503

Vraylar (cariprazine) package insert. U.S Food and Drug Administration, 2022. Available at: https://www.accessdata.fda.gov/spl/data/cb810327–2cd3–412c-a152-ecd66aee191c/cb810327–2cd3–412c-a152-ecd66aee191c.xml. Accessed March 13, 2024.

References

Fergusson D, Doucette S, Glass KC, et al: Association between suicide attempts and selective serotonin reuptake inhibitors: systematic review of randomised controlled trials. BMJ 330(7488):396, 2005 15718539

Roth BL, Driscoll J. PDSP Ki Database. Psychoactive Drug Screening Program (PDSP). University of North Carolina at Chapel Hill and the United States National Institute of Mental Health, 2023

Other Atypical Antipsychotics

Lumateperone

I. **Brand Names**: Caplyta

II. **Therapeutic Class**: Atypical antipsychotic

III. **Mechanism-Based Class**: Serotonin receptor antagonist and dopamine receptor antagonist/agonist

IV. **Mechanism(s) of Action**

A. Serotonin 5-HT_{2A} receptor antagonist; D_2 receptor antagonist (postsynaptic receptor); D_2 receptor agonist (presynaptic autoreceptors)

B. 5-HT_{2A} receptor antagonist (Ki=0.54 nM); serotonin reuptake transport inhibition (SERT; Ki=33 nM)

C. D_2 receptor antagonist/agonist (Ki=32 nM), D_1 receptor (Ki=41 nM)

D. Alpha-1 (α_1) receptor antagonist (Ki <100 nM)

E. Minimal/no affinity for histaminergic or muscarinic receptors

F. Possible activity at *N*-methyl-D-aspartate (NMDA) and α-amino-3-hydroxy-5-methyl-4-isoxazolepropionic acid (AMPA) receptors

V. **Indications**

A. FDA adult:

1. Bipolar depression, as monotherapy or adjunct to lithium or valproate
2. Schizophrenia

B. Evidence-based[1] off-label uses:

1. Multiple indications under investigation

C. FDA pediatric: None

VI. **Major Contraindications and When to Use Caution**:

A. **Contraindications**: Hypersensitivity to lumateperone

B. **Use caution**: Patients with baseline fall risk, hyponatremia or other electrolyte abnormalities, dysrhythmias (including QTc prolongation), leukopenia/neutropenia, hypotension/syncope or on antihypertensive medications, seizures, motor/cognitive impairments or on CNS depressants or anticholinergic agents, temperature dysregulation, aspiration, dysphagia, obesity, hyperglycemia, hyperlipidemia, risk factors for neuroleptic malignant syndrome (NMS) (e.g., dehydration), or dementia-related psychosis (boxed warning), pregnancy/lactation, or Parkinson's disease.

[1]Evidence strength varies; readers are referred to the literature for more detailed information.

VII. **Dosage Formulations**

A. Brand capsule (10.5 mg, 21 mg, 42 mg)

VIII. **Dosage Ranges and Guidelines**

A. **Initial/maximum dosing/titration**:

1. Adults (both younger and older): Recommended dosage is 42 mg PO daily without titration; nightly dosing is recommended due to sedation.
2. Children/adolescents: Safety/efficacy not established.
3. See "Clinically Relevant Drug Interactions" below and adjust dosages accordingly.

B. **Discontinuation**: For patients on long-term treatment, taper slowly to avoid rebound psychosis, withdrawal dyskinesias, and serotonin withdrawal symptoms (e.g., flu-like symptoms, malaise, headache).

IX. **Monitoring**

A. Baseline and periodic:

1. Labs: CBC with differential (rule out hematological changes), LFTs, renal function, electrolytes (especially in older adult patients)
2. Metabolic: Weight, hemoglobin A1c test, lipid panel for metabolic risk
3. Extrapyramidal symptoms (EPS): Monitor for abnormal involuntary movements/parkinsonian signs (via Abnormal Involuntary Movement Scale [AIMS]) at baseline and periodically.
4. Consider obtaining an ECG at baseline and periodically if indicated (cardiac risk factors, concomitant high-risk medication).
5. Other: Visual changes/ocular exam, sexual changes, mental status changes, blood pressure changes, falls.

B. In patients at risk of significant electrolyte disturbances (e.g., diuretic therapy, diarrhea), consider checking serum potassium and magnesium and repleting as needed.

X. **Relevant Pharmacokinetics/Pharmacodynamics**

A. **Metabolism**: Phase I: Cytochrome P450 (CYP) 3A4 (major), CYP1A2 (minor), CYP2C8 (minor). Phase II: human uridine 5′-diphospho-glucuronosyltransferase (UGT) 1A1, UGT1A4, UGT2B15

B. **Time to peak plasma concentration**: 1–2 hours

C. **Half-life**: 18 hours

D. **Time to steady state**: ~5 days

E. **Excretion**: 58% renally (less than 1% unchanged); 29% biliary

F. **Bioavailability**: 4.4% (increased with food)

G. **Distribution**: 97.4% plasma protein bound

H. **Use with food**: Must be taken with food.

I. **Hepatic impairment**:

1. For moderate to severe impairment (Child-Pugh B/C): Reduce dosage to 21 mg once nightly.

J. **Renal impairment**: No dosage adjustments required.

K. **Special populations**: No significant age-, sex-, or race-related differences in metabolism.

XI. **Clinically Relevant Drug Interactions**

A. Metabolized by CYP3A4 (major) and human UGT:

1. Use caution/decrease dose when combined with moderate or strong CYP3A4 inhibitors (e.g., erythromycin, terbinafine, nefazodone). The following recommendations are provided from the manufacturer:
    a. With concomitant moderate CYP3A4 inhibitors: Decrease lumateperone dosage to 21 mg/day.
    b. With concomitant strong CYP3A4 inhibitors: Decrease lumateperone dosage to 10.5 mg/day.
2. Avoid use of lumateperone in combination with CYP3A4 inducers (strong: carbamazepine, St. John's wort, phenytoin, rifampin; moderate: modafinil, thioridazine, efavirenz, nafcillin).
3. Avoid use of lumateperone in combination with UGT inhibitors (e.g., valproic acid, probenecid).

B. Use caution with other drugs known to prolong the QTc interval, antihypertensive drugs, other CNS depressants, and anticholinergic agents.

XII. **Adverse Effects**

A. **See Table 6–1 ("Antipsychotic Class Adverse Effects") at beginning of chapter.**

B. Lumateperone's adverse effects include metabolic syndrome, anticholinergic effects, QTc prolongation, orthostatic hypotension, EPS, prolactin elevation, sexual dysfunction, NMS, temperature dysregulation, hyponatremia/syndrome of inappropriate antidiuretic hormone secretion (SIADH), and seizures.

1. For the full scope of potential adverse effects, see drug labeling (Lumateperone package insert).

C. **Boxed warnings**:

1. Increased mortality in older patients with dementia-related psychosis
2. Potential increased risk of suicidal thoughts/behaviors in pediatric/young adult patients. Monitor closely for emergence of suicidal thoughts. For detailed information, the reader is referred to comprehensive sources in the literature (e.g., Fergusson et al. 2005).

D. **Common**: Nausea/vomiting, dry mouth, headache, sedation, dizziness

E. **Uncommon**: Increased liver enzymes, EPS, dyscrasias

XIII. **Clinical Pearls/Prescribing Tips**

A. Lumateperone has a unique mechanism in that it is an antagonist at postsynaptic D_2 receptors but an agonist at presynaptic autoreceptors, thereby preventing more outflow of dopamine into the synaptic cleft (Cooper and Gupta 2022).

B. Lumateperone has a much higher affinity for the 5-HT_{2A} receptor than for the D_2 receptor, possibly leading to less risk of EPS and NMS.

C. Lumateperone inhibits the SERT receptor, decreasing reuptake of serotonin from the synaptic cleft. This mechanism may be beneficial for augmentation in unipolar or bipolar depression, or for negative symptoms of schizophrenia.

D. Although concomitant use of a monoamine oxidase inhibitor (MAOI) or another serotonergic agent is not a contraindication to use of lumateperone, caution should be exercised because such use increases the risk of serotonin syndrome.
E. The manufacturer recommends taking lumateperone with food for best absorption.

Further Reading

Caplyta (lumateperone) package insert. U.S Food and Drug Administration, 2022. Available at: https://www.accessdata.fda.gov/spl/data/e7101e78-2736-432f-e053-2995a90addec/e7101e78-2736-432f-e053-2995a90addec.xml. Accessed March 13, 2024.

Roth BL, Driscoll J: PDSP Ki Database. Psychoactive Drug Screening Program (PDSP). University of North Carolina at Chapel Hill and the United States National Institute of Mental Health, 2023

References

Cooper D, Gupta V: Lumateperone, in StatPearls. Treasure Island, FL, StatPearls Publishing. 2022. Available at: https://www.ncbi.nlm.nih.gov/books/NBK560844/. Accessed March 13, 2024.

Fergusson D, Doucette S, Glass KC, et al: Association between suicide attempts and selective serotonin reuptake inhibitors: systematic review of randomised controlled trials. BMJ 330(7488):396, 2005 15718539

Pimavanserin

I. **Brand Name(s)**: Nuplazid
II. **Therapeutic Class**: Atypical antipsychotic
III. **Mechanism-Based Class**: Serotonin receptor antagonist and inverse agonist
IV. **Mechanism(s) of Action**

A. Serotonin 5-HT_{2A} receptor antagonist and inverse agonist
B. Minimal to no affinity for dopamine D_2 receptors
C. High affinity for serotonergic receptors: 5-HT_{2A} antagonist (Ki=0.087 nM), 5-HT_{2C} antagonist (Ki=0.44 nM)
D. Minimal to no affinity for muscarinic, histaminergic, and adrenergic receptors

V. **Indications**

A. FDA adult:

1. Hallucinations and delusions associated with Parkinson's disease psychosis

B. Evidence-based[1] off-label uses:

1. Major depressive disorder—Adjunctive agent (under investigation)
2. Negative symptoms of schizophrenia (under investigation)

C. FDA pediatric: None

---

[1]Evidence strength varies; readers are referred to the literature for more detailed information.

VI. **Major Contraindications and When to Use Caution**

A. **Contraindications**: Hypersensitivity to pimavanserin

B. **Use caution**: Patients with baseline fall risk, hyponatremia or other electrolyte abnormalities, dysrhythmias (including QTc prolongation), leukopenia/neutropenia, hypotension/syncope or on antihypertensive medications, seizures, motor/cognitive impairments or on CNS depressants or anticholinergic agents, temperature dysregulation, aspiration, dysphagia, obesity, hyperglycemia, hyperlipidemia, risk factors for NMS (e.g., dehydration), or dementia-related psychosis (boxed warning), pregnancy/lactation.

VII. **Dosage Formulations**

A. Brand tablet (10 mg)

B. Brand capsule (34 mg)

VIII. **Dosage Ranges and Guidelines**

A. **Initial/maximum dosing/titration**:

1. Adults (both younger and older): Recommended dosage is 34 mg PO daily without titration. (With concomitant CYP3A4 inhibitors, maximum pimavanserin dosage is 10 mg/day.)
2. Children/adolescents: Safety/efficacy not established.
3. See "Clinically Relevant Drug Interactions" below and adjust dosages accordingly.

B. **Discontinuation**: For patients on long-term treatment, taper slowly to avoid rebound psychosis and withdrawal dyskinesias.

IX. **Monitoring**

A. Baseline and periodic:

1. Labs: CBC with differential (rule out hematological changes), LFTs (rare liver damage risk, contraindicated in hepatic impairment), renal function, electrolytes
2. Metabolic: Weight, hemoglobin A1c test, lipid panel for metabolic risk
3. Extrapyramidal symptoms (EPS): Monitor for abnormal involuntary movements/parkinsonian signs (via Abnormal Involuntary Movement Scale [AIMS]) at baseline and periodically.
4. Consider obtaining an ECG at baseline and periodically if indicated (cardiac risk factors, high-risk medication).
5. Other: Visual changes/ocular exam, sexual changes, mental status changes, blood pressure changes, falls

B. For individuals at risk of significant electrolyte disturbances (e.g., diuretic therapy, diarrhea), consider checking serum potassium and magnesium and repleting as needed.

C. If there are concerns regarding QTc prolongation, consider obtaining an ECG.

X. **Relevant Pharmacokinetics/Pharmacodynamics**

A. **Metabolism**: Phase I: cytochrome P450 (CYP) 3A4 (major), CYP3A5 (major), CYP2J2 (minor), CYP2D6 (minor)

B. **Time to peak plasma concentration**: 4–24 (median of 6) hours

C. **Half-life**: 57 hours; *N*-desmethylated metabolite (AC-279): 200 hours

D. **Excretion**: Feces, renal (both as less than 1% unchanged drug)
E. **Bioavailability**: 99.7%
F. **Distribution**: 95% plasma protein bound
G. **Hepatic impairment**: No dosage adjustment required.
H. **Renal impairment**: CrCl≥30 mL/minute: No dosage adjustment required. CrCl<30 mL/minute: Although no dosage adjustment is required, caution is advised due to increased pimavanserin exposure.
I. **Special populations**: No significant age-, sex-, or race-related differences in metabolism.

XI. Clinically Relevant Drug Interactions

A. Metabolized primarily by CYP3A4 (major):

1. Use caution/decrease dosage when combined with strong CYP3A4 inhibitors (e.g., erythromycin, terbinafine, nefazodone). The following recommendations are provided by the manufacturer:

    a. With concomitant use of strong CYP3A4 inhibitors, decrease pimavanserin dosage to 10 mg/day.

2. Do not use in combination with moderate or strong CYP3A4 inducers (strong: carbamazepine, St. John's wort, phenytoin, rifampin; moderate: modafinil, thioridazine, efavirenz, nafcillin).

B. Use caution with other drugs known to prolong the QTc, antihypertensive drugs, other CNS depressants, and anticholinergic agents.

XII. Adverse Effects

A. Most D_2 receptor–related adverse effects of antipsychotics do not apply, given pimavanserin's lack of D_2 receptor affinity, but QTc prolongation, orthostatic hypotension, and sexual side effects can still occur.

1. For full scope of potential adverse effects, see drug labeling (Pimavanserin package insert).

B. **Boxed warning**: Increased mortality in older patients with dementia-related psychosis.
C. **Common**: QTc prolongation, peripheral edema, confusional state, nausea
D. **Uncommon/rare**: Constipation, gait disturbance, hallucination, urinary tract infection, fatigue

XIII. Clinical Pearls/Prescribing Tips

A. No dosage adjustment of carbidopa/levodopa is required when used concomitantly with pimavanserin.
B. Pimavanserin is extensively metabolized by CYP3A4; for patients on concomitant strong CYP3A4 inhibitors, pimavanserin dosage should be decreased to 10 mg/day.
C. Although pimavanserin is indicated for delusions/hallucinations in patients with Parkinson's disease psychosis, it still carries a warning of increased mortality in older patients with dementia-related psychosis, and it is not FDA approved for this specific purpose.
D. Data on the efficacy of pimavanserin for its FDA indication have been mixed.

Further Reading

Citrome L, Norton JC, Chi-Burris K, et al: Pimavanserin for the treatment of Parkinson's disease psychosis: number needed to treat, number needed to harm, and likelihood to be helped or harmed. CNS Spectr 23(3):228–238, 2018 29098976

Iketani R, Furushima D, Imai S, et al: Efficacy and safety of atypical antipsychotics for psychosis in Parkinson's disease: a systematic review and Bayesian network meta-analysis. Parkinsonism Relat Disord 78:82–90, 2020 32755800

Mansuri Z, Reddy A, Vadukapuram R, et al: Pimavanserin in the treatment of Parkinson's disease psychosis: meta-analysis and meta-regression of randomized clinical trials. Innov Clin Neurosci 19(1–3):46–51, 2022 35382074

Nuplazid (pimavanserin) package insert. U.S Food and Drug Administration, 2022. Available at: https://www.accessdata.fda.gov/spl/data/812acf7c-c2bd-4833-9d79-66c8f593a01f/812acf7c-c2bd-4833-9d79-66c8f593a01f.xml. Accessed March 13, 2024.

Roth BL, Driscoll J: PDSP Ki Database. Psychoactive Drug Screening Program (PDSP). University of North Carolina at Chapel Hill and the United States National Institute of Mental Health, 2023

7

Stimulants

Michael S. Ziffra, M.D.

A variety of pharmacological treatments are available for the treatment of attention-deficit hyperactivity disorder (ADHD). Psychostimulant medications (including methylphenidate-based agents and amphetamine-based agents) are commonly prescribed, but several alternative options exist. An assortment of factors will influence what specific medication might be recommended to a patient, including the severity and timing of ADHD symptoms, side-effect profiles, and comorbid psychiatric and medical conditions.

Psychostimulants

Amphetamines

I. **Brand Names**: Adderall, Adderall extended-release (XR), Adzenys ER–orally disintegrating tablet (XR-ODT), Dyanavel XR, Evekeo, Evekeo ODT, Mydayis

II. **Therapeutic Class**: CNS stimulant

III. **Mechanism-Based Class**: Dopamine and norepinephrine reuptake inhibitor and releaser

IV. **Mechanism(s) of Action**

A. Blocks reuptake of dopamine and norepinephrine into the presynaptic neuron.

B. Increases release of dopamine and norepinephrine into the extraneuronal space.

V. **Indications**

A. FDA adult:

1. ADHD in adults (Adderall XR, Evekeo, Adzenys XR-ODT)
2. Narcolepsy (Adderall, Evekeo)
3. Exogenous obesity (Evekeo)
    1. Exogenous obesity: Obesity due to energy intake exceeding energy expenditure

B. Evidence-based[1] off-label uses:

1. Treatment-resistant depression
2. Other disorders associated with excessive daytime sleepiness

C. FDA pediatric:

1. ADHD in children age 3 years and older (Adderall, Evekeo, Evekeo ODT)
2. ADHD in children age 6 years and older (Adderall XR, Adzenys XR-ODT, Dyanavel XR)
3. ADHD in children age 13 years and older (Mydayis)

VI. **Major Contraindications and When to Use Caution**

A. Known allergy to amphetamines or brand drugs containing amphetamine

B. Concomitant use of monoamine oxidase inhibitors (MAOIs) (2-week washout required)

C. Avoid use in patients with structural cardiac abnormalities, cardiomyopathy, serious heart arrhythmia, or coronary artery disease.

VII. **Dosage Formulations**—*Note:* Capsules can be opened and beads mixed with food.

A. Brand:

1. Adderall tablet (5 mg, 7.5 mg, 10 mg, 12.5 mg, 15 mg, 20 mg, 30 mg)
2. Adderall XR capsule (5 mg, 10 mg, 15 mg, 20 mg, 25 mg, 30 mg)

---

[1]Evidence strength varies; readers are referred to the literature for more detailed information.

3. Adzenys XR-ODT (3.1 mg, 6.3 mg, 9.4 mg, 12.5 mg, 15.7 mg, 18.8 mg)
4. Dyanavel XR tablet (5 mg, 10 mg, 15 mg, 20 mg); oral suspension (2.5 mg/mL)
5. Evekeo tablet (5 mg, 10 mg)
6. Evekeo ODT (2.5 mg, 5 mg, 10 mg, 15 mg, 20 mg)
7. Mydayis capsule (12.5, 25 mg, 37.5 mg, 50 mg)

B. Generic:

1. Tablet (5 mg, 7.5 mg, 10 mg, 12.5 mg, 15 mg, 20 mg, 30 mg)
2. ER capsule (5 mg, 10 mg, 15 mg, 20 mg, 25 mg, 30 mg)

VIII. **Dosage Ranges and Guidelines**

A. Table 7–1 presents dosage ranges and administration guidelines for amphetamine formulations.

Table 7–1. Amphetamine formulations: dosages and administration

Medication	Dosing instructions
Adderall	**Children age 3–5 years**: Initial dosage 2.5 mg/day. May increase by 2.5 mg/day at weekly intervals. Maximum dosage 40 mg/day. **Patients age ≥6 years**: Initial dosage 5 mg 1–2 times a day. May increase by 5 mg/day at weekly intervals. Maximum dosage 40 mg/day.
Adderall XR	Initial dosage 10 mg once a day. May increase by 5–10 mg/day at weekly intervals. Maximum dosage 60 mg/day.
Adzenys XR-ODT	**Children age 6–12 years**: Initial dosage 6.3 mg/day. Titrate upward as needed/tolerated. Maximum recommended dosage 18.8 mg/day. **Youth age 13–18 years**: Initial dosage 6.3 mg/day. Titrate upward as needed/tolerated. Maximum recommended dosage 12.5 mg/day. **Adults**: Initial dosage 12.5 mg/day. Titrate upward as needed/tolerated. Maximum recommended dosage 18.8 mg/day.
Dyanavel XR	Initial dosage 2.5–5 mg once a day. May increase by 2.5–5 mg/day at weekly intervals. Maximum dosage 40 mg/day.
Evekeo	Initial dosage 2.5 mg/day. May increase by 2.5–10 mg/day every 4–7 days. Maximum dosage 20 mg/day.
Evekeo ODT	**Children age 3–5 years**: Initial dosage 2.5 mg/day. May increase by 2.5 mg/day at weekly intervals. Maximum dosage 40 mg/day. **Patients age ≥6 years**: Initial dosage 5 mg 1–2 times a day. May increase by 2.5–5 mg/day at weekly intervals. Maximum dosage 40 mg/day.

Note. ODT=orally disintegrating tablet; XR=extended release.

IX. **Monitoring**

A. Cardiac: Prior to starting, assess for the presence of a personal or family history of relevant cardiac disease. During treatment, monitor blood pressure and pulse. Consider periodic ECG monitoring.
B. Monitor height and weight in pediatric patients.

X. **Relevant Pharmacokinetics/Pharmacodynamics**

A. **Metabolism**: Hepatic

B. **Time to peak plasma concentration**: Approximately 3 hours for immediate-release formulations. Approximately 7 hours for extended-release formulations

C. **Half-life**: 9–11 hours. Extended-release formulations have delivery systems that release the drug over longer periods of time. For more detailed information, see other sources, including the package inserts of specific formulations.

D. **Use with food**: Can be taken with or without food. Peak effect may be delayed by several hours when taken with food (particularly high-fat meals).

E. **Hepatic impairment**: No dosage adjustment needed.

F. **Renal impairment**: For Adderall XR and Mydayis, use a reduced dosage in individuals with severe renal disease. Do not use Adderall XR or Mydayis in individuals with end-stage renal disease.

XI. **Clinically Relevant Drug Interactions**

A. Metabolized by cytochrome P450 (CYP) 2D6.

1. Serum levels can be increased by CYP2D6 inhibitors.
2. Tricyclic antidepressants can cause striking and sustained increases in brain concentrations of dextroamphetamine and can potentiate cardiovascular effects.

B. Blood levels are decreased by urine-acidifying agents.

C. Blood levels are increased by urine-alkalinizing agents.

D. Potential for serotonin syndrome when combined with antidepressants or other serotonergic agents.

E. Risk for hypertensive crisis when used concomitantly with MAOIs.

XII. **Adverse Effects**

A. **Most common**:

1. Reduced appetite and weight
2. Anxiety
3. Insomnia
4. Tics, exacerbation of tic disorders
5. Headache

B. **Other notable side effects**:

1. Increased blood pressure and heart rate
2. Serious cardiac events (stroke, myocardial infarction, sudden death)
3. Peripheral vasculopathy, including Raynaud's phenomenon
4. Growth suppression in children
5. Psychiatric side effects (mania, psychosis)
6. May lower seizure threshold
7. Visual disturbances

XIII. **Clinical Pearls/Prescribing Tips**

A. Multiple variants are available, including both immediate-release and extended-release formulations. Some trial and error may be required to find the regimen that best suits the patient's needs.
B. Adderall, Evekeo, and Evekeo ODT are immediate-release formulations that are usually taken at least twice a day. Duration of action is about 3–6 hours.
C. Adderall XR, Dyanavel XR, Adzenys XR-ODT, and Mydayis are extended-release formulations that are typically taken once a day. Duration of action is about 8 hours.
D. Patients may find that immediate-release formulations are more likely than extended-release formulations to cause a "crash" (tiredness, headache, mood changes) as the medication is wearing off.
E. In rare cases, an extended-release formulation and an immediate-release formulation can be combined to improve efficacy or tolerability.
F. Taking extended-release amphetamine formulations with a high-fat meal (as opposed to taking after an overnight fast) may result in a delayed peak effect, with lower concentrations (by ~50%) in the first several hours (Auiler et al. 2002; Wang et al. 2019).

Further Reading

Adderall XR package insert. U.S. Food and Drug Administration, 2022. Available at: https://www.accessdata.fda.gov/drugsatfda_docs/label/2022/021303s036lbl.pdf. Accessed March 13, 2024.

Castells X, Blanco-Silvente L, Cunill R: Amphetamines for attention deficit hyperactivity disorder (ADHD) in adults. Cochrane Database Syst Rev 8(8):CD007813, 2018 30091808

Punja S, Shamseer L, Hartling L, et al: Amphetamines for attention deficit hyperactivity disorder (ADHD) in children and adolescents. Cochrane Database Syst Rev 2(2):CD009996, 2016 26844979

References

Auiler JF, Liu K, Lynch JM, et al: Effect of food on early drug exposure from extended-release stimulants: results from the Concerta, Adderall XR Food Evaluation (CAFE) Study. Curr Med Res Opin 18(5):311–316, 2002 12240794

Wang Y, Yu M, Yan B, et al: Effects of food on the bioavailability of amphetamine in healthy adults after administration of SHP465 mixed amphetamine salts extended-release capsules. Drugs R D 19(2):167–175, 2019 30911906

Dextroamphetamine

I. **Brand Names**: Dexedrine (discontinued), Dexedrine Spansule, Xelstrym (transdermal), Zenzedi

II. **Therapeutic Class**: CNS stimulant

III. **Mechanism-Based Class**: Dopamine and norepinephrine reuptake inhibitor and releaser

IV. **Mechanism(s) of Action**

A. Blocks reuptake of dopamine and norepinephrine into the presynaptic neuron

B. Increases release of dopamine and norepinephrine into the extraneuronal space

V. **Indications**

A. FDA adult:

1. ADHD
2. Narcolepsy

B. Evidence-based[1] off-label uses:

1. Treatment-resistant depression
2. Other disorders associated with excessive daytime sleepiness

C. FDA pediatric:

1. ADHD in children age 3 years and older (Zenzedi)
2. ADHD in children age 6 years and older (Dexedrine Spansules, Xelstrym)
3. Narcolepsy

VI. **Major Contraindications and When to Use Caution**

A. Known allergy to dextroamphetamine or any brand drugs containing dextroamphetamine

B. Concomitant use of monoamine oxidase inhibitors (MAOIs) (2-week washout required)

C. Avoid use in patients with structural cardiac abnormalities, cardiomyopathy, serious heart arrhythmia, or coronary artery disease.

VII. **Dosage Formulations**

A. Brand:

1. Dexedrine Spansule (dextroamphetamine sulfate) extended-release (ER) capsule (5 mg, 10 mg, 15 mg)
2. Xelstrym (dextroamphetamine) transdermal patch (4.5 mg/9 hr, 9 mg/9 hr, 13.5 mg/9 hr, 18 mg/9 hr)
3. Zenzedi (dextroamphetamine sulfate) tablet (2.5 mg, 5 mg, 7.5 mg, 10 mg, 15 mg, 20 mg, 30 mg)

---

[1]Evidence strength varies; readers are referred to the literature for more detailed information.

B. Generic:

1. Dextroamphetamine sulfate tablet (2.5 mg, 5 mg, 7.5 mg, 10 mg, 15 mg, 20 mg, 30 mg); oral suspension (5 mg/5 mL)
2. Dextroamphetamine sulfate ER capsule (5 mg, 10 mg, 15 mg)

VIII. **Dosage Ranges and Guidelines**

A. Table 7–2 presents dosage ranges and administration guidelines for dextroamphetamine formulations.

Table 7–2. Dextroamphetamine formulations: dosages and administration

Medication	Dosing instructions
Dexedrine	**Children age 3–5 years**: Initial dosage 2.5 mg/day. May increase by 2.5 mg at weekly intervals. Maximum dosage 40 mg/day. **Patients age ≥6 years**: Initial dosage 5 mg 1–2 times a day. May increase by 5 mg at weekly intervals. Maximum dosage 40 mg/day.
Dexedrine Spansules	Initial dosage 5 mg 1–2 times a day. May increase by 5 mg at weekly intervals. Maximum dosage 40 mg/day.
Xelstrym	**Children age 6–17 years**: Initial dosage 4.5 mg once a day. May increase dosage by 4.5 mg at weekly intervals. Maximum dosage 18 mg/day. **Adults**: Initial dosage 9 mg once a day. May increase dosage by 4.5 mg at weekly intervals. Maximum dosage 18 mg/day. **Administration**: Apply patch 2 hours before an effect is needed. Remove patch 9 hours after application.
Zenzedi	**Children age 3–5 years**: Initial dosage 2.5 mg once a day. May increase by 2.5 mg at weekly intervals. Maximum dosage 40 mg/day. **Patients age ≥6 years**: Initial dosage 5 mg 1–2 times a day. May increase by 5 mg at weekly intervals. Maximum dosage 40 mg/day.

IX. **Monitoring**

A. Cardiac: Prior to starting, assess for presence of relevant personal and family history of cardiac disease. During treatment, monitor blood pressure and pulse. Consider periodic ECG monitoring.
B. Monitor height and weight in pediatric patients.

X. **Relevant Pharmacokinetics/Pharmacodynamics**

A. **Metabolism**: Hepatic
B. **Time to peak plasma concentration**: 3 hours (immediate-release), 8 hours (sustained-release)
C. **Half-life**: 12 hours
D. **Use with food**: Can be taken with or without food. Peak effect may be slightly delayed when taken with food.
E. **Hepatic impairment**: No dosage adjustment needed.
F. **Renal impairment**: For Xelstrym, maximum dosage is 13.5 mg/9 hours in patients with severe renal disease, and 9 mg/9 hours in individuals with end-stage renal disease.

XI. Clinically Relevant Drug Interactions

A. Metabolized by cytochrome P450 (CYP) 2D6.

1. Use with CYP2D6 inhibitors can increase serum levels of dextroamphetamine.
2. Tricyclic antidepressants can cause striking and sustained increases in brain concentrations of dextroamphetamine and can potentiate cardiovascular effects.

B. Blood levels are decreased by urine-acidifying agents.

C. Blood levels are increased by urine-alkalinizing agents.

D. Potential for serotonin syndrome when used concomitantly with an antidepressant or another serotonergic agent.

E. Risk of hypertensive crisis when used concomitantly with an MAOI.

XII. Adverse Effects

A. **Most common**:

1. Reduced appetite and weight
2. Anxiety
3. Insomnia
4. Tics, exacerbation of tic disorders
5. Headache

B. **Other notable side effects**:

1. Increased blood pressure and heart rate
2. Serious cardiovascular events (sudden death, stroke, myocardial infarction)
3. Peripheral vasculopathy, including Raynaud's phenomenon
4. Growth suppression in children
5. Psychiatric side effects (mania, psychosis)
6. May lower seizure threshold.
7. Visual disturbances

XIII. Clinical Pearls/Prescribing Tips

A. Compared with D,L-amphetamine, dextroamphetamine has greater action on dopamine, which may influence efficacy and tolerability.

B. Multiple variants are available, including both immediate-release and extended-release formulations. Some trial and error may be required to find the regimen that best suits the patient's needs.

C. Dexedrine and Zenzedi are immediate-release formulations that are usually taken at least twice a day. Duration of action is about 4 hours.

D. Dexedrine Spansules (oral) and Xelstrym (transdermal) are extended-release formulations that are typically taken once a day. Duration of action is about 8 hours.

E. Patients may find that immediate-release formulations are more likely than extended-release formulations to cause a "crash" (tiredness, headache, mood changes) as the medication is wearing off.

F. In rare cases, an extended-release formulation and an immediate-release formulation can be combined to improve efficacy or tolerability.

Further Reading

Dexedrine Spansule package insert. U.S. Food and Drug Administration, 2022. Available at: https://www.accessdata.fda.gov/drugsatfda_docs/label/2022/017078s054lbl.pdf. Accessed March 13, 2024.

Paterson R, Douglas C, Hallmayer J, et al: A randomised, double-blind, placebo-controlled trial of dexamphetamine in adults with attention deficit hyperactivity disorder. Aust NZ J Psychiatry 33(4):494–502, 1999 10483843

Taylor FB, Russo J: Comparing guanfacine and dextroamphetamine for the treatment of adult attention-deficit/hyperactivity disorder. J Clin Psychopharmacol 21(2):223–228, 2001 11270920

Xelstrym package insert. U.S. Food and Drug Administration, 2022. Available at: https://www.accessdata.fda.gov/drugsatfda_docs/label/2022/215401s000lbl.pdf. Accessed March 13, 2024.

Zenzedi package insert. Available at: https://www.zenzedi.com/docs/Zenzedi_Prescribing_Information_and_Medication_Guide.pdf. Accessed March 13, 2024.

Lisdexamfetamine

I. **Brand Names**: Vyvanse

II. **Therapeutic Class**: CNS stimulant

III. **Mechanism-Based Class**: Dopamine and norepinephrine reuptake inhibitor and releaser

IV. **Mechanism(s) of Action**

- A. Blocks reuptake of dopamine and norepinephrine into the presynaptic neuron.
- B. Increases release of dopamine and norepinephrine into the extraneuronal space.

V. **Indications**

- A. FDA adult:
  1. ADHD
  2. Binge-eating disorder
- B. Evidence-based[1] off-label uses:
  1. Treatment-resistant depression
  2. Narcolepsy, excessive daytime sleepiness
- C. FDA pediatric: ADHD (children age 6 years and older)

VI. **Major Contraindications and When to Use Caution**

- A. Known allergy to lisdexamfetamine or Vyvanse
- B. Concomitant use of monoamine oxidase inhibitors (MAOIs) (2-week washout required)
- C. Avoid use in patients with structural cardiac abnormalities, cardiomyopathy, serious heart arrhythmia, or coronary artery disease.

---

[1]Evidence strength varies; readers are referred to the literature for more detailed information.

VII. **Dosage Formulations**

A. Brand capsule (10 mg, 20 mg, 30 mg, 40 mg, 50 mg, 60 mg, 70 mg)

1. Note: Capsule can be opened and mixed with water, applesauce, or ice cream and given immediately, if needed.

B. Brand chewable tablet (10 mg, 20 mg, 30 mg, 40 mg, 50 mg, 60 mg)

VIII. **Dosage Ranges and Guidelines**

A. ADHD: Start at 30 mg every morning. Titrate upward by 10–20 mg/day at weekly intervals. Recommended dosage is 30–70 mg/day. Maximum dosage is 70 mg/day.

B. Binge-eating disorder: Start at 30 mg every morning. Titrate upward by 20 mg/day at weekly intervals. Recommended dosage is 50–70 mg/day. Maximum dosage is 70 mg/day.

IX. **Monitoring**

A. Cardiac: Prior to starting, assess for presence of relevant personal and family history of cardiac disease. During treatment, monitor blood pressure and pulse. Consider periodic ECG monitoring.

B. Monitor height and weight in pediatric patients

X. **Relevant Pharmacokinetics/Pharmacodynamics**

A. **Metabolism**: Converted to dextroamphetamine and L-lysine in the blood

B. **Time to peak plasma concentration**: 1–4 hours (1 hour for lisdexamfetamine, ~4 hours for dextroamphetamine)

C. **Half-life**: 9–11 hours

D. **Use with food**: Can be taken with or without food. Peak effect may be delayed when taken with food (Krishnan and Zhang 2008).

E. **Hepatic impairments**: No dosage adjustments needed

F. **Renal impairment**: Maximum dosage is 50 mg/day in individuals with severe renal impairment; 30 mg/day in individuals with end-stage renal disease

XI. **Clinically Relevant Drug Interactions**

A. Metabolized by cytochrome P450 (CYP) 2D6.

1. Use with CYP2D6 inhibitors can increase serum levels of dextroamphetamine.
2. Tricyclic antidepressants can cause striking and sustained increases in brain concentrations of dextroamphetamine, and can potentiate cardiovascular effects.

B. Blood levels are decreased by urine-acidifying agents.

C. Blood levels are increased by urine-alkalinizing agents.

D. Potential for serotonin syndrome when combined with antidepressants and other serotonergic agents.

E. Risk for hypertensive crisis when used concomitantly with MAOIs.

XII. **Adverse Effects**

A. **Most common**:

1. Reduced appetite and weight
2. Anxiety

3. Insomnia
4. Tics, exacerbation of tic disorders
5. Headache

B. **Other notable side effects**:

1. Increased blood pressure and heart rate
2. Serious cardiac events (sudden death, stroke, myocardial infarction)
3. Peripheral vasculopathy, including Raynaud's phenomenon
4. Growth suppression in children
5. Psychiatric side effects (e.g., mania, psychosis)
6. May lower seizure threshold.
7. Visual disturbances

XIII. **Clinical Pearls/Prescribing Tips**

A. Lisdexamfetamine is a prodrug of dextroamphetamine and is active after it has been absorbed by the gastrointestinal tract and converted to dextroamphetamine and L-lysine.
B. Lisdexamfetamine has a long duration of action (up to 12 hours) and can be a good choice for individuals with symptoms that persist into the evening.
C. Dose should be taken early in the day to avoid insomnia at night.
D. Lisdexamfetamine can be a good choice for individuals with comorbid ADHD and binge-eating disorder.
E. Because there is no active D-amphetamine in the prodrug (which must be absorbed in the gastrointestinal tract), the abuse potential of lisdexamfetamine is thought to be lower than that of other amphetamine formulations (Jasinski and Krishnan 2009).

Further Reading

Coghill DR, Caballero B, Sorooshian S, et al: A systematic review of the safety of lisdexamfetamine dimesylate. CNS Drugs 28(6):497–511, 2014 24788672

Frampton JE: Lisdesamfetamine: a review in ADHD in adults. CNS Drugs 30(4):343–354, 2016 27048350

Frampton JE: Lisdesamfetamine dimesylate: a review in paediatric ADHD. Drugs 78(10):1025–1036, 2018 29923015

Vyvanse package insert. U.S. Food and Drug Administration, 2022. Available at: https://www.accessdata.fda.gov/drugsatfda_docs/label/2022/021977s048,208510s005lbl.pdf. Accessed March 13, 2024.

References

Jasinski DR, Krishnan S: Human pharmacology of intravenous lisdexamfetamine dimesylate: abuse liability in adult stimulant abusers. J Psychopharmacol 23(4):410–418, 2009 18635707

Krishnan S, Zhang Y: Relative bioavailability of lisdexamfetamine 70-mg capsules in fasted and fed healthy adult volunteers and in solution: a single-dose, crossover pharmacokinetic study. J Clin Pharmacol 48(3):293–302, 2008 18285619

Methylphenidates (Methylphenidate, Dexmethylphenidate)

I. **Brand Names**: Ritalin, Ritalin SR, Ritalin LA, Aptensio XR, Concerta, Daytrana, Focalin, Focalin XR, Metadate CD, Metadate ER, Methylin, Methylin ER, Quilli-Chew ER, Quillivant XR

II. **Therapeutic Class**: Stimulant

III. **Mechanism-Based Class**: Dopamine and norepinephrine reuptake inhibitor and releaser

IV. **Mechanism(s) of Action**

A. Blocks reuptake of dopamine and norepinephrine into the presynaptic neuron.

B. Increases release of dopamine and norepinephrine into the extraneuronal space (minor).

V. **Indications**

A. FDA adult:

1. ADHD
2. Narcolepsy (Ritalin, Ritalin SR, Metadate ER)

B. Evidence-based[1] off-label uses:

1. Treatment-resistant depression
2. Other disorders associated with excessive daytime sleepiness

C. FDA pediatric:

1. ADHD (age 6 years and older; precise age range varies by specific formulation)
2. Narcolepsy

VI. **Major Contraindications and When to Use Caution**

A. Known allergy to methylphenidate or brand drugs containing methylphenidate

B. Concomitant use of monoamine oxidase inhibitors (MAOIs) (2-week washout required)

C. Avoid use in patients with structural cardiac abnormalities, cardiomyopathy, serious heart arrhythmia, or coronary artery disease.

VII. **Dosage Formulations**

A. Table 7–3 presents the available formulations and strengths for methylphenidate preparations.

VIII. **Dosage Ranges and Guidelines**

A. Table 7–4 presents dosage ranges and administration guidelines for methylphenidate formulations.

[1]Evidence strength varies; readers are referred to the literature for more detailed information.

Table 7–3. Methylphenidate: available formulations

Medication	Brand	Generic
Ritalin	Tablet (5 mg, 10 mg, 20 mg)	Tablet (5 mg, 10 mg, 20 mg)
Ritalin SR	N/A	Tablet (20 mg)
Ritalin LA[a]	Capsule (10 mg, 20 mg, 30 mg, 40 mg)	Capsule (10 mg, 20 mg, 30 mg, 40 mg)
Aptensio XR	Capsule (10 mg, 15 mg, 20 mg, 30 mg, 40 mg, 50 mg, 60 mg)	Capsule (10 mg, 15 mg, 20 mg, 30 mg, 40 mg, 50 mg, 60 mg)
Concerta[b]	Tablet (18 mg, 27 mg, 36 mg, 54 mg)	Tablet (18 mg, 27 mg, 36 mg, 54 mg)
Daytrana	Transdermal patch (10 mg/9 hr, 15 mg/9 hr, 20 mg/9 hr, 30 mg/9 hr)	Transdermal patch (10 mg/9 hr, 20 mg/9 hr, 30 mg/9 hr)
Focalin	Tablet (2.5 mg, 5 mg, 10 mg)	Tablet (2.5 mg, 5 mg, 10 mg)
Focalin XR[c]	Capsule (5 mg, 10 mg, 15 mg, 20 mg, 25 mg, 30 mg, 35 mg, 40 mg)	Capsule (5 mg, 10 mg, 15 mg, 20 mg, 25 mg, 30 mg, 35 mg, 40 mg)
Metadate CD[d]	Not available	Capsule (10 mg, 20 mg, 30 mg, 40 mg, 50 mg, 60 mg)
Metadate ER	Not available	Tablet (20 mg)
Methylin	Oral suspension (5 mg/5 mL, 10 mg/5 mL)	Oral suspension (5 mg/5 mL, 10 mg/5 mL)
Methylin ER	Not available	Tablet (10, 20 mg)
QuilliChew ER	Chewable tablet (20 mg, 30 mg, 40 mg)	Not available
Quillivant XR	Oral suspension (5 mg/mL)	Not available

Note. Capsules can be opened and beads mixed with food. CD=controlled delivery; ER=extended release; IR=immediate release; LA=long-acting; SR=sustained release; XR=extended release.

[a]Ritalin LA uses a "spheroidal oral drug absorption system" (SODAS) and consists of 50% IR and 50% ER methylphenidate. It produces two distinct peaks, approximately 4 hours apart.

[b]Concerta uses an "osmotic release oral system" (OROS) in which osmotic pressure activates the "push compartment," causing the system to release methylphenidate through "exit ports." Concerta consists of approximately 22% immediate-release and 78% extended-release methylphenidate.

[c]Focalin XR (or dexmethylphenidate) is a sustained-release capsule consisting of 50% IR and 50% ER methylphenidate.

[d]Metadate CD (methylphenidate controlled delivery) uses a "difficaps" system; each capsule contains 30% immediate-release beads and 70% extended-release beads.

Table 7–4. Methylphenidate formulations: dosages and administration

Medication	Dosing instructions
Ritalin	**Children age 6–17 years**: Initial dosage 5 mg twice a day. May increase by 5–10 mg/day at weekly intervals. Maximum dosage 60 mg/day. **Adults**: Initial dosage 5–10 mg 2–3 times a day. May increase by 5–10 mg/day at weekly intervals. Maximum dosage 60 mg/day.
Ritalin SR	Initial dosage 20 mg/day. May increase dosage at weekly intervals. Maximum dosage 60 mg/day.
Ritalin LA	Start 10–20 mg once a day. May increase dosage at weekly intervals. Maximum dosage 60 mg/day.
Aptensio XR	Initial dosage 10 mg once a day. May increase by 10 mg/day at weekly intervals. Maximum dosage 60 mg/day.
Concerta	**Children and adolescents**: Initial dosage 18 mg once a day. May increase by 18 mg/day at weekly intervals. Maximum dosage is 54 mg/day in children and 72 mg/day in adolescents. **Adults**: Initial dosage 18–36 mg once a day. May increase by 18 mg/day at weekly intervals. Maximum dosage 72 mg/day.
Daytrana	Initial dosage 10 mg once a day. May increase dosage at weekly intervals. Maximum dosage 60 mg/day. Administration: Apply patch to hip area (using alternating sites) 2 hours before an effect is needed. Remove patch 9 hours after application.
Focalin	**Patients naive to methylphenidate**: Start at 2.5 mg twice a day. May increase by 2.5–5 mg/day at weekly intervals. Maximum dosage 20 mg/day. **Patients currently taking methylphenidate**: Initial dosage should be one-half the current daily methylphenidate dosage.
Focalin XR	**Patients naive to methylphenidate**: Start at 5 mg once a day. May increase by 5 mg/day at weekly intervals. Maximum dosage 30 mg/day. **Patients currently taking methylphenidate**: Initial dosage should be one-half the current daily methylphenidate dosage. **Patients currently taking immediate-release dexmethylphenidate**: Initial dosage should be the same total daily dosage, taken once a day.
Metadate CD	Initial dosage 20 mg once a day. May increase by 10–20 mg/day at weekly intervals. Maximum dosage is 60 mg/day.
Metadate ER	Initial dosage 20 mg once a day. May increase by 10–20 mg/day at weekly intervals. Maximum dosage is 60 mg/day.
Methylin	Initial dosage 5 mg twice a day. May increase by 5–10 mg/day at weekly intervals. Maximum dosage is 60 mg/day.
Methylin ER	Initial dosage 10 mg/day. May titrate upward as needed/tolerated. Maximum dosage is 60 mg/day.
QuilliChew ER	Initial dosage 20 mg once a day. May increase by 10–20 mg/day at weekly intervals. Maximum dosage is 60 mg/day.
Quillivant XR	Initial dosage 20 mg once a day. May increase by 10–20 mg/day at weekly intervals. Maximum dosage is 60 mg/day.

Note. CD=controlled delivery; ER=extended release; IR=immediate release; LA=long-acting; SR=sustained release; XR=extended release.

IX. **Monitoring**

A. Cardiac: Prior to starting, assess for the presence of relevant personal and family history of cardiac disease. During treatment, monitor blood pressure and heart rate. Consider periodic ECG monitoring.

B. Monitor height and weight in pediatric patients.

X. **Relevant Pharmacokinetics/Pharmacodynamics**

A. **Metabolism**: Metabolized extrahepatically by nonmicrosomal esterases that are widely distributed throughout the body

B. **Time to peak plasma concentration**: Variable, depending on the specific drug. Approximately 1–3 hours for immediate-release formulations. Approximately 6–8 hours for extended-release formulations

C. **Half-life**: 3.5 hours

D. **Use with food**: Can be taken with or without food. Peak effect may be delayed when taken with food.

E. **Hepatic impairment**: No dosage adjustment needed.

F. **Renal impairment**: No dosage adjustment needed.

XI. **Clinically Relevant Drug Interactions**

A. Potential for serotonin syndrome when combined with antidepressants or other serotonergic agents.

B. Risk for hypertensive crisis when used concomitantly with MAOIs.

C. May inhibit metabolism of several drugs, including certain antidepressants (e.g., SSRIs and TCAs), some anticonvulsants, and coumarin anticoagulants.

D. Effects of centrally acting antihypertensives (e.g., clonidine, methyldopa) can be reduced by methylphenidate.

XII. **Adverse Effects**

A. **Most common**:

1. Reduced appetite and weight
2. Anxiety
3. Insomnia
4. Tics, exacerbation of tic disorders
5. Headache

B. **Other notable side effects**:

1. Increased blood pressure and heart rate
2. Serious cardiac events (sudden death, stroke, myocardial infarction)
3. Peripheral vasculopathy, including Raynaud's phenomenon
4. Growth suppression in children
5. Psychiatric side effects (mania, psychosis)
6. May lower seizure threshold
7. Visual disturbances
8. Priapism (rare)

XIII. **Clinical Pearls/Prescribing Tips**

A. Multiple variants are available, including both immediate-release and extended-release formulations. Some trial and error may be required to find the regimen that best suits the patient's needs.

B. Duration of action of immediate-release formulations is about 4 hours.

C. Metadate CD and Ritalin LA are time-release formulations that have a peak action early in the day. Duration of action is about 8 hours.

D. Concerta is a time-release formulation that has less of an early peak and lasts up to 12 hours.

E. Focalin is the D-enantiomer of racemic methylphenidate. It is considered to be more efficacious than racemic methylphenidate (Focalin is about twice as potent as Ritalin).

F. Patients may find that immediate-release formulations are more likely than extended-release formulations to cause a "crash" (tiredness, headache, mood changes) as the medication is wearing off.

G. In rare cases, an extended-release formulation and an immediate-release formulation can be combined to improve efficacy or tolerability.

H. Methylphenidate products are widely believed to be less potent than mixed-amphetamine-salt products.

Further Reading

Boesen K, Paludan-Müller AS, Gøtzsche PC, et al: Extended-release methylphenidate for attention deficit hyperactivity disorder (ADHD) in adults. Cochrane Database Syst Rev 2(2):CD012857, 2022 35201607

Cândido RCF, Menezes de Padua CA, Golder S, et al: Immediate-release methylphenidate for attention deficit hyperactivity disorder (ADHD) in adults. Cochrane Database Syst Rev 1(1):CD013011, 2021 33460048

Concerta package insert. U.S. Food and Drug Administration, 2021. Available at: https://www.accessdata.fda.gov/drugsatfda_docs/label/2021/021121s044lbl.pdf. Accessed March 13, 2024.

Focalin package insert. U.S. Food and Drug Administration, 2021. Available at: https://www.accessdata.fda.gov/drugsatfda_docs/label/2021/021278s029lbl.pdf. Accessed March 13, 2024.

Ritalin LA package insert. U.S. Food and Drug Administration, 2021. Available at: https://www.accessdata.fda.gov/drugsatfda_docs/label/2021/021284s043lbl.pdf. Accessed March 13, 2024.

Storebo OJ, Pedersen N, Ramstad E, et al: Methylphenidate for attention deficit hyperactivity disorder (ADHD) in children and adolescents: assessment of adverse events in non-randomised studies. Cochrane Database Syst Rev (5):CD012069, 2018 29744873

Wakefulness-Promoting Medications

Modafinil/Armodafinil

I. **Brand Names**: Provigil (modafinil); Nuvigil (armodafinil)
II. **Therapeutic Class**: Wakefulness-promoting agent
III. **Mechanism-Based Class**: Dopamine reuptake inhibitor
IV. **Mechanism(s) of Action**

A. Armodafinil is the longer-lasting *R*-isomer of racemic modafinil.
B. Modafinil and armodafinil bind to dopamine transporter and inhibit dopamine reuptake.
C. Modafinil and armodafinil are presumed to augment activity in regions of the hypothalamus that regulate wakefulness.

V. **Indications**

A. FDA adult:

1. Narcolepsy
2. Obstructive sleep apnea (OSA)
3. Shift work sleep disorder

B. Evidence-based[1] off-label uses:

1. ADHD
2. Jet lag
3. Fatigue associated with depression
4. Fatigue associated with other comorbid medical issues

C. FDA pediatric: None

VI. **Major Contraindications and When to Use Caution**

A. Known allergy to modafinil or Provigil
B. Known allergy to armodafinil or Nuvigil

VII. **Dosage Formulations**

A. Modafinil:

1. Brand (Provigil) tablet (100 mg, 200 mg)
2. Generic tablet (100 mg, 200 mg)

B. Armodafinil:

1. Brand (Nuvigil) tablet (50 mg, 150 mg, 200 mg, 250 mg)
2. Generic tablet (50 mg, 100 mg, 150 mg, 200 mg, 250 mg)

---

[1]Evidence strength varies; readers are referred to the literature for more detailed information.

VIII. **Dosage Ranges and Guidelines**

A. Modafinil:

1. Narcolepsy, obstructive sleep apnea (OSA): Start at 200 mg taken once a day in the morning. Maximum recommended dosage is 400 mg/day.
2. Shift work disorder: Start at 200 mg once a day, taken 1 hour prior to the start of the work shift. Maximum recommended dosage is 400 mg/day.

B. Armodafinil:

1. Narcolepsy, OSA: Start at 150–250 mg taken once a day in the morning.
2. Shift work disorder: Start at 150 mg once a day, taken 1 hour prior to the start of the work shift.

C. No firm dosing guidelines have been established for off-label use in ADHD. Guidelines for use in narcolepsy and OSA can reasonably be applied for use in ADHD.

IX. **Monitoring**

A. No routine monitoring needed for most patients

B. Consider monitoring heart rate and blood pressure in individuals with known cardiovascular disease.

X. **Relevant Pharmacokinetics/Pharmacodynamics**

A. **Metabolism**: Primarily hepatic

B. **Time to peak plasma concentration**: 2–4 hours

C. **Half-life**: 15 hours

1. Modafinil and armodafinil have similar half lives (~13 hours), but after reaching maximum concentrations, modafinil appears to decline more rapidly, whereas armodafinil maintains higher concentrations later in the day. Therefore, armodafinil may be the preferred choice for longer-lasting wakefulness effects (Darwish et al. 2009).

D. **Use with food**: Can be taken with or without food.

E. **Hepatic impairment**: Reduce dosage by 50% in individuals with severe hepatic impairment

F. **Renal impairment**: No dosage adjustment necessary

XI. **Clinically Relevant Drug Interactions**

A. Both metabolized by and inducers of cytochrome P450 (CYP) 3A4.

1. At higher dosages, modafinil and armodafinil may induce their own metabolism.
2. Modafinil and armodafinil may reduce blood levels of drugs metabolized by CYP3A4 (e.g., steroidal contraceptives, cyclosporine).

B. Inhibitors of CYP2C19.

1. May also increase systemic levels of drugs metabolized by CYP2D6, such as some SSRIs and TCAs, as CYP2D6 substrates may take an ancillary route of elimination through CYP2C19 in individuals deficient in the CYP2D6 enzyme.

C. Caution should be exercised if used concomitantly with MAOIs.

XII. **Adverse Effects**

A. **Most common**:

1. Headache
2. Nausea
3. Dizziness
4. Insomnia

B. **Other notable side effects**:

1. Rash, Stevens-Johnson syndrome (rare)
2. Angioedema and anaphylaxis (rare)
3. Multiorgan hypersensitivity reactions (rare)
4. Psychiatric symptoms, including anxiety, insomnia, depression, confusion, agitation
5. Cardiovascular events, including increased blood pressure, chest pain, palpitations

XIII. **Clinical Pearls/Prescribing Tips**

A. Armodafinil maintains a greater plasma concentration later in the day compared with modafinil. Therefore, armodafinil can generally be taken once a day, whereas modafinil may need to be taken twice a day.
B. Modafinil and armodafinil may have less abuse potential than traditional CNS stimulants such as methylphenidate or amphetamines.
C. For treatment of ADHD, modafinil and armodafinil may be reasonable options to consider for individuals for whom traditional CNS stimulants may not be appropriate.

Further Reading

Bogan RK: Armodafinil in the treatment of excessive sleepiness. Expert Opin Pharmacother 11(6):993–1002, 2010 20307223

Nuvigil package insert. U.S. Food and Drug Administration, 2017. Available at: https://www.accessdata.fda.gov/drugsatfda_docs/label/2017/021875s023lbl.pdf. Accessed May 31, 2022.

Provigil package insert. U.S. Food and Drug Administration, 2015. Available at: https://www.accessdata.fda.gov/drugsatfda_docs/label/2015/020717s037s038lbl.pdf. Accessed May 31, 2022.

Wang SM, Han C, Lee SJ, et al: Modafinil for the treatment of attention-deficit/hyperactivity disorder: a meta-analysis. J Psychiatr Res 84:292–300, 2017 27810669

References

Darwish M, Kirby M, Hellriegel ET, et al: Armodafinil and modafinil have substantially different pharmacokinetic profiles despite having the same terminal half-lives: analysis of data from three randomized, single-dose, pharmacokinetic studies. Clin Drug Investig 29(9):613–623, 2009 19663523

Selective Norepinephrine Reuptake Inhibitors

Atomoxetine

I. **Brand Names**: Strattera

II. **Therapeutic Class**: Norepinephrine reuptake inhibitor

III. **Mechanism-Based Class**: Selective norepinephrine reuptake inhibitor

IV. **Mechanism(s) of Action**

A. Inhibition of the presynaptic norepinephrine transporter.

B. Inhibition of norepinephrine reuptake also increases dopaminergic transmission in the frontal cortex.

V. **Indications**

A. FDA adult: ADHD

B. Evidence-based[1] off-label uses:

1. Treatment-resistant depression

C. FDA pediatric: Approved for ADHD in children age 6 years and older

VI. **Major Contraindications and When to Use Caution**

A. Known allergy to atomoxetine or Strattera

B. Concomitant use of monoamine oxidase inhibitors (MAOIs) (2-week washout required)

C. Narrow angle glaucoma

D. Pheochromocytoma or history of pheochromocytoma

E. Severe cardiovascular disorders that might deteriorate with increases in HR and BP

VII. **Dosage Formulations**

A. Brand capsule (10 mg, 18 mg, 25 mg, 40 mg, 60 mg, 80 mg, 100 mg)

B. Generic capsule (10 mg, 18 mg, 25 mg, 40 mg, 60 mg, 80 mg, 100 mg)

VIII. **Dosage Ranges and Guidelines**

A. Children weighing up to 70 kg (154 lb): Start at 0.5 mg/kg/day. Target dosage is 1.2 mg/kg/day. Maximum total dosage is 1.4 mg/kg/day or 100 mg/day (whichever is lower).

B. Children weighing more than 70 kg (154 lb) and adults: Start at 40 mg/day. Target dosage is 80 mg/day. Maximum total dosage is 100 mg/day.

[1]Evidence strength varies; readers are referred to the literature for more detailed information.

IX. **Monitoring**

A. Cardiac: Prior to starting, assess for the presence of relevant personal and family history of cardiac disease. During treatment, monitor blood pressure and pulse. Consider periodic ECG monitoring.
B. Monitor height and weight in pediatric patients.
C. Routine laboratory tests are not required, but check liver function tests if potential signs of liver failure emerge.

X. **Relevant Pharmacokinetics/Pharmacodynamics**

A. **Metabolism**: Hepatic
B. **Time to peak plasma concentration**: 1–2 hours
C. **Half-life**: 5 hours
D. **Use with food**: Can be taken with or without food. Administration with a high-fat meal may delay absorption slightly.
E. **Hepatic impairment**: For moderate impairment, reduce to 50% of normal dosage. For severe impairment, reduce to 25% of normal dosage.
F. **Renal impairment**: Dosage adjustment not necessary

XI. **Clinically Relevant Drug Interactions**

A. Metabolized by cytochrome P450 (CYP) 2D6.
   1. Levels are increased by CYP2D6 inhibitors.
B. Risk for elevated blood pressure with pressor agents.
C. Can potentiate the action of albuterol and other β_2-adrenergic agonists on the cardiovascular system.

XII. **Adverse Effects**

A. **Most common**:
   1. Gastrointestinal (nausea, vomiting, abdominal pain)
   2. Fatigue, sedation
B. **Other notable side effects**:
   1. Increased blood pressure and heart rate
   2. Serious cardiac events (sudden death, stroke, myocardial infarction)
   3. Psychiatric side effects (including anxiety, mania, psychosis)
   4. Urinary hesitancy/retention
   5. Priapism
   6. Liver injury
   7. Growth suppression in children

XIII. **Clinical Pearls/Prescribing Tips**

A. Atomoxetine is a reasonable alternative for individuals for whom stimulants are contraindicated.
B. Although some clinical benefit may be observed within the first few days, it may take several weeks to see the full effect.
C. Given its possible antidepressant effects, atomoxetine may be a good choice for individuals with comorbid depression.

D. In comparison with stimulants, atomoxetine carries a reduced risk of causing and/or exacerbating tics.
E. Atomoxetine is usually prescribed as monotherapy but could potentially be combined with stimulants for treatment-resistant symptoms.

Further Reading

Michelson D, Allen AJ, Busner J, et al: Once-daily atomoxetine treatment for children and adolescents with attention deficit hyperactivity disorder: a randomized, placebo-controlled study. Am J Psychiatry 159(11):1896–1901, 2002 12411225

Ni HC, Lin YJ, Gau SS, et al: An open-label, randomized trial of methylphenidate and atomoxetine treatment in adults with ADHD. J Atten Disord 21(1):27–39, 2017 23475825

Strattera package insert. U.S. Food and Drug Administration, 2022. Available at: https://www.accessdata.fda.gov/drugsatfda_docs/label/2022/021411s050lbl.pdf. Accessed March 13, 2024.

Viloxazine

I. **Brand Names**: Qelbree
II. **Therapeutic Class**: Norepinephrine reuptake inhibitor
III. **Mechanism-Based Class**: Selective norepinephrine reuptake inhibitor
IV. **Mechanism(s) of Action**

A. Inhibition of the presynaptic norepinephrine transporter.
B. Inhibition of norepinephrine reuptake also increases dopaminergic transmission in the frontal cortex.

V. **Indications**

A. FDA adult: ADHD
B. Evidence-based[1] off-label uses:

1. Depression (previously marketed for depression)

C. FDA pediatric: Approved for ADHD in children age 6 years and older

VI. **Major Contraindications and When to Use Caution**

A. Known allergy to viloxazine or Qelbree
B. Concomitant use of monoamine oxidase inhibitors (MAOIs) (2-week washout required)
C. Severe cardiovascular disorders that might deteriorate with increases in heart rate and blood pressure

[1]Evidence strength varies; readers are referred to the literature for more detailed information.

VII. **Dosage Formulations**

A. Brand capsule (100 mg, 150 mg, 200 mg)
B. Generic: Not available

VIII. **Dosage Ranges and Guidelines**

A. Children ages 6–11 years: Start at 100 mg/day. May increase by 100 mg/day at weekly intervals. Maximum total dosage is 400 mg/day.
B. Children ages 12–17 years: Start at 200 mg/day. May increase by 200 mg/day after 1 week. Maximum total dosage is 400 mg/day.
C. Adults: Start at 200 mg/day. May increase by 200 mg/day at weekly intervals. Maximum total dosage is 600 mg/day.

IX. **Monitoring**

A. Cardiac: Prior to starting, assess for the presence of relevant personal and family history of cardiac disease. During treatment, monitor blood pressure and heart rate. Consider periodic ECG monitoring.
B. Monitor height and weight in pediatric patients.

X. **Relevant Pharmacokinetics/Pharmacodynamics**

A. **Metabolism**: hepatic
B. **Time to peak plasma concentration**: 5 hours
C. **Half-life**: 7 hours
D. **Use with food**: Can be taken with or without food. Administration with a high-fat meal may delay peak effects.
E. **Hepatic impairment**: Dosage adjustment not necessary
F. **Renal impairment**: For individuals with severe renal impairment, initial dosage is 100 mg/day. Titrate upward by 50–100 mg/day at weekly intervals. Maximum recommended dosage is 200 mg/day.

XI. **Clinically Relevant Drug Interactions**

A. Strong cytochrome P450 (CYP) 1A2 inhibitor.
B. Weak inhibitor of CYP2D6 and CYP3A4.

XII. **Adverse Effects**

A. **Most common**:

1. Gastrointestinal (nausea, vomiting, reduced appetite)
2. Somnolence, fatigue

B. **Other notable side effects**:

1. Increased blood pressure and heart rate
2. Psychiatric side effects (including anxiety, irritability, mania)
3. Insomnia
4. Headache

XIII. **Clinical Pearls/Prescribing Tips**

A. An immediate-release version of viloxazine was approved as an antidepressant in Europe several decades ago but was eventually discontinued (for reasons unrelated to safety or efficacy).

B. Viloxazine is a reasonable alternative for individuals for whom stimulants are contraindicated.

C. Although some clinical benefit may be observed within the first few days, it may take several weeks to see the full effect.

D. Given its probable antidepressant effects, viloxazine may be a good choice for individuals with comorbid depression.

E. Viloxazine is generally prescribed as monotherapy but could potentially be combined with stimulants for treatment-resistant symptoms; however, data on combined use are limited.

Further Reading

Lorman WJ: Viloxazine (Qelbree): a nonstimulant extended-release capsule for the treatment of attention deficit hyperactivity disorder. J Addict Nurs 33(2):114–115, 2022 35640214

Nasser A, Liranso T, Adewole T, et al: A phase 3, placebo-controlled trial of once-daily viloxazine extended-release capsules in adolescents with attention-deficit/hyperactivity disorder. J Clin Psychopharmacol 41(4):370–380, 2021 34181360

Qelbree package insert. U.S. Food and Drug Administration, 2022. Available at: https://www.accessdata.fda.gov/drugsatfda_docs/label/2022/211964s003lbl.pdf. Accessed March 13, 2024.

Alpha-2 Adrenergic Receptor Agonists

Clonidine[1]

I. **Brand Names**: Kapvay (an extended release formulation), Catapres (immediate release), Catapres-TTS (transdermal therapeutic system)

II. **Therapeutic Class**: Antihypertensive

III. **Mechanism-Based Class**: Centrally acting alpha$_2$-adrenergic receptor agonist

IV. **Mechanism(s) of Action**

A. Binds equally to α_{2A}, α_{2B}, and α_{2C} receptors.

B. Agonist at postsynaptic alpha$_{2A}$ receptors in the CNS, preventing the secretion of norepinephrine in downstream neurons

C. Exact mechanism unknown, but is believed to enhance cognitive functioning in the (pre)frontal cortex

V. **Indications**

A. FDA adult and pediatric:

1. ADHD in children age 6–17 years (Kapvay brand is extended release])
2. Hypertension (immediate-release [IR] clonidine)

B. Evidence-based[2] off-label uses:

1. ADHD in adults (Kapvay; IR clonidine; patch)
2. ADHD in children age 6–17 years (IR clonidine; patch)
3. Substance withdrawal (opiates and related substances)
4. Anxiety disorders
5. Tic disorders

VI. **Major Contraindications and When to Use Caution**

A. Known allergy to clonidine or Kapvay

B. Avoid or use extreme caution in individuals with known cardiac disease

VII. **Dosage Formulations**

A. Brand (Kapvay) extended-release (ER) tablet (0.1 mg)

B. Generic ER tablet (0.1 mg)

C. Generic IR tablet (0.1 mg, 0.2 mg, 0.3 mg)

---

[1]Also see Chapter 4, "Nonbenzodiazepine Hypnotics," and Chapter 10, "Treatment of Substance Use Disorders" for more information regarding clonidine's use for other indications and conditions.

[2]Evidence strength varies; readers are referred to the literature for more detailed information.

D. Generic patch and brand (Catapres TTS) (0.1 mg/day, 0.2 mg/day, 0.3 mg/day x 1 week)

   1. Catapres-TTS is a weekly transdermal patch system available in three patch sizes/dose strengths. A generic patch is available in the same doses.

VIII. Dosage Ranges and Guidelines

A. Start at 0.1 mg/day taken at bedtime. May increase dosage by 0.1 mg/day at weekly intervals.

B. For dosages ≥0.2 mg/day, split dosage and take twice a day, with either an equal or a greater portion of the daily dose taken at bedtime.

C. Maximum recommended dosage is 0.4 mg/day.

IX. Monitoring

A. Check pulse and blood pressure before starting treatment, and monitor periodically, especially after dosage changes.

B. Consider periodic ECG monitoring, especially in patients with known cardiac disease.

X. Relevant Pharmacokinetics/Pharmacodynamics

A. **Metabolism**: Hepatic

B. **Time to peak plasma concentration**: 7 hours (Kapvay); 3 hours (IR clonidine)

C. **Half-life**: 12 hours

D. **Use with food**: Can be taken with or without food.

E. **Hepatic impairment**: Consider dosage reduction in individuals with significant impairment.

F. **Renal impairment**: Consider dosage reduction in individuals with significant impairment.

XI. Clinically Relevant Drug Interactions

A. Use with other CNS depressants can increase risk for sedation.

B. Use with other antihypertensive drugs can increase risk for hypotension.

C. Use with drugs that affect sinus node function or atrioventricular node conduction can increase risk for bradycardia and atrioventricular block.

XII. Adverse Effects

A. **Most common**:

   1. Sedation, somnolence, fatigue
   2. Headache
   3. Gastrointestinal side effects: abdominal pain, nausea

B. **Other notable side effects**:

   1. Cardiovascular: hypotension, bradycardia, syncope, conduction abnormalities (sinus node dysfunction, atrioventricular block)
   2. Rebound hypertension if stopped abruptly

XIII. Risks in Pregnancy and Lactation

A. Fetal loss was shown in animal studies at both low and high dosages. Fetal malformations were not shown in animal studies. However, risk in pregnancy in humans is unknown. Clonidine's use in pregnant women is not recommended.

B. A relatively high amount of clonidine is transmitted in breast milk and may result in adverse reactions in infants. Use while breastfeeding is not recommended.

XIV. **Clinical Pearls/Prescribing Tips**

A. Compared with guanfacine (the other α_2-adrenergic agonist commonly used for ADHD), clonidine carries a higher risk of side effects such as sedation and hypotension.
B. Clonidine can be used as monotherapy or in conjunction with a stimulant.
C. Although Kapvay is approved only for children ages 6–17 years, data have shown its effectiveness in adults as well.
D. Clonidine can be used to treat tic disorder, and may be more tolerable than stimulants, which can worsen tics.
E. Immediate-release clonidine has not been FDA approved for ADHD, but it was used off-label for this indication prior to the approval of Kapvay.

Further Reading

Croxtall JD: Clonidine extended-release: in attention-deficit hyperactivity disorder. Paediatr Drugs 13(5):329–336, 2011 21888447

Kapvay package insert. U.S. Food and Drug Administration, 2020. Available at: https://www.accessdata.fda.gov/drugsatfda_docs/label/2020/022331s021lbl.pdf. Accessed March 13, 2024.

Ming X, Mulvey M, Mohanty S, et al: Safety and efficacy of clonidine and clonidine extended-release in the treatment of children and adolescents with attention deficit and hyperactivity disorders. Adolesc Health Med Ther 2:105–112, 2011 24600280

Guanfacine

I. **Brand Names**: Intuniv (extended release), Tenex (immediate release)

A. Brand-name Tenex is no longer available in the United States, but generic immediate-release guanfacine is available.

II. **Therapeutic Class**: Antihypertensive

III. **Mechanism-Based Class**: Centrally acting alpha$_2$-adrenergic receptor agonist

IV. **Mechanism of Action**

A. Agonist at postsynaptic alpha$_{2A}$ receptors in the CNS, preventing the secretion of norepinephrine in downstream neurons.
B. Exact mechanism unknown, but guanfacine is believed to enhance cognitive functioning in the (pre)frontal cortex.

V. **Indications**

A. FDA adult and pediatric:

1. ADHD in children age 6–17 years (Intuniv)
2. Hypertension (guanfacine immediate-release [IR])

B. Evidence-based[1] off-label uses:

1. ADHD in children (guanfacine IR)
2. ADHD in adults (Intuniv, guanfacine IR)
3. Tic disorders

VI. **Major Contraindications and When to Use Caution**

A. Known allergy to guanfacine, Intuniv, or guanfacine IR

B. Concomitant use of monoamine oxidase inhibitors (MAOIs) (2-week washout required)

VII. **Dosage Formulations**

A. Brand (Intuniv) extended-release (ER) tablet (1 mg, 2 mg, 3 mg, 4 mg)

B. Generic ER tablet (1 mg, 2 mg, 3 mg, 4 mg)

C. Generic IR tablet (1 mg, 2 mg)

VIII. **Dosage Ranges and Guidelines**

A. Intuniv (or guanfacine ER): Start at 1 mg once a day. May increase by 1 mg/day at weekly intervals. Maximum recommended dosage 4 mg/day (children age 6–12 years) and 7 mg/day (adolescents age 13–17 years), weight dependent.

B. Guanfacine IR): Start at 1 mg once a day. May titrate upward as needed/tolerated. Maximum recommended dosage 2–4 mg/day (weight dependent). Dosage can be divided.

IX. **Monitoring**

A. No routine monitoring needed for most patients

B. Consider monitoring pulse and blood pressure in individuals with known cardiovascular disease.

X. **Relevant Pharmacokinetics/Pharmacodynamics**

A. **Metabolism**: hepatic

B. **Time to peak plasma concentration**: 1–4 hours (IR), 4–8 hours (ER)

C. **Half-life**: 16–18 hours

D. **Use with food**: Intuniv should not be taken with high-fat meals, as this increases its effect.

E. **Hepatic impairment**: Dosage reduction advised in patients with severe impairment.

F. **Renal impairment**: Dosage reduction advised in patients with severe impairment.

XI. **Clinically Relevant Drug Interactions**

A. Metabolized by cytochrome P450 (CYP) 3A4.

1. Levels are increased by CYP3A4 inhibitors. Decrease to 50% of target dosage when combined with moderate/strong CYP3A4 inhibitors.
2. Levels are decreased by CYP3A4 inducers. When combined with CYP3A4 inducers, consider titrating dosage upward to double the target dosage.

B. Use with valproic acid can cause increased concentration of valproic acid.

---

[1]Evidence strength varies; readers are referred to the literature for more detailed information.

C. Use with antihypertensive drugs can cause increased risk for hypotension.
D. Use with CNS depressants can cause increased risk for sedation.

XII. **Adverse Effects**

A. **Most common**:

1. Sedation, somnolence, fatigue
2. Headache
3. Gastrointestinal side effects: abdominal pain, nausea

B. **Other notable side effects**:

1. Cardiovascular: hypotension, bradycardia, syncope, conduction abnormalities (sinus node dysfunction, atrioventricular block)
2. Rebound hypertension if stopped abruptly

XIII. **Clinical Pearls/Prescribing Tips**

A. Compared with clonidine (the other α_2-adrenergic receptor agonist commonly used for ADHD), guanfacine carries a lower risk for side effects such as sedation and hypotension.
B. Guanfacine can be used as monotherapy or in conjunction with a stimulant.
C. Although Intuniv is approved by the FDA only for children ages 6–17 years; data have shown its effectiveness in adults as well.
D. Guanfacine can be used to treat tic disorder, and may be more tolerable than stimulants, which can worsen tics.
E. Immediate-release guanfacine has not been FDA approved for ADHD, but it was commonly used off-label for this indication prior to the approval of Intuniv.

Further Reading

Biederman J, Melmed RD, Patel A, et al: Long-term, open-label extension study of guanfacine extended release in children and adolescents with ADHD. CNS Spectr 13(12):1047–1055, 2008 19179940

Faraone SV, McBurnett K, Sallee FR, et al: Guanfacine extended release: a novel treatment for attention-deficit/hyperactivity disorder in children and adolescents. Clin Ther 35(11):1778–1793, 2013 24139092

Intuniv package insert. U.S. Food and Drug Administration, 2019. Available at: https://www.accessdata.fda.gov/drugsatfda_docs/label/2019/022037s019lbl.pdf. Accessed March 13, 2024.

Other Medications With Activating Effects

Bupropion[1]

I. **Brand Names**: Wellbutrin, Wellbutrin SR, Wellbutrin XL, Aplenzin, Forfivo XL

II. **Therapeutic Class**: Atypical antidepressant

III. **Mechanism-Based Class**: Norepinephrine-dopamine reuptake inhibitor and releaser

IV. **Mechanism(s) of Action**

A. Inhibits neuronal reuptake of norepinephrine and dopamine.

B. Increases release of dopamine and norepinephrine into the extraneuronal space.

V. **Indications**

A. FDA adult:

1. Major depressive disorder (MDD)
2. Seasonal affective disorder (Wellbutrin XL)
3. Nicotine dependence (Wellbutrin SR)

B. Evidence-based[2] off-label uses:

1. ADHD
2. Other substance dependence
3. Sexual dysfunction associated with antidepressant use

C. FDA pediatric: None

VI. **Major Contraindications and When to Use Caution**

A. Known allergy to bupropion or brand drugs containing bupropion

B. Seizure disorder

C. Abrupt withdrawal of alcohol, benzodiazepines, barbiturates, or antiepileptic drugs (or other sedative drugs whose cessation can predispose to seizures)

D. Current or prior diagnosis of bulimia or anorexia nervosa

E. Any condition that lowers the seizure threshold

F. Concomitant use of monoamine oxidase inhibitors (MAOIs) (2-week washout required)

VII. **Dosage Formulations**

A. Brand:

1. Wellbutrin sustained-release (SR) tablet (100 mg, 150 mg, 200 mg)
2. Wellbutrin extended-release (XL) brand tablet (150 mg, 300 mg)

---

[1]See Chapter 2, "Antidepressants," for more information regarding bupropion.

[2]Evidence strength varies; readers are referred to the literature for more detailed information.

3. Forfivo XL tablet (450 mg)
4. Aplenzin tablet (174 mg, 348 mg, 522 mg)

B. Generic:

1. Bupropion IR tablet (75 mg, 100 mg)
2. Bupropion SR tablet (100 mg, 150 mg, 200 mg)
3. Bupropion XL tablet (150 mg, 300 mg)

VIII. **Dosage Ranges and Guidelines**

A. MDD:

1. Start at a relatively low dosage (100–200/day total, depending on the specific formulation) and titrate upward as needed.
2. Maximum dosages: 450 mg/day (Bupropion, Bupropion XL, Forfivo); 400 mg/day (Bupropion SR); 522 mg/day (Aplenzin)

B. ADHD (off-label):

1. No firm dosing guidelines for ADHD have been established. Guidelines for use in MDD can reasonably be applied for use in ADHD.

IX. **Monitoring**

A. No routine monitoring is needed for most patients.
B. Consider monitoring pulse and blood pressure in individuals with known cardiovascular disease.

X. **Relevant Pharmacokinetics/Pharmacodynamics**

A. **Metabolism**: hepatic
B. **Time to peak plasma concentration**: 3–5 hours
C. **Half-life**: 21 hours
D. **Use with food**: Can be taken with or without food.
E. **Hepatic impairment**: For mild impairment, consider reducing the dosage and/or the frequency of dosing. For moderate/severe impairment, use dosage of 100–150 mg every other day.
F. **Renal impairment**: Consider reducing the dosage and/or the frequency of dosing.

XI. **Clinically Relevant Drug Interactions**

A. Metabolized by cytochrome P450 (CYP) 2B6.

1. Bupropion levels can be increased by CYP2B6 inhibitors and reduced by CYP2B6 inducers.

B. Bupropion is a potent/strong CYP2D6 inhibitor.
C. Use caution when coadministered with drugs that lower the seizure threshold.
D. Concomitant use with dopamine agonists can lead to adverse reactions (restlessness, agitation, tremor, ataxia).

XII. Adverse Effects

A. **Most common**:

1. Dry mouth
2. Nausea
3. Insomnia
4. Dizziness

B. **Other notable side effects**:

1. Seizures
2. Increased blood pressure
3. Angle-closure glaucoma

XIII. Risks in pregnancy and lactation

A. Bupropion was designated a Category C drug in the prior FDA classification and is present in breast milk. A thorough risk/benefit discussion with the patient is recommended on continuing versus stopping the medication, including consultation with an OB/GYN specialist and/or lactation expert. See Chapter 15 ("Women: Pregnancy, Postpartum, and Breastfeeding") for more information.

XIV. Clinical Pearls/Prescribing Tips

A. Bupropion's benefit for ADHD is believed to be related to its activity at norepinephrine and dopamine receptors.

B. Although bupropion's use for ADHD is off-label, there are substantial published data validating its benefit for that disorder.

C. For treatment of ADHD, bupropion may be a reasonable option to consider for individuals for whom traditional stimulants may not be appropriate.

D. Bupropion could be used as monotherapy for individuals with comorbid ADHD and depression.

E. Bupropion can be useful for patients with comorbid nicotine dependence or other substance use disorders.

F. Bupropion is often prescribed as monotherapy for ADHD, but can be combined with stimulants.

G. Bupropion is less likely than stimulants to cause and/or exacerbate tics.

Further Reading

Deang KT, Sidi H, Zakaria H, et al: The novelty of bupropion as a dopaminergic antidepressant for the treatment of adult attention deficit hyperactive disorder. Curr Drug Targets 20(2):210–219, 2019 28494748

Verbeeck W, Bekkering GE, Van den Noortgate W, et al: Bupropion for attention deficit hyperactivity disorder (ADHD) in adults. Cochrane Database Syst Rev (10):CD009504, 2017 28965364

Wellbutrin XL package insert. U.S. Food and Drug Administration, 2022. Available at: https://www.accessdata.fda.gov/drugsatfda_docs/label/2022/021515s044lbl.pdf. Accessed March 13, 2024.

Desipramine/Imipramine[1]

I. **Brand Names**: Norpramin (desipramine); Tofranil (imipramine)
II. **Therapeutic Class**: Tricyclic antidepressants
III. **Mechanism-Based Class**: Norepinephrine reuptake inhibitor (desipramine); serotonin/norepinephrine reuptake inhibitor (imipramine)
IV. **Mechanism(s) of Action**

A. Inhibits neuronal reuptake of norepinephrine (desipramine)
B. Inhibits neuronal reuptake of norepinephrine and serotonin (imipramine)

V. **Indications**

A. FDA adult: Major depressive disorder
B. Evidence-based[2] off-label uses:

1. ADHD
2. Anxiety
3. Insomnia
4. Pain

C. FDA pediatric: Childhood enuresis (imipramine)

VI. **Major Contraindications and When to Use Caution**

A. Known allergy to desipramine, imipramine, Norpramin, or Tofranil
B. Concomitant use of monoamine oxidase inhibitors (MAOIs) (2-week washout required); see Chapter 2, "Antidepressants," for detailed information and comprehensive guidelines regarding washout.
C. Known cardiac disease
D. Patients on anticholinergic medications or who may otherwise be susceptible to anticholinergic side effects (e.g., urinary retention, angle-closure glaucoma)

VII. **Dosage Formulations**

A. Desipramine:

1. Brand (Norpramin) tablet (10 mg, 25 mg, 50 mg, 75 mg, 100 mg, 150 mg)
2. Generic tablet (10 mg, 25 mg, 50 mg, 75 mg, 100 mg, 150 mg)

B. Imipramine:

1. Brand (Tofranil) tablet (10 mg, 25 mg, 50 mg)
2. Generic tablet (10 mg, 25 mg, 50 mg) and capsule (75 mg, 100 mg, 125 mg, 150 mg)

VIII. **Dosage Ranges and Guidelines**

A. MDD:

1. Adults: Start at a lower dosage (25–50 mg/day). The typical target dosage is 100–200 mg/day. Dosages higher than 300 mg/day are not recommended.

---

[1]See Chapter 2, "Antidepressants," for more information regarding desipramine/imipramine.
[2]Evidence strength varies; readers are referred to the literature for more detailed information.

(See Chapter 2, "Antidepressants," for further information, including guidelines on therapeutic drug monitoring of desipramine and imipramine.)

2. Adolescent and geriatric patients: "Start low and go slow." Dosages higher than 100 mg/day are not recommended.
3. Children: With imipramine, do not exceed a dosage of 2.5 mg/kg/day. No firm dosing recommendations have been published for desipramine.

B. ADHD (off-label):

1. No firm dosing guidelines for ADHD have been established. Guidelines for use in MDD can reasonably be applied for use in ADHD.

IX. **Monitoring**

A. Cardiac: Prior to starting, assess for the presence of cardiac disease. During treatment, monitor blood pressure and heart rate. Consider periodic ECG monitoring, especially for patients older than 50 years.

B. Serum drug levels of desipramine can be monitored.

X. **Relevant Pharmacokinetics/Pharmacodynamics**

A. **Metabolism**: Hepatic
B. **Time to peak plasma concentration**: 4–6 hours
C. **Half-life**: 7–12 hours (15–24 hours)
D. **Use with food**: Can be taken with or without food.
E. **Hepatic impairment**: Consider dosage reduction in individuals with significant impairment.
F. **Renal impairment**: Consider dosage reduction in individuals with significant impairment.

XI. **Clinically Relevant Drug Interactions**

A. Metabolized by cytochrome P450 (CYP) 2D6.

1. Levels can be increased by CYP2D6 inhibitors and reduced by CYP2D6 inducers.

B. Use with CNS depressants can increase risk for sedation.
C. Anticholinergic side effects can be exacerbated when combined with other agents with anticholinergic properties.

XII. **Adverse Effects**

A. **Most common**:

1. Anticholinergic effects (dry mouth, urinary retention, blurred vision, constipation)
2. Sedation
3. Weight gain

B. **Other notable side effects**:

1. Cardiovascular (orthostatic hypotension, tachycardia, arrhythmia, QTc prolongation)
2. Can reduce seizure threshold.

XIII. **Clinical Pearls/Prescribing Tips**

A. Desipramine's and imipramine's benefit for ADHD is believed to be related to their activity at norepinephrine and dopamine receptors.
B. Both agents were used off-label for ADHD for many years, until newer nonstimulants such as atomoxetine were developed.
C. Nowadays, TCAs are less preferred than other nonstimulants, given their risk for drug interactions, adverse effects, and toxicity.
D. Desipramine or imipramine could be used as monotherapy for individuals with comorbid ADHD and depression.
E. Desipramine and imipramine are less likely than stimulants to cause and/or exacerbate tics.

Further Reading

Gualtieri CT, Keenan PA, Chandler M: Clinical and neuropsychological effects of desipramine in children with attention deficit hyperactivity disorder. J Clin Psychopharmacol 11(3):155–159, 1991 2066453

Norpramin package insert. U.S. Food and Drug Administration, 2018. Available at: https://www.accessdata.fda.gov/drugsatfda_docs/label/2018/014399s071lbl.pdf. Accessed March 13, 2024.

Otasowie J, Castells X, Ehimare UP, et al: Tricyclic antidepressants for attention deficit hyperactivity disorder (ADHD) in children and adolescents. Cochrane Database Syst Rev (9):CD006997, 2014 25238582

Tofranil package insert. U.S. Food and Drug Administration, 2014. Available at: https://www.accessdata.fda.gov/drugsatfda_docs/label/2014/087846s028,087844s027,087845s027lbl.pdf. Accessed March 13, 2024.

Tranylcypromine[1]

I. **Brand Names**: Parnate
II. **Therapeutic Class**: Monoamine oxidase (MAO) inhibitor
III. **Mechanism-Based Class**: Multimodal: serotonin, norepinephrine dopamine enzyme inhibitor (MAO-A, MAO-B); serotonin, norepinephrine, dopamine enzyme releaser (SERT, DAT, NET)
IV. **Mechanism(s) of Action**

A. Irreversibly inhibits MAO, which enhances serotonergic, noradrenergic, and dopaminergic neurotransmission.
B. Increases release of dopamine and norepinephrine into the extraneuronal space.

V. **Indications**

A. FDA adult: Major depressive disorder (MDD)

---

[1]See Chapter 2, "Antidepressants," for more information regarding tranylcypromine.

B. Evidence-based[1] off-label uses:

  1. ADHD
  2. Anxiety

C. FDA pediatric: None; use not approved or recommended for individuals younger than 18 years.

VI. Major Contraindications and When to Use Caution

A. Known allergy to tranylcypromine or Parnate
B. Concomitant use with another serotonergic agent (e.g., SSRI, SNRI, TCA).
C. Concomitant use with a high-tyramine diet
D. Pheochromocytoma and other catecholamine-releasing paragangliomas

VII. Dosage Formulations

A. Brand tablet (10 mg)
B. Generic tablet (10 mg)

VIII. Dosage Ranges and Guidelines

A. For MDD, start at 30 mg/day, in divided doses. Dosage can be increased by 10 mg/day every 3 weeks. Maximum dosage is 60 mg/day.
B. No firm dosing guidelines for use in ADHD have been established. Guidelines for tranylcypromine's use in MDD can reasonably be applied for use in ADHD (see Chapter 2, "Antidepressants," for dosage guidelines for tranylcypromine).

IX. Monitoring

A. Check blood pressure prior to starting, and monitor regularly.
B. Check liver function tests prior to starting, and monitor regularly.

X. Relevant Pharmacokinetics/Pharmacodynamics

A. **Metabolism**: Hepatic
B. **Time to peak plasma concentration**: 1–2 hours
C. **Half-life**: 2 hours (however, pharmacodynamic effects can last weeks because of the irreversible inhibition of MAO)
D. **Use with food**: Can be taken with or without food, but patients must adhere to a low-tyramine diet.
E. **Hepatic impairment**: Stop if there are any signs of hepatitis or liver function test (LFT) abnormalities.
F. **Renal impairment**: Consider use of a lower dosage.

XI. Clinically Relevant Drug Interactions

A. High risk for serotonin syndrome when used concomitantly with other agents with serotonergic activity.
B. High risk for hypertensive crisis when high levels of dietary tyramine are consumed or when tranylcypromine is used concomitantly with other drugs that can increase blood pressure.

---

[1]Evidence strength varies; readers are referred to the literature for more detailed information.

XII. **Adverse Effects**

A. **Most common**:

1. Hypotension
2. Dizziness
3. Dry mouth
4. Headache

B. **Other notable side effects**:

1. Hypertension, hypertensive crisis
2. Hepatitis, elevated liver function tests

XIII. **Clinical Pearls/Prescribing Tips**

A. Tranylcypromine's benefit for ADHD is believed to be related mostly to release of dopamine and norepinephrine into the extraneuronal space.

B. Tranylcypromine is structurally related to amphetamine (of note, amphetamine is a weak, reversible MAO inhibitor).

C. Data on tranylcypromine's use in ADHD are very limited. Use should be considered only in cases in which ADHD symptoms have not responded to more established evidence-based interventions.

D. Tranylcypromine could be used as monotherapy for individuals with comorbid ADHD and depression.

E. Tranylcypromine's use is limited by its significant risks for drug interactions and adverse reactions.

F. Concomitant use with stimulants carries a high risk for hypertensive crisis and serotonin syndrome; therefore, such use is rarely advisable. For severe treatment-resistant depression, coadministration of tranylcypromine with a stimulant can be considered if extreme caution is exercised and the patient is closely monitored.

Further Reading

Bortolato M, Chen K, Shih JC: Monoamine oxidase inactivation: from pathophysiology to therapeutics. Adv Drug Deliv Rev 60(13–14):1527–1533, 2008 18652859

Feinberg SS: Combining stimulants with monoamine oxidase inhibitors: a review of uses and one possible additional indication. J Clin Psychiatry 65(11):1520–1524, 2004 15554766

Parnate package insert. U.S. Food and Drug Administration, 2018. Available at https://www.accessdata.fda.gov/drugsatfda_docs/label/2018/012342s064lbl.pdf. Accessed May 31, 2022.

Zametkin A, Rapoport JL, Murphy DL, et al: Treatment of hyperactive children with monoamine oxidase inhibitors. I. Clinical efficacy. Arch Gen Psychiatry 42(10):962–966, 1985 3899047

PART III

Medications Used to Treat Specific Disorders/Conditions

8

Treatment of Neurocognitive Disorders

Matthew J. Ehrlich, M.D.
M. Bates Redwine, M.D.

Overview

- Major neurocognitive disorders (NCDs), formerly and colloquially termed *dementias*, are of growing concern as our population ages and the number of patients with this disorder increases. Treatments until recent years have largely been symptomatic or ameliorative, without addressing the underlying mechanisms of neural damage. By the time patients are symptomatic, the neuropathological process has usually been under way for years or even decades (in the case of Alzheimer's disease), limiting pharmacological treatments' efficacy and durability.
- The mainstay of treatment has been acetylcholinesterase inhibitors, which have been shown to slow the rate of cognitive decline, reduce the amount of behavioral disturbance, and delay nursing home placement. Memantine has been shown to have similar effects on the symptoms of major NCD, with evidence that it may have additive benefit when combined with acetylcholinesterase inhibitors.
- The strength of benefit of all these agents, possibly including even the newer disease-modifying monoclonal antibodies, is modest, but a trial of these drugs is often worthwhile, since NCDs usually progress and only very rarely appear to stabilize or improve.
- In addition to agents that target the disease process or ameliorate symptoms via neurotransmitter modulation, agents discussed in other chapters of this Handbook are frequently used to target symptoms or syndromes associated with major NCDs, including depression, anxiety, apathy, agitation, sleep-cycle disruption, and dementia-related psychosis. The presence of an NCD may modify efficacy (usually making treatments less effective) or safety (note the black box warning for increased mortality in patients with dementia using antipsychotic medications). Despite having efficacy for collateral conditions, none of these agents have a clear evidence base for treating the core symptoms of cognitive impairment.

Acetylcholinesterase Inhibitors

Donepezil

I. **Brand Names**: Aricept, Aricept ODT, Namzaric (combination with memantine)

II. **Therapeutic Class**: Cognitive enhancer

III. **Mechanism-Based Class**: Cholinesterase inhibitor (acetylcholinesterase and butyrylcholinesterase); acetylcholinesterase inhibitor (AChEI)

IV. **Mechanism(s) of Action**

A. CNS inhibition of acetylcholinesterase (reversible), prevents hydrolysis of acetylcholine.

B. "[O]ther mechanisms of action of donepezil are possible, including the opposition of glutamate-induced excitatory transmission via downregulation of NMDA [*N*-methyl-D-aspartate] receptors and the regulation of amyloid proteins, which have demonstrated significant effects on the disease process of Alzheimer's [disease]. Other possible targets for donepezil may also include the inhibition of various inflammatory signaling pathways, exerting neuroprotective effects" (PubChem 2022).

V. **Indications**

A. FDA adult:

1. Dementia of the Alzheimer's type (mild, moderate, severe)
   a. Donepezil is the only AChEI that is FDA approved in severe Alzheimer's disease.

B. Evidence-based[1] off-label uses:

1. Non-Alzheimer's neurocognitive disorders: some evidence for efficacy in major neurocognitive disorders due to mixed vascular, Parkinson's disease, and Lewy body etiologies. No evidence for efficacy in mild cognitive impairment/mild neurocognitive disorder.

C. FDA pediatric: None

VI. **Major Contraindications and When to Use Caution**

A. Known allergy to donepezil/Aricept or piperidine derivatives

VII. **Dosage Formulations**

A. Brand tablet (5 mg, 10 mg, 23 mg)

B. Generic tablet (5 mg, 10 mg, 23 mg)

C. Generic orally dissolving tablet (5 mg, 10 mg)

---

[1]Evidence strength varies; readers are referred to the literature for more detailed information.

VIII. **Dosage Ranges and Guidelines**

A. Start at 5 mg nightly and increase to 10 mg nightly after 4–6 weeks (Table 8–1). For severe Alzheimer's disease dementia (major neurocognitive disorder due to Alzheimer's disease), the dosage may be increased to the 23-mg tablet after 3 months, as tolerated and based on clinical judgment.

B. Donepezil's benefits over placebo may not be easily distinguished until 12–26 weeks after initiation, if at all. Effect sizes are small.

Table 8–1. Donepezil indications and dosage ranges

Indications	Usual dosage range
Dementia (major neurocognitive disorder) due to Alzheimer's disease, mild or moderate	5–10 mg/day
Dementia (major neurocognitive disorder) due to Alzheimer's disease, severe	5–23 mg/day
Dementia (major neurocognitive disorder) due to mixed vascular/ Alzheimer's disease (off-label)	5–10 mg/day
Dementia (major neurocognitive disorder) due to Parkinson's disease (off-label)	5–10 mg/day
Dementia (major neurocognitive disorder) with Lewy bodies (off-label)	5–10 mg/day

IX. **Monitoring**: Not applicable

X. **Relevant Pharmacokinetics/Pharmacodynamics**

A. **Metabolism**: hepatic (cytochrome P450 [CYP] 2D6/CYP3A4/glucuronidation; two active metabolites) and renal

B. **Time to peak plasma concentration**: 3 hours (8 hours for 23-mg tablet)

C. **Half-life**: ~70 hours (steady state reached in 15 days)

D. **Protein binding**: 96%

E. **Hepatic impairment**: No recommendations (studies in stable alcoholic cirrhosis showed 20% decrease in clearance [Donepezil package insert]).

F. **Renal impairment**: No recommendations (a study in moderate to severe renal disease showed no difference in clearance [Donepezil package insert]).

XI. **Clinically Relevant Drug Interactions**

A. Metabolized by CYP3A4 and CYP2D6.

1. CYP3A4 and CYP2D6 inhibitors/inducers (as well as CYP polymorphisms) could have clinically significant interactions within the range of about 20%–30% variance in clearance/blood levels.

B. Protein binding/displacement studies did not indicate clinically significant interactions.

C. May exacerbate succinylcholine's paralytic effect during anesthesia.

D. May increase risk of gastrointestinal ulcers if used concomitantly with NSAIDs.

E. May increase risk of bradycardia or heart block if used with beta-blockers.

F. Avoid use with anticholinergic medications which may compromise efficacy.

XII. **Adverse Effects**

A. **Most common**:

1. Gastrointestinal: Anorexia, diarrhea, nausea/vomiting, dyspepsia, increased gastric acid secretion. Can result in clinically significant weight loss, leading to discontinuation. May improve spontaneously within 1–2 weeks.
2. Cardiovascular: Dizziness. Taking donepezil at night can reduce risk of syncope.
3. Behavioral: Hostility
4. Neurological: Headache

B. **Other notable side effects**:

1. Cardiovascular: syncope, bradycardia, heart block
2. Rhabdomyolysis (case reports)
3. Neuroleptic malignant syndrome (case reports)
4. QTc prolongation and torsades de pointes (case reports)

C. **Risks in pregnancy and lactation**: Donepezil was designated a Category C drug in the prior FDA classification, but no information is available on its use in pregnancy or breastfeeding.

XIII. **Clinical Pearls/Prescribing Tips**

A. Studies have shown clinically relevant differences in activities of daily living and clinician-rated rating scales, as well as delays in institutional placement of between 6 and 12 months (Donepezil package insert).

B. A Cochrane Review found no clinical benefit and increased adverse effects with the 23-mg slow-release formulation (Birks and Harvey 2018).

C. Gastrointestinal effects are common. Another AChEI, rivastigmine, has a patch formulation that can avoid some gastrointestinal adverse effects.

D. In general, adverse effects and discontinuation due to adverse effects were seen more frequently in individuals weighing less than 55 kg (121 lbs).

E. Although some expert opinion suggests that withdrawal of AChEIs is a viable option after placement in an institutional setting, there is limited evidence to support that strategy, and it may lead to worsening in cognition (Parsons et al. 2021).

Further Reading

Adlimoghaddam A, Neuendorff M, Roy B, et al: A review of clinical treatment considerations of donepezil in severe Alzheimer's disease. CNS Neurosci Ther 24(10):876–888, 2018 30058285

Aricept package insert. U.S. Food and Drug Administration, 2018. Available at: https://www.accessdata.fda.gov/drugsatfda_docs/label/2018/020690s042,021720s014,022568s011lbl \.pdf. Accessed March 13, 2024.

Arvanitakis Z, Shah RC, Bennett DA: Diagnosis and management of dementia: review. JAMA 322(16):1589–1599, 2019 31638686

Hansen RA, Gartlehner G, Webb AP, et al: Efficacy and safety of donepezil, galantamine, and rivastigmine for the treatment of Alzheimer's disease: a systematic review and meta-analysis. Clin Interv Aging 3(2):211–225, 2008 18686744

O'Brien JT, Holmes C, Jones M, et al: Clinical practice with anti-dementia drugs: a revised (third) consensus statement from the British Association for Psychopharmacology. J Psychopharmacol 31(2):147–168, 2017 28103749
Parsons C, Lim WY, Loy C, et al: Withdrawal or continuation of cholinesterase inhibitors or memantine or both, in people with dementia. Cochrane Database Syst Rev (2):CD009081, 2021 35608903
Rolinski M, Fox C, Maidment I, et al: Cholinesterase inhibitors for dementia with Lewy bodies, Parkinson's disease dementia and cognitive impairment in Parkinson's disease. Cochrane Database Syst Rev (3):CD006504, 2012 22419314
Taylor JP, McKeith IG, Burn DJ, et al: New evidence on the management of Lewy body dementia. Lancet Neurol 19(2):157–169, 2020 31519472

References

Birks JS, Harvey RJ: Donepezil for dementia due to Alzheimer's disease. Cochrane Database Syst Rev 6(6):CD001190, 2018 29923184
PubChem: PubChem Compound Summary for CID 3152, Donepezil. Bethesda, MD, National Library of Medicine, National Center for Biotechnology Information, 2022. Available at: https://pubchem.ncbi.nlm.nih.gov/compound/Donepezil. Accessed March 13, 2024.

Galantamine

I. **Brand Names**: Razadyne, Razadyne ER
II. **Therapeutic Class**: Cognitive enhancer
III. **Mechanism-Based Class**: Cholinesterase inhibitor (acetylcholinesterase and butyrylcholinesterase); acetylcholinesterase inhibitor (AChEI)
IV. **Mechanism(s) of Action**

A. CNS inhibition of acetylcholinesterase (reversible); prevents hydrolysis of acetylcholine.
B. CNS modulation of cholinergic nicotinic receptors.

V. **Indications**

A. FDA adult:
   1. Dementia (major neurocognitive disorder [NCD] of the Alzheimer's type), mild or moderate
B. Evidence-based[1] off-label uses:
   1. Non-Alzheimer's neurocognitive disorders: Major NCDs due to mixed vascular, Parkinson's disease, or Lewy body etiologies. No evidence for efficacy in mild cognitive impairment/mild NCD.
   2. Major NCD due to severe Alzheimer's disease
C. FDA pediatric: None

---

[1]Evidence strength varies; readers are referred to the literature for more detailed information.

VI. **Major Contraindications and When to Use Caution**

A. Known allergy to galantamine/Razadyne

VII. **Dosage Formulations**

A. Brand extended-release (ER) capsule (8 mg, 16 mg, 24 mg)
B. Generic ER capsule (8 mg, 16 mg, 24 mg)
C. Generic tablet (4 mg, 8 mg, 12 mg)
D. Generic oral solution (4 mg/mL)

VIII. **Dosage Ranges and Guidelines**

A. Start at 8 mg total daily dosage (4 mg BID or 8 mg once a day of ER formulation) and increase to 16 mg total daily dosage after a minimum of 4 weeks (Table 8–2). Some patients may benefit from an additional increase to 24 mg total daily dosage after an additional 4 weeks, based on tolerability and response at the lower dosage as well as on clinical judgment.
B. Need to restart/re-titrate from the starting dosage if galantamine is discontinued for more than 3 consecutive days.
C. Galantamine's benefits over placebo may not be easily distinguished until 12–26 weeks after initiation, if at all. Effect sizes are small.

Table 8–2. Galantamine indications and dosage ranges

Indication	Usual dosage range
Dementia (major neurocognitive disorder) due to Alzheimer's disease, mild or moderate	4–12 mg BID 8–24 mg/day (ER)
Dementia (major neurocognitive disorder) due to mixed vascular/ Alzheimer's disease (off-label)	4–12 mg BID 8–24 mg/day (ER)
Dementia (major neurocognitive disorder) with Lewy bodies (off-label)	4–12 mg BID 8–24 mg/day (ER)
Dementia (major neurocognitive disorder) due to Alzheimer's disease, severe (off-label)	4–12 mg BID 8–24 mg/day (ER)
Dementia due to Parkinson's disease (off-label)	4–12 mg BID 8–24 mg/day (ER)

IX. **Monitoring**: Not applicable

X. **Relevant Pharmacokinetics/Pharmacodynamics**

A. **Metabolism**: Hepatic cytochrome P450 (CYP) 2D6 and 3A4, glucuronidation, and renal elimination
B. **Time to peak plasma concentration**: 1 hour; 4.5–5 hours (ER formulation)
C. **Half-life**: 7 hours
D. **Effect of food**: Food delays blood level peaks by 90 minutes and decreases peak concentrations, but does not affect area under the curve (AUC). The ER formulation is not affected by administration with food.
E. **Protein binding**: 18%

F. **Hepatic impairment**: Do not exceed 16 mg/day.
G. **Renal impairment**: Should not exceed 16 mg/day for creatinine clearance 9–59 mL/minute; do not use in patients with creatinine clearance <9 mL/minute.

XI. **Clinically Relevant Drug Interactions**

A. Metabolized by CYP3A4 and CYP2D6.

1. Strong CYP3A4 and CYP2D6 inhibitors/inducers (as well as CYP polymorphisms) could have clinically significant interactions within the range of about 20%–40% variance in clearance/blood levels.

B. Protein binding/displacement studies did not indicate clinically significant interactions.
C. May exacerbate succinylcholine's paralytic effect during anesthesia.
D. May increase risk of gastrointestinal ulcers if used in concert with NSAIDs.
E. May increase risk of bradycardia or heart block if used with beta-blockers.
F. Avoid use with anticholinergic medications, which may compromise efficacy.

XII. **Adverse Effects**

A. **Most common**:

1. Gastrointestinal: Anorexia, diarrhea, nausea/vomiting, dyspepsia, increased gastric acid secretion. Can result in clinically significant weight loss, resulting to discontinuation. May improve spontaneously within 1–2 weeks.
2. Cardiovascular: Dizziness. Taking galantamine at night can reduce risk of syncope.
3. Neurological: Headache

B. **Other notable side effects**:

1. Cardiovascular: Syncope, bradycardia, heart block
2. Skin reactions: Rash, including Stevens-Johnson syndrome and acute generalized exanthematous pustulosis
3. Increased mortality risk: In two trials of patients with mild cognitive impairment, there was a significant difference in mortality rates between those who received placebo and those who received galantamine (Winblad et al. 2008). Although this finding appears to have been due to an unusually low placebo mortality rate , the possibility of drug effects cannot be excluded.

C. **Risks in pregnancy and lactation**: Some evidence of teratogenicity in studies in pregnant rats or rabbits was found at galantamine dosage equivalents higher than the approved dosage range. No information is available on use during breastfeeding.

XIII. **Clinical Pearls/Prescribing Tips**

A. Galantamine studies have shown clinically relevant differences in activities of daily living and clinical rating scales, as well as delays in institutional placement of between 6 and 12 months.
B. Approval studies found no significant difference in efficacy between galantamine 16 mg/day and 24 mg/day dosages. Some patients may benefit from higher dosages, but such dosages are also associated with increased adverse effects.

C. Although galantamine's nicotinic modulation theoretically offers benefit, no clinically relevant difference from other acetylcholinesterase inhibitors (AChEIs) has been noted in efficacy.
D. Gastrointestinal effects are common. Another AChEI, rivastigmine, has a patch formulation that can avoid some gastrointestinal adverse effects.
E. In general, adverse effects and discontinuation due to adverse effects were seen more frequently among individuals weighing less than 50 kg (110 lb).
F. Although some expert opinion suggests that withdrawal of AChEIs is a viable option after placement in an institutional setting, there is limited evidence to support that strategy, and it may lead to worsening in cognition (Parsons et al. 2021).
G. No dosage adjustment is necessary when converting between galantamine formulations.

Further Reading

Arvanitakis Z, Shah RC, Bennett DA: Diagnosis and management of dementia: review. JAMA 322(16):1589–1599, 2019 31638686

Galantamine package insert. U.S. Food and Drug Administration, 2015. Available at: https://www.accessdata.fda.gov/drugsatfda_docs/label/2015/021615s021lbl.pdf. Accessed March 13, 2024.

Hansen RA, Gartlehner G, Webb AP, et al: Efficacy and safety of donepezil, galantamine, and rivastigmine for the treatment of Alzheimer's disease: a systematic review and meta-analysis. Clin Interv Aging 3(2):211–225, 2008 18686744

Heinrich M: Galanthamine from galanthus and other amaryllidaceae—chemistry and biology based on traditional use, in The Alkaloids: Chemistry and Biology, Vol. 68. Edited by Cordell GA. Cambridge, MA, 2010, pp. 157–165. Available at: https://www.sciencedirect.com/science/article/abs/pii/S1099483110068045. Accessed September 11, 2022.

Loy C, Schneider L: Galantamine for Alzheimer's disease and mild cognitive impairment. Cochrane Database Syst Rev (1):CD001747, 2006 16437436

O'Brien JT, Holmes C, Jones M, et al: Clinical practice with anti-dementia drugs: a revised (third) consensus statement from the British Association for Psychopharmacology. J Psychopharmacol 31(2):147–168, 2017 28103749

PubChem: PubChem Compound Summary for CID 9651, Galantamine. Bethesda, MD, National Library of Medicine, National Center for Biotechnology Information, 2024. Available at: https://pubchem.ncbi.nlm.nih.gov/compound/Galantamine. Accessed June 16, 2024.

Rolinski M, Fox C, Maidment I, et al: Cholinesterase inhibitors for dementia with Lewy bodies, Parkinson's disease dementia and cognitive impairment in Parkinson's disease. Cochrane Database Syst Rev (3):CD006504, 2012 22419314

Taylor JP, McKeith IG, Burn DJ, et al: New evidence on the management of Lewy body dementia. Lancet Neurol 19(2):157–169, 2020 31519472

References

Parsons C, Lim WY, Loy C, et al: Withdrawal or continuation of cholinesterase inhibitors or memantine or both, in people with dementia. Cochrane Database Syst Rev (2):CD009081, 2021 35608903

Winblad B, Gauthier S, Scinto L, et al; GAL-INT-11/18 Study Group: Safety and efficacy of galantamine in subjects with mild cognitive impairment. Neurology 70(22):2024–2035, 2008 18322263

Rivastigmine

I. **Brand Names**: Exelon; Exelon patch

II. **Therapeutic Class**: Cognitive enhancer

III. **Mechanism-Based Class**: Cholinesterase inhibitor (acetylcholinesterase and butyrylcholinesterase); acetylcholinesterase inhibitor (AChEI)

IV. **Mechanism(s) of Action**

A. CNS inhibition of acetylcholinesterase (reversible), prevents hydrolysis of acetylcholine.

V. **Indications**

A. FDA adult:

1. Dementia (major neurocognitive disorder) of the Alzheimer's type (mild or moderate)
2. Dementia (major neurocognitive disorder) associated with Parkinson's disease (mild or moderate)

B. Evidence-based[1] off-label uses:

1. Non-Alzheimer's neurocognitive disorders: Major neurocognitive disorder due to mixed vascular or Lewy body etiologies. No evidence for efficacy in mild cognitive impairment/mild neurocognitive disorder.

C. FDA pediatric: None

VI. **Major Contraindications and When to Use Caution**

A. Known allergy to rivastigmine/Exelon, carbamates

B. Known history of sensitivity to rivastigmine patch components

VII. **Dosage Formulations**

A. Brand tablet (1.5 mg, 3 mg, 4.5 mg, 6 mg)

B. Generic tablet (1.5 mg, 3 mg, 4.5 mg, 6 mg)

C. Brand patch (4.6 mg/24 hours, 9.5 mg/24 hours, 13.3 mg/24 hours)

D. Generic patch (4.6 mg/24 hours, 9.5 mg/24 hours, 13.3 mg/24 hours)

---

[1]Evidence strength varies; readers are referred to the literature for more detailed information.

VIII. **Dosage Ranges and Guidelines**

A. Start at 1.5 mg BID and increase in 1.5-mg BID increments every 4 weeks (oral) (Table 8–3).

B. Start at 4.6 mg/24 hour patch and increase to 9.5 mg/24 hours after 4 weeks. For severe Alzheimer's dementia (major neurocognitive disorder), the dosage may be increased to 13.3 mg/24 hours after 4 weeks at 9.5 mg/24 hours.

C. Need to restart/re-titrate from the starting dosage if rivastigmine is discontinued for more than 3 consecutive days.

D. Switching from oral to patch: Start patch on day after last oral dose. For a total dosage <6 mg/day, use the 4.6 mg/24 hour patch. For a total dosage of 6–12 mg/day, use the 9.5 mg/24 hour patch.

E. Rivastigmine's benefits over placebo may not be easily distinguished until 12–26 weeks after initiation, if at all. Effect sizes are small.

Table 8–3. Rivastigmine indications and dosage ranges

Indication	Usual dosage range
Dementia due to Alzheimer's disease, mild or moderate	1.5–6 mg BID (oral) 4.6–9.5 mg patch
Dementia due to Alzheimer's disease, severe	4.6–13.3 mg patch
Dementia due to Parkinson's disease	1.5–6 mg BID (oral) 4.6–9.5 mg patch
Dementia due to mixed vascular/Alzheimer's disease (off-label)	1.5–6 mg BID (oral) 4.6–13.3 mg patch
Dementia with Lewy bodies (off-label)	1.5–6 mg BID (oral) 4.6–13.3 mg patch

IX. **Monitoring**: Not applicable

X. **Relevant Pharmacokinetics/Pharmacodynamics**

A. **Metabolism**: Largely renal elimination after tissue catabolism

B. **Time to peak plasma concentration**: 3 hours (oral); time to peak enzyme inhibition: 5 hours (oral).

C. **Half-life**: ~1.5 hours (oral); 3 hours (patch, after removal)

D. **Effect of food.** Food delays absorption by 90 minutes and decreases peak concentration, but increases AUC.

E. **Protein binding**: 40%

F. **Hepatic impairment**: No recommendations

G. **Renal impairment**: No recommendations

XI. **Clinically Relevant Drug Interactions**

A. Minimal cytochrome P450 (CYP) or other drug interactions

B. Protein binding/displacement studies did not indicate clinically significant interactions.

C. Smoking may increase clearance by 23%.

D. May exacerbate succinylcholine's paralytic effect during anesthesia.
E. May increase risk of gastrointestinal ulcers if used in concert with NSAIDs (theoretically decreased with patch formulation).
F. May increase risk of bradycardia or heart block if used with beta-blockers.
G. Avoid use with anticholinergic medications, which may compromise efficacy.

XII. **Adverse Effects**

A. **Most common**:

1. Gastrointestinal: Anorexia, diarrhea, nausea/vomiting, dyspepsia, increased gastric acid secretion. Can result in clinically significant weight loss, leading to discontinuation. May improve spontaneously within 1–2 weeks. Rates are somewhat higher than donepezil with oral dosing.
2. Cardiovascular: Dizziness. Taking rivastigmine at night can reduce the risk of syncope.
3. Skin reactions (patch)
4. Neurological: Headache

B. **Other notable side effects**:

1. Cardiovascular: Syncope, bradycardia, heart block

C. **Risks in pregnancy and lactation**: No evidence of teratogenicity was found for rivastigmine in studies in pregnant rats or rabbits; some decreased birth weights. No information is available on breastfeeding use.

XIII. **Clinical Pearls/Prescribing Tips**

A. Rivastigmine studies have shown clinically relevant differences in activities of daily living and clinical rating scales, as well as delays in institutional placement of between 6 and 12 months.
B. Gastrointestinal effects are common with rivastigmine, and possibly worse than with other AChEIs in the oral form. The patch formulation can avoid some gastrointestinal adverse effects.
C. In general, adverse effects and discontinuation due to adverse effects were seen more frequently among individuals weighing less than 50 kg (110 lb).
D. Although some expert opinion suggests that withdrawal of AChEIs is a viable option after placement in an institutional setting, there is limited evidence to support that strategy, and it may lead to worsening in cognitive outcomes (Parsons et al. 2021).

Further Reading

Arvanitakis Z, Shah RC, Bennett DA: Diagnosis and management of dementia: review. JAMA 322(16):1589–1599, 2019 31638686

Birks JS, Grimley Evans J: Rivastigmine for Alzheimer's disease. Cochrane Database Syst Rev (4):CD001191, 2015 25858345

Hansen RA, Gartlehner G, Webb AP, et al: Efficacy and safety of donepezil, galantamine, and rivastigmine for the treatment of Alzheimer's disease: a systematic review and meta-analysis. Clin Interv Aging 3(2):211–225, 2008 18686744

O'Brien JT, Holmes C, Jones M, et al: Clinical practice with anti-dementia drugs: a revised (third) consensus statement from the British Association for Psychopharmacology. J Psychopharmacol 31(2):147–168, 2017 28103749

PubChem: PubChem Compound Summary for CID 77991, Rivastigmine. Bethesda, MD, National Library of Medicine, National Center for Biotechnology Information, 2004. Available at: https://pubchem.ncbi.nlm.nih.gov/compound/Rivastigmine. Accessed September 11, 2022.

Rivastigmine package insert. U.S. Food and Drug Administration, 2018. Available at: https://www.accessdata.fda.gov/drugsatfda_docs/label/2018/020823s036,021025s024lbl.pdf. Accessed March 13, 2024.

Rivastigmine patch package insert. U.S. Food and Drug Administration, 2015. Available at: https://www.accessdata.fda.gov/drugsatfda_docs/label/2015/022083s020lbl.pdf. Accessed June 15, 2024.

Rolinski M, Fox C, Maidment I, et al: Cholinesterase inhibitors for dementia with Lewy bodies, Parkinson's disease dementia and cognitive impairment in Parkinson's disease. Cochrane Database Syst Rev (3):CD006504, 2012 22419314

Taylor JP, McKeith IG, Burn DJ, et al: New evidence on the management of Lewy body dementia. Lancet Neurol 19(2):157–169, 2020 31519472

References

Parsons C, Lim WY, Loy C, et al: Withdrawal or continuation of cholinesterase inhibitors or memantine or both, in people with dementia. Cochrane Database Syst Rev (2):CD009081, 2021 35608903

NMDA Receptor Antagonist

Memantine

I. **Brand Names**: Namenda; Namenda XR; Namzaric (combination with donepezil)

II. **Therapeutic Class**: Cognitive enhancer

III. **Mechanism-Based Class**: Reversible *N*-methyl-D-aspartate (NMDA) receptor antagonist

IV. **Mechanism(s) of Action**

A. CNS inhibition of magnesium site of NMDA receptor (reversible, noncompetitive antagonist).

B. Also antagonizes nicotinic acetylcholine receptors and 5-HT_3 serotonin receptors.

V. **Indications**

A. FDA adult:

1. Dementia (major neurocognitive disorder) of the Alzheimer's type (moderate, severe)

B. Evidence-based[1] off-label uses:

1. Non-Alzheimer's neurocognitive disorders: Some evidence for efficacy in major neurocognitive disorders due to mixed vascular, Parkinson's disease, and Lewy body etiologies.
2. Treatment-resistant depression. Supporting evidence is weak and extremely limited.

C. FDA pediatric: None

VI. **Major Contraindications and When to Use Caution**

A. Known hypersensitivity to memantine/Namenda

VII. **Dosage Formulations**

A. Brand tablet (5 mg, 10 mg)

B. Brand extended-release (XR) capsule (7 mg, 14 mg, 21 mg, 28 mg)

C. Generic tablet (5 mg, 10 mg)

D. Generic XR capsule (7 mg, 14 mg, 21 mg, 28 mg)

E. Generic oral solution (2 mg/mL)

VIII. **Dosage Ranges and Guidelines**

A. Start at 5 mg/day and increase in 5-mg increments to 10 mg twice daily (BID), with at least 1 week between increases (Table 8–4).

B. XR formulation: Start at 7 mg/day and increase in 7-mg increments to 28 mg/day, with at least 1 week between increases.

---

[1]Evidence strength varies; readers are referred to the literature for more detailed information.

C. Re-titration (starting again at the starting dosage and titrating upward) may be required after sustained nonadherence.
D. Memantine's benefits over placebo may not be easily distinguished until 12–26 weeks after initiation, if at all. Effect sizes are small.

Table 8–4. Memantine indications and dosage ranges

Indication	Usual dosage range
Dementia due to Alzheimer's disease, moderate or severe	5–10 mg BID 7–28 mg/day (XR)
Dementia due to mixed vascular/Alzheimer's disease (off-label)	5–10 mg BID
Dementia due to vascular disease (off-label)	5–10 mg BID
Dementia due to Parkinson's disease (off-label)	5–10 mg BID
Dementia with Lewy bodies (off-label)	5–10 mg BID

IX. **Monitoring**: Not applicable

X. **Relevant Pharmacokinetics/Pharmacodynamics**

A. **Metabolism**: Largely renal (active tubular secretion) moderated by pH-dependent reabsorption
B. **Time to peak plasma concentration**: 3–7 hours (delayed with XR form; no significant difference if taken with/without food)
C. **Half-life**: 60–80 hours (steady state reached in 15 days)
D. **Protein binding**: Low (<45%)
E. **Hepatic impairment**: Caution in severe hepatic impairment.
F. **Renal impairment**: Caution in severe renal impairment.

XI. **Clinically Relevant Drug Interactions**

A. Urine alkalinization may decrease clearance by up to 80%; use care with carbonic anhydrase inhibitors, bicarbonate.
B. Protein binding/displacement studies did not indicate clinically significant interactions.

XII. **Adverse Effects**

A. **Most common**:

1. In approval trials, discontinuation due to adverse effects was no more common than in the placebo group. No individual adverse effects with frequency of less than 1% were significantly more common in the memantine group than in the placebo group.
2. Gastrointestinal: Constipation.
3. Cardiovascular: Dizziness
4. Behavioral: Confusion, irritability, agitation
5. Neurological: Headache

B. **Other notable side effects**: Rare postmarketing reports of uncertain causality of agranulocytosis, leukopenia (including neutropenia), pancytopenia, thrombocytopenia, thrombotic thrombocytopenic purpura, congestive heart failure, pancreatitis, hepatitis, suicidal ideation, acute renal failure, and Stevens-Johnson syndrome.

C. **Risks in pregnancy and lactation**: No adequate human data are available.

XIII. **Clinical Pearls/Prescribing Tips**

A. There is no evidence that memantine prevents or slows neurodegeneration, despite its theoretical prevention of glutamatergic excitotoxicity.

B. Memantine appears to be no more effective than placebo in mild or major neurocognitive disorder due to Alzheimer's disease.

C. Memantine appears to be equally effective for major neurocognitive disorder due to Alzheimer's disease whether co-prescribed with an acetylcholinesterase inhibitor or not.

D. In major neurocognitive disorder due to vascular disease (mild to moderate), memantine appears to be effective for cognitive outcomes and may also improve mood and behavior.

E. XR capsules may be opened and granules poured out, but contents should not be crushed or chewed.

F. Although some expert opinion suggests that withdrawal of memantine is a viable option in severe disease after placement in an institutional setting, there is limited evidence to support that strategy, and it may lead to worsening in cognition (Parsons et al. 2021). Given memantine's benign side-effect profile, continuation may be preferred.

Further Reading

Arvanitakis Z, Shah RC, Bennett DA: Diagnosis and management of dementia: review. JAMA 322(16):1589–1599, 2019 31638686

Davies SR (on behalf of Cochrane Clinical Answers Editors): How does memantine compare with placebo for treating adults with mild to moderate vascular dementia? Cochrane Clinical Answers, 2019. Available at: https://www.cochranelibrary.com/cca/doi/10.1002/cca.2647/full. Accessed June 15, 2024.

Kirkman MA, Day J, Gehring K, et al: Interventions for preventing and ameliorating cognitive deficits in adults treated with cranial irradiation. Cochrane Database Syst Rev (11):CD011335, 2022 36427235

McShane R, Westby MJ, Roberts E, et al: Memantine for dementia. Cochrane Database Syst Rev (3):CD003154, 2019 30891742

Memantine package insert. U.S. Food and Drug Administration. Available at: https://www.accessdata.fda.gov/drugsatfda_docs/label/2005/021627lbl.pdf. Accessed March 13, 2024.

Memantine XR package insert. U.S. Food and Drug Administration. Available at: https://www.accessdata.fda.gov/drugsatfda_docs/label/2010/022525s000lbl.pdf. Accessed March 13, 2024.

O'Brien JT, Holmes C, Jones M, et al: Clinical practice with anti-dementia drugs: a revised (third) consensus statement from the British Association for Psychopharmacology. J Psychopharmacol 31(2):147–168, 2017 28103749
PubChem: PubChem Compound Summary for CID 4054, Memantine. Bethesda, MD, National Library of Medicine, National Center for Biotechnology Information, 2004. Available from: https://pubchem.ncbi.nlm.nih.gov/compound/Memantine. Accessed November 14, 2022.
Verdijk JPAJ, van Kessel MA, Oud M, et al: Pharmacological interventions to diminish cognitive side effects of electroconvulsive therapy: a systematic review and meta-analysis. Acta Psychiatr Scand 145(4):343–356, 2022 35075641

References

Parsons C, Lim WY, Loy C, et al: Withdrawal or continuation of cholinesterase inhibitors or memantine or both, in people with dementia. Cochrane Database Syst Rev (2):CD009081, 2021 35608903

Amyloid-Specific Monoclonal Antibodies

Lecanemab[1]

I. **Brand Name**: Leqembi (lecanemab-irmb)

II. **Therapeutic Class**: Cognitive enhancer targeting amyloid beta pathology

III. **Mechanism-Based Class**: Amyloid beta–specific humanized monoclonal antibody of immunoglobulin G (IgG)

IV. **Mechanism(s) of Action**

A. Binds to, and accelerates clearance of, soluble aggregated forms (protofibrils) of amyloid beta, reducing amyloid plaque burden in the brain.

V. **Indications**

A. FDA adult: Treatment of Alzheimer's disease (mild cognitive impairment or mild dementia)

B. Off-label: None

C. FDA pediatric: None

VI. **Major Contraindications and When to Use Caution**

A. Caution in patients with apolipoprotein E epsilon 4 homozygosity (increases risk of edema and hemorrhage).

B. Caution in patient with cerebral amyloid angiopathy, superficial siderosis, or vasogenic cerebral edema.

C. Caution in patients with intracranial aneurysms or other CNS vascular malformations.

D. Caution in patients with cerebral hemorrhage risk or hemorrhages numbering 4 or more or greater than 1 cm.

E. Caution in patients on anticoagulant therapy.

VII. **Dosage Formulations**

A. Infusion (100 mg/mL)

VIII. **Dosage Ranges and Guidelines**

A. Dementia due to Alzheimer's disease, mild: 10 mg/kg/dose IV every 2 weeks (Table 8–5).

B. Mild cognitive impairment due to Alzheimer's disease: 10 mg/kg/dose IV every 2 weeks (Table 8–5).

---

[1] In July 2024, the FDA approved donanemab (Kisunla), a similar monoclonal antibody, with administration every 4 weeks. Another monoclonal antibody, aducanumab (Aduhelm), has received only limited FDA approval, has fewer available data on clinical/outcome efficacy, and appears to carry a greater risk of adverse effects. Aducanumab is not approved for Medicare coverage outside of clinical studies. Our discussion here will be limited to lecanemab, which has full FDA approval and Medicare coverage.

Table 8–5. Lecanemab indications and dosage ranges

Indication	Usual dosage range
Dementia due to Alzheimer's disease, mild	10 mg/kg/dose IV every 2 weeks
Mild cognitive impairment due to Alzheimer's disease	10 mg/kg/dose IV every 2 weeks

IX. **Monitoring**

A. Presence of amyloid beta pathology must be confirmed prior to prescribing.

B. A baseline brain MRI must be obtained within 1 year prior to starting treatment.

C. Interval brain MRIs must be obtained prior to the 5th, 7th, and 14th infusions.

D. The prescribing information (Eisai 2023) contains detailed guidelines on suspension or continuation of dosing based on radiological and clinical findings of amyloid-related imaging abnormalities—edema (ARIA-E [Esai 2023, Table 1]) or amyloid-related imaging abnormalities—hemorrhage (ARIA-H [Esai 2023, Table 2]).

X. **Relevant Pharmacokinetics/Pharmacodynamics**

A. **Metabolism**: Monoclonal antibodies are degraded by proteolytic enzymes that metabolize native immunoglobulins

B. **Time to peak plasma concentration**: N/A

C. **Half-life**: 5–7 days; steady state reached in 6 weeks

D. **Protein binding**: Not applicable

E. **Hepatic impairment**: Not hepatically cleared.

F. **Renal impairment:** Not renally cleared.

XI. **Clinically Relevant Drug Interactions**

A. Patients on anticoagulant or antiplatelet therapies may be at greater risk of microhemorrhage or hemorrhage. Patients on anticoagulant therapies were initially excluded from trials, although antiplatelet therapies were allowed. If patients required anticoagulants, lecanemab was paused for 4 weeks. There did not appear to be a higher risk of ARIA-H in patients exposed to antithrombotic therapies in the treatment versus placebo arms.

XII. **Adverse Effects**

A. **Most common**:

1. Infusion reactions (fever, flu-like symptoms, nausea, vomiting, hypotension, hypertension, oxygen desaturation) occurred in about 20% of lecanemab patients. May require pretreatment with antihistamine, acetaminophen, or a corticosteroid.
2. **Boxed warning: amyloid-related imaging abnormalities**: In preapproval trials and their open-label extensions for lecanemab, about 12%–13% of participants had radiographic ARIA-E, and 2%–3% had symptomatic ARIA-E (Eisai 2023). The placebo group had very low rates of ARIA-E. Lecanemab was also associated with a near-doubling of the rate of ARIA-H (from 8%–9% to 16%–17%, depending on anticoagulant/antiplatelet use). Refer to the full prescribing information (Eisai 2023) for the complete boxed warning.

3. Cardiovascular: Atrial fibrillation occurred more frequently in the treatment group than in the placebo group (4% vs. 1%) (Eisai 2023).
4. Hematological: Lymphopenia occurred more frequently in the treatment group than in the placebo group (4% vs. 1%) (Eisai 2023).

B. **Risks in pregnancy and lactation**: No information available.

XIII. **Clinical Pearls/Prescribing Tips**

A. In one large study (van Dyck et al. 2023), patients receiving lecanemab showed about a 27% reduction in cognitive decline on the Clinical Dementia Rating scale—sum of boxes (CDR-SB) over 18 months (a difference of about 0.45 point on an 18-point scale).

B. Even for patients with Medicare coverage, the annual expense could be upward of $6,600, and the $26,500 yearly cost of medication alone would add a significant burden to the Medicare budget (Arbanas et al. 2023).

C. A real-world assessment of eligibility in the Mayo Clinic Study of Aging, based on clinical trial inclusion/exclusion criteria, found that between 53% (using only inclusion criteria) and 92% (using both inclusion and exclusion criteria) of patients with mild cognitive impairment or mild dementia and positive amyloid scans would not have been eligible for the lecanemab preapproval trials (Pittock et al. 2023).

D. Patients with moderate or severe Alzheimer's dementia, as well as those with non-Alzheimer's or mixed-Alzheimer's dementias, are not eligible for treatment with anti-amyloid therapy, given the limited clinical benefit and greater risk of adverse outcomes in these patients.

Further Reading

Hampel H, Elhage A, Cho M, et al: Amyloid-related imaging abnormalities (ARIA): radiological, biological and clinical characteristics. Brain 146(11):4414–4424, 2023 37280110

Honig LS, Sabbagh MN, et al. Updated safety results from phase 3 lecanemab study in early Alzheimer's disease. Alzheimers Res Ther 16(1):105, 2024 38730496

Knight Alzheimer Disease Research Center: CDR Scoring Table. St. Louis, MO, Washington University School of Medicine, 2024. Available at: https://knightadrc.wustl.edu/professionals-clinicians/cdr-dementia-staging-instrument/cdr-scoring-table/. Accessed June 10, 2024.

Terao I, Kodama W: Comparative efficacy, tolerability and acceptability of donanemab, lecanemab, aducanumab and lithium on cognitive function in MCI and Alzheimer's disease: a systematic review and network meta-analysis. Ageing Res Rev 94:102203, 2024 38253184

References

Arbanas JC, Damberg CL, Leng M, et al: Estimated annual spending on lecanemab and its ancillary costs in the US Medicare program. JAMA Intern Med 183(8):885–889, 2023 37167598

Eisai: Leqembi (lecanemab-irmb) injection, for intravenous use [package insert]. U.S. Food and Drug Administration website. Revised July 2023. Available at: https://www.accessdata.fda.gov/drugsatfda_docs/label/2023/761269Orig1s001lbl.pdf. Accessed June 21, 2024.

Pittock RR, Aakre JA, Castillo AM, et al: Eligibility for anti-amyloid treatment in a population-based study of cognitive aging. Neurology 101(19):e1837–e1849, 2023 37586881

van Dyck CH, Swanson CJ, Aisen P, et al: Lecanemab in early Alzheimer's disease. N Engl J Med 388(1):9–21, 2023 36449413

9

Treatment of Eating Disorders

Alexandra F. Muratore, Ph.D.
B. Timothy Walsh, M.D.

Pharmacological Treatment of Eating Disorders

- The pathophysiology of eating disorders remains unclear. As a result, research investigating pharmacological treatment of eating disorders has frequently tested the efficacy of medications useful in treating other psychiatric disorders frequently comorbid with eating disorders. For example, high rates of comorbidity between eating and mood disorders prompted initial investigation of antidepressants as a potential treatment for eating disorder symptoms. Medication classes subsequently investigated included antipsychotics, anticonvulsants, and mood stabilizers, among others, with different levels of efficacy identified for different eating disorder diagnoses.
- Of the eating disorders sufficiently studied, anorexia nervosa remains the most resistant to pharmacological treatment. Although trials of pharmacological interventions for this diagnosis remain limited, the only medication that appears to confer some benefit (increased rate of weight gain but no improvement in psychological symptoms) is the second-generation antipsychotic olanzapine. All other antidepressants, antipsychotics, anxiolytics, and other medication classes studied have been largely unsuccessful in treating the symptoms of anorexia nervosa. As a result, the first-line treatment for anorexia nervosa is behavioral weight restoration.
- Results of pharmacological research for bulimia nervosa and binge-eating disorder are more promising. Among patients with bulimia nervosa, virtually all antidepressants have outperformed placebo, although fluoxetine (at a dosage of 60 mg/day) is still the selective serotonin reuptake inhibitor (SSRI) with the most substantial evidence of efficacy and is the only medication currently FDA approved for treatment of bulimia nervosa. Cognitive-behavioral therapy (CBT) remains the first-line treatment for bulimia nervosa, and there is evidence to suggest that combining CBT with medications such as fluoxetine is superior to medication alone.

- Several antidepressant medications are also effective in reducing the symptoms of binge-eating disorder. However, the stimulant medication lisdexamfetamine is the most effective pharmacological intervention both for reducing binge-eating frequency and for aiding weight loss, and is currently the only FDA-approved medication for treatment of binge-eating disorder. Behavioral approaches are still first-line treatments for binge-eating disorder, and limited research suggests that combining psychotherapy with medications does not improve outcomes.

Further Reading

Crow SJ: Pharmacologic treatment of eating disorders. Psychiatr Clin North Am 42(2):253–262, 2019 31046927

Muratore AF, Attia E: Psychopharmacologic management of eating disorders. Curr Psychiatry Rep 24(7):345–351, 2022 35576089

Reas DL, Grilo CM: Psychotherapy and medications for eating disorders: better together? Clin Ther 43(1):17–39, 2021 33342555

Treatment of Anorexia Nervosa

Overview

- A wide range of medications have been examined for efficacy in the treatment of anorexia nervosa (Table 9–1). The psychopharmacological agents investigated were selected for testing because 1) they showed efficacy in improving symptoms commonly experienced by individuals with anorexia nervosa (e.g., depression, anxiety, obsessional thinking, weight-related thought disturbance) and/or 2) they had side effects that could improve physical (e.g., weight loss) or psychological symptoms (e.g., anxiety) of this disorder.
- The medications studied most extensively in anorexia nervosa are antidepressants and antipsychotics.
  - Although second-generation antidepressants (e.g., SSRIs) are generally safer and better-tolerated than first-generation antidepressants (i.e., tricyclic antidepressants [TCAs] and monoamine oxidase inhibitors [MAOIs]), evidence from antidepressant trials indicates that overall, these medications confer no therapeutic benefit for patients with anorexia nervosa.
  - In common with antidepressants, first-generation antipsychotics have not been found to be effective for patients with anorexia nervosa.
  - Research on the effects of second-generation antipsychotics has found that olanzapine provides modest benefit for weight gain in outpatients with anorexia nervosa.
  - Bupropion is an antidepressant medication (a norepinephrine and dopamine reuptake inhibitor [NDRI]) that is contraindicated in anorexia nervosa because of its association with increased risk of drug-induced seizures. There is currently insufficient evidence supporting the use of any other medications in anorexia nervosa.

Table 9–1. Evidence for benefit of various agents in anorexia nervosa

Class/Medication	Overall level of evidence*
Antidepressants	
Amitriptyline	N
Bupropion	X
Citalopram	I
Clomipramine	N
Fluoxetine	N
Mirtazapine	I
Sertraline	I
Antipsychotics	
Aripiprazole	N
Olanzapine	E
Pimozide	N
Sulpiride	N
Anxiolytic	
Alprazolam	N
Mood stabilizer	
Lithium	I
Psychedelics	
Ayahuasca	I
Psilocybin	I

***Level of evidence**: I=insufficient research; N=no evidence of efficacy; E=evidence of efficacy; X=use contraindicated.

Medication for Anorexia Nervosa

Olanzapine (Anorexia Nervosa)[1]

- Studies of olanzapine in patients with anorexia nervosa have used dosages of 2.5–15 mg/day.
- Olanzapine was originally considered as a potential medication for anorexia nervosa due, in part, to its effects of weight gain in other populations with mental disorders. Although smaller early studies found conflicting evidence of olanzapine's utility, the largest trial to date (Attia et al. 2019) found that outpatients with anorexia nervosa who received olanzapine treatment for 16 weeks showed greater weight gain than did those

[1] See Chapter 6, "Antipsychotics," for more detailed information regarding olanzapine.

who received placebo. However, there was no evidence to suggest that olanzapine significantly reduced the core psychological symptoms of anorexia nervosa.

Further Reading

Cassioli E, Sensi C, Mannucci E, et al: Pharmacological treatment of acute-phase anorexia nervosa: evidence from randomized controlled trials. J Psychopharmacol 34(8):864–873, 2020 32448045

Çöpür S, Çöpür M: Olanzapine in the treatment of anorexia nervosa: a systematic review. Egypt J Neurol Psychiatr Neurosurg 56:60, 2020

Muratore AF, Attia E: Current therapeutic approaches to anorexia nervosa: state of the art. Clin Ther 43(1):85–94, 2021 33293054

Walsh BT, Xu T, Wang Y, et al: Time course of relapse following acute treatment for anorexia nervosa. Am J Psychiatry 178(9):848–853, 2021 34154394

References

Attia E, Steinglass JE, Walsh BT, et al: Olanzapine versus placebo in adult outpatients with anorexia nervosa: a randomized clinical trial. Am J Psychiatry 176(6):449–456, 2019 30654643

Treatment of Bulimia Nervosa

Overview

- Numerous clinical trials have investigated various medication classes for efficacy in the treatment of bulimia nervosa, and have yielded findings more promising than those in research on anorexia nervosa. Table 9–2 presents a review of the evidence for medications studied in the treatment of bulimia nervosa.
- Virtually all antidepressants have been shown to be effective in reducing binge-eating and purging frequency. Of these, the strongest evidence is for fluoxetine (at a dosage of 60 mg/day), which is the only currently FDA-approved medication for bulimia nervosa.
- Preliminary research investigating the anticonvulsant topiramate and the 5-HT_3 receptor agonist ondansetron suggests that these medications may also be effective in reducing bingeing/purging symptoms.
- As with anorexia nervosa, the antidepressant bupropion is contraindicated in patients with bulimia nervosa because of the risk of drug-induced seizures.

Table 9–2. Evidence for benefit of various agents in bulimia nervosa

Class/Medication	Overall level of evidence*
Antidepressants	
Amitriptyline	N
Brofaromine	N
Bupropion	X
Desipramine	E
Fluoxetine	S
Fluvoxamine	M
Imipramine	E
Phenelzine	E
Sertraline	E
Trazodone	E
Anticonvulsant	
Topiramate	E
5-HT_3 receptor antagonist	
Ondansetron	M

***Level of evidence**: N=no evidence of efficacy; E=evidence of efficacy; M=mixed evidence; S=substantial evidence of efficacy; X=use contraindicated.

Medications for Bulimia Nervosa

Fluoxetine (Bulimia Nervosa)[1]

- For treatment of bulimia nervosa, fluoxetine should be administered at 60 mg/day.
- Fluoxetine is the only medication that is FDA approved for the treatment of bulimia nervosa.
- In clinical trials examining patients with bulimia nervosa, fluoxetine dosages of 20 mg/day and 60/mg day were compared with placebo. The 60 mg/day dosage was significantly more effective than placebo in reducing symptoms and was associated with reduced likelihood of relapse, whereas the 20 mg/day dosage was not (Fluoxetine Bulimia Nervosa Collaborative Study Group 1992). Therefore, the recommended dosage for patients with bulimia nervosa is 60 mg/day, taken in the morning. It is advisable to begin at 20 mg/day but to quickly titrate upward to 60 mg/day over a brief time (e.g., a week). Higher dosages of fluoxetine for bulimia nervosa have not been systematically studied.

[1] See Chapter 2, "Antidepressants," for more detailed information regarding fluoxetine.

Further Reading

Goldstein DJ, Wilson MG, Ascroft RC, al-Banna M: Effectiveness of fluoxetine therapy in bulimia nervosa regardless of comorbid depression. Int J Eat Disord 25(1):19–27, 1999 9924649

Hagan KE, Walsh BT: State of the art: the therapeutic approaches to bulimia nervosa. Clin Ther 43(1):40–49, 2021 33358256

Walsh BT, Agras WS, Devlin MJ, et al: Fluoxetine for bulimia nervosa following poor response to psychotherapy. Am J Psychiatry 157(8):1332–1334, 2000 10910801

References

Fluoxetine Bulimia Nervosa Collaborative Study Group: Fluoxetine in the treatment of bulimia nervosa: a multicenter, placebo-controlled, double-blind trial. Arch Gen Psychiatry 49(2):139–147, 1992 1550466

Sertraline (Bulimia Nervosa)[1]

- For adults with bulimia nervosa, studies have examined sertraline dosages of 50–200 mg/day.
- Virtually all of the trials examining patients with bulimia nervosa have found antidepressant treatments to be associated with greater improvement in the symptoms of bulimia nervosa than placebo (e.g., reduced binge-eating frequency). Sertraline is one such example of an antidepressant that has demonstrated efficacy, although there are several other medications that also show promise (e.g., fluvoxamine). However, fluoxetine is the only SSRI with substantial evidence of efficacy and is the only medication that is FDA approved for the treatment of bulimia nervosa.

Further Reading

Hagan KE, Walsh BT: State of the art: the therapeutic approaches to bulimia nervosa. Clin Ther 43(1):40–49, 2021 33358256

Milano W, Petrella C, Sabatino C, et al: Treatment of bulimia nervosa with sertraline: a randomized controlled trial. Adv Ther 21(4):232–237, 2004 15605617

Sloan DM, Mizes JS, Helbok C, et al: Efficacy of sertraline for bulimia nervosa. Int J Eat Disord 36(1):48–54, 2004 15185271

---

[1] See Chapter 2, "Antidepressants," for more detailed information regarding sertraline.

Treatment of Binge-Eating Disorder

Overview

- As with bulimia nervosa, pharmacotherapy research for binge-eating disorder has yielded promising findings. Table 9–3 presents a review of the evidence for medications studied in the treatment of binge-eating disorder.
- Antidepressants, particularly SSRIs, tend to outperform placebo in reducing binge-eating behaviors, but they are generally not effective for weight loss.
- The anticonvulsant topiramate and the stimulant lisdexamfetamine are effective in reducing both binge eating and weight. Thus far, lisdexamfetamine has received the most substantial support, and remains the only FDA-approved medication for binge-eating disorder at the time of this writing. However, research findings suggest that other medications may show promise, including certain SSRIs and anticonvulsants.

Table 9–3. Evidence for benefit of various agents in binge-eating disorder

Class/Medication	Overall level of evidence*
Antidepressants	
Citalopram	E
Desipramine	E
Duloxetine	N
Escitalopram	E
Fluoxetine	E
Fluvoxamine	E
Sertraline	E
Anticonvulsants	
Topiramate	E
Zonisamide	M
Stimulant	
Lisdexamfetamine	S

***Level of evidence**: N=no evidence of efficacy; E=evidence of efficacy; M=mixed evidence; S=substantial evidence of efficacy.

Medications for Binge-Eating Disorder

Fluoxetine (Binge-Eating Disorder)[1]

- Fluoxetine is used off-label for binge-eating disorder.
- The usual dosage range is 20–80 mg/day.

[1] See Chapter 2, "Antidepressants," for more detailed information regarding fluoxetine.

- Fluoxetine is one of several medications, including certain antidepressants (e.g., fluvoxamine, sertraline) and anticonvulsants (e.g., topiramate), that demonstrate some efficacy in reducing the frequency of binge-eating episodes.

Further Reading

Arnold LM, McElroy SL, Hudson JI, et al: A placebo-controlled, randomized trial of fluoxetine in the treatment of binge-eating disorder. J Clin Psychiatry 63(11):1028–1033, 2002 12444817

Greeno CG, Wing RR: A double-blind, placebo-controlled trial of the effect of fluoxetine on dietary intake in overweight women with and without binge-eating disorder. Am J Clin Nutr 64(3):267–273, 1996 8780333

Heal DJ, Gosden J: What pharmacological interventions are effective in binge-eating disorder? Insights from a critical evaluation of the evidence from clinical trials. Int J Obes (Lond) 46(4):677–695, 2022 34992243

Lisdexamfetamine (Binge-Eating Disorder)[1]

- Lisdexamfetamine is approved for use in the treatment of moderate to severe binge-eating disorder in adults.
- Lisdexamfetamine is the only medication currently FDA approved for binge-eating disorder.
- The recommended dosage for binge-eating disorder is 50–70 mg/day, with a maximum dosage of 70 mg/day. The recommended initial dosage is 30 mg every morning, with upward titration of 20 mg/day at weekly intervals.
- The most common adverse effects of lisdexamfetamine in adults include dry mouth, insomnia, decreased appetite, and increased heart rate. Lisdexamfetamine should be taken earlier in the day to minimize the likelihood of insomnia at night.
- Lisdexamfetamine is associated with modest weight loss when used to treat binge-eating disorder. Although antidepressant treatment reduces binge-eating episodes, such treatment is not generally associated with weight loss.

Further Reading

Heal DJ, Gosden J: What pharmacological interventions are effective in binge-eating disorder? Insights from a critical evaluation of the evidence from clinical trials. Int J Obes (Lond) 46(4):677–695, 2022 34992243

Hudson JI, McElroy SL, Ferreira-Cornwell MC, et al: Efficacy of lisdexamfetamine in adults with moderate to severe binge-eating disorder: a randomized clinical trial. JAMA Psychiatry 74(9):903–910, 2017 28700805

Schneider E, Higgs S, Dourish CT: Lisdexamfetamine and binge-eating disorder: a systematic review and meta-analysis of the preclinical and clinical data with a focus on mechanism of drug action in treating the disorder. Eur Neuropsychopharmacol 53:49–78, 2021

---

[1] See Chapter 7, "Stimulants," for more detailed information on lisdexamfetamine.

10

Treatment of Substance Use Disorders

Andrew T. Olagunju, M.B.B.S., M.Sc., Ph.D., FMCPsych, FWACP
Claire Slavin-Stewart, M.Sc., M.D.

In this chapter we provide information on the effective use of medications to treat substance use disorders (SUDs): those related to alcohol, opioids, and tobacco/nicotine. In addition to covering medications with FDA indications for treating SUDs (i.e., acamprosate and naltrexone for alcohol use disorder; buprenorphine, buprenorphine-naloxone, methadone, and naltrexone for opioid use disorder, and varenicline for tobacco use disorder), we also cover an array of evidence-based off-label medications that are used clinically to decrease withdrawal symptoms and/or cravings associated with specific SUDs—for example, the antihypertensive clonidine; the anticonvulsants carbamazepine, gabapentin, and topiramate; and the antidepressant bupropion. Patients with SUDs have diverse needs and may benefit from access to a variety of medications while undergoing SUD treatment.

Multi-Use Medications for Substance Use Disorders

Clonidine (Alcohol Withdrawal, Opioid Withdrawal, Smoking Cessation)[1]

I. **Brand Names**: Catapres, Catapres-TTS (transdermal therapeutic system), Kapvay (extended-release), Jenloga (extended-release), Nexiclon XR

II. **Therapeutic Class**: Antihypertensive

III. **Mechanism-Based Class**: Centrally acting α_2-adrenergic receptor agonist

IV. **Mechanism(s) of Action**:

A. Blockade/activation of norepinephrine α_1 and α_2 receptors

B. α_2-Adrenergic receptor activation reduces sympathetic outflow from the CNS, decreases peripheral vascular resistance and renal vascular resistance, and lowers heart rate and blood pressure.

C. When used acutely, clonidine stimulates the release of growth hormones, but it does not do so with prolonged use.

V. **Indications**:

A. FDA adult and pediatric:

1. Hypertension
2. Cancer pain (when injected epidurally)
3. Clonidine extended-release (Kapvay): ADHD, age ≥6 years as monotherapy or as adjunctive therapy to stimulant medications.

B. Evidence-based off-label uses (Table 10–1)

VI. **Major Contraindications and When to Use Caution**:

A. **Contraindications**:

1. Hypersensitivity to the drug or any ingredients in the formulation
2. Severe bradycardia due to sick sinus syndrome, sinus node dysfunction, or second- or third-degree atrioventricular block
3. Galactose intolerance

---

[1]Also see Chapter 4, "Nonbenzodiazepine Hypnotics," and Chapter 7, "Stimulants," for further information regarding clonidine's use for other indications.

Table 10–1. Clonidine: evidence-based off-label uses

Analgesia/anesthesia	**Psychiatry**
Anesthesia (pediatric)	**Alcohol withdrawal**
Antiemetic (pediatric)	**Opioid withdrawal**
Chronic headache	**Smoking cessation**
Cluster headache prophylaxis	Acute anorexia nervosa
Migraines	Akathisia
Postoperative pain (pediatric)	Bipolar disorder
Reflex sympathetic dystrophy	Conduct disorder
Sedation (intensive care setting)	Korsakoff psychosis (memory enhancement)
Spinal cord injury pain	Narcolepsy
	Panic disorder
Cardiovascular	PTSD
Acute hypertension	Restless legs syndrome
Atrial fibrillation	Schizophrenia
Congestive heart failure	Sleep disorders
Orthostatic hypotension	Social anxiety disorder
Portal pressure	Tourette's syndrome
Gastrointestinal	**Neurology**
Carcinoid-associated diarrhea	Diabetic gastroparesis
High intestinal output after SBT	Essential tremor
Ulcerative colitis and proctitis	HIV-1 encephalopathy (behavioral symptoms)
	Hyperkinetic movement disorders
Endocrine	Hypertonicity
Hyperthyroidism	Neuropathic orofacial pain
Growth delay	Peripheral neuropathy
	Postanesthesia shivering
Miscellaneous	Postepidural shivering
Cyclosporine-induced nephrotoxicity	Postherpetic neuralgia
Menopausal flushing	Tetanus-induced autonomic dysfunction
Dysmenorrhea	

Note. Evidence strength varies; readers are referred to the literature for more detailed information. SBT=small bowel transplant.
Source. Adapted from Fagan et al. 2016.

B. **Use caution**:

1. Mild to moderate bradycardia
2. Recent myocardial infarction
3. Severe coronary insufficiency
4. Congestive heart failure
5. Cerebrovascular disease
6. Chronic renal failure
7. Poor cerebral or peripheral perfusion
8. Polyneuropathy
9. Thromboangiitis obliterans
10. Raynaud's disease
11. Constipation
12. Depression (reports of increased risk of relapse in patients with depression)

VII. **Dosage Formulations**:

A. Generic tablet (0.1 mg, 0.2 mg, 0.3 mg [*most are scored*])
B. Generic and brand (Kapvay) 12-hour extended-release (ER) tablet (0.1 mg)
C. Brand (Nexiclon) 24-hour ER tablet (0.17 mg [*scored*])
D. Brand (Duraclon) epidural solution/continuous infusion (100 μg/mL [10-mL vials])
E. Generic epidural solution (100 μg/mL [10-mL vials], 500 μg/mL [10 mL vials])
F. Generic and brand (Catapres-TTS) weekly transdermal patch (0.1 mg/24 hour, 0.2 mg/24 hour, 0.3 mg/24 hour)

VIII. **Dosage Ranges and Guidelines**:

A. **Alcohol withdrawal**: (off-label; no official evidence-based recommendations available)

1. Suggested dosage is 0.1 mg PO TID in addition to benzodiazepines.

B. **Opioid withdrawal**: (See Clinical Pearls/Prescribing Tips for evidence supporting off-label use.)

1. Day 1: Take 0.1 mg every 45–60 minutes for up to 4 doses (0.4 mg), then 0.1–0.3 mg every 6–8 hours (maximum dosage 1.2 mg/day)
2. Days 2–4: Total daily dose given on day 1 divided into 3–4 equal doses.
3. Day 5: Start taper by 0.1–0.2 mg/day.

C. **Smoking cessation**: (off-label; no official evidence-based recommendations available)

1. Suggested dosage range: 0.15–0.75 mg/day PO for 3–10 weeks.

D. **Drug information/dosing**:

1. When reducing clonidine dosages, taper the dosage over 2–4 days to avoid withdrawal reactions.
2. Tolerance may develop in some patients.
3. Clonidine's hypotensive and sedating effects may limit its usefulness, especially at high dosages.

E. **Psychoeducation**:

1. Caution patients about the risk of pronounced withdrawal symptoms if clonidine is abruptly discontinued (especially dosages higher than 1.2 mg/day).

F. **Missed doses**:

1. If a dose missed, take the dose as soon as possible and then return to regular dosing schedule.

G. **Special populations**:

1. Older adults: Dosage reduction is suggested.

IX. **Monitoring**:

A. Consider obtaining blood pressure and ECG prior to initiation.
B. Monitor blood pressure and heart rate periodically, especially in the presence of dizziness. Consider monitoring orthostatic vitals.
C. Periodic eye exams are suggested, given risk of dry eye.

X. **Relevant Pharmacokinetics/Pharmacodynamics**:

A. **Onset of action**: 30–60 minutes
B. **Time to peak plasma concentration**: 7 hours (Kapvay); 3 hours (IR clonidine)
C. **Half-life**: 5–25.5 hours
D. **Active metabolites**: None
E. **Effect of food**: N/A
F. **Hepatic impairment**: No dosage instructions for this population.
G. **Renal impairment**: Use with caution (half-life increases to as high as 41 hours in severe renal impairment).

XI. **Clinically Relevant Drug Interactions**:

A. CNS depressants (analgesics, sedatives, opioids): Effect potentiated
B. Local anesthetics: Epidural clonidine can prolong effects of anesthesia.
C. Tricyclic antidepressants: Hypotensive effect of clonidine may be blocked.
D. Beta-blockers, guanethidine, cardiac glycosides: bradycardia
E. Hypotensive agents: May enhance clonidine's hypotensive effect.
F. Methylphenidate: Serious interactions in children; can be fatal.

XII. **Adverse Effects**:

A. **Common**: (Side effects tend to be mild and to diminish over time.)

1. Dry mouth, dry eyes, drowsiness, dizziness, sedation, constipation, headache, orthostatic hypotension

B. **Less common**:

1. Sleep disorders, erectile dysfunction

C. **Potentially serious**:

1. Bradycardia and hypotension: Use caution with patients with cardiac risk factors and with concomitant use of other antihypertensive medications.
2. Rebound hypertension with abrupt discontinuation. Other withdrawal symptoms may include diaphoresis, flushing, insomnia, headache. Risk factors include higher dosages (>1 mg/day) and longer duration of use (>1 month).

D. **Risks in pregnancy and lactation**:
   1. Pregnancy: Clonidine should only be used in pregnancy when clearly indicated.
   2. Lactation: Clonidine does pass into the breast milk. There is not sufficient evidence to confirm that clonidine is safe during breastfeeding.

XIII. **Clinical Pearls/Prescribing Tips**:

A. Clonidine is effective in reducing opioid-related withdrawal symptoms, including sweating, intestinal cramps, diarrhea, nausea, anxiety, and irritability.
B. Clonidine has recently been approved for the treatment of ADHD in patients age ≥6 year. According to the Canadian ADHD Resource Alliance (CADDRA) guidelines, clonidine is a third-line medication choice for ADHD (CADDRA 2020).
C. Clonidine is less effective for cravings, muscle aches, restlessness, and insomnia.
D. One study indicated that clonidine increased the duration of abstinence from opioids when used as an adjunct to buprenorphine maintenance treatment (Kowalczyk et al. 2015).
E. When clonidine is being discontinued after long-term use, taper slowly to avoid rebound hypertension.
F. As an alternative to clonidine, lofexidine (which is also an alpha-2 agonist) has a lower risk of sedative and hypotensive effects compared with clonidine (Washton et al. 1983). During trials for opioid detoxification, lofexidine was titrated to a maximum dosage of 1.6–3.2 mg/day in divided doses (Gish et al. 2010).
G. In addition to its use in opioid withdrawal, clonidine has also been used for numerous other indications, including alcohol withdrawal and nightmares/sleep disorders (see Chapter 4, "Nonbenzodiazepine Hypnotics").

Further Reading

Charney DS, Sternberg DE, Kleber HD, et al: The clinical use of clonidine in abrupt withdrawal from methadone: effects on blood pressure and specific signs and symptoms. Arch Gen Psychiatry 38(11):1273–1277, 1981 7305608

CRISM National Guideline Review Committee: CRISM National Guidelines for the Clinical Management of Opioid Use Disorder. Canada, Canadian Research Initiative in Substance Misuse, 2018

Cunningham C, Edlund FMJ, Fishman M, et al: The ASAM National Practice Guideline for the Treatment of Opioid Use Disorder: 2020 focused update. J Addict Med 14(2S Suppl 1):1–91, 2020 32511106

Jasinski DR, Johnson RE, Kocher TR: Clonidine in morphine withdrawal: differential effects on signs and symptoms. Arch Gen Psychiatry 42(11):1063–1066, 1985 2413818

National Library of Medicine: Compound summary: clonidine. PubChem, 2022. Available at: https://pubchem.ncbi.nlm.nih.gov/compound/Clonidine. Accessed March 13, 2024.

Sevarino KA: Opioid withdrawal: medically supervised withdrawal during treatment for opioid use disorder, in UpToDate (Saxon AJ, Friedman M [Eds]). Updated October 23, 2023. Available at: https://www.uptodate.com/contents/opioid-withdrawal-medically-supervised-withdrawal-during-treatment-for-opioid-use-disorder. Accessed July 2, 2024.

Teva Canada Limited: Product monograph: Teva—clonidine. Teva Canada, 2014. Available at: https://pdf.hres.ca/dpd_pm/00024986.PDF. Accessed March 13, 2024.

References

CADDRA—Canadian ADHD Resource Alliance: Canadian ADHD Practice Guidelines, 4.1 Edition. Toronto, ON, Canada, 2020. Available at: https://adhdlearn.caddra.ca/wp-content/uploads/2022/08/Canadian-ADHD-Practice-Guidelines-4.1-January-6-2021.pdf. Accessed July 31, 2024.

Fagan NL, Wargo KA, Malone PM, et al: The clinical utility of clonidine. US Pharmacist 5:HS-2-HS-16, 2016. Available at: https://www.uspharmacist.com/article/the-clinical-utility-of-clonidine#:~:text=The%20only%20FDA%2Dapproved%20indication,uses%20described%20are%20off%2Dlabel. Accessed March 6, 2024.

Gish EC, Miller JL, Honey BL, et al: Lofexidine, an alpha2-receptor agonist for opioid detoxification. Ann Pharmacother 44(2):343–351, 2010 20040696

Kowalczyk WJ, Phillips KA, Jobes ML, et al: Clonidine maintenance prolongs opioid abstinence and decouples stress from craving in daily life: a randomized controlled trial with ecological momentary assessment. Am J Psychiatry 172(8):760–767, 2015 25783757

Washton AM, Resnick RB, Geyer G: Opiate withdrawal using lofexidine, a clonidine analogue with fewer side effects. J Clin Psychiatry 44(9):335–337, 1983 6355070

Gabapentin (Alcohol Use Disorder, Opioid Use Disorder)[1]

I. **Brand Names**: Neurontin, Gralise

II. **Therapeutic Class**: Anticonvulsant

III. **Mechanism-Based Class**: GABA analog, glutamate channel blocker

IV. **Mechanism(s) of Action**

A. The precise mechanism of action of gabapentin is largely unknown. Gabapentin is similar in structure to GABA but does not affect GABA binding, uptake, or degradation. It is possible that gabapentin binds to $\alpha_2\delta$ voltage-gated calcium channels, but it is unclear whether this binding relates to its therapeutic effects. There is evidence that gabapentin binds in the outer layers of the cerebral cortex and in other brain regions (e.g., hippocampus, cerebellum), which likely contributes to its anticonvulsant properties.

V. **Indications**

A. FDA adult (and pediatric where shown):

1. Postherpetic neuralgia
2. Adjunctive therapy, treatment of epilepsy with partial-onset seizures with and without secondary generalization (adults; pediatric patients age >3 years and older)

---

[1]Also see Chapter 3, "Anxiolytics: Benzodiazepines and Nonbenzodiazepines," for further information regarding gabapentin's use for other indications.

B. Evidence-based[1] off-label uses:

1. Diabetic neuropathy, neuropathic pain
2. Fibromyalgia
3. Acute postoperative pain
4. Migraine prophylaxis
5. Treatment-resistant partial epilepsy
6. Social anxiety disorder
7. Alcohol use disorder
8. Opioid use disorder
9. Insomnia
10. Restless legs syndrome

VI. Major Contraindications and When to Use Caution

A. **Contraindications**:

1. Known hypersensitivity to medication or class

B. **Use caution**:

1. Use of gabapentin with opioids can result in life-threatening respiratory depression; therefore, limit dosages and monitor closely.
2. Gabapentin can increase suicidal thoughts and behavior.

VII. Dosage Formulations

A. Generic: capsule (100 mg, 300 mg, 400 mg); tablet (600 mg, 800 mg); concentrate (50 mg/mL)

B. Brand: capsule (100 mg, 300 mg, 400 mg); tablet (600 mg, 800 mg); extended-release (ER) tablet (300 mg, 600 mg); concentrate (50 mg/mL)

1. Do not chew, break, or crush ER form. The ER tablet must be taken with food.

VIII. Dosage Ranges and Guidelines

A. **Alcohol use disorder**:

1. Initial:
   a. Day 1: 300 mg/day
   b. Day 2: 300 mg BID
   c. Day 3: 300 mg TID
2. Maintenance: 300 mg TID → 600 mg TID
3. Maximum dosage: 1,800 mg/day

B. **Opioid use disorder**:

1. Initial:
   a. Day 1: 800 mg/day
   b. Day 2: 1,200 mg/day
   c. Day 3: 1,600 mg/day
2. Maintenance: 1,600 mg/day

---

[1]Evidence strength varies; readers are referred to the literature for more detailed information.

C. **Drug information/dosing**:

1. Gabapentin's abuse potential has been documented (Peckham et al. 2018), prompting a Schedule V controlled substance classification in certain states.
2. If discontinuing gabapentin, gradually taper over at least 1 week to reduce risk of withdrawal-precipitated seizures.

D. **Psychoeducation**:

1. Counsel patients to monitor for fever and lymphadenopathy, which are preliminary symptoms of drug reaction with eosinophilia and systemic symptoms (DRESS). If detected, stop gabapentin and seek immediate evaluation.
2. Counsel patients to monitor for signs of anaphylaxis and angioedema. If detected, stop gabapentin and seek immediate evaluation.
3. Counsel patients to contact their health care provider if they experience an increase in suicidal ideation or behavior, depression, anxiety, irritability, or aggression.
4. Counsel patients to avoid driving, operating heavy machinery, or other tasks requiring sustained attention until a stable dosage is established.

E. **Missed doses**:

1. Take missed dose as soon as possible if time until next dose is longer than 4 hours. If time until next dose is less than 4 hours, continue with regular dosing schedule.

F. **Special populations**:

1. Older adult patients: Caution and dosage reduction is suggested because of poorer renal function in older adults.

IX. **Monitoring**

A. No indications for routine monitoring.

X. **Relevant Pharmacokinetics/Pharmacodynamics**

A. **Metabolism**: Gabapentin is cleared renally (100% unchanged); it has no hepatic metabolism.

1. Gabapentin is highly lipid soluble, making it readily distributed across the blood-brain barrier.

B. **Onset of action**: 2–3 hours
C. **Half-life**: 5–7 hours
D. **Active metabolites**: None
E. **Effect of food**: N/A
F. **Hepatic impairment**: No adjustment required.
G. **Renal impairment**: Gabapentin can be removed by hemodialysis. Adjust dosage according to estimated glomerular filtration rate (eGFR):

1. eGFR >60: 300 mg TID → 1,200 mg TID
2. eGFR 30–59: 200 mg BID → 700 mg BID
3. eGFR: 15–29: 200–700 mg once daily
4. eGFR: <15: 100–300 mg once daily
5. Hemodialysis: 125–350 mg once daily plus an additional dose 4 hours after hemodialysis.

XI. **Clinically Relevant Drug Interactions**

A. Concomitant use of opioids, benzodiazepines, or alcohol produces additive CNS depressant effects.
B. Gabapentin decreases levels of hydrocodone.
C. Naproxen increases gabapentin absorption.
D. Maalox (aluminum hydroxide/magnesium hydroxide) reduces the bioavailability of gabapentin. Take gabapentin 2 hours after taking Maalox.

XII. **Adverse Effects**

A. **Common**:

1. Dizziness, fatigue, somnolence, peripheral edema, diarrhea, dry mouth, ataxia, nystagmus, tremor

B. **Rare**:

1. DRESS, anaphylaxis/angioedema

C. **Risks in pregnancy and lactation**:

1. Pregnancy: Risks are unknown in humans. Animal studies indicate an increase in fetal skeletal and visceral abnormalities and increased embryofetal mortality.
2. Lactation: Gabapentin is secreted into the breast milk.

XIII. **Clinical Pearls/Prescribing Tips**

A. **Evidence supporting gabapentin use for treatment of alcohol use disorder**:

1. Gabapentin is a third-line choice in the pharmacological treatment of alcohol use disorder. Studies indicate that it significantly reduces rates of heavy drinking, increases rates of abstinence (NNT=5), and reduces cravings (Mason et al. 2014).

B. **Evidence supporting gabapentin use for treatment of opioid use disorder**:

1. Gabapentin has been shown to be effective in reducing some symptoms of opioid withdrawal in patients undergoing opioid detoxification (Sanders et al. 2013).

Further Reading

Goodman CW, Brett AS: A clinical overview of off-label use of gabapentinoid drugs. JAMA Intern Med 179(5):695–701, 2019 30907944

National Collaborating Centre for Mental Health (UK): Alcohol Use Disorders: Diagnosis, Assessment and Management of Harmful Drinking and Alcohol Dependence. Leicester, UK, British Psychological Society, 2011 22624177

Neurontin (gabapentin) [package insert]. U.S Food and Drug Administration, 2022. Available at: https://www.accessdata.fda.gov/spl/data/20876c74-5c0b-472c-a19a-d79987402df2/20876c74-5c0b-472c-a19a-d79987402df2.xml. Accessed March 13, 2024.

Peckham AM, Evoy KE, Ochs L, et al: Gabapentin for off-label use: evidence-based or cause for concern? Subst Abuse 12:1178221818801311, 2018 30262984

Salehi M, Kheirabadi GR, Maracy MR, et al: Importance of gabapentin dose in treatment of opioid withdrawal. J Clin Psychopharmacol 31(5):593–596, 2011 21869694

Winslow BT, Onysko M, Hebert M: Medications for alcohol use disorder. Am Fam Physician 93(6):457–465, 2016 26977830

References

Mason BJ, Quello S, Goodell V, et al: Gabapentin treatment for alcohol dependence: a randomized clinical trial. JAMA Intern Med 174(1):70–77, 2014 24190578

Peckham AM, Ananickal MJ, Sclar DA: Gabapentin use, abuse, and the US opioid epidemic: the case for reclassification as a controlled substance and the need for pharmacovigilance. Risk Manag Healthc Policy 11:109–116, 2018 30154674

Sanders NC, Mancino MJ, Gentry WB, et al: Randomized, placebo-controlled pilot trial of gabapentin during an outpatient, buprenorphine-assisted detoxification procedure. Exp Clin Psychopharmacol 21(4):294–302, 2013 23855333

Naltrexone (Alcohol Use Disorder, Opioid Use Disorder)

I. **Brand Names**: Depade, Revia, Vivitrol (IM)

II. **Therapeutic Class**: Opioid antagonist

III. **Mechanism-Based Class**: Opioid antagonist

IV. **Mechanism(s) of Action**

A. Pure opioid antagonist. Competitive antagonist at mu (μ), kappa (κ), and delta (δ) opioid receptors in the CNS, with the highest affinity for the mu receptors. By binding to opioid receptors, naltrexone reduces the euphoric effects of alcohol or opioids and decreases cravings.

V. **Indications**

A. FDA adult:

1. Opioid dependence (PO and IM)
   a. IM formulation is indicated in the prevention of relapse following opioid detoxification.
   b. PO formulation for opioid dependence: As per the product monograph, there are no data that "unequivocally" demonstrate that PO naltrexone reduces the rate of recidivism among "detoxified formerly opioid-dependent individuals" (Teva Canada Limited 2015).
2. Alcohol dependence (PO and IM)
   a. Abstinence from alcohol is recommended prior to starting IM formulation.

B. Evidence-based[1] off-label uses:

1. Chronic pain
2. Compulsive behavior/impulse-control disorders

---

[1]Evidence strength varies; readers are referred to the literature for more detailed information.

VI. Major Contraindications and When to Use Caution

A. **Contraindications:**

1. Hypersensitivity to naltrexone or any other ingredients
2. Opioid agonist therapy or concurrent opioid use/positive urine drug screen for opioids
3. Failure of naloxone challenge (0.5 mL IV, then 1.5 mL IV after 30 seconds, or 0.8 mg IM and observe for 20 minutes)
4. Acute opioid withdrawal
5. Acute hepatitis or liver failure

B. **Use caution:**

1. Risk of precipitated opioid withdrawal if short-acting opioids have been used in the past 7–10 days or if long-acting opioids (e.g., methadone, fentanyl) have been used in the past 10–14 days.
2. Increased vulnerability to opioid overdose after stopping naltrexone treatment.
3. Possible dosage-related hepatocellular injury.
4. Can increase depressive symptoms and suicidal ideation.
5. IM formulation: Use with caution in individuals with bleeding disorders.

VII. Dosage Formulations

A. Generic tablet (50 mg)
B. Brand (Vivitrol) suspension (IM) (380 mg)

VIII. Dosage Ranges and Guidelines

A. **Alcohol use disorder:**

1. PO formulations:
   a. Induction: Naltrexone 25 mg for 3 days, then increase to 50 mg (can start at 50 mg if low risk of gastrointestinal side effects)
   b. Maintenance: 50–150 mg/day. There is flexibility in the dosing regimen (see "Drug information/dosing" for details regarding the Sinclair method).
2. IM formulations:
   a. Patient must be abstinent from alcohol.
   b. Naltrexone 380 mg IM every 4 weeks administered in upper lateral area of the gluteal muscle
   c. Steady state achieved 3–4 weeks after first injection.

B. **Opioid use disorder:**

1. PO formulations:
   a. Use in opioid dependence: Listed as an indication in full prescribing information, although evidence of efficacy for this indication is less than robust.
   b. Induction: Naltrexone 25 mg for 3 days, then increase to 50 mg (can start at 50 mg if low risk of gastrointestinal side effects).
   c. Maintenance: 50 mg/day. Can also prescribe as a dose taken every 2–3 days (e.g., 100 mg taken every 2 days; 150 mg taken every 3 days; 100 mg taken twice weekly, 150 mg taken once a week) if there is concern about noncompliance, although clinical effectiveness may be reduced.

2. IM formulations:
   a. Naltrexone 380 mg IM every 4 weeks administered in the upper lateral area of the gluteal muscle
   b. Steady state is achieved 3–4 weeks after first injection.
3. If switching from naltrexone to buprenorphine, buprenorphine can be started approximately 1 day after stopping PO naltrexone and approximately 1 month after stopping IM naltrexone.

C. **Drug information/dosing**:
1. Opioids:
   a. Patient should be abstinent from opioids for at least 7–10 days before starting naltrexone (7 days for short-acting opioids and 10–14 days for long-acting opioids such as methadone).
2. Alcohol:
   a. Patients do not need to be abstinent from alcohol while taking the PO formulation, and there are no adverse effects related to drinking alcohol while taking naltrexone.
   b. For patients who do not have coverage and/or do not have the financial means to take naltrexone daily, and/or individuals who are not medication compliant, use the Sinclair method, wherein naltrexone is taken approximately 1 hour before the patient enters an environment in which they are concerned about drinking or drinking to excess.
3. No evidence or guidelines are available regarding switching from PO to IM formulations or vice versa.
4. IM administration can be initiated without starting with PO (can consider a PO naltrexone challenge beforehand).
5. IM formulation should be refrigerated.
6. Naltrexone is covered by the Ontario Drug Benefit (ODB) Program (limited use [LU] code: 532) if the patient 1) meets clinical criteria for alcohol use disorder (AUD), 2) expresses a desire to reduce consumption or abstain from alcohol, and 3) is participating in AUD treatment.

D. **Psychoeducation**:
1. Counsel patients to continue to take naltrexone even if they relapse on alcohol.
2. Counsel patients to discontinue oral naltrexone at least 48 hours before—and IM naltrexone at least 30 days before—elective surgery requiring analgesia with an opioid.
3. Counsel patients about increased sensitivity to opioids and increased vulnerability to opioid overdose.

E. **Missed doses**:
1. PO: Take missed dose as soon as possible.
2. IM: Reschedule dose as soon as possible.

IX. Monitoring

A. Baseline serum liver function tests (LFTs), then monthly during the first 6 months and intermittently thereafter.

B. Consider intermittent urine naltrexone/6-β-naltrexol test and/or UDS.

C. Monitor for depressive symptoms and suicidal ideation.

X. Relevant Pharmacokinetics/Pharmacodynamics

A. **Time to peak plasma concentration**: PO: 1 hour; IM: 48–72 hours

B. **Half-life**:

1. PO: Naltrexone: 4 hours; 6-β-naltrexol: 13 hours
2. IM: 5–10 days

C. **Active metabolites**: Noroxymorphone (minor metabolite potentially responsible for transient elevations in liver enzymes), 6-β-naltrexol

1. Oral formulation has substantial first-pass metabolism.
2. IM formulation does not have significant first-pass metabolism and, as a result, has a substantially lower concentration of 6-β-naltrexol than the PO formulation.

D. **Effect of food**: Take with food.

E. **Hepatic impairment**: No adjustment needed for mild hepatic impairment. Individuals with moderate hepatic impairment may require lower dosages.

F. **Renal impairment**: Use with caution in patients with moderate to severe renal impairment.

XI. Clinically Relevant Drug Interactions

A. **Serious interactions**:

1. All medications that act on the opioid receptors, including opioid analgesics and opioid agonist therapy.
2. Disulfiram: Increased risk of hepatotoxicity
3. Phenothiazines: Increased lethargy, somnolence

B. **Moderate interactions**:

1. Acamprosate
2. Dronabinol
3. Nabilone
4. Duloxetine: Increased risk of hepatotoxicity
5. Bupropion: Increased risk of hepatotoxicity

XII. Adverse Effects

A. **PO formulations**:

1. Precipitated opioid withdrawal
2. Nausea, vomiting
3. Headache
4. Dizziness
5. Anxiety
6. Fatigue, somnolence
7. Insomnia

8. Transient increase in liver enzymes thought to be dosage dependent and time limited
9. Decreased platelet count but not associated with increased bleeding-related adverse events

B. **IM formulation**:

1. See above; IM formulation has the same adverse effects as the PO formulation.
2. The IM formulation is not associated with increases in liver enzymes.
3. Injection site reactions:

   a. Common: Tenderness, induration, pain, pruritus, bruising, swelling
   b. Rare: Cellulitis, hematoma, abscess, necrosis
   c. Alternating injection sites is recommended.

4. Eosinophilic pneumonia: Rare

C. **Both PO and IM formulations**: Risk of analgesia failure for patients taking naltrexone (especially IM formulation) in the case of unforeseen surgery or accident, given high-level opioid blockade.

D. **Risks in pregnancy and lactation**:

1. Naltrexone was designated a Category C drug in the prior FDA classification, and naltrexone and 6-β-naltrexol (naltrexone's active metabolite) are present in breast milk. A thorough risk/benefit discussion with the patient is recommended on continuing versus stopping the medication, including consultation with an OB/GYN specialist and/or a lactation expert. See Chapter 15 ("Women: Pregnancy, Postpartum, and Breastfeeding") for more information.

XIII. Clinical Pearls/Prescribing Tips

A. **Evidence supporting naltrexone use for treatment of alcohol use disorder**:

1. Naltrexone and acamprosate are the first-line choices for anticraving medications for alcohol use disorder.
2. The quality of the evidence is high. Naltrexone decreases cravings, reduces overall consumption, decreases number of drinking days, maintains abstinence, and prevents and decreases the severity of relapses.
3. Meta-analyses of randomized controlled trials (RCTs) have demonstrated naltrexone's efficacy in reducing alcohol intake and relapse rate (heavy drinking reduced by 83%; NNT=9) (Kim et al. 2018).

   a. Naltrexone has been shown to be more effective than acamprosate in reducing cravings and improving outcomes related to heavy drinking.
   b. Naltrexone may be superior to acamprosate when the target is controlled use rather than abstinence.

B. **Evidence supporting naltrexone use for treatment of opioid use disorder**:

1. Naltrexone reduces cravings for opioids 3–5 weeks after starting oral naltrexone, although sometimes a reduction can be noted within 1 week.
2. Evidence of effectiveness is primarily from highly motivated patients, when treatment is mandated and/or under supervision.

Further Reading

Alkermes Inc: Highlights of prescribing information: Vivitrol. October 2010. Available at: https://www.vivitrol.com/content/pdfs/prescribing-information.pdf. Accessed March 13, 2024.

Bouza C, Angeles M, Muñoz A, et al: Efficacy and safety of naltrexone and acamprosate in the treatment of alcohol dependence: a systematic review. Addiction 99(7):811–828, 2004 15200577

CRISM National Guideline Review Committee: CRISM National Guidelines for the Clinical Management of Opioid Use Disorder. Canada, Canadian Research Initiative in Substance Misuse, 2018

Cunningham C, Edlund FMJ, Fishman M, et al: National Practice Guideline for the Treatment of Opioid Use Disorder: 2020 focused update. J Addict Med 14(2S Suppl 1):1–91, 2020 32487948

Fontenelle LF, Oostermeijer S, Harrison BJ, et al: Obsessive-compulsive disorder, impulse control disorders and drug addiction: common features and potential treatments. Drugs 71(7):827–840, 2011 21568361

Heinälä P, Alho H, Kiianmaa K, et al: Targeted use of naltrexone without prior detoxification in the treatment of alcohol dependence: a factorial double-blind, placebo-controlled trial. J Clin Psychopharmacol 21(3):287–292, 2001 11386491

Kampman K, Jarvis M: American Society of Addiction Medicine (ASAM) National Practice Guideline for the Use of Medications in the Treatment of Addiction Involving Opioid Use. J Addict Med 9(5):358–367, 2015 26406300

Kim SW: Opioid antagonists in the treatment of impulse-control disorders. J Clin Psychiatry 59(4):159–164, 1998 9590665

Maisel NC, Blodgett JC, Wilbourne PL, et al: Meta-analysis of naltrexone and acamprosate for treating alcohol use disorders: when are these medications most helpful? Addiction 108(2):275–293, 2013 23075288

Minozzi S, Amato L, Vecchi S, et al: Oral naltrexone maintenance treatment for opioid dependence. Cochrane Database Syst Rev (4):CD001333, 2011 21491383

Patten DK, Schultz BG, Berlau DJ: The safety and efficacy of low-dose naltrexone in the management of chronic pain and inflammation in multiple sclerosis, fibromyalgia, Crohn's disease, and other chronic pain disorders. Pharmacotherapy 38(3):382–389, 2018 29377216

Sinclair JD: Evidence about the use of naltrexone and for different ways of using it in the treatment of alcoholism. Alcohol Alcohol 36(1):2–10, 2001 11139409

Younger J, Parkitny L, McLain D: The use of low-dose naltrexone (LDN) as a novel anti-inflammatory treatment for chronic pain. Clin Rheumatol 33(4):451–459, 2014 24526250

References

Kim Y, Hack LM, Ahn ES, et al. Practical outpatient pharmacotherapy for alcohol use disorder. Drugs Context 7:212308, 2018 29445407

Teva Canada Limited: Product monograph: Revia. 2015. Available at: https://www.drugs.com/dosage/naltrexone.html. Accessed March 13, 2024.

Medications for Alcohol Use Disorder

Acamprosate

I. **Brand Name**: Campral

II. **Therapeutic Class**: GABA analogs

III. **Mechanism-Based Class**: Unclear; glutamate-acting

IV. **Mechanism(s) of Action**

A. Mechanism of action is unclear. It is hypothesized that acamprosate reestablishes homeostatic levels of GABA and glutamate in the brain that are altered in long-term alcohol use.

V. **Indications**

A. FDA adult: Maintenance of abstinence from alcohol in individuals with alcohol dependence (alcohol use disorder).

B. Off-label uses: None

VI. **Major Contraindications and When to Use Caution**

A. **Contraindications**:

1. Hypersensitivity to acamprosate or any ingredients in the formulation
2. Severe renal impairment (creatinine clearance [CrCl] ≤30 mL/minute)

B. **Use caution**:

1. Moderate renal impairment (see "Relevant Pharmacokinetics/Pharmacodynamics" section below).
2. Monitor for depression and suicidality.

   a. Suicidal ideation and behavior were found to be more common with acamprosate than with placebo, although these episodes typically occurred following a relapse on alcohol. As a result, it is unclear whether there is a direct link between acamprosate and suicidality (Mylan Pharmaceuticals 2011).

VII. **Dosage Formulations**

A. Generic delayed-release tablet (333 mg)

VIII. **Dosage Ranges and Guidelines**

A. **Alcohol use disorder**:

1. Initiation: Start after alcohol withdrawal symptoms have resolved or there has been a period of abstinence from alcohol.
2. Start at the maintenance dosage of 666 mg TID.

B. **Drug information/dosing**:

1. Steady state is achieved on day 5 after initiation.
2. Unlike disulfiram (which has a different mechanism of action), acamprosate does not induce an adverse reaction when alcohol is consumed.
3. Acamprosate does not affect anxiety, mood, or seizure activity.
4. TID dosing is a significant drawback in patients with a history of noncompliance.

C. **Psychoeducation**:

1. Counsel patients to continue to take acamprosate even if they relapse on alcohol.

D. **Missed doses**:

1. Counsel patients that if they miss a dose, they should take the next dose at the regularly scheduled time.

E. **Special populations**:

1. Elderly patients: Dosage reduction may be necessary because of reduced renal function in older individuals.

IX. **Monitoring**

A. Baseline renal function

X. **Relevant Pharmacokinetics/Pharmacodynamics**

A. **Time to peak plasma concentration**: 3–8 hours
B. **Half-life**: 20–33 hours
C. **Active metabolites**: Acamprosate is not metabolized hepatically and is renally excreted.
D. **Effect of food**: N/A
E. **Hepatic impairment**: No dosage adjustment necessary.
F. **Renal impairment**: For moderate impairment (CrCl 30–50 mL/minute), recommended acamprosate dosage is 333 mg TID.

XI. **Clinically Relevant Drug Interactions**

A. Naltrexone increases levels of acamprosate, but dosage adjustment is not recommended.

XII. **Adverse Effects**

A. **Common**:

1. Gastrointestinal: Diarrhea (most common), nausea, flatulence, anorexia
2. CNS: Insomnia, anxiety, depression, dizziness

B. **Other**: Asthenia, pruritus

C. **Risks in pregnancy and lactation**:

1. Fertility: Acamprosate has no effect on fertility.
2. Pregnancy: Acamprosate should be used with caution in pregnant patients. Risks and benefits should be carefully weighed. Consider consultation with an OB/GYN specialist.
3. Lactation: Acamprosate is excreted in the breast milk. Caution is advised. Consider consultation with an OB/GYN specialist or a lactation expert.

XIII. **Clinical Pearls/Prescribing Tips**

A. Acamprosate, along with naltrexone, is the first-line choice for treatment of alcohol use disorder in individuals who have a goal of reducing alcohol consumption or achieving abstinence.
B. The quality of the evidence is high. Acamprosate has a small but significantly greater therapeutic effect in promoting abstinence from alcohol compared with placebo.
C. Acamprosate and naltrexone appear to be similar in effectiveness across the main alcohol-related outcome measures. The choice of naltrexone or acamprosate should be determined on the basis of side-effect profile, ease of administration, medical comorbidity (hepatic or renal impairment), and specific features of the patient's alcohol use disorder (e.g., presence of craving).
D. Acamprosate may be superior to naltrexone when the target is abstinence rather than controlled or reduced alcohol use.

Further Reading

Anton RF, O'Malley SS, Ciraulo DA, et al; COMBINE Study Research Group: Combined pharmacotherapies and behavioral interventions for alcohol dependence: the COMBINE study: a randomized controlled trial. JAMA 295(17):2003–2017, 2006 16670409

Bouza C, Angeles M, Muñoz A, et al: Efficacy and safety of naltrexone and acamprosate in the treatment of alcohol dependence: a systematic review. Addiction 99(7):811–828, 2004 15200577

Glöckner-Rist A, Lémenager T, Mann K; PREDICT Study Research Group: Reward and relief craving tendencies in patients with alcohol use disorders: results from the PREDICT study. Addict Behav 38(2):1532–1540, 2013 23148916

Jonas DE, Amick HR, Feltner C, et al: Pharmacotherapy for adults with alcohol use disorders in outpatient settings: a systematic review and meta-analysis. JAMA 311(18):1889–1900, 2014 24825644

Maisel NC, Blodgett JC, Wilbourne PL, et al: Meta-analysis of naltrexone and acamprosate for treating alcohol use disorders: when are these medications most helpful? Addiction 108(2):275–293, 2013 23075288

Palpacuer C, Duprez R, Huneau A, et al: Pharmacologically controlled drinking in the treatment of alcohol dependence or alcohol use disorders: a systematic review with direct and network meta-analyses on nalmefene, naltrexone, acamprosate, baclofen and topiramate. Addiction 113(2):220–237, 2018 28940866

Rösner S, Hackl-Herrwerth A, Leucht S, et al: Acamprosate for alcohol dependence. Cochrane Database Syst Rev (9):CD004332, 2010 20824837

References

Mylan Pharmaceuticals: Campral (acamprosate) product monograph: acamprosate. Mylan Pharmaceuticals, 2011. Available at: https://www.drugs.com/monograph/acamprosate.html. Accessed March 13, 2024.

Carbamazepine for Alcohol Use Disorder[1]

I. **Brand Names**: Carbatrol, Carnexiv (discontinued), Epitol, Equetro, Tegretol, Tegretol XR, Teril

II. **Therapeutic Class**: Anticonvulsant; antimanic agent

III. **Mechanism-Based Class**: Sodium channel blocker

IV. **Mechanism(s) of Action**

A. Largely unknown

B. Inhibits voltage-gated sodium channels and potentiates GABAergic neurotransmission

C. In animal studies, carbamazepine is thought to reduce seizure activity by reducing polysynaptic responses and blocking postsynaptic potentiation.

D. Carbamazepine is chemically unrelated to other anticonvulsant agents.

V. **Indications**

A. FDA adult (age >18 years) and pediatric (age >6 years):

1. Epilepsy: monotherapy or in combination with other anticonvulsants
2. Trigeminal neuralgia
3. Bipolar disorder
   a. Acute mania (monotherapy or adjunct to lithium)
   b. Maintenance (in treatment-resistant illness)

B. Evidence-based[2] off-label uses:

1. Restless legs syndrome
2. Postherpetic neuralgia
3. Alcohol use disorder
   a. Acute withdrawal
   b. Long-term treatment

VI. **Major Contraindications and When to Use Caution**

A. **Contraindications**:

1. Hypersensitivity to carbamazepine and its components or related drugs (e.g., tricyclic antidepressants [TCAs])
2. Liver disease
3. Hepatic porphyria
4. Bone marrow suppression
5. Hematological disorder
6. Atrioventricular block
7. Concurrent use of a monoamine oxidase inhibitor (MAOI) or of itraconazole or voriconazole

---

[1]Also see Chapter 5, "Mood Stabilizers," for further information regarding carbamazepine's use for other indications.

[2]Evidence strength varies; readers are referred to the literature for more detailed information.

B. **Use caution**:

1. Older adults (age >65 years)
2. HLA-A*31:01 and HLA-B*15:02: Increased risk for Stevens-Johnson syndrome (SJS), toxic epidermal necrolysis (TEN), and other severe dermatological conditions in certain populations. See the package insert and published literature for full details.
3. Raised intraocular pressure
4. Urinary retention
5. Hypothetical risk of activating latent psychosis due to chemical structure similar to TCAs.
6. Monitor for increase in suicidal ideation and behavior (relative risk: 1.8 [Novartis Pharmaceuticals Canada 2021])
7. Mixed seizures (typical, atypical, absence): Risk of exacerbation of seizures.
8. Carbamazepine withdrawal: Risk of precipitating seizures. Gradual withdrawal over 6 months is recommended.
9. Carbamazepine significantly decreases the efficacy of hormonal contraceptive methods, and if a pregnancy were to occur, has significant teratogenic risks.

VII. Dosage Formulations

A. Brand or generic immediate-release (IR) capsule (100 mg, 200 mg, 300 mg)
B. Brand or generic extended-release (ER) capsule (100 mg, 200 mg, 300 mg)
C. Brand or generic chewable tablet (100 mg)
D. Brand or generic oral suspension (100 mg/5 mL)

VIII. Dosage Ranges and Guidelines

A. **Alcohol use disorder**:

1. Initial: 200 mg BID
2. Maintenance: 800–1,200 mg/day in divided doses
3. Maximum dosage: 1,600 mg/day
4. Studies examining the use of carbamazepine for alcohol use disorder have used dosages of 600–800 mg/day (Barrows and Roberts 2010; Hammond et al. 2015).

B. **Drug information/dosing**:

1. Carbamazepine suspension has a higher peak concentration and reaches peak concentrations more rapidly than the tablet form.
2. Tolerance can develop after a few months of treatment.

C. **Psychoeducation**:

1. Counsel patients to stop carbamazepine as soon as they see a rash.
2. Counsel patients to seek immediate medical attention for symptoms of blood dyscrasias, including fever, sore throat, oral ulcers, rash, easy bruising, or petechial or purpuric hemorrhage.
3. Counsel patients to monitor for suicidal ideation or behavior.

D. **Missed doses**:

1. Take as soon as possible. If close to the next dose, do not take the missed dose; instead, take the next dose as scheduled.

E. **Special populations**:

1. Older adult patients: Start at a lower dosage range because of age-related reduction in liver, renal, and cardiac functioning.

IX. **Monitoring**

A. Regular clinical and laboratory monitoring should be maintained throughout treatment.
B. Baseline: Cardiac, renal, hepatic, and hematological functioning
C. Periodic monitoring: Complete blood count (white blood cells, platelets, reticulocytes). Stop if leukopenia is progressive or symptomatic. Serum iron, liver function tests, urinalysis, blood urea nitrogen. Eye exams, including slit lamp fundoscopy and tonometry.
D. Although carbamazepine plasma levels are not highly correlated with dosage, therapeutic drug-level monitoring can be useful for verifying a patient's adherence to medication, treating a patient during pregnancy, treating pediatric patients, or investigating possible problems with absorption or toxicity.

X. **Relevant Pharmacokinetics/Pharmacodynamics**

A. **Onset of action**: 2–24 hours
B. **Half-life**: 36 hours

1. Repeated administration results in autoinduction, leading to a reduction in the half-life to 16–24 hours. If patient is using other anticonvulsants with enzyme-inducing properties, the half-life is further reduced to 9–10 hours.

C. **Active metabolites**: Carbamazepine-10,11-epoxide, which is further metabolized into carbamazepine-10,11-transdiol and 9-hydroxymethyl-10-carbamoyl-acridan.
D. **Effect of food**: Avoid grapefruit juice (increases carbamazepine levels).
E. **Hepatic impairment**: No data
F. **Renal impairment**: No data. Some sources recommend 75% dosage reduction if estimated glomerular filtration rate (eGFR) is <10 mL/minute.

XI. **Clinically Relevant Drug Interactions**

A. Metabolized by cytochrome P450 (CYP) 3A4.

1. CYP3A4 inhibitors (e.g., antihistamines, azoles, danazol, diltiazem, fluoxetine, fluvoxamine, macrolides, nefazodone, nicotinamide, protease inhibitors, valproate) inhibit carbamazepine metabolism and increase plasma levels.
2. CYP3A4 inducers (e.g., cisplatin, doxorubicin HCl, felbamate, phenytoin, phenobarbital, primidone, rifampin) can increase the rate of carbamazepine metabolism.

B. Inducer of CYP3A4

1. Increases levels of clomipramine, phenytoin, primidone.
2. Decreases levels of acetaminophen, alprazolam, clonazepam, anticonvulsants (lamotrigine, phenytoin, oxcarbazepine, valproate), antipsychotics (clozapine, haloperidol, olanzapine, risperidone, ziprasidone), calcium channel blockers, cyclosporine, corticosteroids, hormonal contraceptives, protease inhibitors, levothyroxine, methadone, topiramate, TCAs, warfarin

C. Carbamazepine is also metabolized by CYP2C8, CYP3A5, CYP2B6, and uridine 5′-diphospho-glucuronosyltransferase (UGT) 2B7, but to lesser extent than CYP3A4.
D. Carbamazepine significantly inhibits the efficacy of hormonal contraception. Use extreme caution in patients who may become pregnant.
E. Use caution with concomitant use of lithium, as such use is associated with an increased risk of neurotoxic effects.
F. Carbamazepine oral suspension should not be coadministered with liquid formulations of chlorpromazine or thioridazine, as the mixture produces an unknown orange precipitant.

XII. **Adverse Effects**

A. **Common:** (*Note.* Effects marked with an asterisk [*] usually occur during initiation.)
1. Drowsiness*
2. Headache*
3. Ataxia*
4. Diplopia/blurred vision*
5. Dizziness*
6. Gastrointestinal upset*
7. Mild skin reactions*
   a. Isolated macular or maculopapular exanthem can occur when starting carbamazepine but usually resolves within a few days to weeks.
8. Dry mouth
9. Edema/fluid retention
10. Hyponatremia

B. **Potentially serious:**
1. Agranulocytosis and aplastic anemia
2. Leukopenia: usually transient
3. Thrombocytopenia: usually transient
4. Hepatocellular and cholestatic jaundice
5. Syndrome of inappropriate antidiuretic hormone secretion (SIADH)
6. Stevens-Johnson syndrome (SJS) and toxic epidermal necrolysis (TEN): Ten times higher risk in Asian populations
7. Cardiac conduction disorders: Second- or third-degree heart block

C. **Risks in pregnancy and lactation:**
1. Very rare reports of impaired spermatogenesis and male fertility. Counsel women of childbearing age to use contraception up to 2 weeks after the last dose.
2. Carbamazepine significantly reduces the efficacy of hormonal contraceptive methods, and if a pregnancy were to occur, has significant teratogenic risks (Crawford et al. 1990; Davis et al. 2011). Consider copper IUD for contraception in these patients.
3. Pregnancy: In animal studies, carbamazepine was associated with a potentially significant teratogenic risk. Fetal exposure within the first 3 months of pregnancy is associated with the highest risk of congenital anomalies. Risk can be reduced/minimized with folic acid supplementation.

4. Lactation: 25%–60% of the maternal plasma level of carbamazepine passes into the breast milk.

XIII. Clinical Pearls/Prescribing Tips

A. Evidence indicates carbamazepine's effectiveness in managing alcohol withdrawal.
   1. In the postwithdrawal period, individuals treated with carbamazepine drank less compared with individuals treated with lorazepam (Malcolm et al. 2002).

B. Carbamazepine significantly decreases the efficacy of hormonal contraceptives, and if a pregnancy were to occur, has significant teratogenic risks.

Further Reading

Amato L, Minozzi S, Davoli M: Efficacy and safety of pharmacological interventions for the treatment of the alcohol withdrawal syndrome. Cochrane Database Syst Rev 2011(6):CD008537, 2011 21678378

Berglund M, Thelander S, Salaspuro M, et al: Treatment of alcohol abuse: an evidence-based review. Alcohol Clin Exp Res 27(10):1645–1656, 2003 14574236

Butler D, Messiha FS: Alcohol withdrawal and carbamazepine. Alcohol 3(2):113–129, 1986 2872902

Hammond CJ, Niciu MJ, Drew S, et al: Anticonvulsants for the treatment of alcohol withdrawal syndrome and alcohol use disorders. CNS Drugs 29(4):293–311, 2015 25895020

Malcolm R, Myrick H, Roberts J, et al: The effects of carbamazepine and lorazepam on single versus multiple previous alcohol withdrawals in an outpatient randomized trial. J Gen Intern Med 17(5):349–355, 2002 12047731

Minozzi S, Amato L, Vecchi S, et al: Anticonvulsants for alcohol withdrawal. Cochrane Database Syst Rev (3):CD005064, 2010 20238337

Mueller TI, Stout RL, Rudden S, et al: A double-blind, placebo-controlled pilot study of carbamazepine for the treatment of alcohol dependence. Alcohol Clin Exp Res 21(1):86–92, 1997 9046378

Stuppaeck CH, Pycha R, Miller C, et al: Carbamazepine versus oxazepam in the treatment of alcohol withdrawal: a double-blind study. Alcohol Alcohol 27(2):153–158, 1992 1524606

References

Barrons R, Roberts N: The role of carbamazepine and oxcarbazepine in alcohol withdrawal syndrome. J Clin Pharm Ther 35(2):153–167, 2010 20456734

Crawford P, Chadwick DJ, Martin C, et al: The interaction of phenytoin and carbamazepine with combined oral contraceptive steroids. Br J Clin Pharmacol 30(6):892–896, 1990 2126946

Davis AR, Westhoff CL, Stanczyk FZ: Carbamazepine coadministration with an oral contraceptive: effects on steroid pharmacokinetics, ovulation, and bleeding. Epilepsia 52(2):243–247, 2011 21204827

Hammond CJ, Niciu MJ, Drew S, et al: Anticonvulsants for the treatment of alcohol withdrawal syndrome and alcohol use disorders. CNS Drugs 29(4):293–311, 2015 25895020

Malcolm R, Myrick H, Roberts J, et al: The effects of carbamazepine and lorazepam on single versus multiple previous alcohol withdrawals in an outpatient randomized trial. J Gen Intern Med 17(5):349–355, 2002 12047731

Novartis Pharmaceuticals Canada: Tegretol (carbamazepine): product monograph including patient medication information. Novartis Pharmaceuticals Canada, 2021. Available at: https://www.ask.novartispharma.ca. Accessed March 13, 2024.

Clonidine for Alcohol Withdrawal

See "Clonidine" in the "Multi-Use Medications for Substance Use Disorders" section at the beginning of this chapter.

Disulfiram

I. **Brand Name**: Antabuse (discontinued)
II. **Therapeutic Class**: Alcohol deterrent
III. **Mechanism-Based Class**: Aldehyde dehydrogenase inhibitor
IV. **Mechanism(s) of Action**

A. When alcohol is ingested, disulfiram (tetraethylthiuram disulfide) inhibits the enzyme acetaldehyde dehydrogenase, resulting in an accumulation of the toxic by-product aldehyde. The buildup of aldehyde causes symptoms of headache, flushing, tachycardia, nausea, vomiting, shortness of breath, and hypotension. Mild reactions can begin after ingestion of 5–10 mg per 100 mL of alcohol; full symptoms develop after 50 mg per 100 mL. Symptom duration is approximately 30–60 minutes but may be up to a few hours or beyond in some patients.

V. **Indications**

A. FDA adult: Maintenance of abstinence from alcohol in individuals with alcohol dependence (alcohol use disorder)
B. Evidence-based[1] off-label uses:

1. Parasitic infections
2. Lyme disease
3. Cancer
4. HIV latency-reversing agent
5. Cocaine dependence

VI. **Major Contraindications and When to Use Caution**

A. **Contraindications**:

1. Hypersensitivity to disulfiram or products containing thiuram derivatives
2. Acute alcohol intoxication
3. Severe myocardial disease/coronary occlusion
4. Psychosis
5. Concurrent use of dichloralphenazone or chloral hydrate
6. Concurrent use of azole antifungal agents (increased risk of psychosis)
7. Concurrent use of amprenavir or ixabepilone (contain alcohol)

---

[1]Evidence strength varies; readers are referred to the literature for more detailed information.

B. **Use caution**:
   1. Diabetes mellitus
   2. Hypothyroidism
   3. Epilepsy
   4. Cerebral damage
   5. Acute/chronic nephritis
   6. Liver cirrhosis or insufficiency

VII. **Dosage Formulations**

A. Generic tablet (250 mg, 500 mg [*scored*])

VIII. **Dosage Ranges and Guidelines** (*Note.* **Patient must be abstinent from alcohol for at least 12 hours before starting disulfiram.)**

A. **Alcohol use disorder**:
   1. Initiation: Maximum of 500 mg/day for 1–2 weeks
   2. Maintenance: 125–500 mg/day

B. **Drug information/dosing**:
   1. **Testing of the reaction with alcohol is not recommended, especially in patients older than 50 years.**
   2. **The adverse reaction following ingestion of alcohol is proportional to the amount of alcohol ingested and the dose of disulfiram used.**
   3. **Less severe symptoms can be elicited up to 1–2 weeks after the last dose of disulfiram when alcohol is consumed.**
   4. **In severe adverse reactions to alcohol, treatment includes supportive measures to control blood pressure and monitoring of ventilation and potassium levels.**
   5. **Availability of disulfiram is limited in some locations; physicians should ensure that a local pharmacy can supply compounded disulfiram before prescribing it.**
   6. There is no specific duration of treatment recommended for disulfiram.

C. **Psychoeducation**:
   1. **Fully inform patients of the disulfiram-elicited adverse reactions if alcohol is ingested; counsel them to avoid alcohol and alcohol-containing foods/products.**

D. **Missed doses**:
   1. **Counsel patients to take the missed dose as soon as possible. If almost time for the next dose, skip the missed dose and continue with regular dosing schedule.**

IX. **Monitoring**

A. Baseline: Complete blood count, liver function tests (LFTs)
B. Days 10–14: LFTs

X. **Relevant Pharmacokinetics/Pharmacodynamics**

A. **Onset of action**: 3–12 hours
B. **Time to peak plasma concentration**: 4 hours
C. **Half-life**: 60–120 hours
D. **Active metabolites**: S-methyl N, N-diethylthiocarbamate sulfoxide; S-methyl N, N-diethylthiocarbamate sulfone

E. **Effect of food**: N/A

F. **Hepatic impairment**: The manufacturer recommends extreme caution in prescribing disulfiram to individuals with liver cirrhosis or insufficiency, but exact dosage adjustments are not available.

G. **Renal impairment**: N/A; no dosage adjustment information provided.

XI. **Clinically Relevant Drug Interactions** (*Note.* This is not an exhaustive list. For a more complete list of known interactions with disulfiram, see ScriptSave WellRx 2024. It is additionally recommended that clinicians consult other available resources [e.g., drug interaction software, applications, textbooks/handbooks].)

A. **Increased levels of disulfiram**: Proton pump inhibitors, ciprofloxacin, protease inhibitors

B. **Increased levels of other agent**: Anticoagulants, caffeine, antipsychotics (pimozide, clozapine), monoamine oxidase inhibitors, benzodiazepines, phenytoin

C. **Contains alcohol**: Sertraline, IV trimethoprim/sulfamethoxazole, lithium (some formulations), cyclosporines

D. **Other**: Isoniazid (monitor for gait or changes in mental status), tricyclic antidepressants (risk of transient delirium), bupropion (additive hepatotoxicity), naltrexone (additive hepatotoxicity)

XII. **Adverse Effects**

A. **Boxed warning**: Disulfiram should NEVER be administered to a patient who is in a state of alcohol intoxication, or without the patient's full knowledge. The physician should instruct relatives accordingly.

B. **Serious**:

1. Gastrointestinal: Diarrhea (most common), nausea, flatulence, anorexia
2. Rare deaths have been reported, usually involving high disulfiram doses and co-ingestion of three or more alcoholic beverages.

C. **Moderate**:

1. Acute generalized exanthematous pustulosis (AGEP): Monitor for sudden onset of nonfollicular, pustular erythematous rash/fever.

D. **Mild**:

1. The following typically occur during the first 2 weeks after initiation and generally resolve spontaneously (but may require dosage reduction): Drowsiness, fatigability, impotence, headache, acneiform eruptions, allergic dermatitis
2. Psychosis: Reported only with higher disulfiram dosages, disulfiram toxicity, or alcohol withdrawal

E. **Reactions after ingestion of alcohol**:

1. Common: Headache, dyspnea, flushing, syncope, nausea/vomiting, hyperhidrosis, chest pain, tachycardia, hypotension, anxiety, weakness, vertigo, blurred vision, confusion
2. Less common: Severe respiratory depression, cardiac arrhythmias, cardiovascular collapse, acute congestive heart failure, myocardial infarction, seizures

F. **Risks in pregnancy and lactation**:

1. Pregnancy: Disulfiram's safety in pregnancy has not been established. Consult with an OB/GYN specialist.
2. Lactation: It is not known whether disulfiram is excreted in breast milk. Consult with an OB/GYN specialist or lactation expert.

XIII. **Clinical Pearls/Prescribing Tips**

A. Disulfiram is not considered a first-line choice in the treatment of alcohol use disorder. It is maximally effective when prescribed to a highly motivated patient with a support system to promote accountability (i.e., directly observed therapy, such as monitoring by a family member or friend).

B. Modest evidence indicates that disulfiram increases the time to first drink, time to first heavy drinking day, amount of alcohol consumed, and number of abstinent days (Laaksonen et al. 2008).

Further Reading

Cvek B: Nonprofit drugs as the salvation of the world's healthcare systems: the case of Antabuse (disulfiram). Drug Discov Today 17(9–10):409–412, 2012 22192884

Gao J, Gong Z, Montesano D, et al: "Repurposing" disulfiram in the treatment of Lyme disease and babesiosis: retrospective review of first 3 years' experience in one medical practice. Antibiotics (Basel) 9(12):868, 2020 33291557

National Collaborating Centre for Mental Health (UK): Alcohol-Use Disorders: Diagnosis, Assessment and Management of Harmful Drinking and Alcohol Dependence. Leicester (UK), British Psychological Society (UK), 2011 22624177

Reus VI, Fochtmann LJ, Bukstein O, et al: The American Psychiatric Association practice guideline for the pharmacological treatment of patients with alcohol use disorder. Am J Psychiatry 175(1):86–90, 2018 29301420

Shirley DA, Sharma I, Warren CA, et al: Drug repurposing of the alcohol abuse medication disulfiram as an anti-parasitic agent. Front Cell Infect Microbiol 11:633194, 2021 33777846

Sigmapharm Laboratories: Disulfiram tablets. Revised August 2024. Available at: https://dailymed.nlm.nih.gov/dailymed/fda/fdaDrugXsl.cfm?setid=40f5497f-fe84-43b2-8ff4-32d59edf3917&type=display. Accessed September 7, 2024.

Traccis F, Minozzi S, Trogu E, et al: Disulfiram for the treatment of cocaine dependence. Cochrane Database Syst Rev (1):CD007024, 2024 38180268

References

Laaksonen E, Koski-Jännes A, Salaspuro M, et al: A randomized, multicentre, open-label, comparative trial of disulfiram, naltrexone and acamprosate in the treatment of alcohol dependence. Alcohol Alcohol 43(1):53–61, 2008 17965444

ScriptSave WellRx: Disulfiram (Generic for Antabuse) Monographs. Tucson, AZ, Medical Security Card Company LLC, 2024. Available at: https://www.wellrx.com/disulfiram/monographs/. Accessed September 7, 2024.

Gabapentin for Alcohol Use Disorder

See "Gabapentin" in the "Multi-Use Medications for Substance Use Disorders" section at the beginning of this chapter.

Naltrexone for Alcohol Use Disorder

See "Naltrexone" in the "Multi-Use Medications for Substance Use Disorders" section at the beginning of this chapter.

Topiramate for Alcohol Use Disorder

I. **Brand Names**: Eprontia, Topamax, Trokendi XR, Qudexy XR

II. **Therapeutic Class**: Antiepileptic/anticonvulsant; migraine prophylaxis/antimigraine

III. **Mechanism-Based Class**: Unclear; GABA and glutamate-acting

IV. **Mechanism(s) of Action**

A. Mechanism of action is largely unknown. Three potential mechanisms have been proposed that contribute to its anticonvulsant properties. Topiramate inhibits voltage-dependent sodium channels, increases inhibitory activity of GABA (most likely $GABA_A$ receptors), and inhibits the activation of kainate/AMPA receptors (a subtype of glutamate receptors). Topiramate is also a weak carbonic anhydrase inhibitor, but this is unrelated to its anticonvulsant properties.

V. **Indications**

A. FDA adult:

1. Epilepsy
2. Migraine
3. Lennox-Gastaut syndrome

B. Evidence-based[1] off-label uses:

1. Cluster headache prophylaxis
2. Alcohol use disorder

VI. **Major Contraindications and When to Use Caution**

A. **Contraindications**:

1. Hypersensitivity to topiramate or any of its ingredients
2. Use of the extended-release formulation is contraindicated if patient has consumed alcohol within the past 6 hours, shows evidence of metabolic acidosis, or is concurrently taking metformin.

---

[1]Evidence strength varies; readers are referred to the literature for more detailed information.

B. **Use caution:**

1. Avoid abrupt discontinuation, which can increase the risk of seizures.
2. Hyperammonemia and encephalopathy:
    a. Rare. Usually occurs when topiramate is used in combination with other anticonvulsants, especially valproic acid. Symptoms resolve after discontinuation of topiramate.
3. Oligohidrosis and hyperthermia:
    a. Extremely rare. There have been cases resulting in hospitalization and mortality. Occurs more commonly in children. Risk is reduced with adequate hydration and symptom monitoring.
4. Hyperchloremic non–anion gap metabolic acidosis:
    a. Most commonly occurs early in treatment but can occur throughout treatment. Those with the following conditions/circumstances may be at increased risk: renal disease, severe respiratory dysfunction, status epilepticus, diarrhea, surgery, keto diet.
5. Because of the side effects of somnolence, dizziness, and confusion, patients initiating treatment with topiramate should be counseled to avoid operating motor vehicles or heavy machinery until a stable dosage is established.

VII. Dosage Formulations

A. Generic and brand (Topamax) tablet (25 mg, 50 mg, 100 mg, 200 mg)
B. Brand (Trokendi XR) 24-hour extended-release (ER) capsule (24 mg, 50 mg, 100 mg, 200 mg)
C. Generic and brand (Topamax) sprinkle capsule (15 mg, 25 mg)
D. Generic and brand (Qudexy XR) 24-hour ER sprinkle capsule (25 mg, 50 mg, 100 mg, 150 mg, 200 mg)
E. Brand (Eprontia) oral solution (25 mg/mL [473-mL bottle])

VIII. Dosage Ranges and Guidelines

A. **Alcohol use disorder**:

1. Initiation: 25 mg/day for 1 week; increase weekly by 25 mg and take in divided doses, as follows:
    a. Week 2: 25 mg BID
    b. Week 3: 25 mg every morning, 50 mg every night at bedtime
    c. Week 4: 50 mg BID
2. Maintenance: 200–300 mg/day; can be divided and taken every 12 hours or every 8 hours.

B. **Drug information/dosing**:

1. Monitor for signs of hyperammonemic encephalopathy (vomiting, lethargy, confusion, change in level of consciousness) and psychiatric/cognitive disturbances.

C. **Psychoeducation**:

1. Counsel patients to call their family doctor immediately or go to the emergency department if they experience blurry vision or eye pain.

2. Given the risk of CNS depressant effects, counsel patients to avoid operating a motor vehicle or heavy machinery until a stable dosage has been reached.

D. **Missed doses**:

1. Should be taken as soon as possible. If the next scheduled dose is imminent, do not take the missed dose. Instead, take the next dose at the regular time.

E. **Special populations**:

1. Older adult patients: No specific recommendations. Dosage reduction is suggested due to reduced renal function in older adults.

IX. **Monitoring**

A. Baseline and periodic serum bicarbonate levels (average reduction of serum bicarbonate and sodium is 4 mmol/L)
B. Consider monitoring serum chloride, ammonia, and phosphorus.
C. Monitor for cognitive and psychiatric disturbances.

X. **Relevant Pharmacokinetics/Pharmacodynamics**

A. **Half-life**: 21 hours (IR); 31 hours (ER)
B. **Steady state**: 4–8 days
C. **Active metabolites**: None
D. **Effect of food**: N/A
E. **Hepatic impairment**: Will likely need lower dosages given poorer drug clearance.
F. **Renal impairment**: Creatinine clearance <70 mL/minute; 50% of the usual dose.

XI. **Clinically Relevant Drug Interactions**

A. Hydrochlorothiazide: Hypokalemia; can increase serum levels of topiramate
B. Carbonic anhydrase inhibitors: Increased risk of hyperthermia, oligohidrosis, and nephrolithiasis
C. Anticholinergic medications: Increased risk of hyperthermia, oligohidrosis
D. Valproic acid: Increased risk of hyperammonemia, hypothermia
E. Digoxin: Topiramate can decrease digoxin levels.
F. CNS depressants (including alcohol): Use with caution due to additive effects.
G. Metformin: Topiramate may increase serum levels of metformin, and metformin may reduce clearance of topiramate.
H. Topiramate may potentially decrease the efficacy of hormonal contraceptives (Rosenfeld et al. 1997); therefore, use caution with patients who may become pregnant, even if they are using these methods.

XII. **Adverse Effects**

A. **Common**:

1. Gastrointestinal: Nausea, anorexia, weight loss, abdominal pain, diarrhea
   a. Weight loss may be significant. Use caution in patients with a history of eating disorders and/or a low baseline body mass index.
2. Dizziness, headache, fatigue
3. Paresthesias (see "CNS side effects" below)
4. Hyperammonemia, decreased serum bicarbonate
5. Upper respiratory tract infection

B. **CNS side effects**: Dizziness, headache, drowsiness, fatigue, somnolence, short-/long-term cognitive dysfunction, attention disturbances, memory/language impairment, psychiatric disturbances, paresthesias. Usually dosage dependent.

1. Cognitive dysfunction occurs in approximately 10% of individuals and may include effects on working memory, verbal fluency, processing speed, and psychomotor speed (Sommer et al. 2013). Risk factors include a higher initial dosage or rapid escalation, use in pediatric patients or older adults, and higher drug concentrations/dosages.
2. Psychiatric disturbances may include aggression, mood/anxiety disorder, depression, suicidal ideation/behavior. Topiramate has both been used for depression and thought to worsen or induce depression. Psychiatric disturbances may not occur until later in treatment. Risk factors include higher initial dosage or rapid escalation and prior psychiatric history, including psychosis.
3. Paresthesias usually remit after 2–3 months. Risk factors include female sex and higher dosage.

C. **Less common**:

1. Fever
2. Hyperchloremic non–anion gap metabolic acidosis
3. Acute myopia associated with secondary angle-closure glaucoma:
   a. Usually appears within the first few days to 1 month of treatment.
   b. Other ocular effects may include choroidal effusion, visual field defects, maculopathy, or scotoma; these are usually reversible with discontinuation.
4. Suicidal ideation and behavior
5. Kidney stones:
   a. Higher risk among men and patients taking other carbonic anhydrase inhibitors
6. Stevens-Johnson syndrome (SJS), toxic epidermal necrolysis (TEN):
   a. Rare. In the majority of cases, there has been concomitant use of other medications associated with SJS and TEN.
7. Hypohidrosis, decreased sweat production, hyperthermia

D. **Risks in pregnancy and lactation**:

1. Topiramate has been shown to decrease the efficacy of hormonal contraceptives (Rosenfeld et al. 1997) and also has clear teratogenic risks.
2. Because of teratogenicity risk, topiramate is contraindicated for use in migraine prophylaxis in pregnancy and in women of child-bearing age who are not using contraception.
3. Pregnancy: Animal studies indicate that topiramate is teratogenic and is associated with increased risk of congenital malformations (e.g., cleft palate, hypospadias). For patient taking topiramate while pregnant, encourage registration in the North American Antiepileptic Drug (AED) Pregnancy Registry (www.aedpregnancyregistry.org). Also consider consultation with an OB/GYN specialist.
4. Lactation: Topiramate does not enter the breast milk.

XIII. **Clinical Pearls/Prescribing Tips**

A. Topiramate is generally considered a third-line choice in the pharmacological treatment of alcohol use disorder.

B. Moderate evidence indicates that topiramate decreases number of drinking days, number of heavy-drinking days, and number of drinks per day (Guglielmo et al. 2015).

Further Reading

Johnson BA, Ait-Daoud N, Bowden CL, et al: Oral topiramate for treatment of alcohol dependence: a randomised controlled trial. Lancet 361(9370):1677–1685, 2003 12767733

Johnson BA, Rosenthal N, Capece JA, et al; Topiramate for Alcoholism Advisory Board; Topiramate for Alcoholism Study Group: Topiramate for treating alcohol dependence: a randomized controlled trial. JAMA 298(14):1641–1651, 2007 17925516

National Collaborating Centre for Mental Health, National Institute for Health, and Clinical Excellence (Great Britain): Alcohol use disorders: the NICE guideline on the diagnosis, assessment and management of harmful drinking and alcohol dependence, 2011

Nu-Pharm Inc: Product monograph: Nu-Topiramate. 2011. Available at: https://pdf.hres.ca/dpd_pm/00013816.PDF. Accessed March 13, 2024.

Palpacuer C, Duprez R, Huneau A, et al: Pharmacologically controlled drinking in the treatment of alcohol dependence or alcohol use disorders: a systematic review with direct and network meta-analyses on nalmefene, naltrexone, acamprosate, baclofen and topiramate. Addiction 113(2):220–237, 2018 28940866

Pani PP, Trogu E, Pacini M, et al: Anticonvulsants for alcohol dependence. Cochrane Database Syst Rev 2014(2):CD008544, 2014 24523233

Paparrigopoulos T, Tzavellas E, Karaiskos D, et al: Treatment of alcohol dependence with low-dose topiramate: an open-label controlled study. BMC Psychiatry 11(1):41, 2011 21401921

Reus VI, Fochtmann LJ, Bukstein O, et al: The American Psychiatric Association practice guideline for the pharmacological treatment of patients with alcohol use disorder. Am J Psychiatry 175(1):86–90, 2018 29301420

Winslow BT, Onysko M, Hebert M: Medications for alcohol use disorder. Am Fam Physician 93(6):457–465, 2016 26977830

References

Guglielmo R, Martinotti G, Quatrale M, et al: Topiramate in alcohol use disorders: review and update. CNS Drugs 29(5):383–395, 2015 25899459

Rosenfeld WE, Doose DR, Walker SA, et al: Effect of topiramate on the pharmacokinetics of an oral contraceptive containing norethindrone and ethinyl estradiol in patients with epilepsy. Epilepsia 38(3):317–323, 1997 9070594

Sommer BR, Mitchell EL, Wroolie TE: Topiramate: effects on cognition in patients with epilepsy, migraine headache and obesity. Ther Adv Neurol Disord 6(4):211–227, 2013 23858325

Medications for Opioid Use Disorder

Buprenorphine

I. **Brand Names**: Belbuca, Buprenex, Butrans, Probuphine, Sublocade, Subutex

II. **Therapeutic Class**: Analgesic

III. **Mechanism-Based Class**: Opioid partial agonist

IV. **Mechanism(s) of Action**

A. Buprenorphine is a partial agonist at the mu and delta opioid receptors and an antagonist at the kappa opioid receptor. Because of its high receptor affinity, buprenorphine displaces other synthetic opioids. Partial agonism of the receptor minimizes risk of respiratory depression and overdose.

V. **Indications**

A. FDA adult:

1. Opioid dependence (tablet, extended-release (ER) injection, implant)
2. Chronic pain (patch)

B. Evidence-based[1] off-label uses:

1. Chronic pain (tablet)
2. Treatment-resistant depression

VI. **Major Contraindications and When to Use Caution**

A. **Absolute contraindications**:

1. Hypersensitivity to buprenorphine. Anaphylactic shock has been reported.

B. **Relative contraindications**:

1. Severe hepatic impairment
2. Severe respiratory distress
3. Acute intoxication from a CNS depressant

C. **Use caution**:

1. Concomitant use of benzodiazepines, alcohol, or other CNS depressants due to the risk of respiratory and CNS depression. However, in comparison with other opioids, buprenorphine has a lower risk of overdose and respiratory depression.
2. Chronic obstructive pulmonary disease, cor pulmonale, decreased respiratory reserve, hypoxia, hypercapnia, preexisting respiratory depression, or central sleep apnea due to risk of respiratory depression.
3. Moderate hepatic impairment. Start on buprenorphine without naloxone and then transition to buprenorphine-naloxone.

---

[1]Evidence strength varies; readers are referred to the literature for more detailed information.

4. Biliary tract dysfunction due to risk of increasing intracholedochal pressure.
5. Adrenal insufficiency due to risk of worsening adrenal function.
6. Head injury, intracranial lesions, and other conditions associated with elevations in cerebrospinal fluid (CSF) pressure due to risk of further elevation in pressure.
7. Older adult patients due to risk of respiratory depression.
8. Pregnancy due to risk of neonatal opioid withdrawal syndrome.

VII. Dosage Formulations

A. There is no clinical difference between films and tabs, and these can be used interchangeably, depending on factors such as patient preference and cost.
B. Generic and brand (Subutex) sublingual tablet (2 mg, 8 mg)
C. Generic and brand (Butrans) weekly patch (5 µg/hour, 7.5 µg/hour, 10 µg/hour, 15 µg/hour, 20 µg/hour)
D. Brand (Belbuca) buccal film (75 µg, 150 µg, 300 µg, 450 µg, 600 µg, 750 µg)
E. Brand (Sublocade) subcutaneous injection (100 mg/0.5 mL, 300 mg/1.5 mL)
F. Brand (Probuphine) subcutaneous implant (74.2 mg)
G. Generic and brand (Buprenex) intravenous injection (0.3 mg/mL [1 mL])

VIII. Dosage Ranges and Guidelines

A. **Drug information/dosing**:

1. For traditional induction, start buprenorphine when Clinical Opiate Withdrawal Scale (COWS) score is ≥13, or at least 12 hours after immediate-release opioids.
    a. For fentanyl withdrawal, it would be appropriate to wait 24–72 hours after last use. Microdosing is the dominant form of induction in some practices.
    b. Consider microdosing if a patient is not in withdr.awal or is not willing to go through withdrawal (META:PHI 2021).
2. Traditional induction:
    a. Day 1: Start at 2–4 mg (2 mg for the older adult or patient using benzodiazepines). Increase by 2–4 mg every 2 hours to 8 mg–12 mg (8 mg for the older adult or patient using benzodiazepines)
    b. Day 2: Increase up to 16 mg/day
3. How to administer: Counsel patients to place the tablet or film under their tongue and allow it to absorb. Swallowing the buprenorphine tabs will lead to little effect.
4. Maintenance:
    a. A buprenorphine to buprenorphine-naloxone switch is recommended unless naloxone hypersensitivity or moderate/severe liver impairment is present.
    b. Therapeutic range: 2–24 mg/day (once daily or divided if preferred)
    c. Maximum dosage: 24 mg/day
    d. Dosage adjustments can be made in 2- to 4-mg increments every 1–3 days or less frequently as clinically indicated/tolerated.
    e. There is no maximum recommended duration of treatment. Treatment can be indefinite as long as there is clinical benefit.
5. When switching to naltrexone, wait 7–14 days after stopping buprenorphine before starting naltrexone.

B. **Psychoeducation**:

1. Caution patients about the risk of CNS depressant effects of buprenorphine, which may impair the ability to drive or operate heavy machinery, particularly during the induction stage.

C. **Missed doses**:

1. For doses ≥4 mg, patients can resume their previous dose if less than 7 days were missed.

D. **Special populations**:

1. Older adult patients: Use with caution. Monitor for respiratory depression and sedation. Consider consultation with a geriatric medicine or psychiatry specialist.

E. **ER subcutaneous (Sublocade) administration**:

1. Establish the patient on a stable dosage of the sublingual tablet or film prior to switching to the ER subcutaneous injection. The manufacturer recommends at least 7 days of PO administration before the Sublocade shot.
2. For patients on buprenorphine 8–18 mg: Give a 300-mg injection followed by a 100-mg injection ≥26 days thereafter (can give 300 mg for the second dose if the patient is experiencing continued cravings/withdrawal). Maintenance dosage: 100 mg once monthly thereafter.
3. For patients on buprenorphine 20–24 mg: Give a 300-mg injection followed by another 300-mg injection ≥26 days thereafter. Maintenance dosage: 100 mg once monthly thereafter. Delays of up to 2 weeks should not affect treatment.
4. On rare occasions (e.g., extended travel), can give a 300-mg dose for 2 months in lieu of monthly doses.

F. **Weekly patch (Butrans)**:

1. Primarily used for chronic pain. Not indicated for OUD and cannot be prescribed for this.
2. For opioid naive patients, start at 5 μg/hour, applied once every 7 days; can increase in 5, 7.5, or 10 μg/hour increments no faster than every 72 hours. Maximum dosage: 20 μg/hour.
3. See full prescribing information for guidelines regarding conversion from other opioids to buprenorphine.

G. **Buccal film (Belbuca)**:

1. Primarily used for chronic pain. Not indicated for OUD and cannot be prescribed for this.
2. For opioid naive patients, start at 75 μg 1–2 times daily. Can increase to 150 μg after 4 days. Continue to titrate in 150 μg increments no sooner than every 4 days until adequate analgesia is achieved. Maximum dosage: 900 μg BID (every 12 hours).
3. See full prescribing information for guidelines regarding dosage titration and conversion from other opioids to buprenorphine.

H. **Intravenous injection**:

1. Used for acute pain only. See full prescribing information for dosing.

IX. Monitoring

A. **Baseline**:

1. CBC, electrolytes, renal function, liver function tests, hepatitis A/B/C serology, sexually transmitted infections (STI) panel, and urine drug screen are recommended, although not required to commence treatment. Use clinical judgment.

B. **Induction phase**:

1. Weekly monitoring of withdrawal symptoms, cravings, and ongoing opioid and other substance use is recommended. Assess for changes in mood, sleep. and overall functioning.
2. A urine drug screen is recommended at each visit to assess compliance and other substance use.
3. Intermittent monitoring of liver function is suggested.

C. **Maintenance phase**:

1. Once stable dose is achieved and there is no evidence of illicit substance use, monthly monitoring (with a urine drug screen at each visit) is recommended.

X. Relevant Pharmacokinetics/Pharmacodynamics

A. **Onset of action**: 1.5–1.7 hours (tablet)
B. **Time to peak plasma concentration**: 30 minutes to 1 hour (SL tablet); 24 hours (ER injection); 3 days to steady state (patch)
C. **Half-life**: 24–42 hours (tablet), 26 hours (patch), 43–60 days (ER injection)
D. **Active metabolites**: Norbuprenorphine
E. **Effect of food**: No food or drink 15–30 min before and 15–30 min after dosing.
F. **Hepatic impairment**: Dosage reduction recommended for moderate to severe hepatic impairment.
G. **Renal impairment**: Limited data; no indication for dosage adjustment.

XI. Clinically Relevant Drug Interactions

A. Metabolized by cytochrome P450 (CYP) 3A4.

1. CYP3A4 inhibitors or inducers: Can increase or decrease drug levels, respectively.
2. Antiretrovirals: Monitor buprenorphine dosage when non-nucleoside reverse transcriptase inhibitors (NNRTIs) are initiated. Atazanavir (with and without ritonavir) can increase blood levels of buprenorphine.

B. **Anticholinergic agents**: Monitor for urinary retention, constipation.
C. **Benzodiazepines**: Lowest effective dosage should be considered, and ideally benzodiazepines should be discontinued.
D. **Diuretics**: Buprenorphine can reduce the efficacy of diuretics.
E. **QTc-prolonging agents**: Additive/synergistic risk of further QTc prolongation.
F. **Serotonergic agents**:

1. Monitor for serotonin syndrome. Discontinue buprenorphine if serotonin syndrome is suspected.
2. Buprenorphine is not recommended for individuals concomitantly taking monoamine oxidase inhibitors (MAOIs). Consider an MAOI washout, which requires clinical judgment and decision making.

XII. Adverse Effects

A. Hypersensitivity/allergic reaction

B. Oral hypoesthesia, glossodynia, oral mucosal erythema:

1. Contact MedWatch (FDA Safety Information and Adverse Event Reporting Program): 1-877-782-6966 or www.fda.gov/medwatch

C. Peripheral edema:

1. Contact MedWatch (1-877-782-6966 or www.fda.gov/medwatch)

D. CNS depression:

1. Avoid use of other CNS depressants, including alcohol and benzodiazepines.

E. Precipitated opioid withdrawal:

1. Counsel patients not to administer parenterally.
2. Patient should have a Clinical Opiate Withdrawal Scale (COWS) score ≥13 prior to initiation of buprenorphine, unless using microdosing method.

F. Addiction, abuse, misuse:

1. Use appropriate precautions to minimize the risk of misuse, abuse, or diversion.

G. Hepatitis:

1. Unclear whether buprenorphine directly causes hepatitis or if elevations in liver enzymes are due to preexisting abnormalities. Recommend baseline liver function tests prior to initiation, as well as periodic monitoring. If marked elevation with initiation, consider dose reduction. Careful risk-benefit analysis must be weighed before discontinuation.

H. Elevation in intracholedochal pressure

I. Opioid-induced sleep apnea

J. Constipation:

1. Recommend laxatives such as polyethylene glycol (PEG) or senna.

K. Adrenal insufficiency or opioid-induced androgen deficiency (OPIAD):

1. Treat with physiological replacement and gradually taper off.

L. Orthostatic hypotension

M. Elevation of cerebrospinal fluid pressure:

1. Slow titration is suggested.

N. **Risks in pregnancy and lactation**:

1. Pregnancy: Limited data indicate that buprenorphine is not associated with an increased risk of malformations or complications. During pregnancy, dosage adjustments may be necessary. During labor and delivery, increased anesthesia may be required. Monitor for neonatal withdrawal symptoms during the first days of life.
2. Lactation: Buprenorphine enters breast milk. No adverse events have been reported. Close monitoring of the infant for respiratory depression and sedation is suggested.

XIII. **Clinical Pearls/Prescribing Tips**

A. Consider using buprenorphine monotherapy in the induction phase (days 1 and 2) for patients dependent on methadone or long-acting opioids, then switch to buprenorphine-naloxone due to the potential elevated risk of precipitated withdrawal with buprenorphine-naloxone as compared with buprenorphine monotherapy (Suboxone package insert). Also consider using buprenorphine monotherapy in the induction phase for patients with moderate to severe hepatic impairment due to the elevated risk of precipitated withdrawal.

B. If patient is experiencing ongoing withdrawal symptoms despite having been on an adequate dose for 2–3 months, consider referral to an addiction specialist.

C. Extra caution is recommended with the use of buprenorphine-naloxone compared with buprenorphine monotherapy because there are extremely limited data on the risk of naloxone to the fetus.

D. The Sublocade injectable form of buprenorphine (extended release) is given once per month (every 28–30 days) and requires the appropriate clinical infrastructure to administer.

E. Buprenorphine has a ceiling effect (at 16 mg/day, 97% opioid receptor occupation).

F. Buprenorphine is metabolized by CYP3A4, so be aware of potential drug interactions. Also exercise caution with concomitant use of benzodiazepines, alcohol, or other CNS depressants.

G. Sublingual buprenorphine films and tabs can be used interchangeably.

Further Reading

See readings and references for Buprenorphine-Naloxone.

Buprenorphine-Naloxone

I. **Brand Names**: Suboxone, Zubsolv, Bunavail, Cassipa

II. **Therapeutic Class**: Analgesics

III. **Mechanism-Based Class**:

A. Buprenorphine: Opioid partial agonist

B. Naloxone: Opioid antagonist

IV. **Mechanism(s) of Action**

A. Buprenorphine

1. Partial agonist at the mu and delta opioid receptors, and kappa opioid antagonist. Due to high receptor affinity, buprenorphine displaces other synthetic opioids. Partial agonism of the receptor minimizes risk of respiratory depression and overdose.

B. Naloxone

1. Potent antagonist at the mu opioid receptor.

2. If buprenorphine-naloxone is administered parenterally, naloxone attenuates the effect of buprenorphine but should not cause precipitated withdrawal, given the small relative amount of naltrexone to buprenorphine.
3. In each tablet, the naloxone dose is one-quarter of the buprenorphine dose.

V. Indications

A. FDA adult:

1. Opioid use disorder

B. Evidence-based[1] off-label uses:

1. Chronic pain

VI. Major Contraindications and When to Use Caution

A. **Absolute contraindications**:

1. Hypersensitivity to buprenorphine or naloxone; anaphylactic shock

B. **Relative contraindications**:

1. Severe hepatic impairment
2. Severe respiratory distress
3. Acute intoxication from a CNS depressant

C. **Use caution**:

1. Concomitant use of benzodiazepines, alcohol, or other CNS depressants. However, compared with other opioids, buprenorphine-naloxone carries a lower risk of overdose and respiratory depression.
2. Chronic obstructive pulmonary disease, cor pulmonale, decreased respiratory reserve, hypoxia, hypercapnia, preexisting respiratory depression, or central sleep apnea due to risk of respiratory depression.
3. Moderate hepatic impairment
4. Biliary tract dysfunction due to risk of increasing intracholedochal pressure
5. Adrenal insufficiency due to risk of worsening adrenal function
6. Head injury, intracranial lesions, other conditions with elevations in cerebrospinal pressure due to risk of further elevation of cerebrospinal fluid pressure
7. Older adult populations due to risk of respiratory depression
8. Pregnancy due to risk of neonatal opioid withdrawal syndrome

VII. Dosage Formulations

A. There is no clinical difference between films and tabs; these can be used interchangeably, depending on factors such as patient preference and cost.
B. Generic and brand (Suboxone) sublingual film (2 mg/0.5 mg, 4 mg/1 mg, 8 mg/2 mg, 12 mg/3 mg)
C. Generic sublingual tablets (2 mg/0.5 mg, 8 mg/2 mg)
D. Brand (Zubsolv) sublingual tablets (11.4 mg/2.9 mg [equivalent to 16 mg/4 mg], 8.6 mg/2.1 mg [equivalent to 12 mg/3 mg], 5.7 mg/1.4 mg [equivalent to 8 mg/2 mg], 2.9 mg/0.71 mg [equivalent to 4 mg/1 mg], 0.7 mg/0.18 mg)

---

[1]Evidence strength varies; readers are referred to the literature for more detailed information.

VIII. Dosage Ranges and Guidelines

A. **Drug information/dosing**:

1. Traditional induction: Start buprenorphine-naloxone when Clinical Opiate Withdrawal Scale (COWS) score is ≥13, or at least 12 hours after immediate-release opioids
    a. Day 1: Start at 2–4 mg (2 mg in the older adult or patient using benzodiazepines. Increase by 2–4 mg every 2 hours to 8–12 mg (8 mg for the older adult or patient using benzodiazepines)
    b. Day 2: Increase up to 16 mg/day
2. Microdosing:
    a. For fentanyl withdrawal, it would be appropriate to wait 24–72 hours after last use. Microdosing is the dominant form of induction in some practices.
    b. Consider microdosing if a patient is not in withdrawal or is not willing to go through withdrawal (META:PHI 2021).

B. **Maintenance**:

1. Therapeutic dosage range: 2–24 mg/day (taken once daily or in divided doses if preferred)
2. Maximum dosage: 24 mg/day
3. Dosage adjustments can be made in 2- to 4-mg increments every 1–3 days or less frequently as clinically indicated/tolerated.
4. There is no maximum recommended duration of treatment. Treatment can be indefinite as long as there is clinical benefit.

C. When switching to naltrexone, wait 7–14 days after stopping buprenorphine-naloxone before starting naltrexone.

D. **Psychoeducation**:

1. Counsel patients that they must place the tablet or film under their tongue and allow it to dissolve. Swallowing the buprenorphine-naloxone tabs produce little effect.
2. Counsel patients not to administer buprenorphine-naloxone parenterally because of the risk of precipitated withdrawal
3. Caution patients about the risk of CNS depressant effects of buprenorphine-naloxone, which may impair the ability to drive or operate heavy machinery, particularly during the induction stage.

E. **Missed doses**:

1. For doses ≥4 mg, patients can resume their previous dose if less than 7 days were missed.

F. **Special populations**:

1. Older adult patients: Use with caution. Monitor for respiratory depression and sedation. Consider consultation with a geriatric medicine or psychiatry specialist.

IX. **Monitoring**

A. **Baseline**:

1. A complete blood count (CBC), electrolytes, renal function, liver function tests, hepatitis A/B/C serology, sexually transmitted infection (STI) panel, and urine drug screen are recommended, although not required to commence treatment. Use clinical judgment.

B. **Induction phase**:

1. Weekly monitoring of withdrawal symptoms, cravings, and ongoing opioid and other substance use; assess for changes in mood, sleep, and functioning.
2. A urine drug screen is recommended at each visit to assess for compliance and other substance use disorders.
3. Intermittent monitoring of liver function is suggested.

C. **Maintenance phase**:

1. Once a stable dosage has been achieved and there is no evidence of illicit substance use, monthly monitoring is recommended. A urine drug screen is recommended at each visit.

X. **Relevant Pharmacokinetics/Pharmacodynamics**

A. **Onset of action**: Buprenorphine: 1.5–1.7 hours; naloxone: 0.8 hour
B. **Half-life**: Buprenorphine: 24–42 hours. Naloxone: 2–12 hours
C. **Active metabolites**: Buprenorphine: Norbuprenorphine. Naloxone: None
D. **Effect of food**: Avoid food or drink 15–30 min before and 15–30 minafter dosing.
E. **Hepatic impairment**:

1. Severe: Use not recommended (given reduced ability to metabolize naloxone, resulting in increased risk of precipitated withdrawal and reduced efficacy).
2. Moderate: Buprenorphine monotherapy suggested.
3. Mild: Close monitoring recommended.

F. **Renal impairment**: Limited data; generally no indication for dosage adjustment.

XI. **Clinically Relevant Drug Interaction**

A. Metabolized by cytochrome P450 (CYP) 3A4.

1. CYP3A4 inhibitors and inducers: Can increase or decrease blood levels of buprenorphine-naloxone.
2. Antiretrovirals: Monitor buprenorphine-naloxone dosage when nonnucleoside reverse transcriptase inhibitors (NNRTIs) are initiated. Atazanavir (with and without ritonavir) can increase drug levels of buprenorphine-naloxone.

B. **Anticholinergic agents**: Monitor for urinary retention, constipation
C. **Benzodiazepines**: Lowest effective dosage should be considered; ideally benzodiazepines should be discontinued.
D. **Diuretics**: Buprenorphine-naloxone can reduce the efficacy of diuretics.
E. **QTc-prolonging agents**: Additive risk of further QTc prolongation (although likely rare)

F. **Serotonergic agents**:

1. Monitor for serotonin syndrome. Discontinue buprenorphine if serotonin syndrome is suspected.
2. Buprenorphine-naloxone is not recommended for individuals concomitantly taking monoamine oxidase inhibitors (MAOIs).

XII. Adverse Effects

A. Hypersensitivity/allergic reaction

B. Oral hypoesthesia, glossodynia, oral mucosal erythema:

1. Contact MedWatch (FDA Safety Information and Adverse Event Reporting Program): 1-877-782-6966 or www.fda.gov/medwatch

C. Peripheral edema:

1. Contact MedWatch (1-877-782-6966 or www.fda.gov/medwatch)

D. CNS depression:

1. Avoid use of other CNS depressants, including alcohol and benzodiazepines.

E. Precipitated opioid withdrawal:

1. Counsel patients not to administer parenterally.
2. Patient should have a COWS score $\geq$13 prior to initiation of buprenorphine-naloxone, unless using microdosing method.

F. Addiction, abuse, misuse:

1. Use appropriate precautions to minimize risk of misuse, abuse, or diversion.

G. Hepatitis:

1. Unclear whether buprenorphine directly causes hepatitis or if elevations in liver enzymes are due to preexisting abnormalities. Recommend baseline liver function tests prior to initiation and periodic monitoring. If marked elevation with initiation, consider dosage reduction. A careful risk-benefit analysis must be done before discontinuation.

H. Elevation in intracholedochal pressure

I. Opioid-induced sleep apnea

J. Constipation:

1. Recommend laxatives such as polyethylene glycol (PEG) or senna.

K. Adrenal insufficiency or opioid-induced androgen deficiency (OPIAD):

1. Treat with physiological replacement and gradually taper off buprenorphine-naloxone.

L. Orthostatic hypotension

M. Elevation of cerebrospinal fluid pressure:

1. Slow titration is suggested.

N. **Risks in pregnancy and lactation**:

1. Pregnancy: Limited data indicate that buprenorphine-naloxone is not associated with an increased risk of malformations or complications. During pregnancy, dosage adjustments may be necessary. During labor and delivery,

increased anesthesia may be required. Monitor for neonatal withdrawal symptoms during the first days of life.

2. Lactation: Buprenorphine enters breast milk. No adverse events have been reported. Close monitoring of the infant for respiratory depression and sedation is suggested.

XIII. **Clinical Pearls/Prescribing Tips**

A. Buprenorphine-naloxone is the first-line treatment for opioid use disorder. One of the main advantages of buprenorphine-naloxone is its safety profile, including a lower risk of overdose compared with full-agonist opioid-assisted treatment. As a result, a clinician can give weekly supplies of buprenorphine-naloxone earlier in the treatment process compared with other medications used in opioid agonist therapy.

B. If patients is experiencing ongoing withdrawal symptoms despite being on an adequate dose for 2–3 months, consider referral to an addiction specialist.

C. Buprenorphine-naloxone has a ceiling effect. At 16 mg, 97% of opioid receptors are occupied.

D. Buprenorphine-naloxone is metabolized by CYP3A4, so be aware of potential drug interactions. Also use caution in combination with benzodiazepines, alcohol, or other CNS depressants.

E. Sublingual buprenorphine-naloxone films and tabs can be used interchangeably.

Further Reading

Bruneau J, Ahamad K, Goyer MÈ, et al; CIHR Canadian Research Initiative in Substance Misuse: Management of opioid use disorders: a national clinical practice guideline. CMAJ 190(9):E247–E257, 2018 29507156

Buprenorphine/naloxone microdosing: the Bernese method: a brief summary for primary care clinicians. London, ON, Canada, METEA:PHI, September 2019. Available at: https://www.metaphi.ca/wp-content/uploads/Guide_Microdosing.pdf. Accessed March 13, 2024.

Caddy P, Smith K: A quick-reference guide for prescribing buprenorphine/naloxone (Suboxone) in the outpatient setting. BC Med J 60(8):392–397, 2018

Canadian Research Initiative in Substance Misuse (CRISM) National Guideline Review Committee: Buprenorphine/naloxone: recommended practice manual, in CRISM National Guidelines for the Clinical Management of Opioid Use Disorder. Manitoba, Canada, College of Physicians and Surgeons Manitoba, 2018. Available at: https://cpsm.mb.ca/assets/PrescribingPracticesProgram/Micro-dosing%20Guidance.pdf. Accessed March 13, 2024.

Chen KY, Chen L, Mao J: Buprenorphine-naloxone therapy in pain management. Anesthesiology 120(5):1262–1274, 2014 24509068

Cunningham C, Edlund FMJ, Fishman M, et al: National Practice Guideline for the Treatment of Opioid Use Disorder: 2020 focused update. J Addict Med 14(2S Suppl 1):1–91, 2020 32487948

Edwards FJ, Wicelinski R, Gallagher N, et al: Treating opioid withdrawal with buprenorphine in a community hospital emergency department: an outreach program. Ann Emerg Med 75(1):49–56, 2020 31732373

Kampman K, Jarvis M: American Society of Addiction Medicine (ASAM) National Practice Guideline for the Use of Medications in the Treatment of Addiction Involving Opioid Use. J Addict Med 9(5):358–367, 2015 26406300

Malinoff HL, Barkin RL, Wilson G: Sublingual buprenorphine is effective in the treatment of chronic pain syndrome. Am J Ther 12(5):379–384, 2005 16148422

Serafini G, Adavastro G, Canepa G, et al: The efficacy of buprenorphine in major depression, treatment-resistant depression and suicidal behavior: a systematic review. Int J Mol Sci 19(8):2410, 2018 30111745

Wong B, Semaka A: The Rxfiles: drug comparison chart updates 2021 (13th collected edition). Saskatoon, Canada, Saskatoon Health Region, 2019. Available at: https://www.rxfiles.ca/rxfiles/uploads/documents/books/charts.html. Accessed March 13, 2024.

References

Indivior UK: Suboxone (buprenorphine [as buprenorphine hydrochloride] and naloxone [as naloxone hydrochloride dihydrate]) sublingual tablets: product monograph. Revised August 31, 2017. Available at: https://pdf.hres.ca/dpd_pm/00041074.PDF. Accessed February 15, 2024.

META:PHI: Primary Care Management of Substance Use, 2nd Edition. Toronto, ON, Canada, Mentoring, Education, and Clinical Tools for Addiction: Partners in Health Integration (META:PHI), 2021. Available at: https://www.metaphi.ca/wp-content/uploads/Guide_PrimaryCareManagement.pdf. Accessed March 27, 2024.

Clonidine for Opioid Withdrawal

See “Clonidine” in the “Multi-Use Medications for Substance Use Disorders” section at the beginning of this chapter.

Gabapentin for Opioid Use Disorder

See “Gabapentin” in the “Multi-Use Medications for Substance Use Disorders” section at the beginning of this chapter.

Methadone

I. **Brand Names**: Dolophine, Methadose, Metadol

II. **Therapeutic Class**: Opioid analgesic

III. **Mechanism-Based Class**: Opioid agonist

IV. **Mechanism(s) of Action**

A. Methadone is a synthetic opioid analgesic that works primarily at the mu opioid receptor in the CNS and smooth muscle. Research has also indicated that methadone is an *N*-methyl-D-aspartate (NMDA) receptor antagonist which is unrelated to its analgesic effects.

B. Derivatives of methadone are being studied for depression, but these are not approved treatments and there is not sufficient evidence to support their use at the time of this writing.

V. **Indications**

A. FDA adult:

1. Severe pain
2. Detoxification from opioid dependence
3. Maintenance treatment of opioid use disorder

B. Off-label uses: None

VI. **Major Contraindications and When to Use Caution**

A. **Contraindications**: (*Note*. Package labeling differs between the United States and Canada; consult local prescribing guidelines/labeling.)

1. Hypersensitivity to methadone
2. Acute respiratory depression, elevated serum carbon dioxide levels or cor pulmonale
3. Acute or severe bronchial asthma
4. Uncontrolled alcohol use disorder; delirium tremens
5. Suspected/known mechanical gastrointestinal obstruction
6. Suspected surgical abdomen
7. Diarrhea secondary to pseudomembranous colitis or patients having diarrhea caused by poisoning
8. Patients who are currently taking monoamine oxidase inhibitors (MAOIs) or have taken MAOIs within the last 14 days

B. **Use caution**:

1. Concomitant use of benzodiazepines, alcohol, or other CNS depressants due to the risk of respiratory and CNS depression
2. Baseline hypotension
3. Head injury and increased intracranial pressure
4. Methadone may affect cognition. Recommend caution in operating a car or heavy machinery.
5. Use caution in convulsive disorders (relative contraindication).
6. Use caution with individuals naive to opioids.

VII. Dosage Formulations

A. Generic tablet (5 mg, 10 mg [*both scored*])
B. Generic and brand (Methadose) soluble tablet (40 mg [*scored*])
C. Powder:
   1. Generic solution (5 mg/5 mL, 10 mg/5 mL)
   2. Generic or brand concentrate (10 mg/mL):
      a. Unflavored (methadone HCl Intensol), cherry (Methadose), or sugar-free unflavored (Methadose Sugar-Free)

VIII. Dosage Ranges and Guidelines

A. **Administration**:
   1. Methadone can be dispensed only by certified treatment programs.
   2. Methadone is typically administered as a combination of Metadol (1 mg/mL or 10 mg/mL) dissolved in 100 mL of grape-flavored Kool-Aid, orange-flavored Tang, Allen's Apple Juice, Crystal Light tangerine-grapefruit flavor, or Crystal Light lemonade flavor.

B. **Initiation**:
   1. Day 1:
      a. Low tolerance: 5–10 mg
      b. Moderate opioid use: 10–20 mg
      c. Significant tolerance: 20–30 mg
   2. Titrate cautiously, watching for oversedation.
      a. Dosage increases can be in increments of ~ 10–15 mg every 3–5 days. Some sources recommend upward titration no faster than 10 mg every 5 days.
      b. Methadone should not be increased daily (after just 1 day of dosing at a specific dose) because of the risk of potentially fatal drug accumulation.
   3. Patients should be seen at least weekly during the initiation phase.

C. **Maintenance**:
   1. Therapeutic dosage range: 60–120 mg:
      a. Lower dosages may help with withdrawal but often are not sufficient to suppress cravings (Cunningham et al. 2020).
   2. Maximum dosage is unclear. Some resources recommend dosages of 120–200 mg or even greater with close monitoring.
   3. Dosage increases can be in 5- to 10-mg increments every 5–7 days.

D. **Take-home dosing**: Criteria for take-home dosing varies substantially internationally and in the United States, and varies by state as well. Refer to SAMHSA guidelines for U.S. patients (Substance Abuse and Mental Health Services Administration 2024).

E. **Tapering**

1. Dosage reductions should be less than 10% of the current daily dosage at least every 10–14 days, with a more gradual reduction toward the end of the taper.
   a. Switching to buprenorphine (or buprenorphine-naloxone): Decrease methadone to a low dosage (30–40 mg or less) for about 1 week prior to stopping. Prior to starting buprenorphine, the patient should be in mild to moderate withdrawal (i.e., Clinical Opiate Withdrawal Scale [COWS] score of 11–12 or more), a level that may not be reached until 24–48 hours after the last dose of methadone. Consider starting a low dosage of buprenorphine (2–4 mg) and repeating as needed to treat withdrawal symptoms (Cunningham et al. 2020).
   b. Switching to naltrexone: Prior to switching to naltrexone, the patient must be completely withdrawn from methadone and all other opioids (for 7–14 days after the last dose of methadone). Consider a naloxone challenge (0.4–0.8 mg) to test for precipitated withdrawal prior to initiating naltrexone treatment.

F. **Drug information/dosing**:

1. Methadone is a Schedule II drug in the United States (according to the Controlled Substances Act [CSA]) and a Schedule I drug in Canada (according to the Controlled Drugs and Substances Act [CDSA]).
2. Methadone should not be stored for more than 14 days.
3. Optimal dosing is patient-specific and depends on tolerance, metabolism, comorbid substance use, recovery environment, and side effects; however, 60–80 mg is a common target dosage.

G. **Psychoeducation**:

1. After initiation of treatment and after dosage increases, patients should be counseled to avoid operating motor vehicles or heavy machinery until a stable dosage of methadone is established.
2. Counsel patients to avoid other CNS depressants (e.g., alcohol, benzodiazepines) because of the risk of excessive sedation and respiratory depression.
3. Dispelling myths:
   a. In itself, methadone does not cause tooth decay. A common side effect is dry mouth, which can increase the risk of plaque buildup and cause gum disease and/or tooth decay. Methadone also has a high acid content, which can cause enamel erosion. It is recommended that patients brush their teeth a minimum of twice per day, floss once per day, and rinse their mouth after taking methadone.
   b. Methadone does not "rot your bones." If a patient is experiencing body aches, the dosage of methadone could be too low, in which case a dosage increase would be required.
   c. Methadone does not directly cause weight gain. Weight gain may be attributable to a healthier lifestyle and appetite as the patient becomes more stable clinically. Methadone can also cause water retention, which can increase body weight.

H. **Protocol for managing missed doses** (Table 10–2):

Table 10–2. Protocol for managing missed doses of methadone

Number of missed days	Dose	Dose adjustment
1–2	N/A	Continue home dose
3–4	30 mg	No change
	31–60 mg	Restart at 30 mg
	>60 mg	50% of home dose
5 or more	N/A	Restart at initial dose (5–30 mg)

Source. Adapted from British Columbia Centre on Substance Use 2023.

I. **Special populations**:

1. Older adults: Extreme caution should be used in adjusting dosages. Due to age-related changes in hepatic, renal, and cardiac functioning, start at a lower dosage.

IX. **Monitoring**

A. **Baseline lab measurements**:

1. Complete blood count, urine drug screen, renal function, liver function tests, hepatitis A/B/C serology, HIV (with consent), STI panel, pregnancy test (in women of childbearing age), tuberculosis, rapid plasma reagin are recommended tests, but are generally not required. Use clinical judgment.
2. Obtain an ECG if indicated (cardiac history or risk factors for QTc prolongation).

B. **Initiation phase**:

1. Weekly monitoring of withdrawal symptoms, cravings, and ongoing opioid and other substance use. Assess for changes in mood, sleep and general/overall functioning.
2. A weekly UDS is recommended to assess for compliance and other substance use.
3. Blood pressure and heart rate monitoring
4. Monitor for symptoms of QTc prolongation
5. Monitor for respiratory depression

C. **Maintenance phase**:

1. Scheduled and random urine drug screenings
2. Repeat ECG if methadone dosage is ≥120 mg/day.

D. **Duration of treatment**:

1. There is no recommended time limit for treatment. Generally, 12 months is considered the minimum duration of treatment.

X. **Relevant Pharmacokinetics/Pharmacodynamics**

A. **Onset of action**: 2.5 hours (range: 1–7.5 hours)

B. **Half-life**: 37 hours (range: 8–59 hours)

1. Methadone is lipophilic. One proposed mechanism for the variable and prolonged half-life is that methadone can be retained in the liver and other fatty tissue despite low serum levels.

C. Duration of action for analgesia is 4–8 hours with single dosing and 22–48 hours with long-term dosing. For treatment of cravings, duration varies from 24 to 36 hours (Cunningham et al. 2020).

D. **Active metabolites**: None

E. **Effect of food**: Not studied

F. **Hepatic impairment**: Has not been comprehensively studied.

G. **Renal impairment**: Has not been comprehensively studied. Caution is recommended because of the potential for impaired metabolism of methadone, resulting in increased accumulation.

XI. **Clinically Relevant Drug Interaction**

A. Metabolized primarily by cytochrome P450 (CYP) 2B6 and CYP3A4 and, to a lesser extent, CYP2C19 and CYP2C9:

1. CYP3A4 inducers (e.g., rifampin, phenytoin) can decrease methadone levels.
2. CYP3A4 inhibitors (e.g., azole antifungals, macrolides) can increase methadone levels.

B. Weak CYP2D6 inhibitor:

1. Methadone may increase levels of tricyclic antidepressants (e.g., desipramine).

C. **Antiretrovirals**: Bidirectional effects; when combined, methadone levels may be decreased, or serum levels of antiretrovirals may be increased.

D. **Protease inhibitors**: Methadone may decrease levels of protease inhibitors; protease inhibitors may increase levels of methadone.

E. **QTc-prolonging agents**: Additive risk of further QTc prolongation (synergistic effect)

F. **Anticholinergic agents**: Monitor for urinary retention and constipation.

G. **Benzodiazepines**: Lowest effective dosage should be considered, and ideally benzodiazepines should be discontinued.

XII. **Adverse Effects**

A. **Boxed warnings**:

1. Risk of addiction, abuse, misuse
2. Respiratory depression:
   a. These effects occur later than analgesic effects and lasts longer.
   b. Consider providing all patients on methadone with a Narcan kit in the event of respiratory depression.
3. Accidental ingestion (potentially resulting in death)
4. QTc prolongation (and torsades de pointes):
   a. Risk factors include high dosage, multiple-day dosing, cardiac hypertrophy, electrolyte abnormalities, history of cardiac conduction abnormalities, and high baseline QTc (≥500 ms).
   b. Monitor QTc at baseline and periodically.
5. Neonatal opioid withdrawal syndrome when used in pregnancy

B. **Common**:

1. Sedation, CNS depression, hypotension, lightheadedness, gastrointestinal (nausea/vomiting, constipation, dry mouth), hyperhidrosis
2. Opioid withdrawal if stopped abruptly:
   a. Withdrawal with methadone may not occur until 1–3 days after the last dose, often peaks at days 3–5, and can last for several weeks—a protracted withdrawal syndrome (Cunningham et al. 2020).
3. Opioid-induced sleep apnea
4. Adrenal insufficiency or opioid-induced androgen deficiency (OPIAD):
   a. Treat with physiological replacement and gradually taper off.

C. **Less common**:

1. Weakness, headache, edema, abdominal pain, hypokalemia, hypomagnesemia, weight gain, urinary retention, decreased libido
2. CNS/psychiatric: Agitation, confusion, dysphoria, insomnia

D. **Severe and rare**:

1. Respiratory depression; increased risk of respiratory arrest
2. Cardiac arrest and death have been reported.
3. Cardiac arrhythmias
4. Hypersensitivity/allergic reaction
5. Seizures
6. Serotonin syndrome

E. **Risks in pregnancy and lactation**:

1. Pregnancy: Generally methadone is considered safe during pregnancy. Use caution in pregnancy given the risk of neonatal opioid withdrawal syndrome. If benefits outweigh risks, the dosage may need to be increased or split during pregnancy because of pregnancy-induced physiological changes.
   1. Infants: Monitor for neonatal opioid withdrawal syndrome from day 2 through day 28.
2. Lactation: Generally, women taking methadone should not be discouraged from breastfeeding. However, methadone does enter the breast milk. Use caution in breastfeeding. Consider consultation with an OB/GYN specialist or lactation expert.

XIII. **Clinical Pearls/Prescribing Tips**

A. Both methadone and buprenorphine-naloxone are considered first-line choices for treatment of opioid use disorder, but recommendations for which to use depend on patient- and clinician-specific factors (e.g., cost, accessibility, induction risks, analgesic requirements).

B. Methadone has a narrow therapeutic window and a long half-life, which increases the risk of toxicity and adverse effects.

C. Methadone has been shown to be significantly more effective than nonpharmacological treatment in improving treatment retention, decreasing illicit opioid use, and reducing high-risk injection behaviors, thereby reducing the risk of acquiring hepatitis C and HIV.
D. Methadone is a good option for patients who would benefit from daily supervision with dosing or who have been unsuccessful with buprenorphine treatment.

Further Reading

Bruneau J, Ahamad K, Goyer MÈ, et al; CIHR Canadian Research Initiative in Substance Misuse: management of opioid use disorders: a national clinical practice guideline. CMAJ 190(9):E247–E257, 2018 29507156

CRISM National Guideline Review Committee: CRISM National Guidelines for the Clinical Management of Opioid Use Disorder. Canada, Canadian Research Initiative in Substance Misuse, 2018

Kampman K, Jarvis M: American Society of Addiction Medicine (ASAM) National Practice Guideline for the Use of Medications in the Treatment of Addiction Involving Opioid Use. J Addict Med 9(5):358–367, 2015 26406300

Paladin Labs Inc: Metadol: product monograph including patient medication information. Paladin Labs, 2014. Available at: https://www.paladin-labs.com/our_products/Metadol-D_En.pdf. Accessed March 13, 2024.

META:PHI: Primary care management of substance use, 2nd edition. Toronto, ON, Canada, Mentoring, Education, and Clinical Tools for Addiction: Partners in Health Integration (META:PHI), 2021. Available at: https://www.metaphi.ca/wp-content/uploads/Guide_PrimaryCareManagement.pdf. Accessed March 27, 2024.

Ontario Dental Hygienists' Association (ODHA): Dental hygiene facts: methadone. Available at: https://odha.on.ca/wp-content/uploads/2016/08/Methadone-Fact-Sheet-FINAL.pdf. Accessed March 13, 2024.

References

British Columbia Centre on Substance Use: A Guideline for the Clinical Management of Opioid Use Disorder, 2023 Update. Victoria, BC, Canada, British Columbia Ministry of Health, November 2023. Available at: https://www.bccsu.ca/opioid-use-disorder/. Accessed July 7, 2024.

Cunningham C, Edlund FMJ, Fishman M, et al: National Practice Guideline for the Treatment of Opioid Use Disorder: 2020 focused update. J Addict Med 14(2S Suppl 1):1–91, 2020 32487948

Substance Abuse and Mental Health Services Administration: Methadone Take-Home Flexibilities Extension Guidance. Last updated 01/23/2024. Available at: https://www.samhsa.gov/medications-substance-use-disorders/statutes-regulations-guidelines/methadone-guidance. Accessed July 31, 2024.

Naltrexone for Opioid Dependence

See "Naltrexone" in the "Multi-Use Medications for Substance Use Disorders" section at the beginning of this chapter.

Medications for Tobacco Use Disorder

Bupropion for Smoking Cessation[1]

I. **Brand Names**: Aplenzin (extended release), Budeprion SR, Buproban, Forfivo XL, Wellbutrin SR, Wellbutrin XL, Zyban

II. **Therapeutic Class**: Atypical antidepressant

III. **Mechanism-Based Class**: Aminoketone class; norepinephrine and dopamine reuptake inhibitor (NDRI)

IV. **Mechanism(s) of Action**

A. NDRI; bupropion's specific pharmacodynamics are unknown.

V. **Indications**

A. FDA adult:

1. Major depressive disorder
2. Seasonal affective disorder
3. Smoking cessation

B. Evidence-based[2] off-label uses:

A. Sexual dysfunction secondary to antidepressants
B. ADHD
C. Obesity

D. FDA pediatric: None

VI. **Major Contraindications and When to Use Caution**

A. **Contraindications**:

1. Hypersensitivity to bupropion or other ingredients
2. Concurrent use of another formulation of bupropion
3. Seizure disorder or epilepsy (or any condition or concomitant treatment that lowers the seizure threshold)
4. Eating disorder (current or past diagnosis of anorexia nervosa, bulimia) due to risk of seizures

B. **Use caution**:

1. Avoid consumption of significant amounts of alcohol while taking bupropion. Counsel patients who consume alcohol regularly to use moderation and refrain from abrupt discontinuation of alcohol to avoid increased risk of seizures.

---

[1]Also see Chapter 2, "Antidepressants," and Chapter 7, "Stimulants," for further information regarding bupropion's use for other indications.
[2]Evidence strength varies; readers are referred to the literature for more detailed information.

2. Use with extreme caution in individuals with liver cirrhosis.
3. Counsel patients to avoid operating a motor vehicle or heavy machinery until they are aware of how bupropion affects their level of consciousness and cognition.
4. In children, adolescents, and young adults with major depressive disorder and/or other psychiatric disorders, monitor for suicidal ideation and behavior.
5. Antidepressants (including bupropion) may trigger manic/hypomania/mixed episodes in individuals with bipolar disorder, or they may unmask bipolar disorder. Antidepressants may also increase risk of psychosis in at-risk individuals.
6. Concomitant use of monoamine oxidase inhibitors (MAOIs) should be undertaken with caution, although risk of serotonin syndrome is likely low, given the weaker serotonergic action of bupropion (see the 'Monoamine Oxidase Inhibitors" section in Chapter 2, "Antidepressants").

VII. **Dosage Formulations** (*Note.* For SR/XL/ER forms, do not break, cut, or crush.)

A. Generic immediate-release (IR) tablets (75 mg, 100 mg [*not scored*])
B. Brand sustained-release (SR) tablets (100 mg, 150 mg, 300 mg)
C. Generic SR tablets (100 mg, 150 mg, 300 mg)
D. Brand extended-release (ER/XL) tablets (150 mg, 300 mg)
E. Generic ER tablets (150 mg, 300 mg)

VIII. **Dosage Ranges and Guidelines**

A. Wellbutrin SR:

1. Set quit date 10 days after starting Wellbutrin.
2. Initial: 150 mg every morning for 3–5 days
3. Maintenance: 150 mg BID for 7–12 weeks (doses should be taken ≥8 hours apart)
4. Maximum: 150 mg BID
5. Can consider long-term use with Wellbutrin SR 150 mg/day every 6 months after quit date.

B. **Drug information/dosing**:

1. Smoking does not affect drug levels of bupropion.
2. Duration between doses should be at least 8 hours.
3. It is possible that patients taking bupropion may show a positive urine drug screen for amphetamines.
4. When administered at recommended daily dosages and in divided doses, bupropion is unlikely to be reinforcing to individuals with amphetamine or stimulant use disorders.

C. **Psychoeducation**:

1. Advise patients and caregivers to monitor for agitation, depressed mood, changes in behavior, or suicidality. If these are observed, advise patient to stop bupropion immediately.
2. If an overdose on bupropion occurs, advise patients to call a local emergency department or poison control center immediately.

D. **Missed doses**:

1. Wait until the next scheduled dose.

E. **Special populations**:

1. Older adults: Dosage reduction is recommended.

IX. **Monitoring**

A. Monitor blood pressure periodically, especially if used in combination with nicotine replacement therapy (NRT).

X. **Relevant Pharmacokinetics/Pharmacodynamics**

A. **Onset of action**: 2 hours (IR); 3 hours (SR); 3 hours (active metabolite)
B. **Half-life**: 8–24 hours (IR); 14–28 hours (SR); 15–25 hours (active metabolite)
C. **Steady state**: 8 days
D. **Active metabolites**: Hydroxybupropion (50% potency of parent compound and 10 times greater peak plasma concentration), threohydrobupropion, erythrohydrobupropion
E. **Effect of food**: N/A
F. **Hepatic impairment**:

1. Mild to moderate: Consider dosage reduction. Use of Forfivo XL is not recommended.
2. Moderate to severe: Buproban, Wellbutrin XL dosage not to exceed 150 mg every 2 days. Aplenzin dosage not to exceed 174 mg every 2 days. Wellbutrin SR dosage not to exceed 100 mg/day or 150 mg every 2 days.

G. **Renal impairment**: Consider dosage reduction.

XI. **Clinically Relevant Drug Interactions**

A. Metabolized by cytochrome P450 (CYP) 2B6:

1. Drugs that are metabolized by or inhibit CYP2B6 (clopidogrel, cyclophosphamide, orphenadrine, thiotepa, ticlopidine, thioefavirenz, ritonavir)
2. Bupropion levels can be reduced by carbamazepine, phenobarbital, and phenytoin.

B. Inhibitor of CYP2D6:

1. Bupropion may increase concentrations of drugs metabolized by CYP2D6 (e.g., paroxetine, sertraline, norfluoxetine, fluvoxamine, tricyclic antidepressants, beta-blockers, antiarrhythmics, antipsychotics)

C. Drugs that lower the seizure threshold
D. Levodopa/amantadine: Increase in adverse effects.

XII. **Adverse Effects**

A. **Common**: Dry mouth, agitation, insomnia, migraine/headache, nausea/vomiting, constipation, tremor, dizziness, excessive sweating
B. **Less common**: Nocturia, ataxia/discoordination, hypertension, myoclonus, dyskinesia, dystonia, mania/hypomania, hallucinations, stomatitis, flu-like symptoms
C. **Potentially serious**: Seizure (dose-dependent). Incidence is approximately 0.4% for doses ≤450 mg.

D. **Risks in pregnancy and lactation:**

1. Pregnancy: Effects on pregnancy and the fetus are unknown.
2. Lactation: Bupropion does enter breast milk. The amount and impact on infants are not known.

XIII. **Clinical Pearls/Prescribing Tips**

A. Bupropion has been shown to significantly increase the likelihood of abstinence from smoking for 6 months compared with placebo (Hajizadeh et al. 2023).

B. Bupropion could be a good first-line choice for some patients with comorbid depression and tobacco use (tobacco use disorder).

Further Reading

Centre for Addiction and Mental Health: Canadian Smoking Cessation Clinical Practice Guideline. CAN-ADAPTT, 2011. Available at: https://www.nicotinedependence-clinic.com/en/canadaptt/PublishingImages/Pages/CAN-ADAPTT-Guidelines/CAN-ADAPTT%20Canadian%20Smoking%20Cessation%20Guideline_website.pdf. Accessed March 13, 2024.

Centre for Addiction and Mental Health: Smoking Cessation: Tools and Resources, 2021. Available at: https://www.camh.ca/en/professionals/treating-conditions-and-disorders/smoking-cessation/smoking-cessation---tools-and-resources. Accessed March 13, 2024.

GlaxoSmithKline: Wellbutrin prescribing information, 2017. Available at: https://www.accessdata.fda.gov/drugsatfda_docs/label/2011/018644s043lbl.pdf. Accessed March 13, 2024.

Greenway FL, Dunayevich E, Tollefson G, et al; NB-201 Study Group: Comparison of combined bupropion and naltrexone therapy for obesity with monotherapy and placebo. J Clin Endocrinol Metab 94(12):4898–4906, 2009 19846734

Verbeeck W, Bekkering GE, Van den Noortgate W, et al: Bupropion for attention deficit hyperactivity disorder (ADHD) in adults. Cochrane Database Syst Rev (10):CD009504, 2017 28965364

U.S. Department of Health and Human Services: Helping Smokers Quit: A Guide for Clinicians. Revised May 2008. Available at: https://www.ahrq.gov/sites/default/files/wysiwyg/professionals/clinicians-providers/guidelines-recommendations/tobacco/clinicians/references/clinhlpsmkqt/clinhlpsmksqt.pdf. Accessed March 13, 2024.

References

Hajizadeh A, Howes S, Theodoulou A, et al: Antidepressants for smoking cessation. Cochrane Database Syst Rev (5):CD000031, 2023 37230961

Clonidine for Smoking Cessation

See “Clonidine” in the “Multi-Use Medications for Substance Use Disorders” section at the beginning of this chapter.

Varenicline

I. **Brand Names**: Champix, Chantix

II. **Therapeutic Class**: Smoking cessation aid

III. **Mechanism-Based Class**: Acetylcholine partial agonist

IV. **Mechanism(s) of Action**

A. Varenicline is a partial agonist at $\alpha_4\beta_2$ and $\alpha_3\beta_4$ nicotinic acetylcholine receptors. The partial activation of these receptors triggers the mesolimbic dopaminergic pathway associated with reward.

B. Varenicline prevents nicotine from binding to nicotinic receptors via its higher affinity to nicotinic receptors.

C. Varenicline is also a full agonist at 5-HT_3 receptors.

V. **Indications**

A. FDA adult: Smoking cessation aid (in conjunction with counseling)

B. Evidence-based off-label uses: None

VI. **Major Contraindications and When to Use Caution**

A. **Contraindications**:

1. Hypersensitivity to varenicline or any other component compounds

B. **Relative contraindications**:

1. Pregnancy (teratogenicity found in animal studies)
2. End-stage renal disease

C. **Use caution**:

1. Psychiatric disorders: Can exacerbate symptoms (see "Adverse Effects").
2. Seizure disorder/epilepsy: Can increase risk of seizures.
3. Diabetes: Can alter glycemic control.

VII. **Dosage Formulations**

A. Generic and brand (Chantix) tablet (0.5 mg, 1 mg)

1. Chantix starting pack (0.5 mg [11 tabs], 1 mg [42 tabs])

VIII. **Dosage Ranges and Guideline**

A. Initial: 0.5 mg/day for 3 days, then increase to 0.5 mg BID for 4 days

B. Maintenance: 0.5 mg–1.0 mg BID

C. Three approaches to use of varenicline for smoking cessation are available:

1. Scenario 1: Set quit date. Start varenicline 1–2 weeks before the quit date. Treatment duration is typically 12 weeks total.
2. Scenario 2: Start varenicline and quit between weeks 2–5. Treatment duration is 12 weeks total in this scenario.
3. Scenario 3: Start varenicline and quit by week 11. Recommend at least a 50% reduction in smoking by week 4 and at least a 75% reduction by week 8. Treatment duration is 12–24 weeks total in this scenario.

D. Consider tapering varenicline after week 12 to reduce the risk for relapse following abrupt discontinuation of varenicline.

E. **Drug information/dosing**:

1. Screen for seizure history or other factors that could lower seizure threshold.
2. Combination therapy with other forms of NRT may be more effective than varenicline alone, but this is not definitively known, and combination treatment may be associated with more adverse events.
3. If able to successfully quit smoking, an additional 12 weeks of treatment could be considered. For patients who have not quit by week 12, there are no data indicating additional benefit from continuing treatment after 12 weeks.
4. The absence of smoking could increase drug levels of medications that are metabolized through cytochrome P450 (CYP) 1A2 isoenzymes.

F. **Psychoeducation**:

1. Counsel patients to avoid operating a motor vehicle or heavy machinery until they are aware of how varenicline affects them.
2. Counsel patients that varenicline may exacerbate psychiatric symptoms. Instruct patients to monitor themselves for signs of relapse or worsening of symptoms.
3. Counsel patients that varenicline may increase the risk of cardiovascular events or stroke in individuals with or without a prior history.
4. Encourage patients to tell loved ones about their quit date for support and side-effect monitoring.

G. **Missed doses**:

1. Take as soon as missed dose is remembered.

H. **Special populations**:

1. Older adults: Safe

IX. Monitoring

A. For patients with a psychiatric disorder, monitor for relapse/worsening of symptoms.

1. Symptoms may include anxiety, psychosis, depressed mood, agitation, aggression, mood swings, suicidal ideation, and suicidal behavior.

B. Counsel diabetic patients to monitor blood sugar more frequently.

X. Relevant Pharmacokinetics/Pharmacodynamics

A. **Onset of action**: 3–4 hours
B. **Steady state**: 96 hours
C. **Half-life**: 24 hours
D. **Active metabolites**: Not applicable; varenicline undergoes minimal metabolism.
E. **Effect of food**: Take after food with water.
F. **Hepatic impairment**: No dosage adjustment is necessary.
G. **Renal impairment**: Dosage reduction is recommended in moderate to severe renal disease. For severe renal disease, the recommended dosage is 0.5 mg BID. Varenicline is not recommended in end-stage renal disease.

XI. Clinically Relevant Drug Interactions

A. Nicotine replacement therapy (NRT): Can increase risk of adverse reactions (nausea, vomiting, headache, dizziness, dyspepsia, fatigue).

XII. Adverse Effects

A. **Common**:

1. Gastrointestinal effects: Nausea (up to 40% [Pfizer Canada 2019], although transient and dosage dependent), constipation, flatulence, vomiting, irritable bowel syndrome, abdominal pain, fecal incontinence
2. Sleep disorder: May include abnormal dreams, nightmares, sleepwalking; onset is varied.
   a. Nightmares can be managed by nighttime dose reduction, dosing earlier in the night, or eliminating nighttime dosing altogether.
3. Headache, irritability, insomnia

B. **Less common**:

1. Psychiatric: Depression, suicidal ideation, suicidal behavior, irritability, agitation, anxiety. There was a prior boxed warning for serious neuropsychiatric events such as depression and suicidality, but this was subsequently removed after risks were found to be lower than previously suspected (Thomas et al. 2015).
2. Hypertension, rash, diarrhea, toothache, chest pain, bronchitis, sinusitis, nasopharyngitis, cough, respiratory disorders, elevation in alanine aminotransferase (ALT), weight gain, arthralgia, myalgia, menstrual disorder

C. **Rare**:

1. Severe cutaneous reactions (Stevens-Johnson syndrome, erythema multiforme): Discontinue treatment and seek immediate medical attention.
2. Seizures:
   a. If seizures develop, discontinue treatment immediately, and seek prompt medical attention.
   b. Likely dosage related; possibly related to activation of nicotinic acetylcholine receptors, increasing intracellular calcium and epileptic activity; likely to occur early in treatment.
3. Severe cardiovascular events (risk is less than previously thought/reported):
   a. A higher incidence of major cardiovascular events (e.g., cardiovascular-related death, nonfatal heart attack, nonfatal stroke) has been found in patients taking varenicline versus those taking placebo in some studies (1.06% with varenicline vs. 0.82% with placebo) (Singh et al. 2011), although other studies have indicated no significant risk (Prochaska and Hilton 2012; Rigotti et al. 2010). While this risk is notable, smoking is a known major cardiovascular risk factor, so the benefits of quitting may greatly outweigh this small risk. Clinicians should discuss risks/benefits with patients, advise them of signs/symptoms of cardiovascular disease, and exercise greater caution in patients with current unstable cardiovascular disease.
   b. In December of 2012, the FDA released an updated Drug Safety Communication on the cardiovascular risks associated with varenicline (U.S. Food and Drug Administration 2012). The risks were considered to be small (and largely statistically insignificant) in comparison with the benefits of smoking cessation for long-term cardiovascular outcomes.

D. **Risks in pregnancy and lactation**:

1. Pregnancy: Varenicline use is not recommended during pregnancy. It was found to be teratogenic in animal studies.
2. Lactation: It is unknown whether varenicline is excreted into breast milk.

XIII. **Clinical Pearls/Prescribing Tips**

A. Varenicline is considered a first-line option for treatment supporting smoking cessation.

B. Varenicline significantly increases the rates of long-term abstinence.

Further Reading

Centre for Addiction and Mental Health: Canadian Smoking Cessation Clinical Practice Guideline. CAN-ADAPTT, 2011. Available at: https://www.nicotinedependenceclinic.com/en/canadaptt/PublishingImages/Pages/CAN-ADAPTT-Guidelines/CAN-ADAPTT%20Canadian%20Smoking%20Cessation%20Guideline_website.pdf. Accessed March 13, 2024.

Centre for Addiction and Mental Health: Smoking Cessation: Tools and Resources, 2021. Available at: https://www.camh.ca/en/professionals/treating-conditions-and-disorders/smoking-cessation/smoking-cessation---tools-and-resources. Accessed March 13, 2024.

Fiore MC, Jaén CR, Baker TB, et al: Treating tobacco use and dependence: 2008 update. Rockville, MD, U.S. Department of Health and Human Services, 2008

U.S. Department of Health and Human Services: Helping Smokers Quit: A Guide for Clinicians. Revised May 2008. Available at: https://www.ahrq.gov/sites/default/files/wysiwyg/professionals/clinicians-providers/guidelines-recommendations/tobacco/clinicians/references/clinhlpsmkqt/clinhlpsmksqt.pdf. Accessed March 13, 2024.

References

Pfizer Canada: Product monograph: Champix (varenicline). 2019. Available at: https://pdf.hres.ca/dpd_pm/00049350.PDF. Accessed March 13, 2024.

Prochaska JJ, Hilton JF: Risk of cardiovascular serious adverse events associated with varenicline use for tobacco cessation: systematic review and meta-analysis. BMJ 344:e2856, 2012

Rigotti NA, Pipe AL, Benowitz NL, et al: Efficacy and safety of varenicline for smoking cessation in patients with cardiovascular disease: a randomized trial. Circulation 121(2):221–229, 2010 20048210

Singh S, Loke YK, Spangler JG, et al: Risk of serious adverse cardiovascular events associated with varenicline: a systematic review and meta-analysis. CMAJ 183(12):1359–1366, 2011 21727225

Thomas KH, Martin RM, Knipe DW, et al: Risk of neuropsychiatric adverse events associated with varenicline: systematic review and meta-analysis. BMJ 350:h1109, 2015

U.S. Food and Drug Administration: FDA Drug Safety Communication: Safety review update of Chantix (varenicline) and risk of cardiovascular adverse events. December 12, 2012. Available at: https://www.fda.gov/drugs/drug-safety-and-availability/fda-drug-safety-communication-safety-review-update-chantix-varenicline-and-risk-cardiovascular. Accessed March 13, 2024.

11

Treatment of Agitation

William M. Webb, M.D., Ph.D.
Angela Mayorga, M.D.

Pharmacological Treatment of Agitation

- Agitation occurs when a patient's feelings of irritability, restlessness, or mental distress manifest as aggressive, violent, or unsafe behaviors in a clinical setting. The etiology of agitation is diverse and can be multifactorial, but common causes include substance intoxication and withdrawal, delirium, neurocognitive disorders, other mental disorders, and numerous other medical conditions that can result in altered mental status.
- Agitation can often be managed with verbal de-escalation techniques and behavioral interventions, and the initial management of the agitated patient should always favor these less-invasive methods (Spencer et al. 2018).
  - While some de-escalation techniques require special training, others are simple: respect the agitated patient's space, maintain a calm voice and a nonthreatening body posture, identify the patient's feelings and desires, and offer clear choices while setting appropriate limits (Richmond et al. 2012).
  - If agitation has a suspected origin in delirium or a neurocognitive disorder (e.g., sundowning behaviors), the following standard delirium precautions should be employed (Mattison 2020):
    - Reorient patients frequently. Involve family members if possible.
    - Ensure that patients with sensory impairments (e.g., vision, hearing) have access to their regular assistive devices (e.g., glasses, hearing aids).
    - Encourage early mobilization and provide cognitively stimulating activities for patients during the day.
    - Employ a nonpharmacological sleep protocol; promote sleep by avoiding unnecessary assessments and lab draws overnight. Minimize unnecessary noise and other stimuli.
    - Remove catheters and other restraints in a timely fashion.
    - Control pain and other common causes of delirium in older adults (e.g., ensure adequate hydration and avoid constipation).

- When verbal de-escalation techniques and preventive behavioral interventions fail to keep the patient or health care workers safe, use of medications and/or physical restraints becomes necessary. Physical restraints should be used as a last resort, if at all, and only to maintain safety, as they are apt to increase the patient's agitation or cause harm.
  - Because of the risk of neurovascular damage, pressure sores, and even rhabdomyolysis (Mohr et al. 2003), physical restraints should be used only temporarily (e.g., while medications are allowed to take effect).
  - All patients in physical restraints should have their positions changed frequently and should be evaluated regularly to reassess their need for continued restraint.
- Medications for agitation have traditionally included benzodiazepines, antipsychotics, or a combination of the two, although other pharmacotherapies can be employed as well.
  - In general, oral formulations of medications for agitation should be offered before intramuscular or intravenous formulations are administered.

Benzodiazepines

Overview

- Alongside antipsychotics, benzodiazepines are a reasonable first-line therapy for acute agitation because of their calming and sedating effects. The benzodiazepines most commonly used in acute agitation share several features:
  - Rapid onset of action
  - Clinically convenient half-life and/or duration of action
  - Multiple modes of administration (PO, IM, and IV)
- Given their characteristic side effects (**respiratory depression**, **somnolence**, **ataxia**, and worsening of **delirium**), benzodiazepines may be the preferred choice for younger, healthier, nondelirious patients, for whom medical comorbidities and fall risk are of less concern. Clinicians should monitor the respiratory function of patients receiving benzodiazepines (either alone or in combination with other drugs). Providers should also be aware of the rare but well-documented phenomenon of "paradoxical reaction" (i.e., experiencing the opposite of the intended effect) to benzodiazepines, which disproportionately affects older adults (Champion et al. 2021).
- Benzodiazepines are likewise the preferred choice in cases in which agitation stems from acute intoxication with stimulants, or from syndromes of substance withdrawal (e.g., from alcohol or benzodiazepines) characterized by activating sympathetic symptoms (see Chapter 3, "Anxiolytics: Benzodiazepines and Nonbenzodiazepines," in this Handbook for additional/full details).

Diazepam

- Diazepam is favored for control of agitation and seizure prevention in stimulant intoxication, for which a slower onset of action is acceptable (15–60 minutes IM, but < 5 minutes IV) and a longer half-life/duration of action is desired (> 12 hours) (Connors et al. 2019). Diazepam is hepatically metabolized to the active metabolite temazepam, which is further metabolized to oxazepam. Caution should be taken in patients with compromised liver function; consider lorazepam as an alternative:
  - **IV**: 2–10 mg every 3–10 minutes PRN, up to 20 mg/day
  - **IM**: 2–10 mg every 3–6 hours PRN, up to 20 mg/day
  - **PO**: 2–10 mg every 3–6 hours PRN, up to 40 mg/day

Lorazepam

- Lorazepam is preferred for its rapid onset of action (10–15 minutes), convenient duration of action (6–8 hours), and safety (requiring no dosage adjustments for renal or hepatic impairment):
  - **PO, IM, IV**: 0.5–2 mg every 4–6 hours PRN
  - **For severe agitation,** IM lorazepam 2 mg is frequently combined with IM diphenhydramine 50 mg and IM haloperidol 5 mg (i.e., the infamous "B-52"). Benztropine 1 mg may also be used in place of diphenhydramine 50 mg

Midazolam

- Midazolam is notable for its extremely rapid onset of action (~5 minutes IV, ~10 minutes IM). Its short duration of action (60–90 minutes) is particularly suited for acute agitation; however, repeat doses may be required. Although no dosage adjustments are recommended, the presence of active metabolites may be prolonged in patients with renal and/or hepatic impairment (Zaporowska-Stachowiak et al. 2019):
  - **IV**: 2.5–5 mg every 3–5 minutes until sedation is adequate.
  - **IM**: 2.5–5 mg every 5–10 minutes until sedation is adequate.

Antipsychotics

Overview

- With benzodiazepines, antipsychotics make up the mainstay of treatment for acute agitation. In general, antipsychotics cause sedation quickly and offer a clinically useful range of administration options (oral, intramuscular, intravenous, oral disintegrating) while avoiding the typical side effects of benzodiazepines (respiratory depression, ataxia, and delirium).

- Antipsychotics are associated with their own set of characteristic adverse effects. While some of these (e.g., tardive dyskinesia, hyperprolactinemia) are associated with scheduled, longer-term use, others (e.g., **neuroleptic malignant syndrome, dystonia, orthostatic hypotension**) can occur at any time, even with infrequent PRN use. Patients who frequently receive PRN antipsychotics for agitation should be examined periodically for rigidity and should undergo routine assessment of their vital signs.
- In general, antipsychotics may be preferred in patients whose agitation occurs in the setting of psychosis, neurocognitive disorders, or advanced age (given the latter group's particular susceptibility to the side effects of benzodiazepines).
- A word of caution: large-scale clinical trials and meta-analyses have consistently linked antipsychotics to sudden cardiac death (Anyamba et al. 2009), stroke (Fife et al. 2021), and increased mortality in dementia (Gill et al. 2007)—effects that are thought to be mediated by antipsychotics' induction of dyslipidemia, and by prolongation of the QTc interval, leading to increased risk of fatal cardiac arrhythmias such as torsades de pointes. All antipsychotics, both first-generation and second-generation, carry an FDA boxed warning about the risk of increased mortality in "elderly dementia patients."
- As with other medications used for acute agitation, an oral (PO) alternative should first be offered before resorting to intramuscular or intravenous formulations. **The following antipsychotics are commonly used IM or IV when PO options are declined by or are not practical/safe for an agitated patient.**

Antipsychotics for Acute Agitation

Haloperidol

- The use of haloperidol for severe, acute agitation and aggression is technically off-label; however, both IM and IV administration of haloperidol for this purpose is well established in the literature, commonplace, and well studied (Battaglia 2005). Because haloperidol is less sedating (Klein et al. 2018) and less likely to cause orthostasis and respiratory depression compared with other antipsychotics, it is commonly supplemented with benzodiazepines when used for agitation.
- Onset of action is 15 minutes (IM), with peak sedation by 30 minutes. Haloperidol is hepatically metabolized and is a major substrate of the cytochrome P450 (CYP) 1A2 and CYP2D6 enzymes, so care should be taken when using haloperidol in patients with known hepatic impairment, patients concomitantly taking CYP1A2 or CYP2D6 inhibitors, and patients who are known to be poor metabolizers of these enzymes.
- Of note, all IV administration of haloperidol is off-label, and haloperidol carries an FDA boxed warning for increased mortality in elderly patients. IV haloperidol is associated with dosage-dependent QTc prolongation at dosages higher than 2 mg (Meyer-Massetti et al. 2010).
  - **PO**: 1–5 mg every 6 hours PRN
  - **IM**: 1–5 mg every 2–4 hours PRN, up to 10 mg/day. **For severe agitation**, IM lorazepam 2 mg is frequently combined with IM diphenhydramine 50 mg and IM haloperidol 5 mg. Benztropine 1 mg may also be used in place of diphenhydramine 50 mg.

- **IV**: 1–5 mg every 2 hours PRN. *Note*: IV haloperidol has been associated with significant degrees of QTc interval prolongation (Xiong et al. 2020). Use with extreme caution and consider continuous ECG monitoring in patients with known QTc prolongation at baseline and/or those taking other QTc-prolonging medications. For additional information on this topic, readers are referred to the medical literature (Beach et al. 2013, 2018).

Chlorpromazine

- Chlorpromazine is useful for its wide therapeutic window (ranging from an initial dosage of 25 mg/day up to 800 mg/day) and its shorter duration of action (4–6 hours). Like haloperidol, chlorpromazine carries an FDA boxed warning for increased mortality in "elderly dementia patients." Compared with haloperidol, chlorpromazine is associated with a greater risk of orthostatic hypotension; blood pressure should be monitored regularly following administration.
  - **PO**: 25 mg every 4–6 hours PRN
  - **IM**: Initial dose of 25 mg followed by an additional 25–50 mg every 1–4 hours as needed, up to 800 mg/day.

Olanzapine

- Among second-generation (atypical) antipsychotics, olanzapine should be considered the first-line choice in acute agitation because of its strong sedative effects (Klein et al. 2018), which are likely attributable to the drug's antagonism of central H_1 histamine receptors. Additionally, olanzapine acts as an antagonist at the (α_1)-adrenergic receptor, which can result in significant orthostatic hypotension, dizziness, and fall risk (Jana et al. 2015).
- When combined with benzodiazepines, parenteral olanzapine has been linked to worsening respiratory depression (Wilson et al. 2012), and postmarketing case reports have described fatalities (Marder et al. 2010); therefore, care should be taken in patients who are intoxicated with CNS depressants, and coadministration of parenteral olanzapine and benzodiazepines (as well as other CNS depressants) should be avoided within 2–4 hours of one another. Because olanzapine is a substrate of the CYP1A2 enzyme, higher dosages may be required in cigarette smokers, who exhibit increased activity of this enzyme, and lower dosages may be needed when olanzapine is combined with known CYP1A2 inhibitors or prescribed for individuals known to be poor metabolizers.
  - **PO (and oral disintegrating tablet [ODT])**: 5–10 mg every 4 hours PRN, up to 20 mg/day. Keep in mind that time to peak concentration can be as long as 6 hours for PO/disintegrating formulations of olanzapine.
  - **IM**: Initial dose of 5–10 mg, followed by an additional dose 2 hours later if needed; repeat every 4 hours PRN, up to a maximum of 20 mg/day.
  - **IV**: Initial dose of 5–10 mg every 4 hours PRN, up to a maximum of 20 mg/day. *Note:* IV use of olanzapine is off-label and is controversial (given the absence of clear evidence evaluating safety and efficacy [Khorassani and Saad 2019]). Care should be taken to monitor patients for respiratory depression. Do not exceed 20 mg/day.

Ziprasidone

- A second-line atypical antipsychotic for acute agitation (Klein et al. 2018), ziprasidone should be considered for patients who cannot tolerate first-generation antipsychotics for whatever reason or those for whom the risks of respiratory depression and orthostasis make olanzapine an unsafe alternative. Ziprasidone is among the worst offenders for QTc interval prolongation (Xiong et al. 2020); therefore, care should be taken in patients with known QTc prolongation at baseline and/or those taking other QTc-prolonging medications.
  - **IM**: 10 mg every 2 hours or 20 mg every 4 hours PRN, up to 40 mg/day.

Antipsychotics With Oral Disintegrating or Sublingual Options

- Conveniently for acute agitation, a number of atypical antipsychotics are available in ODT formulations that dissolve rapidly in saliva. These medications are easy to administer, require less cooperation on the part of agitated patients, and are difficult to "cheek," and administration may be less traumatic for patients than IM injections. Unfortunately, evidence guiding their use is limited, and none of these medications are FDA-approved to treat agitation.
- Most currently marketed ODT formulations are not absorbed transmucosally and **must be swallowed** to take effect. Accordingly, absorption and time to onset of action for these formulations are not significantly different from absorption and onset of action for their conventional oral counterparts. An exception is asenapine, which is available in a sublingual formulation that reaches peak blood concentration more quickly than its PO counterpart; however, the necessary patient cooperation with sublingual dosing makes it poorly suited for severe agitation. In such cases, IM antipsychotics may be preferred.

Aripiprazole (Abilify Discmelt)

- Time to peak concentration is 3–5 hours, which may limit use in the severely agitated patient:
  - **ODT**: 10–15 mg every 2 hours PRN, up to a maximum of 30 mg/day.

Olanzapine (Zyprexa Zydis)

- The considerations that apply to conventional PO and IM olanzapine are similarly relevant for its ODT formulation. The time to peak concentration for PO/disintegrating formulations of olanzapine is ~6 hours, which may limit its use in severely agitated patients.
  - **ODT**: 5–10 mg every 2 hours PRN.

Risperidone (Risperdal M-Tab)

- Like its first-generation analog haloperidol, risperidone is less sedating than other second-generation antipsychotics. Accordingly, it may be preferred in less agitated patients or those whose psychotic symptoms or familiarity with the drug make risperidone an otherwise more acceptable option. Time to peak concentration is approximately 1 hour.
  - **ODT**: 1–2 mg every 30 minutes PRN, up to a maximum of 6–8 mg/day.

Asenapine (Saphris, Sycrest)

- Although rapid-acting and transmucosally absorbed (with a time to peak concentration of 30 minutes), sublingual asenapine is not recommended for severe agitation, given the high level of patient cooperation required for sublingual use (the tablet must be held under the tongue until it dissolves). Use of sublingual asenapine could be considered in mildly agitated patients who are accepting PO medication.
  - **Sublingual**: 5–10 mg BID, scheduled or PRN

Antipsychotics for Patients With Parkinson's Disease or Neurocognitive Disorder With Lewy Bodies

- Special consideration should be given to patients with Parkinson's disease or neurocognitive disorder with Lewy bodies, because antipsychotics can dramatically worsen preexisting parkinsonian symptoms by way of dopamine blockade and are associated with increased mortality in these patients (Weintraub et al. 2016). Although antipsychotics have been used in patients with Parkinson's disease who experience psychosis, initial treatment normally consists of reducing antiparkinsonian and anticholinergic medications. In the case of acute agitation, benzodiazepines may be favored, with the following second-generation (atypical) antipsychotics being employed as a last resort.

Quetiapine

- Limited evidence suggests that quetiapine may be at least as efficacious as clozapine in preventing psychosis in Parkinson's disease, but without the hematological monitoring concerns presented by clozapine, and without the adverse effects carried by other antipsychotics in Parkinson's disease, such as abnormal movements or worsening of parkinsonism (Seppi et al. 2019).
  - **PO**: 12.5–25 mg every night at bedtime, with dosage increasing in 12.5-mg increments weekly, to a maximum of 200 mg every night at bedtime.

Pimavanserin

- A selective serotonin $5\text{-}HT_{2A}$ receptor inverse agonist without dopaminergic activity, pimavanserin was shown to be efficacious in treating psychosis in Parkinson's disease without causing significant adverse events (Cummings et al. 2014). Pimavanserin has not been studied in acute agitation specifically, and thus should be considered a scheduled medication prescribed to treat psychosis in Parkinson's disease after the acutely agitated patient has been stabilized).
  - **PO**: 34 mg once daily.

Other Agents

Valproate (Valproic Acid) and Divalproex

- Valproate (valproic acid), along with its longer-acting formulations (divalproex), is commonly used off-label to treat agitation in neurocognitive disorders (Meyer and Schuyler 2015) as well as aggressive or impulsive behaviors in patients with traumatic brain injury or developmental or personality disorders (Williamson et al. 2019). Valproate is also commonly used as an augmentation strategy with antipsychotics in patients with psychotic disorders, including schizophrenia. In these contexts, valproate is typically scheduled for longer-term ongoing use as opposed to being used PRN for acute agitation; however, some studies have examined valproate use for acute agitation in psychosis (Olivola et al. 2022).
- Short-term side effects of valproate (in all of its forms) include CNS depression with sedation, cognitive slowing, and gastrointestinal distress. Toxicity (associated with serum levels > 100 μg/mL) manifests as extreme CNS depression, encephalopathy, hyperammonemia, and myoclonus. Side effects with long-term use include alopecia, weight gain, pancreatitis, and dosage-dependent thrombocytopenia.
- Caution should be taken in patients with hepatic disease, and valproate can be hepatotoxic even in healthy patients. Serum liver function tests should be obtained before initiating scheduled therapy and at regular intervals with long-term use. Valproate is safe in patients with renal impairment (see Chapter 5, "Mood Stabilizers," in this Handbook for additional details).
- Because of its association with neural tube defects and neurodevelopmental disorders, valproate should be avoided in pregnant women or individuals with the potential to become pregnant whose use of contraception is unknown.
- With scheduled use, serum valproic acid levels should be assessed periodically, although there is no consensus on the optimal serum level for agitation or behavioral dyscontrol associated with neurocognitive disorders. The therapeutic ranges used for epilepsy (50–100 μg/mL) and mania (50–125 μg/mL) can be used as a guide; however, lower serum levels are often adequate to prevent agitation in neurocognitive disorders, and the lowest clinically efficacious dosage should be used (Dolder et al. 2012). In general, the total

daily dosage should not exceed 30 mg/kg or 2.5 g, although clinical response is often a more reliable indicator of appropriate dosing than serum valproic acid levels.

- Valproate has multiple formulations, including immediate-release (valproate) and delayed- and extended-release products (divalproex sodium).

Valproate (Valproic Acid)

- The immediate-release preparations of valproate are available as PO capsule, syrup (trade name Depakene), and IV (Depacon) formulations. The liquid formulation may be considered for patients with dysphagia. Use PO when the agitated patient is willing to take medications. Onset of action occurs within 15–60 minutes, with a variable half-life of 6–16 hours, depending on the patient's hepatic metabolism. The IV formulation has been studied for the prevention of agitation and delirium in the intensive care setting and has been shown to significantly reduce these complications as well as to decrease the requirement for as-needed dosing to treat behavioral symptoms (Crowley et al. 2020).
  - **PO**: 250–500 mg every 8 hours PRN. Do not exceed 30 mg/kg daily.
  - **IV**: 500–1,000 mg every 12 hours. Do not exceed 30 mg/kg daily.
  - Consider divalproex formulations (see below) when scheduling valproic acid daily, from once a day at bedtime up to three times a day in the case of ongoing agitation associated with a neurocognitive disorder or impulse-control issues.

Divalproex

- Preferred for scheduled dosing because of its longer duration of action, divalproex (trade name Depakote) comes in a variety of formulations, including delayed-release (DR), extended-release (ER), and delayed-release "sprinkles" that can be added to soft food. Use of sprinkles should be considered for patients with dysphagia, or to facilitate adherence in patients with neurocognitive disorders. Time to onset of action may be up to 2 hours, with a variable duration of action up to 18 hours or more (ER). Steady state is usually achieved after 3–5 days at a given dosage.
  - **DR PO**: 250 mg every night at bedtime or BID, up to 2,500 mg/day split BID.
  - **ER PO**: 250 mg every night at bedtime, up to 2,500 mg/day.
  - **DR PO Sprinkles**: 250 mg/day taken before a meal, up to 750 mg TID taken before meal.

Dexmedetomidine

Overview

- Historically used as an IV medication for sedation in intensive care and preprocedural settings, the α_2-adrenergic receptor agonist dexmedetomidine has been studied in recent trials examining the utility of an oral dissolving formulation for treatment of acute agitation in the context of psychosis (SERENITY I and SERENITY II) (Citrome et al. 2022).

- For acute agitation in a critically ill or delirious patient, IV administration of dexmedetomidine remains practical and may even have an anti-delirium effect in intensive care (Boyer 2010) and palliative care settings (Gaertner and Fusi-Schmidhauser 2022).
- When administered as an orally dissolving film (ODF), dexmedetomidine avoids some of the risks and adverse effects of benzodiazepines and antipsychotics in favor of mild to moderate somnolence without unarousable sedation or respiratory depression. The SERENITY trials (Citrome et al. 2022) recorded no treatment-emergent adverse events. Dexmedetomidine ODF also avoids the need for traumatic IM administration and thus can be self-administered.
- Caution should be exercised in patients taking beta-blockers and in those with known bradycardia. A CYP2D6 substrate, dexmedetomidine is safe in patients with renal impairment and has a half-life of 2 hours in healthy patients; however, an increased duration of action has been noted in patients with hepatic impairment (Cunningham et al. 1999). Clinicians should also exercise caution when using dexmedetomidine in patients who are taking concomitant CYP2D6 inhibitors or who are known to be poor metabolizers of CYP2D6.

Considerations and Administration

- Consider use of ODF in psychotic patients who 1) are willing to accept an oral medication for agitation; 2) should avoid the side effects of antipsychotic medications (QTc prolongation) and benzodiazepines (worsening of delirium, respiratory depression); and/or 3) have significant renal impairment. When dexmedetomidine is administered as an ODF, onset of action occurs within 20 minutes, with a duration of action of 60–120 minutes.
- Consider IV administration for the critically ill or delirious patient with agitation in the intensive care unit, for whom the risks of sudden cardiac death (with antipsychotics) or worsening delirium and respiratory depression (with benzodiazepines) are significant. When administered intravenously, dexmedetomidine has an onset of action of 5–10 minutes, and its effects last 60–120 minutes
  - **PO**: 25 mg every 4–6 hours PRN
  - **IM**: Initial dose of 25 mg followed by an additional 25–50 mg every 1–4 hours as needed, up to 800 mg/day.

Dextromethorphan and Quinidine Sulfate

Overview

- Historically used as an antitussive agent, dextromethorphan can be combined with quinidine to treat agitation and aggression in patients with neurocognitive disorders as well as those with inappropriate behaviors associated with pseudobulbar affect (Cummings et al. 2015). This special formulation (trade name Nuedexta) uses quinidine to inhibit the hepatic metabolism of dextromethorphan through CYP2D6 and to increase dextromethorphan's activity as an *N*-methyl-D-aspartate (NMDA) receptor antagonist and a sigma-1 receptor agonist.

- Common side effects include gastrointestinal distress. Quinidine prolongs the QTc interval, so caution should be exercised in patients with known QTc prolongation and those receiving polypharmacy with multiple QTc-prolonging agents or medications that inhibit CYP3A4 enzymes, which is the pathway responsible for metabolizing quinidine.

Considerations and Administration

- The combination dextromethorphan 20 mg/quinidine 10 mg capsule should be considered only for scheduled, long-term treatment of agitation in patients with neurocognitive disorders or for pseudobulbar affect in patients who are able and willing to take medications PO. Accordingly, there is little role for this combination in acute agitation.
  - **PO**: 20 mg/10 mg daily; increase to BID, if tolerated, for 7 days

References

Anyamba A, Chretien JP, Small J, et al: Prediction of a Rift Valley fever outbreak. Proc Natl Acad Sci USA 106(3):955–959, 2009 19144928

Battaglia J: Pharmacological management of acute agitation. Drugs 65(9):1207–1222, 2005 15916448

Beach SR, Celano CM, Noseworthy PA, et al: QTc prolongation, torsades de pointes, and psychotropic medications. Psychosomatics 54(1):1–13, 2013 23295003

Beach SR, Celano CM, Sugrue AM, et al: QTc prolongation, torsades de pointes, and psychotropic medications: a 5-year update. Psychosomatics 59(2):105–122, 2018 29275963

Boyer J: Calming patient agitation with dexmedetomidine. Nursing Critical Care. 5:30–34, 2010

Champion C, Novais T, Dorey JM, et al: Paradoxical reactions to benzodiazepines in the elderly [in French]. Gériatr Psychol Neuropsychiatr Vieil 19(3):305–312, 2021 34526288

Citrome LL, Preskorn SH, Rajachandran L, et al: Dexmedetomidine orally dissolving film for acute agitation associated with schizophrenia or bipolar disorder: SERENITY I and SERENITY II trials. CNS Spectr 27(2):242, 2022

Connors NJ, Alsakha A, Larocque A, et al: Antipsychotics for the treatment of sympathomimetic toxicity: a systematic review. Am J Emerg Med 37(10):1880–1890, 2019 30639129

Crowley KE, Urben L, Hacobian G, et al: Valproic acid for the management of agitation and delirium in the intensive care setting: a retrospective analysis. Clin Ther 42(4):e65–e73, 2020 32273047

Cummings J, Isaacson S, Mills R, et al: Pimavanserin for patients with Parkinson's disease psychosis: a randomised, placebo-controlled phase 3 trial. Lancet 383(9916):533–540, 2014 24183563

Cummings JL, Lyketsos CG, Peskind ER, et al: Effect of dextromethorphan-quinidine on agitation in patients with Alzheimer disease dementia: a randomized clinical trial. JAMA 314(12):1242–1254, 2015 26393847

Cunningham FE, Baughman VL, Tonkovich L, et al: Pharmacokinetics of dexmedetomidine (DEX) in patients with hepatic failure (HF). Clin Pharmacol Ther 65:128, 1999

Dolder CR, Nealy KL, McKinsey J: Valproic acid in dementia: does an optimal dose exist? J Pharm Pract 25(2):142–150, 2012 22095580

Fife D, Blacketer C, Knight RK, et al: Stroke risk among elderly users of haloperidol and typical antipsychotics versus atypical antipsychotics: a real-world study from a US health insurance claims database. Am J Geriatr Psychiatry 29(5):499–510, 2021 33097389

Gaertner J, Fusi-Schmidhauser T: Dexmedetomidine: a magic bullet on its way into palliative care—a narrative review and practice recommendations. Ann Palliat Med 11(4):1491–1504, 2022 35400162

Gill SS, Bronskill SE, Normand SL, et al: Antipsychotic drug use and mortality in older adults with dementia. Ann Intern Med 146(11):775–786, 2007 17548409

Jana AK, Praharaj SK, Roy N: Olanzapine-induced orthostatic hypotension. Clin Psychopharmacol Neurosci 13(1):113–114, 2015 25912545

Khorassani F, Saad M: Intravenous olanzapine for the management of agitation: review of the literature. Ann Pharmacother 53(8):853–859, 2019 30758221

Klein LR, Driver BE, Miner JR, et al: Intramuscular midazolam, olanzapine, ziprasidone, or haloperidol for treating acute agitation in the emergency department. Ann Emerg Med 72(4):374–385, 2018 29885904

Marder SR, Sorsaburu S, Dunayevich E, et al: Case reports of postmarketing adverse event experiences with olanzapine intramuscular treatment in patients with agitation. J Clin Psychiatry 71(4):433–441, 2010 20156413

Mattison MLP: Delirium. Ann Intern Med 173(7):ITC49–ITC64, 2020 33017552

Meyer RP, Schuyler D: Calming the agitated demented patient. Prim Care Companion CNS Disord 17(1): 2015 26137362

Meyer-Massetti C, Cheng CM, Sharpe BA, et al: The FDA extended warning for intravenous haloperidol and torsades de pointes: how should institutions respond? J Hosp Med 5(4):E8–E16, 2010 20394022

Mohr WK, Petti TA, Mohr BD: Adverse effects associated with physical restraint. Can J Psychiatry 48(5):330–337, 2003 12866339

Olivola M, Civardi S, Damiani S, et al: Effectiveness and safety of intravenous valproate in agitation: a systematic review. Psychopharmacology (Berl) 239(2):339–350, 2022 34783884

Richmond JS, Berlin JS, Fishkind AB, et al: Verbal de-escalation of the agitated patient: consensus statement of the American Association for Emergency Psychiatry Project BETA De-escalation Workgroup. West J Emerg Med 13(1):17–25, 2012 22461917

Seppi K, Ray Chaudhuri K, Coelho M, et al: Update on treatments for nonmotor symptoms of Parkinson's disease—an evidence-based medicine review. Mov Disord 34(2):180–198, 2019 30653247

Spencer S, Johnson P, Smith IC: De-escalation techniques for managing non-psychosis induced aggression in adults. Cochrane Database Syst Rev (7):CD012034, 2018 30019748

Weintraub D, Chiang C, Kim HM, et al: Association of antipsychotic use with mortality risk in patients with Parkinson disease. JAMA Neurol 73(5):535–541, 2016 26999262

Williamson D, Frenette AJ, Burry LD, et al: Pharmacological interventions for agitated behaviours in patients with traumatic brain injury: a systematic review. BMJ Open 9(7):e029604, 2019 31289093

Wilson MP, MacDonald K, Vilke GM, et al: A comparison of the safety of olanzapine and haloperidol in combination with benzodiazepines in emergency department patients with acute agitation. J Emerg Med 43(5):790–797, 2012 21601409

Xiong GL, Pinkhasov A, Mangal JP, et al: QTc monitoring in adults with medical and psychiatric comorbidities: expert consensus from the Association of Medicine and Psychiatry. J Psychosom Res 135:110138, 2020 32442893

Zaporowska-Stachowiak I, Szymański K, Oduah MT, et al: Midazolam: safety of use in palliative care: a systematic critical review. Biomed Pharmacother 114:108838, 2019 30981104

12

Treatment of Psychotropic Medication-Induced Adverse Effects

Shailesh (Bobby) Jain, M.D.

Psychotropic medications, while beneficial for managing mental disorders, often come with a variety of side effects that can significantly impact a patient's quality of life. These side effects can range from mild, such as dry mouth or drowsiness, to more severe, such as weight gain, metabolic changes, or movement disorders. However, with few exceptions (e.g., increased risk of dermatological reactions to carbamazepine in Han Chinese), we have no way of knowing which patients will experience specific side effects or what the severity of those effects will be with specific drugs. Addressing these side effects is crucial for ensuring patients' adherence to their medication regimen and patients' overall well-being.

Psychopharmacological interventions are tailored strategies employed to mitigate these adverse effects. One common approach is dosage adjustment, wherein the medication dosage is carefully calibrated to find a balance between therapeutic benefits and tolerable side effects. Additionally, switching to a different medication within the same class, or to another class entirely, may be necessary if the side effects are particularly troublesome. Another important intervention is the use of adjunctive medications to counteract specific side effects. For instance, anticholinergic drugs can be prescribed to alleviate extrapyramidal symptoms caused by antipsychotics, while medications such as metformin may be used to manage weight gain associated with certain antidepressants. Lifestyle modifications, including dietary changes and exercise, are also recommended to help mitigate side effects such as weight gain and metabolic disturbances. Regular monitoring through follow-up appointments and laboratory tests is essential to detect and manage side effects promptly. By employing these psychopharmacological interventions, health care providers can optimize treatment outcomes, enhance patient comfort, and improve patient adherence to psychotropic medications, thereby ensuring that their patients receive the full benefits of their prescribed therapies without being hindered by adverse effects.

Akathisia

Overview

Akathisia, meaning "inability to sit," comprises both an objective restless movement and a subjective feeling of restlessness that is experienced as the need to move. Patients may display akathisia without experiencing subjective distress, a condition that has been termed *pseudoakathisia* (Barnes 1990).

In addition to being associated with antipsychotics, akathisia affects some patients treated with selective serotonin reuptake inhibitors (SSRIs), calcium channel blockers, antibiotics, antiemetics, and anti-vertigo agents.

Akathisia may also arise with dosage reduction or cessation of antipsychotic medications (referred to as *withdrawal akathisia*). Similar to tardive dyskinesia, tardive akathisia develops later in the course of medication treatment, can be exacerbated or provoked by antipsychotic dosage reduction or withdrawal, and improves at least temporarily when the antipsychotic dosage is increased. However, increasing an antipsychotic dosage can worsen parkinsonian side effects, which could mask tardive dyskinesia. Persistent akathisia is disabling and often refractory to treatment (Barnes and Braude 1985). Akathisia may be misinterpreted as agitation or aggression by an observer.

An imbalance between dopaminergic and serotonergic/noradrenergic neurotransmitter systems has been most commonly considered as the basis for akathisia, although other theories—such as overstimulation of the locus coeruleus, leading to a mismatch between the core and the shell of the nucleus accumbens—have also been proposed (Adler et al. 1985; Lonnen and Stahl 2011).

References

Adler L, Angrist B, Peselow E, et al: Efficacy of propranolol in neuroleptic-induced akathesia. J Clin Psychopharmacol 5(3):164–166, 1985 2860136

Barnes TM: Movement disorder associated with antipsychotic drugs: the tardive syndromes. Int Rev Psychiatry 2(3–4):355–366, 1990

Barnes TRE, Braude WM: Akathisia variants and tardive dyskinesia. Arch Gen Psychiatry 42(9):874–878, 1985 2864031

Lonnen AJM, Stahl SM: The mechanism of drug-induced akathisia. CNS Spectr 16(1):7–10, 2011. Available at: https://www.cambridge.org/core/journals/cns-spectrums/article/abs/mechanism-of-druginduced-akathisia/7F12D2E0454720632BD1A957D29167F0. Accessed February 15, 2024.

Benzodiazepines (for Medication-Induced Akathisia)

I. **Mechanism of Action:**

A. Benzodiazepines, specifically clonazepam, reduce the overall CNS excitatory state by an agonist action at the $GABA_A$ receptors, indirectly increasing dopamine levels, and likely addressing the hypodopaminergic state (Thippaiah et al. 2021).

II. **Data:**

A. Clonazepam: Two trials ($n=27$) comparing clonazepam (0.5–2.5 mg/day) and placebo for the treatment (7–14 days) of antipsychotic-induced akathisia in patients with psychosis reported significantly greater improvement in akathisia symptoms with clonazepam in comparison with placebo (Pringsheim et al. 2018).

B. Lorazepam: In a study of 16 patients with antipsychotic-induced akathisia treated with lorazepam, a marked improvement in symptoms was observed in 9 of the patients and moderate improvement in 5 patients. Symptoms remained unchanged among 2 patients. The decrease in the Akathisia Rating Scale score—from 1.81 at pretreatment to 0.5 after 7 days and to 0.32 after 14 days—was statistically significant. No severe side effects were observed (Bartels et al. 1987). The mean dosage used in the study was 2.34 ± 1.22 mg/day.

III. **Dosing:**

A. The studies described above indicate that the optimal dosing for clonazepam is 0.5–2.5 mg/day, and that for lorazepam is 2.34 (± 1.22) mg/day.

B. Benzodiazepines are started low and slowly uptitrated to the lowest effective dosage. Clonazepam (0.5–2.5 mg/day) and lorazepam (1–2 mg/day) have been utilized to manage antipsychotic-induced akathisia, with limited evidence supporting their use (Salem et al. 2017; Thippaiah et al. 2021). Once the akathisia symptoms stabilize, a gradual taper of the benzodiazepine is recommended (Lima et al. 2002).

IV. **Cautions/Monitoring:**

A. Benzodiazepines can produce CNS depression, particularly when combined with other CNS depressants such as opioids or alcohol. Clonazepam should be used with caution, as it can increase the risk of suicidal thoughts or behaviors.

B. Benzodiazepines are categorized as FDA Category D in pregnancy and are relatively contraindicated in breastfeeding.

Further Reading

Adler LA, Angrist B, Reiter S, et al: Neuroleptic-induced akathisia: a review. Psychopharmacology (Berl) 97(1):1–11, 1989 2565586

Arora N, Dhiman P, Kumar S, et al: Recent advances in synthesis and medicinal chemistry of benzodiazepines. Bioorg Chem 97:103668, 2020 32106040

Bateup HS, Santini E, Shen W, et al: Distinct subclasses of medium spiny neurons differentially regulate striatal motor behaviors. Proc Natl Acad Sci USA 107(33):14845–14850, 2010 20682746

Bausch Health US: Ativan (lorazepam) package insert. Revised February 2021. Available at: https://www.accessdata.fda.gov/drugsatfda_docs/label/2021/017794s048lbl.pdf. Accessed July 8, 2024.

Clonazepam package insert. Available at: http://www.accessdata.fda.gov%2Fdrugsatfda_docs% 2Flabel%2F2013%2F017533s053%2C020813s009lbl.pdf. Accessed February 2, 2022.

Demir B, Sancaktar M, Altindag A: Lithium-induced treatment-resistant akathisia: a case report and literature overview. Clin Neuropharmacol 44(3):112–113, 2021 33811193

Lonnen AJM, Stahl SM: The mechanism of drug-induced akathisia. CNS Spectr 16(1):7–10, 2011. Available at: https://www.cambridge.org/core/journals/cns-spectrums/article/abs/mechanism-of-druginduced-akathisia/7F12D2E0454720632BD1A957D29167F0. Accessed February 15, 2024.

Lorman WJ: Pharmacology update: benzodiazepines. J Addict Nurs 28(2):96–97, 2017 28582356

Pujalte D, Bottaï T, Huë B, et al: A double-blind comparison of clonazepam and placebo in the treatment of neuroleptic-induced akathisia. Clin Neuropharmacol 17(3):236–242, 1994 9316669

Sabioni P, Bertram J, Le Foll B: Off-label use of medications for treatment of benzodiazepine use disorder. Curr Pharm Des 21(23):3306–3310, 2015 26088120

Shuen JA, Chen M, Gloss B, et al: Drd1a-tdTomato BAC transgenic mice for simultaneous visualization of medium spiny neurons in the direct and indirect pathways of the basal ganglia. J Neurosci 28(11):2681–2685, 2008 18337395

Sienaert P, van Harten P, Rhebergen D: The psychopharmacology of catatonia, neuroleptic malignant syndrome, akathisia, tardive dyskinesia, and dystonia. Handb Clin Neurol 165:415–428, 2019 31727227

Walther S, Stegmayer K, Wilson JE, et al: Structure and neural mechanisms of catatonia. Lancet Psychiatry 6(7):610–619, 2019 31196794

References

Bartels M, Heide K, Mann K, et al: Treatment of akathisia with lorazepam: an open clinical trial. Pharmacopsychiatry 20(2):51–53, 1987 2884681

Lima AR, Soares-Weiser K, Bacaltchuk J, et al: Benzodiazepines for neuroleptic-induced acute akathisia. Cochrane Database Syst Rev (1):CD001950, 2002 11869614

Pringsheim T, Gardner D, Addington D, et al: The assessment and treatment of antipsychotic-induced akathisia. Can J Psychiatry 63(11):719–729, 2018 29685069

Salem H, Nagpal C, Pigott T, et al: Revisiting antipsychotic-induced akathisia: current issues and prospective challenges. Curr Neuropharmacol 15(5):789–798, 2017 27928948

Thippaiah SM, Fargason RE, Birur B: Struggling to find effective pharmacologic options for akathisia? B-CALM! Psychopharmacol Bull 51(3):72–78, 2021 34421146

Propranolol (for Medication-Induced Akathisia)

I. **Mechanism of Action**:

A. Propranolol is a beta-blocker, also known as a β-adrenergic blocking agent. β-Blockers work by blocking the effects of epinephrine. The exact mechanism of action of β-blockers in the treatment of extrapyramidal symptoms (EPS) is unclear. Lipid solubility and the corresponding ability to enter the CNS are the most important factors determining the efficacy of propranolol in treating akathisia (Adler et al. 1991). A noradrenergic pathway from the locus coeruleus to the limbic system has been proposed as a modulator involved in symptoms of tardive dyskinesia, akathisia, and tremor (Adler et al. 1991; Wilbur et al. 1988). An imbalance between dopaminergic and noradrenergic/serotonergic neurotransmitter systems seems to be involved in the etiology of antipsychotic-induced akathisia that responds to b-adrenergic and 5-HT_{2A} antagonists (Kapur and Remington 1996; Poyurovsky and Weizman 2001; Thippaiah et al. 2021).

II. **Data**:

A. A blinded study showed propranolol to be more efficacious than lorazepam in treating antipsychotic-induced akathisia. The low dosages of propranolol used to treat akathisia did not significantly affect blood pressure (Adler et al. 1985). Six of seven clinical trials ($n = 194$), ranging in duration from 2 to 12 days, that compared propranolol (20–120 mg) and placebo in the treatment of akathisia in patients with schizophrenia reported improvement in akathisia symptoms with propranolol (Pringsheim et al. 2018).

III. **Dosing**:

A. Oral propranolol dosage range: 20–120 mg/day: Initiate at a low dosage (10 mg oral BID), with upward titration every few days to a maximum of 90–120 mg/day (Fleischhacker et al. 1990; Poyurovsky and Weizman 2020).

IV. **Cautions/Monitoring**:

A. Careful assessment of cardiac functioning before initiating propranolol is recommended. Propranolol hydrochloride is contraindicated in the context of cardiogenic shock, sinus bradycardia, significant cardiac conduction abnormalities, bronchial asthma, and certain forms of congestive heart failure.

B. Recent studies have not substantiated the previous notion that propranolol precipitates clinical depression (Kessing et al. 2020).

Further Reading

Akrimax Pharmaceuticals: Inderal (propranolol hydrochloride) package insert. Revised November 2010. Available at: https://www.accessdata.fda.gov/drugsatfda_docs/label/2011/016418s080,016762s017,017683s008lbl.pdf. Accessed July 8, 2024.

Barnes TR: Movement disorder associated with antipsychotic drugs: the tardive syndromes. Int Rev Psychiatry 2(3–4):355–366, 1990

Barnes TR, Braude WM: Akathisia variants and tardive dyskinesia. Arch Gen Psychiatry 42(9):874–878, 1985 2864031

Schatzberg AF, Nemeroff CB (eds): The American Psychiatric Association Publishing Textbook of Psychopharmacology, 6th Edition. Washington, DC, American Psychiatric Association Publishing, 2024

References

Adler L, Angrist B, Peselow E, et al: Efficacy of propranolol in neuroleptic-induced akathesia. J Clin Psychopharmacol 5(3):164–166, 1985 2860136

Adler LA, Angrist B, Weinreb H, et al: Studies on the time course and efficacy of beta-blockers in neuroleptic-induced akathisia and the akathisia of idiopathic Parkinson's disease. Psychopharmacol Bull 27(2):107–111, 1991 1681561

Fleischhacker WW, Roth SD, Kane JM: The pharmacologic treatment of neuroleptic-induced akathisia. J Clin Psychopharmacol 10(1):12–21, 1990 1968470

Kapur S, Remington G: Serotonin-dopamine interaction and its relevance to schizophrenia. Am J Psychiatry 153(4):466–476, 1996 8599393

Kessing LV, Rytgaard HC, Ekstrøm CT, et al: Antihypertensive drugs and risk of depression: a nationwide population-based study. Hypertension 76(4):1263–1279, 2020

Poyurovsky M, Weizman A: Serotonin-based pharmacotherapy for acute neuroleptic-induced akathisia: a new approach to an old problem. Br J Psychiatry 179(JULY):4–8, 2001 11435260

Poyurovsky M, Weizman A: Treatment of antipsychotic-induced akathisia: role of serotonin 5-HT2a receptor antagonists. Drugs 80(9):871–882, 2020 32385739

Pringsheim T, Gardner D, Addington D, et al: The assessment and treatment of antipsychotic-induced akathisia. Can J Psychiatry 63(11):719–729, 2018 29685069

Thippaiah SM, Fargason RE, Birur B: Struggling to find effective pharmacologic options for akathisia? B-CALM! Psychopharmacol Bull 51(3):72–78, 2021 34421146

Wilbur R, Kulik FA, Kulik AV: Noradrenergic effects in tardive dyskinesia, akathisia and pseudoparkinsonism via the limbic system and basal ganglia. Prog Neuropsychopharmacol Biol Psychiatry 12(6):849–864, 1988 2907387

Alopecia

Overview

The development of hair loss and the severity of the same depend on the drug and the individual patient's predisposition. Some drugs cause hair loss in most patients receiving a certain dose, while other drugs are only occasionally responsible for hair loss (Dyall-Smith 2008).

There are two types of drug-induced hair loss: 1) anagen effluvium, the shedding of actively growing hairs, and 2) telogen effluvium, the shedding of resting or bulb hairs. Telogen effluvium is the mechanism of virtually all medication-induced hair loss. Psychotropic medications that are known to cause hair loss include valproic acid (occurring in 12%–28% of patients taking the medication [dose-dependent]), carbamazepine (occurring in up to 6%), and lithium (12%–19%) (Dyall-Smith 2008).

Hair loss because of medications is usually diffuse and nonscarring. The hair loss may be "patterned," as seen in male-pattern (androgenetic) alopecia or female-pattern alopecia. The scalp is the most common site affected, but all body hair, including eyebrows and eyelashes, may be lost, such as occurs with chemotherapy (Dyall-Smith 2008).

Anagen effluvium hair loss may become obvious within days of starting chemotherapy. In contrast, hair loss usually becomes evident after 2–4 months with telogen effluvium (Dyall-Smith 2008).

References

Dyall-Smith D: Alopecia from Drugs. DermNet NZ, 2008. Available at: https://dermnetnz.org/topics/alopecia-from-drugs. Accessed March 13, 2024.

Selenium (for Medication-Induced Alopecia)

I. **Mechanism of Action**:

A. Selenium is a component of an important antioxidase, glutathione peroxidase (Allan et al. 1999). Selenium is also incorporated into iodothyronine deiodinase, catalyzing thyroid hormone production (Rayman 2000). Low serum selenium levels trigger organic oxidative stress, inducing mitochondrial membrane apoptosis. This leads to hair cycle impairment and telogen effluvium (Hwang et al. 2011). Selenium depletion causes hyperplastic epidermis and aberrant morphogenesis of hair follicles, leading to hair loss (Tortelly Costa et al. 2018).

II. **Data**:

A. To prevent cardiomyopathy and skeletal muscle dysfunction, total parenteral nutrition is supplemented by selenium (van Rij et al. 1979). Selenium is used to treat Keshan disease–associated cardiomyopathy, some instances of male infertility, and Kashin-Beck disease–associated arthritis (Institute of Medicine Food and Nutrition Board 2000; Rayman 2008). Selenium is supplemented with iodine to prevent cretinism (Blackman et al. 2010). Lower selenium concentrations in people with HIV are associated with an increased risk of cardiomyopathy-related death. Low selenium in pregnant individuals with HIV facilitates HIV transmission to offspring (Kupka et al. 2005; Twagirumukiza et al. 2007). Selenium is thought to lower cancer risk (Lippman et al. 2009). Because of its antioxidant properties, selenium may play a role in helping with age-related cognitive decline, although this has not been consistently demonstrated in the literature (Perkins et al. 1999). Selenium can reduce the chances of postpartum thyroiditis in women with thyroid peroxidase antibodies (Negro et al. 2007).

III. **Dosing**:

A. Plasma or serum selenium concentrations of 8 µg/dL or higher in healthy people typically meet the body's needs for selenoprotein synthesis (Blackman et al. 2010). The recommended dietary allowance (RDA) for selenium is 55 µg daily for individuals ages 14 years and older (in U.S. populations). Selenium ingestion in an amount exceeding 400 µg daily may cause toxicity (Fan and Kizer 1990).

B. Dosing recommendations (Mayo Clinic 2024) for oral tablets are as follows (*Note*: To prevent deficiency, the amount is based on normal daily recommended intake.):

1. Adult and teenage males—40–70 micrograms (µg) per day
2. Adult and teenage females—45–55 µg/day
3. Pregnant females—65 µg/day
4. Breastfeeding females—75 µg/day
5. Children age 7–10 years—30 µg/day
6. Children age 4–6 years—20 µg/day
7. Children birth to age 3 years—10–20 µg/day

C. To treat selenium deficiency (Mayo Clinic 2024): For adults, teenagers, and children, the treatment dose is determined by the prescriber for each individual based on the severity of the deficiency.

IV. **Cautions/Monitoring**:

A. Long-term excessive dietary intake of selenium (>200 times the labeled amount per day) leads to chronic selenium toxicity, or *selenosis*. Intake can be from either "megadose" supplementation or from diets naturally high in selenium—for example, Brazil nuts contain exorbitant amounts of selenium (68–91 µg per nut). Toxicity initially manifests as a garlic odor with a subjective metallic taste. Other symptoms include hair and nail loss or brittleness, skin and nervous system lesions, nausea, diarrhea, skin rashes, mottled teeth, fatigue, irritability, and nervous system abnormalities (National Institutes of Health 2021).

B. Acute selenium toxicity can also cause severe gastrointestinal and neurological symptoms, acute respiratory distress syndrome, myocardial infarction, hair loss, muscle tenderness, tremors, lightheadedness, facial flushing, kidney failure, cardiac failure, and (rarely) death (Bowman 2006).
C. In one study, long-term consumption of nearly 5 mg/day of selenium from a plant-based diet resulted in hair and nail loss, tooth decay, dermatological lesions, and neurological effects (Yang et al. 1983). A case report of selenium toxicity described clinical manifestations including nausea, emesis, diarrhea, hair loss, nail changes, mental status changes, visual loss, and peripheral neuropathy, with associated abnormalities on brain MRI that resembled reversible posterior encephalopathy syndrome (Rae et al. 2018).
D. Cisplatin has been shown to reduce selenium levels in hair and serum. This interaction is of unknown significance (Dennert and Horneber 2006; Hu et al. 1997).
E. The most commonly used measures of selenium status are plasma and serum selenium concentrations (Ross et al. 2012). Analyses of hair or nail selenium content can be used to monitor longer-term intake over months or years. Quantification of one or more selenoproteins (e.g., glutathione peroxidase, selenoprotein P) is also used as a functional measure of selenium status (Terry and Diamond 2012). Reference values for serum selenium concentration fall in the range of approximately 46–143 μg/L (National Institutes of Health 2021).

Further Reading

Dyall-Smith D: Alopecia from drugs. DermNet NZ, 2008. Available at: https://dermnetnz.org/topics/alopecia-from-drugs. Accessed March 13, 2024.

National Institutes of Health Office of the Dietary Supplements. Available at: https://ods.od.nih.gov/. Accessed March 13, 2024.

References

Allan CB, Lacourciere GM, Stadtman TC: Responsiveness of selenoproteins to dietary selenium. Annu Rev Nutr 19:1–16, 1999 10448514

Blackman MR, Coates PM, Betz JM, eds: Encyclopedia of Dietary Supplements, 2nd Edition. New York, Informa Healthcare, 2010

Bowman RR: Present Knowledge in Nutrition, Ninth Edition. Washington, DC, International Life Sciences Institute, 2006

Dennert G, Horneber M: Selenium for alleviating the side effects of chemotherapy, radiotherapy and surgery in cancer patients. Cochrane Database Syst Rev (3):CD005037, 2006 16856073

Fan AM, Kizer KW: Selenium: nutritional, toxicologic, and clinical aspects. West J Med 153(2):160–167, 1990 2219873

Hu YJ, Chen Y, Zhang YQ, et al: The protective role of selenium on the toxicity of cisplatin-contained chemotherapy regimen in cancer patients. Biol Trace Elem Res 56(3):331–341, 1997 9197929

Hwang SW, Lee HJ, Suh KS, et al: Changes in murine hair with dietary selenium excess or deficiency. Exp Dermatol 20(4):367–369, 2011 21366699

Institute of Medicine Food and Nutrition Board: Dietary Reference Intakes for Vitamin C, Vitamin E, Selenium, and Carotenoids. Washington, DC, National Academy Press, 2000

Kupka R, Msamanga GI, Spiegelman D, et al: Selenium levels in relation to morbidity and mortality among children born to HIV-infected mothers. Eur J Clin Nutr 59(11):1250–1258, 2005 16015252

Lippman SM, Klein EA, Goodman PJ, et al: Effect of selenium and vitamin E on risk of prostate cancer and other cancers: the Selenium and Vitamin E Cancer Prevention Trial (SELECT). JAMA 301(1):39–51, 2009 19066370

Mayo Clinic: Selenium supplement (oral route). Last updated: February 1, 2024. Available at: https://www.mayoclinic.org/drugs-supplements/selenium-supplement-oral-route/proper-use/drg-20063649. Accessed July 8, 2024.

National Institutes of Health: Selenium Fact Sheet for Health Professionals. National Institutes of Health, 2021. Available at: https://ods.od.nih.gov/factsheets/Selenium-HealthProfessional/#h3. Accessed March 13, 2024.

Negro R, Greco G, Mangieri T, et al: The influence of selenium supplementation on postpartum thyroid status in pregnant women with thyroid peroxidase autoantibodies. J Clin Endocrinol Metab 92(4):1263–1268, 2007 17284630

Perkins AJ, Hendrie HC, Callahan CM, et al: Association of antioxidants with memory in a multiethnic elderly sample using the Third National Health and Nutrition Examination Survey. Am J Epidemiol 150(1):37–44, 1999 10400551

Rae W, Kitley J, Pinto A: Selenium toxicity associated with reversible leukoencephalopathy and cortical blindness. JAMA Neurol 75(10):1282–1283, 2018 29971355

Rayman MP: The importance of selenium to human health. Lancet 356(9225):233–241, 2000 10963212

Rayman MP: Food-chain selenium and human health: emphasis on intake. Br J Nutr 100(2):254–268, 2008 18346308

Ross AC, Caballero B, Cousins RJ, et al. (eds): Modern Nutrition in Health and Disease, Eleventh Edition. Philadelphia, Lippincott Williams & Wilkins, 2012

Terry EN, Diamond AM: Present Knowledge in Nutrition, 10th Edition. Edited by Zeisel SH, Erdman JW, Macdonald IA. Washington, DC, Wiley-Blackwell, 2012

Tortelly Costa VD, Melo DF, Matsunaga AM: The relevance of selenium to alopecias. Int J Trichology 10(2):92–93, 2018 29769785

Twagirumukiza M, Nkeramihigo E, Seminega B, et al: Prevalence of dilated cardiomyopathy in HIV-infected African patients not receiving HAART: a multicenter, observational, prospective, cohort study in Rwanda. Curr HIV Res 5(1):129–137, 2007 17266564

van Rij AM, Thomson CD, McKenzie JM, et al: Selenium deficiency in total parenteral nutrition. Am J Clin Nutr 32(10):2076–2085, 1979 114045

Yang GQ, Wang SZ, Zhou RH, et al: Endemic selenium intoxication of humans in China. Am J Clin Nutr 37(5):872–881, 1983 6846228

Zinc (for Medication-Induced Alopecia)

I. **Mechanism of Action**:

A. Zinc plays an essential role in growth, tissue repair, and wound healing. It plays a vital role in lipid and glucose metabolism. Zinc is necessary for cell immunity, and its deficiency causes decreased interleukin-2 production (Dardenne 2002; Haase and Rink 2009; Olechnowicz et al. 2018; Prasad 2007; Shankar and Prasad 1998). Zinc, combined with histidine and cysteine, provides nuclear structural stability.

Zinc-containing proteins play an essential role in gene transcription (Matthews and Sunde 2002; Mehri 2020; Wagner et al. 2011; Zalewski et al. 1993).

B. Zinc sulfate injection is FDA approved for adult and pediatric patients on parenteral nutrition when oral or enteral nutrition is not possible (American Regent 2019). Some reports have suggested zinc supplementation if zinc levels are below 70 μg/dL (Kil et al. 2013).

II. **Data**:

A. Alopecia due to zinc deficiency shows hair regrowth on zinc supplementation (Alhaj et al. 2007; Almohanna et al. 2019). Zinc helps with immune functions by T-lymphocyte activation and bolstering macrophage and neutrophil functions, natural killer cell activity, and complement activity (Beck et al. 1997; Wintergerst et al. 2007). Low zinc levels are associated with recurrent pneumonia in children and older adults (Brooks et al. 2005; Meydani et al. 2007). Skin ulcers improve in response to zinc supplementation, as zinc helps maintain skin and mucosal integrity (Wilkinson 2014; Wilkinson and Hawke 1998). Zinc helps reduce the duration and severity of diarrhea in zinc-deficient or otherwise malnourished children (Lukacik et al. 2008). The World Health Organization has recommended short-term zinc supplementation (20 mg/day of zinc, or 10 mg for infants younger than 6 months, for 10–14 days) to treat acute childhood diarrhea (World Health Organization and United Nations Childrens Fund 2004). Zinc deficiency can cause endemic hypogonadism and dwarfism (Prasad 1985a, 1985b). Zinc deficiency also causes increased mortality from upper respiratory infections and diarrhea (Gibson et al. 2016).

B. Acrodermatitis enteropathica, an autosomal recessive disease, causes zinc malabsorption from infancy onward and responds to lifelong administration of higher dosages of oral zinc supplementation (30–45 mg/day) (King and Klein 2000).

C. Zinc is an essential supplement for a patient taking total parenteral nutrition or long-term diuretics (Filler and Felder 2014; Sutherland et al. 1998; Walter et al. 1991). Zinc has been associated with neuronal excitability, associated excitability disorders, and myelination (Takeuchi et al. 2020).

III. **Dosing**:

A. The current recommended dietary allowance (RDA) for zinc is 11 mg in adult males, 8 mg for females, and 11 mg and 12 mg, respectively, for pregnant and lactating females (Institute of Medicine Food and Nutrition Board 2001). Zinc is safe for most pregnant and breastfeeding women when used in the RDA amounts. However, zinc is unsafe when used at high dosages by breastfeeding women and is considered dangerous when used at high dosages by pregnant women. Pregnant women older than 18 years should not take zinc at dosages higher than 40 mg/day, and pregnant women age 14–18 years should not take dosages higher than 34 mg/day. Breastfeeding women older than 18 years should not take zinc at dosages higher than 40 mg/day, and breastfeeding women age 14–18 years should not take dosages higher than 34 mg/day (RxList.com n.d.).

IV. **Cautions/Monitoring**:

A. Although poorly correlated with tissue zinc levels, plasma zinc levels are still a good measure of body zinc status. Erythrocyte concentrations and alkaline phosphatase activity provide a better standard of zinc status during acute or chronic inflammation (Institute of Medicine Food and Nutrition Board 2001; Oakes et al. 2008).

B. Zinc interacts with quinolone antibiotics and tetracyclines to inhibit the absorption of both zinc and the antibiotics (Lomaestro and Bailie 1995). Similar malabsorption occurs when zinc is combined with penicillamine (Brewer et al. 1993). Zinc supplementation should be taken at least 2 hours before or 6 hours after antibiotic intake. Thiazide diuretics such as hydrochlorothiazide increase zinc excretion by as much as 60%, and prolonged use of thiazides can deplete zinc tissue levels (Wester 1980). Large amounts of supplemental iron (>25 mg) might decrease zinc absorption (Institute of Medicine Food and Nutrition Board 2001). Taking iron supplements between meals helps reduce zinc absorption (Whittaker 1998a). Fortification of foods with iron does not significantly affect zinc absorption. High zinc intake can inhibit copper absorption, sometimes producing copper deficiency and associated anemia.

C. Acute zinc toxicity was reported with an ingestion of more than 570 mg of elemental zinc. Long-term use of 150–500 mg/day of zinc can lead to chronic zinc toxicity (Lewis and Kokan 1998). Acute toxicity effects include nausea, vomiting, loss of appetite, abdominal cramps, diarrhea, and headaches (Institute of Medicine Food and Nutrition Board 2001). Chronic zinc toxicity results in low copper status, altered iron function, reduced immune function, and reduced levels of high-density lipoproteins (Freeland-Graves et al. 1982). Consumption of zinc at doses greater than 60 mg/day for more than five decades was shown to cause genitourinary problems and to reduce the activity of copper-containing enzymes (Johnson et al. 2007).

D. Beans, nuts, certain types of seafood (e.g., crab, lobster), whole grains, fortified breakfast cereals, and dairy products are rich sources of zinc. Oysters, red meat, and poultry are other excellent sources of zinc (Agricultural Research Service 2024; Institute of Medicine Food and Nutrition Board 2001). The population at risk for zinc deficiency includes patients with anorexia nervosa, inflammatory bowel disease, jejunal bypass surgery, or cystic fibrosis. Alcohol use disorder, malignancy, burns, infection, and pregnancy may cause increased zinc metabolism and excretion (Almohanna et al. 2019).

References

Agricultural Research Service: FoodData Central [Internet]. U.S. Department of Agriculture, Beltsville Human Nutrition Research Center. Available at: https://fdc.nal.usda.gov/. Accessed July 8, 2024.

Alhaj E, Alhaj N, Alhaj NE: Diffuse alopecia in a child due to dietary zinc deficiency. Skinmed 6(4):199–200, 2007 17618180

Almohanna HM, Ahmed AA, Tsatalis JP, et al: The role of vitamins and minerals in hair loss: a review. Dermatol Ther (Heidelb) 9(1):51–70, 2019 30547302

American Regent: Prescribing information for zinc sulfate. Revised July 2019. Available at: https://www.accessdata.fda.gov/drugsatfda_docs/label/2019/209377s000lbl.pdf. Accessed January 31, 2020.

Beck FWJ, Prasad AS, Kaplan J, et al: Changes in cytokine production and T cell subpopulations in experimentally induced zinc-deficient humans. Am J Physiol 272(6 Pt 1):E1002–E1007, 1997 9227444

Brewer GJ, Yuzbasiyan-Gurkan V, Johnson V, et al: Treatment of Wilson's disease with zinc, XI: interaction with other anticopper agents. J Am Coll Nutr 12(1):26–30, 1993 8440814

Brooks WA, Santosham M, Naheed A, et al: Effect of weekly zinc supplements on incidence of pneumonia and diarrhoea in children younger than 2 years in an urban, low-income population in Bangladesh: randomised controlled trial. Lancet 366(9490):999–1004, 2005 16168782

Dardenne M: Zinc and immune function. Eur J Clin Nutr 56(Suppl 3):S20–S23, 2002 12142956

Filler G, Felder S: Trace elements in dialysis. Pediatr Nephrol 29(8):1329–1335, 2014 23949629

Freeland-Graves JH, Friedman BJ, Han W-H, et al: Effect of zinc supplementation on plasma high-density lipoprotein cholesterol and zinc. Am J Clin Nutr 35(5):988–992, 1982 7081096

Gibson RS, King JC, Lowe N: A review of dietary zinc recommendations. Food Nutr Bull 37(4):443–460, 2016 27312357

Haase H, Rink L: Functional significance of zinc-related signaling pathways in immune cells. Annu Rev Nutr 29(August):133–152, 2009 19400701

Institute of Medicine Food and Nutrition Board: Dietary reference intakes for Vitamin A, Vitamin K, Arsenic, Boron, Chromium, Copper, Iodine, Iron, Manganese, Molybdenum, Nickel, Silicon, Vanadium, and Zinc. Washington, DC, National Academy Press, 2001

Johnson AR, Munoz A, Gottlieb JL, et al: High dose zinc increases hospital admissions due to genitourinary complications. J Urol 177(2):639–643, 2007 17222649

Kil MS, Kim CW, Kim SS: Analysis of serum zinc and copper concentrations in hair loss. Ann Dermatol 25(4):405–409, 2013 24371385

King JC, Klein CL: Modern Nutrition in Health and Disease. Edited by CL King, JC, Klein. Philadelphia: Lippincott Williams & Wilkins, 2000

Lewis MR, Kokan L: Zinc gluconate: acute ingestion. J Toxicol Clin Toxicol 36(1–2):99–101, 1998 9541053

Lomaestro BM, Bailie GR: Absorption interactions with fluoroquinolones: 1995 update. Drug Saf 12(5):314–333, 1995 7669261

Lukacik M, Thomas RL, Aranda JV: A meta-analysis of the effects of oral zinc in the treatment of acute and persistent diarrhea. Pediatrics 121(2):326–336, 2008 18245424

Matthews JM, Sunde M: Zinc fingers—folds for many occasions. IUBMB Life 54(6):351–355, 2002 12665246

Mehri A: Trace elements in human nutrition (II)—an update. Int J Prev Med 11(1):2, 2020 32042399

Meydani SN, Barnett JB, Dallal GE, et al: Serum zinc and pneumonia in nursing home elderly. Am J Clin Nutr 86(4):1167–1173, 2007 17921398

Oakes EJ, Lyon TD, Duncan A, et al: Acute inflammatory response does not affect erythrocyte concentrations of copper, zinc and selenium. Clin Nutr 27(1):115–120, 2008 18037540

Olechnowicz J, Tinkov A, Skalny A, et al: Zinc status is associated with inflammation, oxidative stress, lipid, and glucose metabolism. J Physiol Sci 68(1):19–31, 2018 28965330

Prasad AS: Clinical manifestations of zinc deficiency. Annu Rev Nutr 5:341–363, 1985a 3896271

Prasad AS: Clinical, endocrinological and biochemical effects of zinc deficiency. Clin Endocrinol Metab 14(3):567–589, 1985b 3905080

Prasad AS: Zinc: mechanisms of host defense. J Nutr 137(5):1345–1349, 2007 17449604

RxList.com: Zinc. n.d. Available at: https://www.rxlist.com/zinc/supplements.htm. Accessed March 8, 2022.

Shankar AH, Prasad AS: Zinc and immune function: the biological basis of altered resistance to infection. Am J Clin Nutr 68(2)(Suppl):447S–463S, 1998 9701160

Sutherland B, Strong P, King JC: Determining human dietary requirements for boron. Biol Trace Elem Res 66(1–3):193–204, 1998 10050920

Takeuchi H, Taki Y, Nouchi R, et al: Succeeding in deactivating: associations of hair zinc levels with functional and structural neural mechanisms. Sci Rep 10(1):12364, 2020 32704167

Wagner K, Moolenaar GF, Goosen N: Role of the insertion domain and the zinc-finger motif of Escherichia coli UvrA in damage recognition and ATP hydrolysis. DNA Repair (Amst) 10(5):483–496, 2011 21393072

Walter RM Jr, Uriu-Hare JY, Olin KL, et al: Copper, zinc, manganese, and magnesium status and complications of diabetes mellitus. Diabetes Care 14(11):1050–1056, 1991 1797486

Wester PO: Urinary zinc excretion during treatment with different diuretics. Acta Med Scand 208(3):209–212, 1980 7001863

Whittaker P: Iron and zinc interactions in humans. Am J Clin Nutr 68(2)(Suppl):442S–446S, 1998 9701159

Wilkinson EAJ: Oral zinc for arterial and venous leg ulcers. Cochrane Database Syst Rev (9):CD001273, 2014

Wilkinson EAJ, Hawke CI: Does oral zinc aid the healing of chronic leg ulcers? A systematic literature review. Arch Dermatol 134(12):1556–1560, 1998 9875193

Wintergerst ES, Maggini S, Hornig DH: Contribution of selected vitamins and trace elements to immune function. Ann Nutr Metab 51(4):301–323, 2007 17726308

World Health Organization and United Nations Childrens Fund: Clinical management of acute diarrhoea. WHO/UNICEF Joint Statement, 2004

Zalewski PD, Forbes IJ, Betts WH: Correlation of apoptosis with change in intracellular labile Zn(II) using zinquin [(2-methyl-8-p-toluenesulphonamido-6-quinolyloxy)acetic acid], a new specific fluorescent probe for Zn(II). Biochem J 296(Pt 2):403–408, 1993 8257431

Dystonia

Overview

Dystonia is a movement disorder characterized by sustained or intermittent muscle contractions causing abnormal (often repetitive) movements, postures, or both. Dystonic movements are typically patterned, twisting, and may be tremulous in nature. Dystonia is often initiated or worsened by voluntary action and is associated with overflow muscle activation (Louis et al. 2022).

References

Louis ED, Mayer SA, Houston HM, et al. (eds): Merritt's Neurology, 14th Edition. Philadelphia: Wolters Kluwer, 2022

Benztropine or Trihexyphenidyl (for Medication-Induced Dystonia)

I. **Mechanism of Action**:

A. Trihexyphenidyl and benztropine are nonselective muscarinic acetylcholine receptor antagonists.

B. Trihexyphenidyl and benztropine have a higher affinity for central muscarinic receptors in the cerebral cortex than peripherally (Lewis and O'Day 2023). Trihexyphenidyl may modify nicotinic acetylcholine receptor neurotransmission, leading indirectly to enhanced dopamine release in the striatum. Trihexyphenidyl produces an atropine-like blocking action on parasympathetic-innervated peripheral structures, including smooth muscle. In addition, trihexyphenidyl exhibits a direct spasmolytic action on smooth muscle and exhibits weak mydriatic, antisialagogue, and cardiovagal blocking effects (Vintage Pharmaceuticals 1997).

C. Benztropine mesylate contains the atropine portion of the atropine molecule and the benzohydryl portion of diphenhydramine resulting in both anticholinergic and antihistaminic effects. However, only the former has been established as therapeutically significant in managing parkinsonism (Pendopharm 2022). Acetylcholine has inhibitory effects on body movement, and dopamine has grossly excitatory effects on movement. Hyperactivity of the cholinergic interneurons may explain the improvement of dystonia with anticholinergics (Deffains and Bergman 2015). More recent evidence has also supported the role of cholinergic interneurons in abnormal corticostriatal synaptic plasticity. Anticholinergics act as antagonists at postsynaptic M_1 receptors. Some medications also act at other receptors (e.g., biperiden at nicotinic receptors; procyclidine at M_2 and M_4 receptors) (Pakkenberg and Pedersen 1985).

D. Benztropine may also prolong the action of dopamine by inhibiting its reuptake and storage (Sridharan and Sivaramakrishnan 2018).

II. **Data**:

A. A prospective double-blind placebo-controlled crossover trial of anticholinergics in children and young adults with torsion dystonia used trihexyphenidyl dosages of up to 120 mg/day. A clinically significant response was seen in 71% of 31 patients, and benefit remained in 42% of the patients after 2.4 years of follow-up. More benefit was demonstrated in children, possibly due to better tolerability, and in patients who received treatment earlier, within 5 years of disease onset (Burke et al. 1986; Greene et al. 1988).

B. Benztropine is FDA approved for use as adjunctive therapy for all forms of parkinsonism, including idiopathic parkinsonism and postencephalitic parkinsonism (Friedman et al. 1997; Paulson and Buffaloe 1965). Benztropine is also used for treatment of drug-induced extrapyramidal symptoms, prevention of dystonic reactions, and treatment of acute dystonic reactions. Benztropine has been used off-label for chronic sialorrhea in developmentally disabled patients (Sridharan and Sivaramakrishnan 2018). Benztropine antagonizes acetylcholine and histamine receptors. Benztropine exerts its action in the CNS and smooth muscle by competing with acetylcholine at muscarinic receptors. It reduces central cholinergic effects by blocking muscarinic receptors, which improves the symptoms of parkinsonism (Friedman et al. 1997).

III. **Dosing**:

A. Trihexyphenidyl should be started with a 1-mg tablet and slowly increased by half-tablets (i.e., half of the 1-mg tablet) until optimal benefit is reached or side effects are encountered.

B. Benztropine therapy may start with the lowest initial dose of 0.5 mg and may increase up to 6 mg over 5–6 days. Benztropine has cumulative action, so the dose should be gradually increased by 0.5 mg until optimal results are obtained.

C. For the symptomatic relief of antipsychotic-induced extrapyramidal side effects (except tardive dyskinesia), the recommended benztropine oral or parenteral dosage is 1–6 mg once or twice daily. The dosage must be individualized according to the patient's response and tolerance. For the symptomatic relief of extrapyramidal side effects that develop shortly after the initiation of antipsychotic (e.g., phenothiazine) therapy, the total daily dosage range for trihexyphenidyl is 5–15 mg for most patients, although there have been reported cases of symptoms being sufficiently controlled at dosages as low as 1 mg/day (Jilani et al. 2024). Because acute extrapyramidal symptoms are generally transient, the need for benztropine should be reevaluated after 1–2 weeks of therapy. There is evidence from animal studies that anticholinergic drugs could cause tardive dyskinesia (Bergman and Soares-Weiser 2018).

D. For acute dystonic reactions, benztropine mesylate 1–2 mg may be given IV (or IM), followed by 1–2 mg PO twice daily to prevent a recurrence.

E. There is no significant clinical difference in the time to onset of action of benztropine between intramuscular and intravenous administration.

IV. **Cautions/Monitoring**:

A. Benztropine is contraindicated during breastfeeding as a cautionary measure (LactMed 2018). Use of benztropine during pregnancy is neither recommended based on evidence nor contraindicated.
B. Common side effects of benztropine in older adults are delirium, confusion, drug-induced dementia, benign prostatic hyperplasia in males, and urinary tract problems (Friedman 2006).
C. Patients should have the iridocorneal angle examined before and intraocular pressure monitored during anticholinergic therapy. For benztropine, patients should be kept under close monitoring, especially at the beginning of treatment or whenever the dosage is changed (Lupu et al. 2017). Older adult patients can have a more intense response to anticholinergic medicines (Friedman et al. 1997).
D. Trihexyphenidyl may cause severe cognitive impairment, including confusion, disorientation, and aggression. Because of this drug's parasympathetic activity, caution is recommended when using trihexyphenidyl in patients with glaucoma or obstructive gastrointestinal or genitourinary tract disease or in elderly male patients with prostatic hypertrophy. Trihexyphenidyl can precipitate glaucoma (Vintage Pharmaceuticals 1997). Benztropine is contraindicated in children younger than 3 years (including infants and neonates).
E. Anticholinergics may slow gastrointestinal motility. Use of anticholinergics (e.g., benztropine) requires caution, as does use of other medications with anticholinergic properties, such as zonisamide, clozapine, topiramate, and certain antipsychotics (e.g., haloperidol) and tricyclic antidepressants (RxList 2023; WebMD 2024).
F. The adverse effects of anticholinergics encompass central and autonomic symptoms. Central side effects include sedation, cognitive slowing, confusion, memory impairment, psychosis, and chorea. Autonomic side effects include blurred vision due to mydriasis, dry mouth, urinary retention, and constipation.
G. Anticholinergics are contraindicated in individuals with a history of acute angle-closure glaucoma. Certain autonomic side effects may be relieved by using pilocarpine eye drops (for blurred vision) or pyridostigmine (Taylor et al. 1991). Abrupt discontinuation of anticholinergics has been reported in rare cases to worsen dystonia and can even trigger life-threatening cholinergic crises (Giménez-Roldán et al. 1989).
H. Side effects reported more rarely with trihexyphenidyl hydrochloride include isolated instances of suppurative parotitis secondary to excessive mouth dryness; skin rashes; dilatation of the colon; paralytic ileus; and specific psychiatric manifestations (e.g., delusions, hallucinations).
I. Patients with arteriosclerosis or a history of idiosyncratic hypersensitivity to other drugs may exhibit mental confusion, agitation, disturbed behavior, or nausea and vomiting in response to trihexyphenidyl hydrochloride. A gradual increase in the dose of anticholinergics should be adhered to. If a severe reaction should occur, administration of the drug should be discontinued for a few days and then resumed at a lower dosage. Psychiatric disturbances can result from indiscriminate use.

J. Potential side effects associated with the use of any atropine-like drugs include constipation, drowsiness, urinary hesitancy or retention, tachycardia, dilation of the pupil, increased intraocular tension, weakness, vomiting, and headache (Drugs.com 2024; Jilani et al. 2024).

K. Benztropine overdose can cause anticholinergic toxicity. In cooperative and alert patients, administering 50 g of activated charcoal is recommended within 2 hours after the benztropine ingestion. Physostigmine is the antidote for benztropine toxicity in the event delirium is not controlled through benzodiazepines, but has central cardiac effects and should be used with caution (Thornton et al. 2016).

L. Anticholinergics should be used cautiously in patients with any cognitive impairment, constipation, and symptoms of prostatism (Taylor et al. 1991).

M. In addition, before prescribing benztropine, it is advisable to rule out toxic megacolon, paralytic ileus, and ocular hypertension (American Society of Health-System Pharmacists 2024).

N. In clinical practice, the issue of anticholinergic withdrawal does not appear to be as much of a concern for benztropine as it is for baclofen or benzodiazepines.

O. Central stimulation with trihexyphenidyl is much higher than with benztropine. The effects of trihexyphenidyl are cumulative and may not be evident until 2 or 3 days after treatment has begun (American Society of Health-System Pharmacists 2024).

Further Reading

Ahuja A, Patel P, Abdijadid S: Benztropine, in StatPearls [Internet]. Treasure Island, FL, StatPearls Publishing, last update January 29, 2024. Available at: https://www.ncbi.nlm.nih.gov/books/NBK560633/. Accessed March 13, 2024.

Lynch MJ, Kotsos A: Fatal benztropine toxicity. Med Sci Law 41(2):155–158, 2001 11368397

McIntyre IM, Mallett P, Burton CG, et al: Acute benztropine intoxication and fatality. J Forensic Sci 59(6):1675–1678, 2014 24697166

References

American Society of Health-System Pharmacists: Benztropine (monograph). Medically reviewed by Drugs.com on February 7, 2024. Available at: https://www.drugs.com/monograph/benztropine.html. Accessed July 29, 2024.

Bergman H, Soares-Weiser K: Anticholinergic medication for antipsychotic-induced tardive dyskinesia. Cochrane Database Syst Rev (1):CD000204, 2018 29341071

Burke RE, Fahn S, Marsden CD: Torsion dystonia: a double-blind, prospective trial of high-dosage trihexyphenidyl. Neurology 36(2):160–164, 1986 3511401

Deffains M, Bergman H: Striatal cholinergic interneurons and cortico-striatal synaptic plasticity in health and disease. Mov Disord 30(8):1014–1025, 2015 26095280

Drugs.com: Trihexyphenidyl: USAGE, forms of parkinsonism with levodopa. Drugs.com; Last updated March 18, 2024. Available at: https://www.drugs.com/pro/trihexyphenidyl.html. Accessed April 11, 2024.

Friedman JH: Anticholinergics in dementia and other confounding problems. Am J Geriatr Psychiatry 14(4):384, 2006 16582052

Friedman JH, Koller WC, Lannon MC, et al: Benztropine versus clozapine for the treatment of tremor in Parkinson's disease. Neurology 48(4):1077–1081, 1997 9109903

Giménez-Roldán S, Mateo D, Martín M: Life-threatening cranial dystonia following trihexyphenidyl withdrawal. Mov Disord 4(4):349–353, 1989 2811895

Greene P, Shale H, Fahn S: Analysis of open-label trials in torsion dystonia using high dosages of anticholinergics and other drugs. Mov Disord 3(1):46–60, 1988 3050472

Jilani TN, Sabir S, Patel P: Trihexyphenidyl, in StatPearls [Internet]. Treasure Island, FL, StatPearls Publishing, last update June 8, 2024. Available at: https://www.ncbi.nlm.nih.gov/books/NBK519488/. Accessed July 31, 2024.

LactMed: Benztropine. National Library of Medicine, 2018. Available at: https://pubmed.ncbi.nlm.nih.gov/30000721/. Accessed March 13, 2024.

Lewis K, O'Day CS: Dystonic reactions, in StatPearls. Treasure Island, FL, StatPearls Publishing, last update May 1, 2023. Available at: https://pubmed.ncbi.nlm.nih.gov/30285361/. Accessed March 13, 2024.

Lupu AM, Clinebell K, Gannon JM, et al: Reducing anticholinergic medication burden in patients with psychotic or bipolar disorders. J Clin Psychiatry 78(9):e1270–e1275, 2017 29178683

Pakkenberg H, Pedersen B: Medical treatment of dystonia. Psychopharmacology Suppl 2:111–117, 1985 2860654

Paulson G, Buffaloe WJ: Some remarks on the treatment of post-encephalitic oculogyric crises with benztropine methanesulfonate. Int J Neuropsychiatry 1:214–215, 1965 14309084

Pendopharm: Pdp-Benztropine package insert. Pendopharm, n.d. Available at: https://pdf.hres.ca/dpd_pm/00029138.PDF. Accessed February 3, 2022.

RxList: Cogentin. Last updated May 6, 2023. Available at: https://www.rxlist.com/cogentin-drug.htm#description. Accessed March 13, 2024.

Sridharan K, Sivaramakrishnan G: Pharmacological interventions for treating sialorrhea associated with neurological disorders: a mixed treatment network meta-analysis of randomized controlled trials. J Clin Neurosci 51:12–17, 2018 29475576

Taylor AE, Lang AE, Saint-Cyr JA, et al: Cognitive processes in idiopathic dystonia treated with high-dose anticholinergic therapy: implications for treatment strategies. Clin Neuropharmacol 14(1):62–77, 1991 2029694

Thornton SL, Farnaes L, Minns A: Prolonged antimuscarinic delirium in a child due to benztropine exposure treated with multiple doses of physostigmine. Pediatr Emerg Care 32(4):243–245, 2016 26383155

Vintage Pharmaceuticals: Trihexyphenidyl package insert. Revised August 1997. Available at: https://www.accessdata.fda.gov/drugsatfda_docs/anda/98/40254_Trihexyphenidyl%20Hydrochloride_Prntlbl.pdf. Accessed July 15, 2024.

WebMD: Benztropine mesylate: uses, side effects, and more. WebMD, n.d. Available at: https://www.webmd.com/drugs/2/drug-8619/benztropine-oral/details. Accessed July 29, 2024.

Hyperprolactinemia

Overview

Prolactin secretion from the pituitary gland is controlled by the hypothalamus mainly through dopamine (prolactin inhibiting factor) and thyrotropin-releasing hormone (TRH) acting as a release factor. Serum prolactin levels may rise in both physiological (pregnancy, lactation, sleep, stress) and pathological conditions (brain and systemic diseases).

Hyperprolactinemia in patients with psychosis is influenced by gender, age (Cookson et al. 2012; Dehelean et al. 2020; Vitiello et al. 2009), overt or subclinical hypothyroidism, psychotropic medications such as antipsychotics, and subtype of psychosis (Meltzer et al. 1974). During antipsychotic treatment, prolactin blood levels may rise up to 10 times the normal average values (Haddad and Wieck 2004). Prolactin levels greater than 250 ng/mL are highly indicative of prolactinomas, whereas levels in drug-induced hyperprolactinemia do not usually exceed 100 ng/mL (Vilar et al. 2019).

References

Cookson J, Hodgson R, Wildgust HJ: Prolactin, hyperprolactinaemia and antipsychotic treatment: a review and lessons for treatment of early psychosis. J Psychopharmacol 26(5)(Suppl):42–51, 2012 22472310

Dehelean L, Romosan AM, Papava I, et al: Prolactin response to antipsychotics: an inpatient study. PLoS One 15(2):e0228648, 2020 32017792

Haddad PM, Wieck A: Antipsychotic-induced hyperprolactinaemia: mechanisms, clinical features and management. Drugs 64(20):2291–2314, 2004 15456328

Meltzer HY, Sachar EJ, Frantz AG: Serum prolactin levels in unmedicated schizophrenic patients. Arch Gen Psychiatry 31(4):564–569, 1974 4422004

Vilar L, Vilar CF, Lyra R, et al: Pitfalls in the diagnostic evaluation of hyperprolactinemia. Neuroendocrinology 109(1):7–19, 2019 30889571

Vitiello B, Correll C, van Zwieten-Boot B, et al: Antipsychotics in children and adolescents: increasing use, evidence for efficacy and safety concerns. Eur Neuropsychopharmacol 19(9):629–635, 2009 19467582

Aripiprazole (for Medication-Induced Hyperprolactinemia)

I. **Mechanism of Action:**

A. Aripiprazole causes prolactin-normalizing effects by being a partial dopamine agonist with a high affinity for dopamine D_2 receptors (Lu et al. 2008). Aripiprazole is a partial agonist at D_2 and 5-HT_{2A} receptors and has an affinity for adrenergic (alpha$_1$-adrenergic blocking activity) and histaminergic, but not cholinergic, receptors. Aripiprazole also has a high affinity for D_2, D_3, 5-HT_{1A}, and 5-HT_{2A} receptors and a moderate affinity for D_4, 5-HT_{2C}, 5-HT_7, alpha$_1$-adrenergic, and H_1 receptors. It also possesses a moderate affinity for the serotonin reuptake transporter (de Bartolomeis et al. 2015).

B. In instances of atypical antipsychotic–induced elevation of prolactin, if changing the antipsychotic is not an option, adding aripiprazole to an existing antipsychotic may be helpful.

II. **Data:**

A. A post hoc subanalysis of an 8-week open-label study in outpatients with schizophrenia examined the short-term effects on prolactin levels during a switch from risperidone or olanzapine to aripiprazole 30 mg/day. Following aripiprazole initiation, mean prolactin levels had decreased significantly ($P<0.001$) at week 1, and decreases were maintained to week 8 in all groups, irrespective of prior treatment. Previously elevated prolactin levels in the risperidone groups were reduced to within normal range within 1 week (Byerly et al. 2009).

B. A study investigated the effects of 8 weeks of adjunctive treatment with aripiprazole in patients with hyperprolactinemia induced either by risperidone or by benzamide antipsychotics (amisulpride or sulpiride). Aripiprazole was administered to 24 patients with antipsychotic-induced hyperprolactinemia. The aripiprazole dosage was 5–20 mg/day during the 8-week study period. Serum prolactin levels were measured at weeks 4 and 8. Mean (standard error) prolactin levels decreased for patients taking risperidone. Adjunctive aripiprazole treatment effectively reversed hyperprolactinemia induced by risperidone (from 77.0±13.3 ng/mL to 18.3±2.1 ng/mL [$P<0.001$ vs. baseline]) but was less effective for hyperprolactinemia induced by a benzamide antipsychotic (amisulpride or sulpiride) (Chen et al. 2010).

C. Another study assessed the time course of changes in antipsychotic-induced hyperprolactinemia during antipsychotic switching to aripiprazole. Assessment scales and serum prolactin levels were measured at baseline, during the combination treatment period, and 4 weeks after the complete discontinuation of the preexisting antipsychotic treatment. Switching antipsychotic drugs to aripiprazole was effective in reducing serum prolactin levels and restoring menstruation in patients with schizophrenia who received prolactin-raising antipsychotics (Lu et al. 2008).

D. In a clinical trial involving 13 patients with schizophrenia or other unspecified psychosis who were being treated with long-acting injectable risperidone and had increased serum prolactin levels, subjects received an additional fixed dosage of 5 mg/day of aripiprazole for 3 months. Twelve of the 13 patients showed a decrease in serum prolactin levels (81±46 μg/L at baseline vs. 42±21 μg/L at 1 month; $P<0.001$, 52% mean reduction). The addition of aripiprazole 5 mg/day was associated with a significant decrease in hyperprolactinemia with no significant additional toxicity in patients with chronic psychosis (Ziadi Trives et al. 2013).

E. In a review of 17 studies, 3,489 psychotic patients were given aripiprazole alone, aripiprazole as an adjuvant to haloperidol or risperidone, or aripiprazole to treat psychosis with a concomitant prolactinoma. Across all studies, aripiprazole lowered prolactin levels by an average of 74.3%, even in psychotic patients with prolactinomas. In contrast, haloperidol and risperidone increased prolactin levels by 272% (Hoffer et al. 2009).

F. A recent systematic review and network analysis indicated that patients with antipsychotic-induced hyperprolactinemia benefit from the strategies of adjunctive aripiprazole or switching to aripiprazole. Patients with initial prolactin levels lower than 50 ng/mL might not need special intervention. Adjunctive use of—or a switch to—aripiprazole has been shown to produce a greater decrease in prolactin levels for levels that were higher than 50 ng/mL. However, only adjunctive aripiprazole (5 mg/day) showed a significant reduction in prolactin when its initial level was greater than 100 ng/mL (Lu et al. 2022).

III. **Dosing**:

A. The recommended dosage range for aripiprazole is 5–10 mg/day (Li et al. 2022; Meng et al. 2015; Shim et al. 2007).

B. Studies have found no relationship between the percentage reduction in prolactin and the aripiprazole dosage or treatment duration. Most studies have found aripiprazole to be helpful in reducing prolactin levels when taken at 5–10 mg/day. The reduction in prolactin level is seen as early as 2 weeks after starting aripiprazole (Raveendranthan et al. 2018). Other studies have also demonstrated a decrease in prolactin levels as early as 2 weeks, with a sustained benefit over time with concomitant aripiprazole (Zhao et al. 2015).

IV. **Cautions/Monitoring**:

A. Aripiprazole is contraindicated in patients with hypersensitivity (e.g., anaphylaxis, pruritus, urticaria) to aripiprazole or to any component of its formulation. Weight/height/BMI should be checked at 8 and 12 weeks after initiation and dosage changes.

B. Adverse cerebrovascular events associated with aripiprazole include stroke in geriatric patients with dementia-related psychosis (Otsuka America Pharmaceutical 2018), neuroleptic malignant syndrome (Srephichit et al. 2006), tardive dyskinesia (Aguilar et al. 2019), metabolic changes (Gupta et al. 2021), dyslipidemia (Bernardo et al. 2021; Hiemke et al. 2018), weight gain (Wu et al. 2022), pathological gambling and other compulsive behaviors (Corbeil et al. 2021), orthostatic hypotension (Takahashi et al. 2021), falls (Layton et al. 2022), leukopenia, neutropenia, and agranulocytosis (Felin et al. 2018).

C. Older adult patients with dementia-related psychosis treated with antipsychotic drugs are at an increased risk of death (Maust et al. 2015; Rubino et al. 2020).

D. During pregnancy, use of an agent other than aripiprazole is preferred (Larsen et al. 2015). Aripiprazole crosses the placenta. Aripiprazole and dehydro-aripiprazole can be detected in the cord blood at delivery (Nguyen et al. 2011; Watanabe et al. 2011). Aripiprazole has been detected in human breast milk (Nordeng et al. 2014).

E. Each aripiprazole 10- or 15-mg orally disintegrating tablet contains aspartame. Patients with phenylketonuria (i.e., homozygous genetic deficiency of phenylalanine hydroxylase) and other individuals who must restrict their intake of phenylalanine should be warned. Following oral administration, aspartame is metabolized in the gastrointestinal tract to phenylalanine, aspartic acid, and methanol (Council on Scientific Affairs 1985).

Further Reading

Aripiprazole prescribing information: 2002. Available at: https://www.accessdata.fda.gov/drugsatfda_docs/label/2014/021436s038,021713s030,021729s022,021866s023lbl.pdf. Accessed March 13, 2024.

Besag FMC, Vasey MJ, Salim I: Is adjunct aripiprazole effective in treating hyperprolactinemia induced by psychotropic medication? A narrative review. CNS Drugs 35(5):507–526, 2021 33880739

Keepers GA, Fochtmann LJ, Anzia JM, et al: The American Psychiatric Association Practice Guideline for the Treatment of Patients With Schizophrenia. Am J Psychiatry 177(9):868–872, 2020 32867516

Labad J, Montalvo I, González-Rodríguez A, et al: Pharmacological treatment strategies for lowering prolactin in people with a psychotic disorder and hyperprolactinaemia: a systematic review and meta-analysis. Schizophr Res 222:88–96, 2020 32507371

References

Aguilar L, Lorenzo C, Fernández-Ovejero R, et al: Tardive dyskinesia after aripiprazole treatment that improved with tetrabenazine, clozapine, and botulinum toxin. Front Pharmacol 10:281, 2019 30949057

Bernardo M, Rico-Villademoros F, García-Rizo C, et al: Real-world data on the adverse metabolic effects of second-generation antipsychotics and their potential determinants in adult patients: a systematic review of population-based studies. Adv Ther 38(5):2491–2512, 2021 33826090

Byerly MJ, Marcus RN, Tran QV, et al: Effects of aripiprazole on prolactin levels in subjects with schizophrenia during cross-titration with risperidone or olanzapine: analysis of a randomized, open-label study. Schizophr Res 107(2–3):218–222, 2009 19038534

Chen CK, Huang YS, Ree SC, et al: Differential add-on effects of aripiprazole in resolving hyperprolactinemia induced by risperidone in comparison to benzamide antipsychotics. Prog Neuropsychopharmacol Biol Psychiatry 34(8):1495–1499, 2010 20732372

Corbeil O, Corbeil S, Dorval M, et al: Problem gambling associated with aripiprazole: a nested case-control study in a first-episode psychosis program. CNS Drugs 35(4):461–468, 2021 33713298

Council on Scientific Affairs: Aspartame: review of safety issues. JAMA 254(3):400–402, 1985 2861297

de Bartolomeis A, Tomasetti C, Iasevoli F: Update on the mechanism of action of aripiprazole: translational insights into antipsychotic strategies beyond dopamine receptor antagonism. CNS Drugs 29(9):773–799, 2015 26346901

Felin T, Naveed S, Chaudhary AM: Aripiprazole-induced neutropenia: case report and literature review. J Psychosoc Nurs Ment Health Serv 56(5):21–24, 2018 29715374

Gupta B, Chee K-S, Neo L-Q, et al: Effect of aripiprazole as an adjunct to atypical antipsychotics on weight and metabolic profile: a 12-week open-label trial. Ther Adv Psychopharmacol 11:20451253211046765, 2021 34646440

Hiemke C, Bergemann N, Clement AHW, et al: Consensus Guidelines for therapeutic drug monitoring in neuropsychopharmacology: update 2017. Pharmacopsychiatry 51(1-02):9–62, 2018 28910830

Hoffer ZS, Roth RL, Mathews M: Evidence for the partial dopamine-receptor agonist aripiprazole as a first-line treatment of psychosis in patients with iatrogenic or tumorogenic hyperprolactinemia. Psychosomatics 50(4):317–324, 2009 19687170

Larsen ER, Damkier P, Pedersen LH, et al; Danish Psychiatric Society; Danish Society of Obstetrics and Gynecology; Danish Paediatric Society; Danish Society of Clinical Pharmacology: Use of psychotropic drugs during pregnancy and breast-feeding. Acta Psychiatr Scand Suppl 132(445):1–28, 2015 26344706

Layton JB, Forns J, Turner ME, et al: Falls and fractures in patients with Parkinson's disease-related psychosis treated with pimavanserin vs atypical antipsychotics: a cohort study. Drugs Real World Outcomes 9(1):9–22, 2022 34718963

Li CB, He YL, Zhang MY: Reasonable application of the consistency test methods [in Chinese]. Shanghai Arch Psychiatry 12(4):228–230, 2000. Available at: http://www.chinadoi.cn/portal/mr.action?doi=10.3969/j.issn.1002-0829.2000.04.016. Accessed February 10, 2022.

Lu ML, Shen WW, Chen CH: Time course of the changes in antipsychotic-induced hyperprolactinemia following the switch to aripiprazole. Prog Neuropsychopharmacol Biol Psychiatry 32(8):1978–1981, 2008 18848860

Lu Z, Sun Y, Zhang Y, et al: Pharmacological treatment strategies for antipsychotic-induced hyperprolactinemia: a systematic review and network meta-analysis. Transl Psychiatry 12(1):267, 2022 35790713

Maust DT, Kim HM, Seyfried LS, et al: Antipsychotics, other psychotropics, and the risk of death in patients with dementia: number needed to harm. JAMA Psychiatry 72(5):438–445, 2015 25786075

Meng M, Li W, Zhang S, et al: Using aripiprazole to reduce antipsychotic-induced hyperprolactinemia: meta-analysis of currently available randomized controlled trials. Shanghai Jingshen Yixue 27(1):4–17, 2015 25852251

Nguyen T, Teoh S, Hackett LP, et al: Placental transfer of aripiprazole. Aust N Z J Psychiatry 45(6):500–501, 2011 21413838

Nordeng H, Gjerdalen G, Brede WR, et al: Transfer of aripiprazole to breast milk: a case report. J Clin Psychopharmacol 34(2):272–275, 2014 24525642

Otsuka America Pharmaceutical: Abilify (aripiprazole) tablets, orally disintegrating tablets, oral solution, and injection prescribing information. Otsuka America Pharmaceutical, 2018

Raveendranthan D, Rao NP, Rao MG, et al: Add-on aripiprazole for atypical antipsychotic-induced, clinically significant hyperprolactinemia. Indian J Psychol Med 40(1):38–40, 2018 29403128

Rubino A, Sanon M, Ganz ML, et al: Association of the US Food and Drug Administration antipsychotic drug boxed warning with medication use and health outcomes in elderly patients with dementia. JAMA Netw Open 3(4):e203630, 2020 32343351

Shim JC, Shin JG, Kelly DL, et al: Adjunctive treatment with a dopamine partial agonist, aripiprazole, for antipsychotic-induced hyperprolactinemia: a placebo-controlled trial. Am J Psychiatry 164(9):1404–1410, 2007 17728426

Srephichit S, Sanchez R, Bourgeois JA: Neuroleptic malignant syndrome and aripiprazole in an antipsychotic-naive patient. J Clin Psychopharmacol 26(1):94–95, 2006 16415717

Takahashi K, Nakamura T, Sasayama D, et al: Orthostatic hypotension: uncommon side effect of aripiprazole. Psychiatr Danub 33(1):63–64, 2021 33857042

Watanabe N, Kasahara M, Sugibayashi R, et al: Perinatal use of aripiprazole: a case report. J Clin Psychopharmacol 31(3):377–379, 2011 21532364

Wu H, Siafis S, Hamza T, et al: Antipsychotic-induced weight gain: dose-response meta-analysis of randomized controlled trials. Schizophr Bull 48(3):643–654, 2022 35137229

Zhao J, Song X, Ai X, et al: Adjunctive aripiprazole treatment for risperidone-induced hyperprolactinemia: an 8-week randomized, open-label, comparative clinical trial. PLoS One 10(10):e0139717, 2015 26448615

Ziadi Trives M, Bonete Llácer JM, García Escudero MA, et al: Effect of the addition of aripiprazole on hyperprolactinemia associated with risperidone long-acting injection. J Clin Psychopharmacol 33(4):538–541, 2013 23775053

Orthostasis

Overview

Orthostatic hypotension is an infrequent adverse effect of most drugs in current use in the treatment of hypertension; however, it is more common with α_1-adrenergic blockers, and specifically with centrally acting drugs. Sudden loss of blood volume, or excess diuresis, may precipitate orthostatic hypotension even in usually hypertensive patients. Many drugs used for the treatment of psychiatric illnesses are associated with a significant incidence of orthostatic hypotension. These medications include phenothiazines (e.g., chlorpromazine, fluphenazine), tricyclic antidepressants, trazodone, alpha-1 blockers (e.g., prazosin, terazosin), benzodiazepines, some second-generation antipsychotics, and monoamine oxidase inhibitors (Bhanu et al. 2021; Schoenberger 1991).

References

Bhanu C, Nimmons D, Petersen I, et al: Drug-induced orthostatic hypotension: a systematic review and meta-analysis of randomised controlled trials. PLoS Med 18(11):e1003821, 2021 34752479

Schoenberger JA: Drug-induced orthostatic hypotension. Drug Saf 6(6):402–407, 1991 1793521

Fludrocortisone (for Medication-Induced Orthostasis)

I. **Mechanism of Action**:

A. Fludrocortisone is a synthetic mineralocorticoid that promotes renal sodium reabsorption, increasing intravascular volume (Freeman et al. 2018; Gibbons et al. 2017). It improves vascular alpha-adrenergic receptor sensitivity, promoting vasoconstriction (Freeman et al. 2018; Gibbons et al. 2017). It is used for adrenal insufficiency, Addison's disease; congenital adrenal hyperplasia classic (salt-losing adrenogenital syndrome); orthostatic hypotension (off-label use), and septic shock (off-label use).

II. **Data**:

A. A 3-week study ($n = 17$) demonstrated an improvement in orthostatic hypotension (Schoffer et al. 2007). To identify and evaluate the benefits and harms of fludrocortisone for orthostatic hypotension, a review was conducted of 13 studies with a total of 513 participants, including 3 crossover randomized controlled trials (RCTs) and 10 observational studies. The included RCTs were small (total of 28 participants in RCTs) and short-term (2–3 weeks), and only examined fludrocortisone for orthostatic hypotension in individuals with two conditions (diabetes and Parkinson's disease). The study found very-low-certainty evidence supporting the benefits of fludrocortisone versus placebo in treating low blood pressure in individuals with diabetes (–26 mm Hg vs. –39 mm Hg systolic; –7 mm Hg vs, –11 mm Hg diastolic). For people with Parkinson's disease, the study found very-low-certainty evidence supporting the beneficial effects of fludrocortisone on low blood pressure compared with pyridostigmine (–14 mm Hg vs. –22.1 mm Hg diastolic; P=0.036) and domperidone. For orthostatic symptoms, the study found very-low-certainty evidence supporting the benefits of fludrocortisone versus placebo in patients with diabetes and of fludrocortisone versus pyridostigmine in patients with Parkinson's disease (Veazie et al. 2021).

B. The evidence is very uncertain regarding the effects of fludrocortisone on blood pressure, orthostatic symptoms, or adverse events in people with orthostatic hypotension and diabetes or Parkinson's disease. Overall, there is a lack of information on long-term fludrocortisone treatment and the treatment of orthostatic hypotension in other disease states (Evidence for Fludrocortisone in Postural Hypotension 2021).

C. A double-blind crossover study that included six people with diabetes and orthostatic hypotension found that fludrocortisone 0.1 mg BID was more effective than placebo in increasing supine and upright blood pressure and improved symptoms of orthostatic hypotension in four patients (Campbell et al. 1975). Subsequent open-label studies reported improvement in symptoms and blood pressure measurements in orthostatic hypotension in 13 of 14 patients with diabetes (Campbell et al. 1976; Cheshire 2018) and 6 of 6 patients with Parkinson's disease (Hoehn 1975).

D. Fludrocortisone is not always sufficiently effective or well tolerated. In a retrospective study of 1,767 patients prescribed fludrocortisone, use was discontinued in 467 (26%), with a median persistence of 254 days (interquartile range: 119–783 days) (Shibao et al. 2013). Patients with orthostatic hypotension related to a neurological condition taking fludrocortisone had higher rates of all-cause hospitalizations than those taking midodrine (Grijalva et al. 2017).

III. **Dosing:**

A. Fludrocortisone is a mineralocorticoid that increases blood volume and blood pressure. Fludrocortisone is considered the first- or second-line pharmacological therapy for orthostatic hypotension, alongside mechanical and positional measures (e.g., increasing fluid and salt intake) and venous compression methods. Initial oral dosing of fludrocortisone is 0.05–0.1 mg once daily (Palma and Kaufmann 2020; Schoffer et al. 2007; Ten Harkel et al. 1992). The fludrocortisone dosing can be adjusted (e.g., in 0.05- to 0.1-mg/day increments) at weekly intervals if needed based on response; usual dosage range: 0.05–0.2 mg/day administered as a single dose or 2 divided doses (Palma and Kaufmann 2020; van Lieshout et al. 2000).

B. Dosages higher than 0.2 mg/day have been associated with an increased risk of adverse effects without any added benefit (Lahrmann et al. 2006; Palma and Kaufmann 2020). When fludrocortisone acetate was used to increase blood pressure in the management of patients with diabetes with postural hypotension, 0.1–0.4 mg of the drug was given daily. In patients with postural hypotension secondary to levodopa therapy, 0.05–0.2 mg of fludrocortisone acetate has been given daily (American Society of Health-System Pharmacists 2019).

IV. **Cautions/Monitoring**:

A. Fludrocortisone is contraindicated in patients with hypersensitivity to fludrocortisone or any component of its formulation. Corticosteroids are contraindicated in patients with systemic fungal infections (Paladin Labs 2019). Regular blood pressure monitoring with fludrocortisone is important.

B. Patients receiving a single large dose should be treated with plenty of water by mouth. In addition, they should undergo monitoring of serum electrolytes, particularly potassium and sodium, and be treated appropriately for any developing imbalances (Drug Bank Online 2022).

C. Corticosteroids (systemic) may enhance the anticoagulant effect of vitamin K antagonists (e.g., warfarin). Corticosteroids (systemic) may diminish the therapeutic effect of the COVID-19 vaccine (mRNA). Therefore, it is suggested that the third dose of the COVID-19 vaccine be administered at least 28 days after completion of the primary two-dose series in patients age 5 years or older taking immunosuppressive therapies (Lexicomp/UpToDate 2024).

D. Combining with estrogen derivatives may increase the serum concentration of corticosteroids. Corticosteroids (systemic) may enhance the hypokalemic effect of thiazide and thiazide-like diuretics. Fludrocortisone can cause hypokalemia, ankle edema, and supine hypertension (Chobanian et al. 1979). Patients receiving fludrocortisone are advised to take potassium supplements (potassium chloride 20 mEq/day) to reduce the risk of hypokalemia. Dependent edema is managed with compression stockings when symptoms are mild. Long-term use of fludrocortisone exacerbates hypertension and organ damage, including left ventricular hypertrophy, congestive heart failure, and renal failure and is associated with a higher risk of all-cause hospitalization in patients with orthostatic hypotension (Grijalva et al. 2017).

E. Fludrocortisone may cause hypercortisolism or suppression of the hypothalamic-pituitary-adrenal (HPA) axis, particularly in younger children or in patients receiving high doses for prolonged periods.

F. Prolonged use increases the risk of infection, masks acute infection (including fungal infections), prolongs or exacerbates viral infections, and limits response to killed or inactivated vaccines. Corticosteroids should not be used in patients with viral hepatitis. Close observation is required in patients with latent tuberculosis and/or tuberculosis reactivity. Prolonged treatment with corticosteroids has been associated with the development of Kaposi's sarcoma (Goedert et al. 2002). An acute myopathy has been reported with high-dose corticosteroids, usually in patients with neuromuscular transmission disorders. Myopathy may involve ocular and/or respiratory muscles. It is recommended that creatine kinase be monitored (Lexicomp/UpToDate 2024).

G. Corticosteroid use may cause psychiatric disturbances, including euphoria, insomnia, mood swings, personality changes, severe depression, and psychotic symptoms. Preexisting psychiatric conditions may be exacerbated by corticosteroid use (Lexicomp/UpToDate 2024). Corticosteroids should be tapered and gradually withdrawn when discontinuing. Patients may require higher doses when subject to stress (e.g., trauma, surgery, severe illness). Systemic use of mineralocorticoids/corticosteroids may necessitate a diet with increased potassium, vitamins A, B_6, C, and D, folate, calcium, zinc, and phosphorus, as well as decreased sodium.

Further Reading

Banda J, Lakshmanan R, Vvs SP, et al: A highly sensitive method for the quantification of fludrocortisone in human plasma using ultra-high-performance liquid chromatography tandem mass spectrometry and its pharmacokinetic application. Biomed Chromatogr 29(8):1213–1219, 2015 25611194

Diederich S, Eigendorff E, Burkhardt P, et al: 11beta-Hydroxysteroid dehydrogenase types 1 and 2: an important pharmacokinetic determinant for the activity of synthetic mineralo- and glucocorticoids. J Clin Endocrinol Metab 87(12):5695–5701, 2002 12466373

Kaufmann H, Freeman R, Biaggioni I, et al; NOH301 Investigators: Droxidopa for neurogenic orthostatic hypotension: a randomized, placebo-controlled, phase 3 trial. Neurology 83(4):328–335, 2014 24944260

Kim MJ, Farrell J: Orthostatic hypotension: a practical approach. Am Fam Physician 105(1):39–49, 2022 35029940

Oelkers W, Buchen S, Diederich S, et al: Impaired renal 11 beta-oxidation of 9 alpha-fluorocortisol: an explanation for its mineralocorticoid potency. J Clin Endocrinol Metab 78(4):928–932, 1994 8157723

Rendic S: Summary of information on human CYP enzymes: human P450 metabolism data. Drug Metab Rev 34(1–2):83–448, 2002 11996015

References

American Society of Health-System Pharmacists: Fludrocortisone acetate tablets. 10/23/2019. Available at: https://www.ashp.org/drug-shortages/current-shortages/drug-shortage-detail.aspx?id=484&loginreturnUrl=SSOCheckOnly. Accessed March 13, 2024.

Campbell IW, Ewing DJ, Clarke BF: 9-Alpha-fluorohydrocortisone in the treatment of postural hypotension in diabetic autonomic neuropathy. Diabetes 24(4):381–384, 1975 1094320

Campbell IW, Ewing DJ, Clarke BF: Therapeutic experience with fludrocortisone in diabetic postural hypotension. BMJ 1(6014):872–874, 1976 769906

Cheshire WP: Chemical pharmacotherapy for the treatment of orthostatic hypotension. Expert Opin Pharmacother 20(2):187–199, 2018

Chobanian AV, Volicer L, Tifft CP, et al: Mineralocorticoid-induced hypertension in patients with orthostatic hypotension. N Engl J Med 301(2):68–73, 1979 449947

Drug Bank Online: Fludrocortisone. Available at: https://go.drugbank.com/drugs/DB00687. Accessed February 14, 2022.

Evidence for fludrocortisone in postural hypotension. Drug Ther Bull 59(12):183, 2021

Freeman R, Abuzinadah AR, Gibbons C, et al: Orthostatic hypotension: JACC State-of-the-Art Review. J Am Coll Cardiol 72(11):1294–1309, 2018 30190008

Gibbons CH, Schmidt P, Biaggioni I, et al: The recommendations of a consensus panel for the screening, diagnosis, and treatment of neurogenic orthostatic hypotension and associated supine hypertension. J Neurol 264(8):1567–1582, 2017 28050656

Goedert JJ, Vitale F, Lauria C, et al; Classical Kaposi's Sarcoma Working Group: Risk factors for classical Kaposi's sarcoma. J Natl Cancer Inst 94(22):1712–1718, 2002 12441327

Grijalva CG, Biaggioni I, Griffin MR, et al: Fludrocortisone is associated with a higher risk of all-cause hospitalizations compared with midodrine in patients with orthostatic hypotension. J Am Heart Assoc 6(10):e006848, 2017 29025750

Hoehn MM: Levodopa-induced postural hypotension: treatment with fludrocortisone. Arch Neurol 32(1):50–51, 1975 1115660

Lahrmann H, Cortelli P, Hilz M, et al: EFNS guidelines on the diagnosis and management of orthostatic hypotension. Eur J Neurol 13(9):930–936, 2006 16930356

Lexicomp/UpToDate: Fludrocortisone: drug information. n.d. Available at: https://pro.uptodatefree.ir/Show/8455#:~:text=Very%20potent%20mineralocorticoid%20with%20high,potassium%20from%20renal%20distal%20tubules. Accessed July 31, 2024.
Paladin Labs: Florinef (fludrocortisone acetate). Paladin Labs, 2019. Available at: https://www.paladin-labs.com/our_products/Florinef_en.pdf. Accessed March 13, 2024.
Palma JA, Kaufmann H: Management of orthostatic hypotension. Continuum (Minneap Minn) 26(1):154–177, 2020 31996627
Schoffer KL, Henderson RD, O'Maley K, et al: Nonpharmacological treatment, fludrocortisone, and domperidone for orthostatic hypotension in Parkinson's disease. Mov Disord 22(11):1543–1549, 2007 17557339
Shibao C, Grijalva CG, Lipsitz LA, et al: Early discontinuation of treatment in patients with orthostatic hypotension. Auton Neurosci 177(2):291–296, 2013 24008021
Ten Harkel AD, van Lieshout JJ, Wieling W: Treatment of orthostatic hypotension with sleeping in the head-up tilt position, alone and in combination with fludrocortisone. J Intern Med 232(2):139–145, 1992 1506810
van Lieshout JJ, ten Harkel ADJ, Wieling W: Fludrocortisone and sleeping in the head-up position limit the postural decrease in cardiac output in autonomic failure. Clin Autonom Res 10(1):35–42, 2000
Veazie S, Peterson K, Ansari Y, et al: Fludrocortisone for orthostatic hypotension. Cochrane Database Syst Rev (5):CD012868, 2021 34000076

Midodrine (for Medication-Induced Orthostasis)

I. **Mechanism of Action**:

A. Midodrine, a short-acting alpha-1-adrenergic agonist that acts via vasoconstriction, has been shown to alleviate symptoms of orthostatic hypotension and elevate blood pressure in multiple randomized placebo-controlled trials (Freeman et al. 2018; Gibbons et al. 2017; Schoffer et al. 2007). It is approved by the FDA for the treatment of orthostatic hypotension and is a recommended first-line medication.

B. Midodrine is a prodrug that forms an active metabolite, desglymidodrine, which is an α_1-adrenoreceptor agonist. Midodrine acts on arteriolar and venous capacitance vessels to increase vascular tone. Desglymidodrine has no effect on cardiac β-adrenergic receptors and diffuses poorly across the blood-brain barrier (American Health Packaging 2022). It is indicated for the treatment of neurogenic orthostatic hypotension.

II. **Data**:

A. A placebo-controlled trial of 97 subjects with moderate to severe orthostatic hypotension randomly assigned patients to either placebo or midodrine at a dosage of 2.5 mg, 5 mg, or 10 mg three times daily for 4 weeks. For those receiving the 10-mg dose of midodrine, there was improvement in standing systolic blood pressure by 22 mm Hg ($P<0.001$) as well as improvement in symptoms of orthostatic lightheadedness ($P<0.05$) and global symptom relief scores (Jankovic et al. 1993).

B. In a second trial, 171 subjects with neurogenic orthostatic hypotension received either placebo or midodrine at a dose of 10 mg three times a day for 4 weeks. Compared with placebo, midodrine was associated with improvement in standing systolic blood pressure at each weekly time point (P<0.001) and improvement in the global symptom relief scores (Low et al. 1997).

C. A subsequent randomized controlled withdrawal study evaluated 33 patients with severe orthostatic hypotension who had been on a stable dose of midodrine for at least 3 months. The outcome measure was the time to syncopal symptoms or near-syncope on a tilt table at 1 hour after receiving of either placebo or their usual dose of midodrine. The mean time to near-syncope for midodrine was 27±3 minutes and for placebo was 18±3 minutes (P=0.013) (Smith et al. 2016).

III. **Dosing**:

A. The recommended dosage of midodrine is 10 mg taken three times daily (TID). Midodrine is supplied as 2.5-mg, 5-mg, and 10-mg tablets. Most patients respond to 5–10 mg TID, taken first thing in the morning, at midday, and in the late afternoon. Doses should be taken during the daytime hours when the patient needs to be upright, pursuing their usual activities of daily living. Doses may be given at 3-hour intervals, if required, to control symptoms. Single doses as high as 20 mg have been given to patients, but severe and persistent systolic supine hypertension occurs at a high rate (about 45%) at these doses. To reduce the potential for supine hypertension during sleep, midodrine should not be given after the evening meal or less than 4 hours before bedtime (Chen et al. 2018; Parsaik et al. 2013). Patients should be instructed not to take midodrine within 5 hours of sleep, because it may exacerbate supine neurogenic hypertension, or if seated or supine blood pressure is greater than 180/110 mm Hg (Smith et al. 2016).

IV. **Cautions/monitoring**:

A. Midodrine hydrochloride is contraindicated in patients with severe organic heart disease, acute renal disease, urinary retention, pheochromocytoma, or thyrotoxicosis. Midodrine hydrochloride should not be used in patients with persistent and excessive supine hypertension (American Health Packaging 2022). Because desglymidodrine is eliminated by the kidneys and the liver has a role in its metabolism, evaluation of the patient should include assessment of renal and hepatic function prior to initiating therapy and periodically after (American Health Packaging 2022). It is essential to monitor supine and sitting blood pressures in patients maintained on midodrine (American Health Packaging 2022).

B. The risk of hypertension increases with concomitant administration of drugs that increase blood pressure (phenylephrine, pseudoephedrine, ephedrine, dihydroergotamine, thyroid hormones, or droxidopa). If concomitant use cannot be avoided, monitor blood pressure closely.

C. Avoid use of MAO inhibitors (including linezolid) with midodrine. Alpha-adrenergic blocking agents, such as prazosin, terazosin, and doxazosin, can antagonize the effects of midodrine. There may be a potential for drug-drug interactions with alpha-adrenergic blocking drugs because active tubular secretion by the base-secreting system is also responsible for the secretion of other drugs including metformin, cimetidine, ranitidine, procainamide, triamterene, flecainide, and quinidine.

D. The most potentially serious adverse reaction associated with midodrine therapy is marked elevation of supine arterial blood pressure (supine hypertension). A systolic pressure of about 200 mm Hg was seen overall in roughly 13.4% of patients given 10 mg of midodrine. Other adverse effects include piloerection, scalp paresthesias, and urinary retention (Smith et al. 2016).

E. Patients receiving midodrine should take their last daily dose of midodrine hydrochloride 3–4 hours before bedtime to minimize nighttime supine hypertension. Patients should be told that certain agents in over-the-counter products, such as cold remedies and diet aids, can elevate blood pressure. Therefore, they should be used cautiously with midodrine hydrochloride, as they may potentiate the pressor effects of midodrine hydrochloride (American Health Packaging 2022). Midodrine was previously labeled as FDA Category C in pregnancy. It is not known whether midodrine is excreted in human breast milk.

Further Reading

Bhanu C, Nimmons D, Petersen I, et al: Drug-induced orthostatic hypotension: a systematic review and meta-analysis of randomised controlled trials. PLoS Med 18(11):e1003821, 2021 34752479

Schoenberger JA: Drug-induced orthostatic hypotension. Drug Saf 6(6):402–407, 1991 1793521

References

American Health Packaging: Midodrine hydrochloride. Revised June 2022. Available at: https://dailymed.nlm.nih.gov/dailymed/fda/fdaDrugXsl.cfm?setid=159cb0cb-4b27-4a1c-8ad4-dc93604c79c7&type=display. Accessed March 13, 2024.

Chen JJ, Han Y, Tang J, et al: Standing and supine blood pressure outcomes associated with droxidopa and midodrine in patients with neurogenic orthostatic hypotension: a Bayesian meta-analysis and mixed treatment comparison of randomized trials. Ann Pharmacother 52(12):1182–1194, 2018 29972032

Freeman R, Abuzinadah AR, Gibbons C, et al: Orthostatic hypotension: JACC State-of-the-Art Review. J Am Coll Cardiol 72(11):1294–1309, 2018 30190008

Gibbons CH, Schmidt P, Biaggioni I, et al: The recommendations of a consensus panel for the screening, diagnosis, and treatment of neurogenic orthostatic hypotension and associated supine hypertension. J Neurol 264(8):1567–1582, 2017 28050656

Jankovic J, Gilden JL, Hiner BC, et al: Neurogenic orthostatic hypotension: a double-blind, placebo-controlled study with midodrine. Am J Med 95(1):38–48, 1993 7687093

Low PA, Gilden JL, Freeman R, et al: Efficacy of midodrine vs placebo in neurogenic orthostatic hypotension. A randomized, double-blind multicenter study. Midodrine Study Group. JAMA 277(13):1046–1051, 1997 9091692

Parsaik AK, Singh B, Altayar O, et al: Midodrine for orthostatic hypotension: a systematic review and meta-analysis of clinical trials. J Gen Intern Med 28(11):1496–1503, 2013 23775146

Schoffer KL, Henderson RD, O'Maley K, et al: Nonpharmacological treatment, fludrocortisone, and domperidone for orthostatic hypotension in Parkinson's disease. Mov Disord 22(11):1543–1549, 2007 17557339

Smith W, Wan H, Much D, et al: Clinical benefit of midodrine hydrochloride in symptomatic orthostatic hypotension: a phase 4, double-blind, placebo-controlled, randomized, tilt-table study. Clin Auton Res 26(4):269–277, 2016 27372462

Parkinsonism

Overview

Drug-induced parkinsonism is likely the most common drug-induced movement disorder and one of the most common nondegenerative causes of parkinsonism. Any medication that interferes with dopamine transmission may cause parkinsonism. The prototypical drugs are dopamine receptor blocking agents, specifically those that block D_2 receptors (Wyant and Chou 2022).

The most common mechanism for drug-induced parkinsonism is a structural or functional blockade of the dopamine D_2 receptor in the striatum by dopamine D_2 receptor–blocking drugs. This D_2 blockade changes the output of the indirect pathway of the basal ganglia–thalamocortical motor loop, similar to changes seen in Parkinson's disease (Wyant and Chou 2022).

The prevalence of drug-induced parkinsonism ranges from 0.09% to 1.7%, with the highest incidence in patients ages 60–80 years (Wyant and Chou 2022).

References

Wyant KJ, Chou KL: Drug-induced parkinsonism. UpToDate, 2022. Available at: https://www.uptodate.com/contents/drug-induced-parkinsonism. Accessed March 13, 2024.

Amantadine (for Medication-Induced Parkinsonism)

I. **Mechanism of Action**:

A. Amantadine blocks dopamine reuptake into presynaptic neurons, causing an accumulation of dopamine in the presynaptic clefts of dopaminergic neurons in the basal ganglia. Amantadine may also cause direct stimulation of postsynaptic receptors (Chang and Ramphul 2023). Amantadine also blocks monoaminoxidase A and *N*-methyl-D-aspartate (NMDA) receptors and seems to raise beta-endorphin/beta-lipotropin levels (Huber et al. 1999).

B. Amantadine is a synthetic adamantane derivative indicated in the treatment of idiopathic Parkinson's disease, postencephalitic parkinsonism, and carbon monoxide intoxication–induced symptomatic parkinsonism. Amantadine is indicated in elderly patients with cerebral arteriosclerosis–induced parkinsonism and in the prevention and symptomatic treatment of influenza caused by influenza A virus strains (Chang and Ramphul 2023).

C. Amantadine has shown efficacy in improving post–traumatic brain injury arousal and cognition (Sawyer et al. 2008). Amantadine has also proved beneficial in drug-induced parkinsonism, Parkinson's disease, traumatic head injury, dementia, multiple sclerosis, and cocaine withdrawal (Huber et al. 1999; Ma and Zafonte 2020).

D. Recently, the putative activity of amantadine against severe acute respiratory syndrome coronavirus 2 (SARS-CoV-2, the virus that causes COVID-19) has been described and widely discussed (Butterworth 2020; Grieb et al. 2021). Patients treated with amantadine also showed more pronounced restoration of consciousness and regression of neurological deficits poststroke (Danysz et al. 2021; Zhong et al. 2020).

II. **Data**:

A. Amantadine is used in the symptomatic treatment of all forms of the parkinsonian syndrome, including the postencephalitic, idiopathic, and arteriosclerotic types, and to relieve parkinsonian signs and symptoms of carbon monoxide poisoning and antipsychotic agent–induced (e.g., phenothiazines) extrapyramidal effects. There is no evidence that the drug alters the course of parkinsonian syndromes.

B. Amantadine may be especially useful in treating drug-induced extrapyramidal symptoms when drugs with anticholinergic properties should be avoided (e.g., in patients with glaucoma or urinary retention) (Chang and Ramphul 2023). Improvement in extrapyramidal symptoms is apparent within 4–48 hours following initiation of amantadine therapy, and optimum results are achieved within 2 weeks to 3 months. Sustained improvement may last up to 30 months with amantadine treatment; however, some patients experience a reduction in benefit after 1–3 months of amantadine therapy.

C. If loss of effectiveness occurs, the benefit may be regained by increasing the dosage of amantadine to 300 mg/day (Chang and Ramphul 2023); or, alternatively, temporary discontinuation of amantadine for several weeks, followed by reinstitution of amantadine, may result in regained benefit in some patients (Chang and Ramphul 2023). The high-dose 274-mg amantadine extended-release capsule (equivalent to 340 mg amantadine HCl) effectively treats dyskinesia in patients with Parkinson's disease who are receiving levodopa-based therapy, with or without concomitant dopaminergic medications (Adamas Pharma 2021). With some success, amantadine has been used to treat spastic pseudosclerosis (Jakob-Creutzfeldt disease).

D. Amantadine has also been shown to have neuroprotective benefits (Wang et al. 2014). Amantadine has a role in the prophylaxis and symptomatic treatment of influenza A virus infection (Chang and Ramphul 2023).

III. **Dosing**:

A. The usual dosage of amantadine in patients without recognized renal disease is 100 mg twice daily (Endo Laboratories 2003). When patients receive other antiparkinsonian drugs or have other serious illnesses, the initial dosage is 100 mg/day.

B. The onset of action of amantadine usually occurs within 48 hours (Endo Laboratories 2003). After 1–2 weeks, the dosage may be increased to 100 mg twice daily. Patients with drug-induced extrapyramidal reactions whose responses are not optimal with a dosage of 200 mg/day may benefit from a dosage increase to 300 mg/day in divided doses. Patients with parkinsonian syndromes may benefit from a dosage increase up to 400 mg/day in divided doses (Endo Laboratories 2003).

C. Patients with creatinine clearances less than 15 mL/minute/1.73 m^2 and hemodialysis patients should receive 200 mg of amantadine every 7 days, according to the package insert (Endo Laboratories 2003).

IV. **Cautions/Monitoring**:

A. Amantadine is used with caution in patients with liver disease or a history of recurrent eczematoid dermatitis, uncontrolled psychosis or severe psychoneurosis, or epilepsy or other seizures, and in those receiving drugs with CNS activity (Endo Laboratories 2003). Patients with seizures should be observed closely for possible increased seizure activity.

B. Caution is recommended in individuals with untreated angle-closure glaucoma. Older adult patients with cerebrovascular disease and/or renal impairment should be monitored for amantadine toxicity. Amantadine should not be abruptly discontinued in patients with parkinsonian syndromes because of the risk of exacerbations of parkinsonian symptoms within 24 hours after discontinuing the drug and risk of developing parkinsonian crises (Chang and Ramphul 2023).

C. Close observation is recommended when the amantadine dose is reduced or stopped or when amantadine is combined with an antipsychotic due to concern for a neuroleptic malignant syndrome (Endo Laboratories 2003). Patients should be monitored for the development of psychosis, depression, and suicidal ideation during treatment. Rapid dose reduction, if unavoidable, needs close observation for withdrawal-induced hyperpyrexia (Adamas Pharma 2021). Amantadine combined with anticholinergic medications may result in increased adverse anticholinergic effects (Chang and Ramphul 2023). Amantadine combined with thioridazine can worsen tremors in elderly patients with Parkinson's disease (Endo Laboratories 2003).

D. Amantadine should be administered with caution to patients receiving other CNS stimulant drugs. Concomitant administration of quinidine or quinine with amantadine may reduce renal clearance of amantadine (Endo Laboratories 2003).

E. Amantadine is contraindicated in patients with creatinine clearance below 15 mL/minute/1.73 m^2 (Adamas Pharma 2021). Patients on amantadine may experience urges (e.g., gambling, sexual, money spending, binge eating) and the inability to control them. Prescribers need to ask patients or caregivers about the development of new or increased urges/compulsions. Consider reducing the dosage or stopping medications (Adamas Pharma 2021).

Further Reading

Crosby N, Deane KH, Clarke CE: Amantadine in Parkinson's disease. Cochrane Database Syst Rev (1):CD003468, 2003 12535476

References

Adamas Pharma: Gocovri package insert. Emeryville, CA, Adamis Pharma, 2021. Available at: https://www.gocovri.com/GOC_PI_01_2021.pdf. Accessed March 13, 2024.

Butterworth RF. Amantadine, Parkinson's disease and COVID19. Covid Perspect Res Rev 1:1–6, 2020

Chang C, Ramphul K: Amantadine, in StatPearls [Internet]. Treasure Island, FL, StatPearls Publishing, last update April 24, 2023. Available at: https://www.ncbi.nlm.nih.gov/books/NBK499953/. Accessed July 31, 2024.

Danysz W, Dekundy A, Scheschonka A, et al: Amantadine: reappraisal of the timeless diamond-target updates and novel therapeutic potentials. J Neural Transm 128(2):127–169, 2021

Endo Laboratories: Symmetrel (amantadine hydrochloride) tablets and syrup prescribing information. Endo Laboratories, 2003

Grieb P, ?wi?tkiewicz M, Rs K, et al: Amantadine for COVID-19. J Clin Pharmacol 61(3):412–413, 2021 33350472

Huber TJ, Dietrich DE, Emrich HM: Possible use of amantadine in depression. Pharmacopsychiatry 32(2):47–55, 1999 10333162

Ma HM, Zafonte RD: Amantadine and memantine: a comprehensive review for acquired brain injury. Brain Inj 34(3):299–315, 2020 32078407

Sawyer E, Mauro LS, Ohlinger MJ: Amantadine enhancement of arousal and cognition after traumatic brain injury. Ann Pharmacother 42(2):247–252, 2008 18212258

Wang T, Huang XJ, Van KC, et al: Amantadine improves cognitive outcome and increases neuronal survival after fluid percussion traumatic brain injury in rats. J Neurotrauma 31(4):370–377, 2014 23574258

Zhong J, Li J, Ni C, et al: Amantadine alleviates postoperative cognitive dysfunction possibly by preserving neurotrophic factor expression and dendritic arborization in the hippocampus of old rodents. Front Aging Neurosci 12:605330, 2020 33324197

Sexual Dysfunction

Overview

Psychotropic medications may cause side effects in all three major phases of the human sexual response cycle, including decreased libido, diminished arousal, decreased lubrication in women and erectile dysfunction in men, and delayed time to orgasm/anorgasmia. Some psychotropics may affect one phase more than others—for example, serotonergic antidepressants adversely affect orgasm more than arousal in most cases (Rosen et al. 1999).

There are essential differences between medication classes in terms of both the incidence of adverse sexual effects and the mechanisms of action leading to such effects. Antidepressants with predominantly serotonergic activity, antipsychotics associated with inducing hyperprolactinemia, and mood stabilizers with hormonal effects are often linked to moderate or severe sexual dysfunction, including decreased libido, delayed orgasm, anorgasmia, and sexual arousal difficulties (Montejo et al. 2018).

Risk factors for developing sexual dysfunction during antidepressant treatment include male gender, older age, lower academic achievement, absence of full-time employment, other comorbid health problems, multiple drug treatments, and difficult interpersonal relationships. However, in clinical practice, patients are sometimes reluctant to speak about sexual side effects (Montejo et al. 2018).

Waiting for spontaneous remission of antidepressant-associated sexual side effects is the least effective but most widely used method for managing such effects (Balon and Segraves 2008; Montejo-González et al. 1997). However, most patients (80%) do not report improvement in sexual side effects even after 6 months of continued antidepressant treatment (Montejo-González et al. 1997).

References

Balon R, Segraves RT: Survey of treatment practices for sexual dysfunction(s) associated with antidepressants. J Sex Marital Ther 34(4):353–365, 2008 18576236

Montejo AL, Montejo L, Baldwin DS: The impact of severe mental disorders and psychotropic medications on sexual health and its implications for clinical management. World Psychiatry 17(1):3–11, 2018 29352532

Montejo-González AL, Llorca G, Izquierdo JA, et al: SSRI-induced sexual dysfunction: fluoxetine, paroxetine, sertraline, and fluvoxamine in a prospective, multicenter, and descriptive clinical study of 344 patients. J Sex Marital Ther 23(3):176–194, 1997 9292833

Rosen RC, Lane RM, Menza M: Effects of SSRIs on sexual function: a critical review. J Clin Psychopharmacol 19(1):67–85, 1999 9934946

Bupropion (for Medication-Induced Sexual Dysfunction)

I. **Mechanism of Action**:

A. Preclinical data show that the mechanism of action of bupropion most likely involves its dual reuptake inhibition of dopamine and norepinephrine (Stahl et al. 2004). Bupropion and its primary metabolite, hydroxybupropion, decrease the reuptake of dopamine and norepinephrine in synaptosomes. Bupropion also reduces the firing of dopamine and norepinephrine neurons in the brain stem in a dose-dependent manner, an effect consistent with an increase in synaptic levels of dopamine and norepinephrine that in turn inhibits neuronal firing via an autoreceptor-mediated negative feedback mechanism. Hence extracellular dopamine and norepinephrine concentrations increase in response to bupropion administration, including in the prefrontal cortex (Li et al. 2002).

B. Serotonin appears to be the main neurotransmitter that has negative effects on sex drive and sexual function, both centrally and peripherally (Keks et al. 2014). In particular, the activation of postsynaptic serotonin (5-HT) 2A receptors in the central serotonergic system is considered a significant contributor to antidepressant-induced sexual dysfunction (Safarinejad 2011). In contrast, dopamine and norepinephrine agonism may have positive effects on sex drive and arousal.

II. **Data**:

A. Preclinical data show that the mechanism of action of bupropion most likely involves its dual-reuptake inhibition of dopamine and norepinephrine (Stahl et al. 2004) as discussed above.

B. In an open-label study, 47 patients with SSRI-induced sexual dysfunction were given a trial of bupropion as an adjunct to their SSRI, either as needed or as a fixed-dose scheduled medicine. Patients received 75 mg or 150 mg of bupropion 1–2 hours before sexual activity. If this was insufficient, the dose was increased gradually to 75 mg TID and sustained for 2 weeks. This regimen was then continued if successful. Bupropion successfully reversed a variety of sexual dysfunctions caused by SSRIs in 31 (66%) of 47 patients. Fifty-two (69%) of 75 sexual complaints improved with bupropion treatment. The as-needed use of bupropion assisted 18 (38%) of 47 patients. Side effects of anxiety and tremor led to discontinuation of bupropion in 7 (15%) of 47 patients (Ashton and Rosen 1998).

C. Similarly, 24 subjects with major depressive disorder with SSRI-associated new-onset sexual side effects were treated with escalating doses of bupropion SR up to 300 mg/day for 7 weeks. Global response rates were 46% for women and 75% for men. All sexual side effects improved in response to bupropion SR in both men and women, with no differential effect on any one sexual side effect. Most of the improvement (more than 50%) occurred within the first 2 weeks and at low dosages (100–200 mg/day) (Gitlin et al. 2002).

D. In another study, following a minimum of 6 weeks of antidepressant treatment with an SSRI or venlafaxine (a serotonin-norepinephrine reuptake inhibitor), eligible subjects received a further 8 weeks of monitored SSRI therapy combined with bupropion SR at a dosage of 150 mg/day. Sexual dysfunction, particularly a decrease in orgasmic delay, was significantly improved with combination therapy (Kennedy et al. 2002).

E. An open-label study tested the efficacy of adjunctive bupropion across several measures of sexual function. Patients who were taking SSRIs for various mood or anxiety disorders who reported progressive decline in sexual function after at least 2 months on these medications were offered treatment with bupropion at 75 mg/day. Eight patients were treated, and sexual function was measured through use of a visual analog scale after 1 month of treatment. Four of eight patients experienced marked improvement of sexual dysfunction following adjunctive bupropion treatment (Labbate et al. 1997).

F. In a study of adult outpatients with moderate to severe MDD and normal sexual functioning randomly assigned to receive bupropion XL (300–450 mg/day; N= 276), escitalopram (10–20 mg/day; N=281), or placebo (N=273) for up to 8 weeks, the incidence of orgasm dysfunction at week 8 (primary endpoint) and the incidence of worsened sexual functioning at the end of the treatment period were statistically significantly lower with bupropion XL than with escitalopram ($P < 0.05$), not statistically different between bupropion XL and placebo ($P \geq 0.067$), and statistically significantly higher with escitalopram than with placebo ($P \leq 0.001$). The percentages of patients with orgasm dysfunction at week 8 in study 1, study 2, and the pooled dataset, respectively, were 13%, 16%, and 15% with bupropion XL; 32%, 29%, and 30% with escitalopram; and 11%, 8%, and 9% with placebo (Clayton et al. 2006).

G. Data from three studies in men and women of bupropion 150 mg twice daily indicate a benefit over placebo on rating scale scores (SMD 1.60; 95% CI 1.40–1.81), but response rates in two studies of bupropion 150 mg once daily demonstrated no statistically significant difference in effect (RR 0.62; 95% CI 0.09–4.41). For women with antidepressant-induced sexual dysfunction, the addition of bupropion at higher doses appears to be the most promising approach studied so far (Taylor et al. 2013).

H. A survey of 29 expert psychiatrists in the area of antidepressant-related sexual dysfunction concluded that adding a dopaminergic agent (e.g., dextroamphetamine, methylphenidate, bupropion) was the most common first-line strategy for combating impaired libido, arousal, and orgasm in men and women, followed by decreasing the antidepressant dosage and waiting for spontaneous remission (Balon and Segraves 2008).

III. **Dosing**:

A. Initiate bupropion at 150 mg once daily for the first 3 days; increase to 150 mg twice daily, based on response and tolerability (Safarinejad 2011).

IV. **Cautions/Monitoring**:

A. Bupropion requires close monitoring of body weight for excessive weight loss. As an antidepressant, bupropion carries the same FDA class warnings carried by other antidepressants regarding the potential for neuropsychiatric reactions in youth younger than 24 years. Close monitoring is required for worsening depression, clinical worsening, suicidality, psychosis, or unusual changes in behavior (e.g., anxiety, agitation, panic attacks, insomnia, irritability, hostility, impulsivity, akathisia, hypomania, mania, social functioning), particularly during the initial 1–2 months of therapy or during periods of dosage adjustments (increases or decreases). Blood pressure monitoring is required at baseline and periodically, especially when used in conjunction with nicotine transdermal replacement.

B. When bupropion is used off-label for the treatment of ADHD, patients should be thoroughly evaluated for cardiovascular risk. Monitor heart rate and blood pressure, and consider obtaining ECG prior to initiation (Vetter et al. 2008).

C. Combining bupropion with a dopamine agonist may exacerbate the adverse/toxic effect of bupropion. Bupropion may decrease the serum concentration of digoxin. Iloperidone may enhance the adverse/toxic effect of bupropion. Bupropion may decrease serum concentrations of the active metabolite(s) of iloperidone. Monoamine oxidase inhibitors may worsen the hypertensive effect of bupropion. Bupropion may intensify the adverse/toxic effect of sertraline. Concomitant use of tricyclic antidepressants can worsen the neuroexcitatory and/or seizure-potentiating effects of bupropion. Bupropion may intensify the adverse/toxic effect of vilazodone by increasing the serum concentration of vilazodone (Lexicomp/UpToDate 2024).

D. Antidepressants (especially when used as monotherapy) may precipitate a mixed/manic episode in patients with bipolar disorder (Baldessarini et al. 2013). Bupropion can cause CNS stimulation in patients, including increased energy, insomnia, agitation, nervousness, and, in more significant cases, anxiety or panic.

E. On rare occasions, more significant neuropsychiatric effects, including abnormalities in thinking, paranoid ideation, delusion, hallucination, psychosis, suicidal ideation, and homicidal ideation, may occur (Stahl et al. 2004). Bupropion was associated with an increased risk of acute angle-closure glaucoma in a case-control study, particularly in adults older than age 50 years (Symes et al. 2015). Bupropion is associated with a dosage-related risk of seizures. Seizure risk with bupropion may be the greatest among antidepressants (Kara et al. 2013). Bupropion use was associated with an increased risk of suicidal ideation and suicidal tendencies in pediatric and young adult patients (age 18–24 years) in short-term studies (Friedman and Leon 2007).

F. In investigative studies, bupropion intake has been associated with the following side effects (Lexicomp/UpToDate 2024): tachycardia (reported by 11%), diaphoresis (5%–22%), weight loss (14%–28%), constipation (8%–26%), nausea (9%–18%), nausea and vomiting (23%), xerostomia (10%–28%), agitation (3%–32%), dizziness (6%–22%), headache (≤34%), insomnia (11%–40% [placebo: 6%–21%]), migraine (≤26%), tremor (1%–21%).

G. For SSRI-induced sexual dysfunction, watchful waiting alone is typically not effective (Sadock et al. 2015). A prospective observational study in 156 patients treated with SSRIs found that after waiting 4–6 months, moderate to complete improvement occurred in only 19%. Waiting for patients to adapt to the SSRI may work best for patients with mild sexual dysfunction (Montejo-González et al. 1997). The insoluble tablet shell may remain intact and be visible in the stool. Bupropion may increase the risks associated with electroconvulsive therapy (ECT); consider discontinuing, when possible, before ECT treatment. Using dosages higher than prescribed may increase motor activity, agitation/excitement, and euphoria. Inhalation of crushed tablets or injection of dissolved bupropion has been reported, in some instances resulting in seizures and death (American Psychiatric Association 2010).

H. An overall increased risk of congenital malformations has not been observed following maternal use of bupropion during pregnancy; however, data specific to cardiovascular malformations are inconsistent (Lexicomp/UpToDate 2024).

I. Bupropion and its metabolites cross the placenta (Fokina et al. 2016a). The pharmacokinetics of bupropion are not significantly influenced by pregnancy; the overall maternal exposure to bupropion and its active metabolite hydroxybupropion is not significantly changed in pregnant patients (Fokina et al. 2016a, 2016b).

Further Reading

Montejo AL, Prieto N, de Alarcón R, et al: Management strategies for antidepressant-related sexual dysfunction: a clinical approach. J Clin Med 8(10):1640, 2019 31591339

Rothmore J: Antidepressant-induced sexual dysfunction. Med J Aust 212(7):329–334, 2020 32172535

Zajecka J: Strategies for the treatment of antidepressant-related sexual dysfunction. J Clin Psychiatry 62(Suppl 3):35–43, 2001 11229451

References

American Psychiatric Association: Practice Guideline for the Treatment of Patients With Major Depressive Disorder, 3rd Edition. Arlington, VA, American Psychiatric Association, November 2010. Available at: https://psychiatryonline.org/pb/assets/raw/sitewide/practice_guidelines/guidelines/mdd.pdf. Accessed March 13, 2024.

Ashton AK, Rosen RC: Bupropion as an antidote for serotonin reuptake inhibitor-induced sexual dysfunction. J Clin Psychiatry 59(3):112–115, 1998 9541153

Baldessarini RJ, Faedda GL, Offidani E, et al: Antidepressant-associated mood-switching and transition from unipolar major depression to bipolar disorder: a review. J Affect Disord 148(1):129–135, 2013 23219059

Balon R, Segraves RT: Survey of treatment practices for sexual dysfunction(s) associated with antidepressants. J Sex Marital Ther 34(4):353–365, 2008 18576236

Clayton AH, Croft HA, Horrigan JP, et al: Bupropion extended release compared with escitalopram: effects on sexual functioning and antidepressant efficacy in 2 randomized, double-blind, placebo-controlled studies. J Clin Psychiatry 67(5):736–746, 2006 16841623

Fokina VM, West H, Oncken C, et al: Bupropion therapy during pregnancy: the drug and its major metabolites in umbilical cord plasma and amniotic fluid. Am J Obstet Gynecol 215(4):497.e1–497.e7, 2016a 27180885

Fokina VM, Xu M, Rytting E, et al: Pharmacokinetics of bupropion and its pharmacologically active metabolites in pregnancy. Drug Metab Dispos 44(11):1832–1838, 2016b 27528039
Friedman RA, Leon AC: Expanding the black box—depression, antidepressants, and the risk of suicide. N Engl J Med 356(23):2343–2346, 2007 17485726
Gitlin MJ, Suri R, Altshuler L, et al: Bupropion-sustained release as a treatment for SSRI-induced sexual side effects. J Sex Marital Ther 28(2):131–138, 2002 11894796
Kara H, Ak A, Bayır A, et al: Seizures after overdoses of bupropion intake. Balkan Med J 30(2):248–249, 2013 25207109
Keks NA, Hope J, Culhane C: Management of antidepressant-induced sexual dysfunction. Australas Psychiatry 22(6):525–528, 2014 25335956
Kennedy SH, McCann SM, Masellis M, et al: Combining bupropion SR with venlafaxine, paroxetine, or fluoxetine: a preliminary report on pharmacokinetic, therapeutic, and sexual dysfunction effects. J Clin Psychiatry 63(3):181–186, 2002 11926715
Labbate LA, Grimes JB, Hines A, et al: Bupropion treatment of serotonin reuptake antidepressant-associated sexual dysfunction. Ann Clin Psychiatry 9(4):241–245, 1997 9511948
Lexicomp/UpToDate: Bupropion: drug information. Lexicomp, n.d. Available at: https://pro.uptodatefree.ir/Show/9171#:~:text=Mechanism%3A%20Dose%2Drelated%3B%20bupropion,thinking%20and%20perception%20(Ref). Accessed July 31, 2024.
Li SXM, Perry KW, Wong DT: Influence of fluoxetine on the ability of bupropion to modulate extracellular dopamine and norepinephrine concentrations in three mesocorticolimbic areas of rats. Neuropharmacology 42(2):181–190, 2002 11804614
Montejo-González AL, Llorca G, Izquierdo JA, et al: SSRI-induced sexual dysfunction: fluoxetine, paroxetine, sertraline, and fluvoxamine in a prospective, multicenter, and descriptive clinical study of 344 patients. J Sex Marital Ther 23(3):176–194, 1997 9292833
Sadock BJ, Sadock VA, Ruiz P: Selective Serotonin Reuptake Inhibitors, Eleventh Edition. Philadelphia, Wolters Kluwer, 2015
Safarinejad MR: Reversal of SSRI-induced female sexual dysfunction by adjunctive bupropion in menstruating women: a double-blind, placebo-controlled and randomized study. J Psychopharmacol 25(3):370–378, 2011 20080928
Stahl SM, Pradko JF, Haight BR, et al: A review of the neuropharmacology of bupropion, a dual norepinephrine and dopamine reuptake inhibitor. Prim Care Companion J Clin Psychiatry 6(4):159–166, 2004 15361919
Symes RJ, Etminan M, Mikelberg FS: Risk of angle-closure glaucoma with bupropion and topiramate. JAMA Ophthalmol 133(10):1187–1189, 2015 26158444
Taylor MJ, Rudkin L, Bullemor-Day P, et al: Strategies for managing sexual dysfunction induced by antidepressant medication. Cochrane Database Syst Rev (5):CD003382, 2013 23728643
Vetter VL, Elia J, Erickson C, et al; American Heart Association Council on Cardiovascular Disease in the Young Congenital Cardiac Defects Committee; American Heart Association Council on Cardiovascular Nursing: Cardiovascular monitoring of children and adolescents with heart disease receiving medications for attention deficit/hyperactivity disorder [corrected]: a scientific statement from the American Heart Association Council on Cardiovascular Disease in the Young Congenital Cardiac Defects Committee and the Council on Cardiovascular Nursing. Circulation 117(18):2407–2423, 2008 18427125

Phosphodiesterase-5 Inhibitors (for Medication-Induced Sexual Dysfunction)

I. **Mechanism of Action:**

A. Oral phosphodiesterase type 5 (PDE5) inhibitors cause cyclic guanosine monophosphate (cGMP)–mediated nitric oxide–induced vasodilation that is helpful in initiating and maintaining an erection. PDE5 inhibitors increase the number and duration of erections in men with erectile dysfunction (Boolell et al. 1996).

II. **Data:**

A. PDE5 inhibitors effectively treat erectile dysfunction secondary to psychoactive drugs. The PDE5 inhibitors play a role in treating men with SSRI-induced erectile dysfunction. However, PDE5 does not address difficulties achieving orgasm (Jing and Straw-Wilson 2016).

B. In a systematic review and network analysis, sildenafil improved sexual dysfunction (Luft et al. 2021). In another study involving 14 outpatients with depression (9 men and 5 women; mean age: 46.4±8.4) treated with oral sildenafil, 12 of the 14 patients were treated with an SSRI and 2 with mirtazapine. All patients were prescribed oral sildenafil tablets at the initial dose of 50 mg/day on an as-needed basis, with the possibility of increasing the dosage to 100 mg/day as needed if clinically indicated. The participants with antidepressant-induced sexual dysfunction showed significant improvements in all domains of sexual functioning (Fava et al. 1998).

C. In another prospective randomized, double-blind, placebo-controlled trial with 90 male outpatients (mean [SD] age, 45 [8] years) with major depressive disorder in remission and SSRI-associated sexual dysfunction, patients were randomly assigned to take sildenafil (*n*=45) or placebo (*n*=45) at a flexible dose starting at 50 mg, adjustable to 100 mg taken prior to sexual activity for 6 weeks. Ninety-three percent (83/89) of patients treated with sildenafil experienced improvement of erectile function and other aspects of sexual function (Nurnberg et al. 2003).

D. In a study with 14 male patients who developed sexual dysfunction while receiving SSRIs, participants were screened with the Arizona Sexual Experience (ASEX) scale. Each patient was prescribed sildenafil tablets to be taken at a dosage of 25–100 mg twice a week. Patients were treated for a total of 8 weeks. All but 1 of the 14 patients experienced an improvement of sexual dysfunction, with 9 patients improving at the initial dose of 25 mg and 4 improving at higher doses (3 at 50 mg and 1 at 75 mg). Sildenafil was shown to be helpful in the treatment of SSRI-induced sexual dysfunction. Few patients had continued benefits after discontinuation of sildenafil (Montejo et al. 2019).

E. Onset and duration of action separate one PDE5 inhibitor from another. Sildenafil, vardenafil, and tadalafil should be taken 60 minutes before sexual activity. Avanafil and the orally disintegrating formulation of vardenafil tablet are more rapidly acting and can be taken 30 minutes before sexual activity. The typical duration of action for sildenafil, vardenafil, and avanafil is about 4–5 hours. In contrast, tadalafil is effective for up to 36 hours after dosing (McCullough et al. 2008; Porst et al. 2003).

F. Sildenafil, vardenafil, tadalafil, and avanafil seem to promote similarly high rates of successful sexual intercourse (68%–69% compared with 33%–35% for placebo) and similar side-effect profiles (Tsertsvadze et al. 2009a). Therefore, a Clinical Practice Guideline from the American College of Physicians (ACP) recommended that the choice of PDE5 inhibitor be based on the patient's preferences regarding cost, ease of use, desired duration of action, and adverse effects (Qaseem et al. 2009).

III. **Dosing**:

A. **Sildenafil**: 25–100 mg PO 1 hour before intercourse (Pfizer Inc 1998). Sildenafil should be taken orally on an empty stomach approximately 1 hour before a planned sexual encounter. The initial dose should be 50 mg, which can be reduced to 25 mg if side effects occur. The dose can be increased to 100 mg if lower doses produce unsatisfactory results (Pfizer Inc 1998).

B. **Vardenafil**: 10–20 mg PO 1 hour before intercourse (Bayer Pharma 2014). Vardenafil is available in 10- and 20-mg doses, and it is also available as an orodispersible tablet with a potentially more rapid onset of action (30 minutes) than the standard oral formulation (Bayer Pharma 2014; Debruyne et al. 2011).

C. **Tadalafil**: 5–20 mg PO 1 hour before intercourse (Lilly USA LLC 2003). Tadalafil's recommended starting dose for as-needed use is 10 mg, decreasing to 5 mg or increasing to 20 mg if necessary. Daily tadalafil may be effective in men with "complete" erectile dysfunction, defined as having a persistent failure to achieve an erection satisfactory for intercourse (Lilly USA LLC 2003). The recommended starting dose of vardenafil (Levitra) is 10 mg, taken orally approximately 60 minutes before sexual activity. The dose may be increased to a maximum recommended dose of 20 mg or decreased to 5 mg based on efficacy and side effects. The maximum recommended dosing frequency is once per day. Vardenafil can be taken with or without food. Sexual stimulation is required for a response to treatment.

D. **Avanafil**: 100–200 mg approximately 15 minutes before sexual activity (Vivus Inc 2012). Avanafil is taken on an as-needed basis at a starting dose of 50 mg, increasing to 100 or 200 mg as needed. The 50-mg dose should be taken 30 minutes before sexual activity. In contrast, the 100- or 200-mg dose can be taken just 15 minutes prior to anticipated sexual activity. Avanafil is the only approved PDE5 inhibitor with an anticipated 15-minute onset of action. Avanafil is rapidly absorbed after oral administration (within 30–45 minutes), and absorption is not significantly impacted by food (Vivus Inc 2012).

IV. **Cautions/Monitoring**:

A. PDE5 inhibitors are contraindicated in patients taking nitrates of any form, regularly or intermittently, because of the risk of severe hypotension. Alpha-adrenergic antagonists, which are commonly used to treat benign prostatic hyperplasia, may cause symptomatic hypotension when taken in combination with PDE5 inhibitors (Pomara et al. 2004). PDE5 inhibitors may cause profound hypotension, lightheadedness, and dizziness. In addition, patients with renal insufficiency and hepatic impairment can have higher serum concentrations of PDE5 inhibitors, requiring dose adjustment. Current labeling for all four PDE5 inhibitors recommends that a patient taking an alpha-blocker be on a stable dose before initiating the PDE5 inhibitor. Prolonged erection greater than 4 hours and priapism (painful erections greater than 6 hours in duration) have been reported with PDE5 inhibitors. The patient should seek immediate medical assistance. If not treated immediately, penile tissue damage and permanent loss of potency could result (Vivus Inc 2012).

B. Strong inhibitors of CYP3A4 (e.g., ritonavir, indinavir, saquinavir, erythromycin, ketoconazole) can increase PDE5 inhibitor levels. Grapefruit juice and cimetidine as selective inhibitors of CYP3A4 increase the systemic exposure to sildenafil and vardenafil. As an inhibitor of CYP3A4 and CYP2C19-mediated metabolism, ritonavir had an unusually high effect on vardenafil, increasing systemic exposure of vardenafil on average 49-fold (Gupta et al. 2005). Tadalafil's absorption rate decreases by 30% when coadministered with antacids (Lilly USA LLC 2003; Pfizer Inc 1998; Vivus Inc 2012).

C. Nitrate treatment should be delayed if chest pain develops on a PDE5 inhibitor. The delay of nitrate intake should be at least 12 hours if avanafil is taken, 24 hours if sildenafil or vardenafil is taken, and 48 hours if tadalafil is taken. The delay should be longer for each if the patient has renal or hepatic dysfunction.

D. Side effects associated with sildenafil are related to its vasodilatory properties and are similar to those induced by nitrates. In a meta-analysis of 14 trials, adverse events with sildenafil included flushing, headaches, and dyspepsia in 12%, 11%, and 5% of participants, respectively (Fink et al. 2002). Nasal congestion has been described in other reports (Tsertsvadze et al. 2009b). Side-effect profiles of vardenafil, avanafil, and tadalafil are similar to those of sildenafil (Goldstein et al. 2003; Porst et al. 2003).

E. Sildenafil occasionally causes "blue vision" in men, an effect related to cross-reaction of the PDE5 inhibitor in sildenafil with the PDE6 inhibitor, which is present in the retina and plays a role in color vision. "Blue vision" has been reported in approximately 3% of sildenafil-treated men, lasts 2–3 hours, and disappears spontaneously (Jägle et al. 2005). Blue vision has not been reported with vardenafil, tadalafil, or avanafil. Rare cases of nonarteritic anterior ischemic optic neuropathy (NAION) have been reported with sildenafil and tadalafil (Carter 2007; Thurtell and Tomsak 2008).

F. Sildenafil, vardenafil, and tadalafil have been associated with rare cases of sudden hearing loss (Thakur et al. 2013). The FDA requires that labeling of all PDE5 inhibitors include a warning of this potential risk. The hearing loss is usually unilateral, occurs within the first 24 hours of drug administration, and is temporary in approximately one-third of patients (Maddox et al. 2009).

G. PDE5 inhibitors require sufficient sexual arousal and stimulation to initiate the needed physiological changes to promote penile erection. Recreational use of sildenafil is common. There are case reports of stroke in men taking high-dose sildenafil (Kim et al. 2008). There is a questionable association between PDE5 use and a small increased risk of malignant melanoma (Loeb et al. 2015). It is recommended that β-blockers not be taken within 4 hours of a sildenafil dose greater than 25 mg.

References

Bayer Pharma: Levitra (vardenafil hydrochloride) tablets package insert. Bayer Pharma, 2014. Available at: https://www.accessdata.fda.gov/drugsatfda_docs/label/2014/021400s017lbl.pdf. Accessed March 7, 2024.

Boolell M, Gepi-Attee S, Gingell JC, et al: Sildenafil, a novel effective oral therapy for male erectile dysfunction. Br J Urol 78(2):257–261, 1996 8813924

Carter JE: Anterior ischemic optic neuropathy and stroke with use of PDE-5 inhibitors for erectile dysfunction: cause or coincidence? J Neurol Sci 262(1–2):89–97, 2007 17706972

Debruyne FM, Gittelman M, Sperling H, et al: Time to onset of action of vardenafil: a retrospective analysis of the pivotal trials for the orodispersible and film-coated tablet formulations. J Sex Med 8(10):2912–2923, 2011 2188395

Fava M, Rankin MA, Alpert JE, et al: An open trial of oral sildenafilin antidepressant-induced sexual dysfunction. Psychother Psychosom 67(6):328–331, 1998 9817955

Fink HA, Mac Donald R, Rutks IR, et al: Sildenafil for male erectile dysfunction: a systematic review and meta-analysis. Arch Intern Med 162(12):1349–1360, 2002 12076233

Goldstein I, Young JM, Fischer J, et al; Vardenafil Diabetes Study Group: Vardenafil, a new phosphodiesterase type 5 inhibitor, in the treatment of erectile dysfunction in men with diabetes: a multicenter double-blind placebo-controlled fixed-dose study. Diabetes Care 26(3):777–783, 2003 12610037

Gupta M, Kovar A, Meibohm B: The clinical pharmacokinetics of phosphodiesterase-5 inhibitors for erectile dysfunction. J Clin Pharmacol 45(9):987–1003, 2005 16100293

Jägle H, Jägle C, Sèrey L, et al: Dose-dependency and time-course of electrophysiologic short-term effects of VIAGRA: a case study. Doc Ophthalmol 110(2–3):247–254, 2005 16328933

Jing E, Straw-Wilson K: Sexual dysfunction in selective serotonin reuptake inhibitors (SSRIs) and potential solutions: a narrative literature review. Ment Health Clin 6(4):191–196, 2016 29955469

Kim KK, Kim DG, Ku YH, et al: Bilateral cerebral hemispheric infarction associated with sildenafil citrate (Viagra) use. Eur J Neurol 15(3):306–308, 2008 18290852

Lilly USA LLC: Cialis (tadalafil) tablets package insert. Lilly USA, 2003. Available at: https://www.accessdata.fda.gov/drugsatfda_docs/label/2011/021368s20s21lbl.pdf. Accessed March 13, 2024.

Loeb S, Folkvaljon Y, Lambe M, et al: Use of phosphodiesterase type 5 inhibitors for erectile dysfunction and risk of malignant melanoma. JAMA 313(24):2449–2455, 2015 26103029

Luft MJ, Dobson ET, Levine A, et al: Pharmacologic interventions for antidepressant-induced sexual dysfunction: a systematic review and network meta-analysis of trials using the Arizona sexual experience scale. CNS Spectr :1–10, 2021 33843553

Maddox PT, Saunders J, Chandrasekhar SS: Sudden hearing loss from PDE-5 inhibitors: a possible cellular stress etiology. Laryngoscope 119(8):1586–1589, 2009 19507217

McCullough AR, Steidle CP, Klee B, et al: Randomized, double-blind, crossover trial of sildenafil in men with mild to moderate erectile dysfunction: efficacy at 8 and 12 hours postdose. Urology 71(4):686–692, 2008 18387397

Montejo AL, Prieto N, de Alarcón R, et al: Management strategies for antidepressant-related sexual dysfunction: a clinical approach. J Clin Med 8(10):1640, 2019 31591339

Nurnberg HG, Hensley PL, Gelenberg AJ, et al: Treatment of antidepressant-associated sexual dysfunction with sildenafil: a randomized controlled trial. JAMA 289(1):56–64, 2003 12503977

Pfizer Inc: Viagra (sildenafil citrate) tablets package insert. Pfizer, 1998. Available at: https://www.accessdata.fda.gov/drugsatfda_docs/label/2014/20895s039s042lbl.pdf. Accessed March 13, 2024.

Pomara G, Morelli G, Pomara S, et al: Cardiovascular parameter changes in patients with erectile dysfunction using pde-5 inhibitors: a study with sildenafil and vardenafil. J Androl 25(4):625–629, 2004 15223851

Porst H, Padma-Nathan H, Giuliano F, et al: Efficacy of tadalafil for the treatment of erectile dysfunction at 24 and 36 hours after dosing: a randomized controlled trial. Urology 62(1):121–125, discussion 125–126, 2003 12837435

Qaseem A, Snow V, Denberg TD, et al; Clinical Efficacy Assessment Subcommittee of the American College of Physicians: Hormonal testing and pharmacologic treatment of erectile dysfunction: a clinical practice guideline from the American College of Physicians. Ann Intern Med 151(9):639–649, 2009 19884625

Thakur JS, Thakur S, Sharma DR, et al: Hearing loss with phosphodiesterase-5 inhibitors: a prospective and objective analysis with tadalafil. Laryngoscope 123(6):1527–1530, 2013 23553123

Thurtell MJ, Tomsak RL: Nonarteritic anterior ischemic optic neuropathy with PDE-5 inhibitors for erectile dysfunction. Int J Impot Res 20(6):537–543, 2008 18528398

Tsertsvadze A, Fink HA, Yazdi F, et al: Oral phosphodiesterase-5 inhibitors and hormonal treatments for erectile dysfunction: a systematic review and meta-analysis. Ann Intern Med 151(9):650–661, 2009a 19884626

Tsertsvadze A, Yazdi F, Fink HA, et al: Oral sildenafil citrate (viagra) for erectile dysfunction: a systematic review and meta-analysis of harms. Urology 74(4):831–836.e8, 2009b 19592078

Vivus Inc: Stendra (avanafil) tablets package insert. Vivus, 2012. Available at: https://www.accessdata.fda.gov/drugsatfda_docs/label/2012/202276s000lbl.pdf. Accessed March 13, 2024.

Sweating (Hyperhidrosis)

Overview

Drug-induced hyperhidrosis is the most common type of secondary hyperhidrosis. Drugs can act on the hypothalamus or at spinal thermoregulatory centers, at sympathetic ganglia, or at the eccrine-neuroeffector junction (Cheshire and Fealey 2008).

Hyperhidrosis results from the release of acetylcholine by medications that block the action of acetylcholinesterase. Because of impaired negative feedback to the hypothalamus, acetylcholine causes the body to sweat more than is needed for the core temperature to reach homeostasis (Cheshire and Fealey 2008).

Psychotropics associated with hyperhidrosis include SSRIs, tricyclic antidepressants, and antipsychotics.

Primary hyperhidrosis occurs symmetrically at sites where there are concentrated eccrine glands, such as the armpits, palms, soles of the feet, and face.

Sweating in drug-induced hyperhidrosis is more likely to be unilateral, asymmetrical, or generalized, affecting any body part. While sweating decreases at night in patients with primary hyperhidrosis, increased sweating can often occur during sleep in drug-induced hyperhidrosis (Brackenrich and Fagg 2022).

Drug-induced hyperhidrosis is diagnosed clinically. Other causes of secondary hyperhidrosis should be excluded, such as an underlying infection, malignancy, or neurological or endocrine conditions. A physical examination can help exclude other causes of increased sweating. If hyperhidrosis is active on examination, the location and pattern of sweating can help to differentiate between primary and secondary causes. There is no laboratory test to confirm drug-induced hyperhidrosis. However, Minor's starch-iodine test and gravimetric analysis can be used to confirm localized sweating, which often points toward primary hyperhidrosis (Colvin et al. 2018).

References

Brackenrich J, Fagg C: Hyperhidrosis, in StatPearls. Treasure Island, FL, StatPearls Publishing, 2022. Available at: https://www.ncbi.nlm.nih.gov/books/NBK459227/. Accessed March 31, 2022.

Cheshire WP, Fealey RD: Drug-induced hyperhidrosis and hypohidrosis: incidence, prevention and management. Drug Saf 31(2):109–126, 2008 18217788

Colvin NN, Hayes H Jr, Chisum A, et al: Don't sweat it: an overview of hyperhidrosis. US Pharm 43(6):15–18, 2018. Available at: https://www.uspharmacist.com/article/dont-sweat-it-an-overview-of-hyperhidrosis. Accessed March 31, 2022.

Clonidine (for Medication-Induced Hyperhidrosis)

I. **Mechanism of Action:**

A. Clonidine stimulates alpha-2 adrenoceptors in the brain stem, thus activating an inhibitory neuron, resulting in reduced sympathetic outflow from the CNS. This decreased outflow produces reductions in peripheral resistance, renal vascular resistance, heart rate, and blood pressure. Epidural clonidine may provide pain relief at spinal presynaptic and postjunctional alpha-2 adrenoceptors by preventing pain signal transmission; pain relief occurs only for the body regions innervated by the spinal segments where analgesic concentrations of clonidine are achieved (Boehringer Ingelheim Pharmaceuticals 2022).

B. Postsynaptic alpha-2 agonist stimulation regulates subcortical activity in the prefrontal cortex, the brain area responsible for emotions, attention, and behaviors, and causes reduced hyperactivity, impulsiveness, and distractibility.

II. **Data:**

A. A retrospective chart review involving 13 patients with primary hyperhidrosis treated with clonidine (0.1 mg twice daily) reported a response rate of 46% (6/13). The 7 patients for whom treatment was not effective included 3 patients who were nonresponders and 4 who experienced adverse effects related to decreased blood pressure (Walling 2012).

B. Another report described the case of a patient treated for specific excessive localized sweating of the face and scalp with clonidine hydrochloride (0.3–0.4 mg) taken at bedtime in combination with aluminum chloride. Over 2–3 weeks, the patient achieved complete remission of symptoms while experiencing only mild side effects (Torch 2000).

III. **Dosing:**

A. Clonidine is available as tablets for oral administration in three dosage strengths: 0.1 mg, 0.2 mg, and 0.3 mg. Sparse case reports of clonidine therapy for hyperhidrosis describe use of oral clonidine dosages of up to 0.15 mg twice daily (Albadrani 2017). Other reports describe use of clonidine dosages up to 0.3 mg or 0.4 mg (Torch 2000).

IV. **Cautions/Monitoring:**

A. Clonidine is contraindicated in patients with hypersensitivity to clonidine or any component of its formulation.

B. Epidural administration of clonidine is contraindicated in patients receiving anticoagulant therapy and in those with a bleeding diathesis (Drugs.com 2024). In addition, injection site infection is a potential risk associated with epidural administration.

C. Alpha-2 agonists such as clonidine may enhance the atrioventricular-blocking effect of beta-blockers. Sinus node dysfunction may also be enhanced. Beta-blockers may enhance the rebound hypertensive effect of alpha-2 agonists.

D. Clonidine may enhance the hypotensive effect of second-generation/atypical antipsychotics.
E. Clonidine may enhance the CNS depressant effects of esketamine and of opioid agonists (e.g., buprenorphine, oxycodone) (Boehringer Ingelheim Pharmaceuticals 2022).
F. The clonidine package insert lists the following frequencies for specific adverse effects: Xerostomia (5%–40%), dizziness (2%–16% [placebo: 5%]), drowsiness (12%–38% [placebo: 4%]), fatigue (6%–16% [placebo: 1%]), headache (1%–20% [placebo: 16%]) (UpToDate 2024).
G. Clonidine may cause eye dryness in patients who wear contact lenses (UpToDate 2024).
H. Abrupt discontinuation of clonidine increases the risk of rebound hypertension and other withdrawal symptoms (e.g., nervousness, agitation, headache, tremor). Clonidine should be discontinued slowly over 6–10 days by reducing the dosage by one-third to one-half every 2–3 days. For patients on a beta-blocker and clonidine, withdraw the beta-blocker several days before clonidine, then slowly taper clonidine. Rebound hypertension and withdrawal symptoms are less likely with a clonidine transdermal patch than with oral clonidine therapy (Houston 1981).
    1. Because children commonly have gastrointestinal illnesses that lead to vomiting, they are susceptible to hypertensive episodes resulting from an abrupt discontinuation of clonidine.
I. Clonidine was previously categorized as FDA pregnancy Category C. Clonidine hydrochloride is excreted in human breast milk.

Further Reading

Walling HW, Swick BL: Treatment options for hyperhidrosis. Am J Clin Dermatol 12(5):285–295, 2011

Wolraich M, Brown L, Brown RT, et al; Subcommittee on Attention-Deficit/Hyperactivity Disorder; Steering Committee on Quality Improvement and Management: ADHD: clinical practice guideline for the diagnosis, evaluation, and treatment of attention-deficit/hyperactivity disorder in children and adolescents. Pediatrics 128(5):1007–1022, 2011 22003063

References

Albadrani A: Clonidine is effective for the treatment of primary idiopathic hyperhidrosis and hot flushes: a case report. J Med Case Rep 11(1):16, 2017 28093070

Boehringer Ingelheim Pharmaceuticals: Catapres (clonidine HCl) package insert. Boehringer Ingelheim Pharmaceuticals, n.d. Available at: https://www.accessdata.fda.gov/drugsatfda_docs/label/2009/017407s034lbl.pdf. Accessed February 12, 2022.

Drugs.com: Clonidine, clonidine hydrochloride (monograph). Medically reviewed by Drugs.com on June 10, 2024. Available at: https://www.drugs.com/monograph/clonidine-clonidine-hydrochloride.html. Accessed July 31, 2024.

Houston MC: Clonidine hydrochloride: review of pharmacologic and clinical aspects. Prog Cardiovasc Dis 23(5):337–350, 1981 7012927

Torch EM: Remission of facial and scalp hyperhidrosis with clonidine hydrochloride and topical aluminum chloride. South Med J 93(1):68–69, 2000 10653070

UpToDate: Clonidine: drug information. n.d. Available at: https://pro.uptodatefree.ir/Show/9285#:~:text=For%20patients%20on%20both%20a,to%20oral%20therapy%20(Ref). Accessed July 31, 2024.

Walling HW: Systemic therapy for primary hyperhidrosis: a retrospective study of 59 patients treated with glycopyrrolate or clonidine. J Am Acad Dermatol 66(3):387–392, 2012 21820204

Terazosin (for Medication-Induced Hyperhidrosis)

I. **Mechanism of Action**:

A. Terazosin is an alpha$_1$-specific blocking agent with minimal alpha$_2$ effects. This allows peripheral postsynaptic blockade, with a resultant decrease in arterial tone, while preserving the negative feedback loop, which is mediated by the peripheral presynaptic alpha$_2$ receptors. Terazosin relaxes the smooth muscle of the bladder neck, thus reducing bladder outlet obstruction (Abbott Laboratories 2009).

II. **Data**:

A. Antidepressant-induced excessive sweating (ADIES) occurs in 5%–14% of patients taking antidepressants that work on biogenic amines, usually persists throughout treatment, and causes subjective distress and functional impairment.

B. A study of terazosin in ADIES involved 23 patients with moderate to severe ADIES who were assessed for a 2-week baseline period, followed by 6 weeks of open-label treatment with flexible-dose terazosin, 1–6 mg/day. Improvement in ADIES was measured by the Clinical Global Impressions (CGI) scale and other measures. Twenty-two of the 23 patients responded to terazosin (CGI Improvement [CGI-I] scores of 1 or 2), with CGI Severity (CGI-S) scores improving from a median of 5 to a median of 2 (P<0.0001). In addition, patient-rated daytime and nighttime severity of ADIES and proportion of time experiencing ADIES also improved significantly. The most common adverse effects of terazosin therapy were dizziness/lightheadedness (n=9) and dry mouth (n=4) (Mago et al. 2013).

C. A study was designed to evaluate the effect of terazosin on sertraline-related sweating. All patients diagnosed with major depressive disorder who were taking sertraline and suffered from excessive sweating were enrolled in the study and randomly allocated into two groups receiving either terazosin (1 mg) or placebo. Sweating severity was classified using the Hyperhidrosis Disease Severity Scale. The patients were evaluated regarding the severity of sweating before the beginning of the study and 14 days after beginning either terazosin or placebo. Fourteen days after beginning treatment with terazosin, the severity of sweating reduced to the lowest grade in 46 (68%) and 2 (6%) cases in the terazosin and placebo groups, respectively (P<0.001) (Ghaleiha et al. 2013).

III. **Dosing**:

A. Terazosin is dosed at 1–6 mg orally daily. To decrease the likelihood of syncope or excessive hypotension, treatment should always be initiated with a 1-mg dose at bedtime.

IV. **Cautions/Monitoring**:

A. Monitoring: The use of terazosin does not require plasma/blood drug level monitoring. Orthostatic vital signs should be obtained after the first dose to exclude postural hypotension (Yang and Raja 2023). For up to 24 months, treatment with terazosin had no significant effect on prostate-specific antigen (PSA) levels. In controlled clinical trials, small but statistically significant decreases in hematocrit, hemoglobin, white blood cells, total protein, and albumin were observed. These laboratory findings suggested the possibility of hemodilution (Abbott Laboratories 2009). Terazosin may diminish the vasoconstricting effect of alpha/beta agonists. Terazosin may enhance the hypotensive effect of antipsychotics. Beta-blockers may enhance the orthostatic hypotensive effect of terazosin. Phosphodiesterase 5 inhibitors may enhance the hypotensive effect of terazosin.

B. Dizziness (9%–19%) and myasthenia (7%–11%) are common side effects of terazosin (Lexicomp/UpToDate 2024). Terazosin may cause CNS depression, which may impair physical or mental abilities. Intraoperative floppy iris syndrome has been observed in cataract surgery patients who were actively taking or previously taking terazosin. In addition, terazosin can cause orthostatic hypotension/syncope.

C. Terazosin should be administered at the same time each day. Terazosin is identified in the Beers Criteria as a potentially inappropriate medication in patients age 65 years and older due to its high risk of orthostatic hypotension (American Geriatrics Society Beers Criteria Update Expert Panel 2023). The manufacturer recommends that caution be exercised when administering terazosin to breastfeeding women (Abbott Laboratories 2009) (Ghaleiha et al. 2013). Terazosin and other α_1 antagonists have been associated with priapism (Abbott Laboratories 2009).

Further Reading

Cheah PY, Liong ML, Yuen KH, et al: Terazosin therapy for chronic prostatitis/chronic pelvic pain syndrome: a randomized, placebo controlled trial. J Urol 169(2):592–596, 2003 12544314

Gregoriou O, Vitoratos N, Papadias C, et al: Treatment of idiopathic oligozoospermia with an alpha-blocker: a placebo-controlled double-blind trial. Int J Fertil Womens Med 42(5):301–305, 1997 9406835

López A, Wright JM: Rosuvastatin and the JUPITER trial: critical appraisal of a lifeless planet in the galaxy of primary prevention. Int J Occup Environ Health 18(1):70–78, 2012 22550699

Sridharan K, Sivaramakrishnan G: Efficacy and safety of alpha blockers in medical expulsive therapy for ureteral stones: a mixed treatment network meta-analysis and trial sequential analysis of randomized controlled clinical trials. Expert Rev Clin Pharmacol 11(3):291–307, 2018 29334287

Wilt TJ, Howe RW, Rutks IR, et al: Terazosin for benign prostatic hyperplasia. Cochrane Database Syst Rev (4):CD003851, 2002

References

Abbott Laboratories: Hytrin (terazosin hydrochloride). Revised July 2009. Available at: https://www.accessdata.fda.gov/drugsatfda_docs/label/2009/019057s022lbl.pdf. Accessed March 13, 2024.

American Geriatrics Society Beers Criteria Update Expert Panel: 2023 updated AGS Beers Criteria for potentially inappropriate medication use in older adults. J Am Geriatr Soc 71(7):2052–2081, 2013 37139824

Ghaleiha A, Shahidi KM, Afzali S, et al: Effect of terazosin on sweating in patients with major depressive disorder receiving sertraline: a randomized controlled trial. Int J Psychiatry Clin Pract 17(1):44–47, 2013 22731399

Lexicomp/UpToDate: Terazosin: drug information. n.d. Available at: https://pro.uptodatefree.ir/Show/9975. Accessed July 31, 2024.

Mago R, Thase ME, Rovner BW: Antidepressant-induced excessive sweating: clinical features and treatment with terazosin. Ann Clin Psychiatry 25(3):186–192, 2013 23638448

Yang CH, Raja A: Terazosin, StatPearls. Treasure Island, FL, StatPearls Publishing, 2023. Available at: https://www.ncbi.nlm.nih.gov/books/NBK545208/. Accessed March 13, 2024.

Tardive Dyskinesia

Overview

Tardive dyskinesia (TD) is a disorder involving involuntary movements of the tongue, lips, face, trunk, and extremities that occurs in patients treated with long-term dopaminergic antagonist medications.

People with schizophrenia and other neuropsychiatric disorders are especially vulnerable to the development of TD after exposure to conventional antipsychotics, certain antidepressants, metoclopramide, anticholinergics, toxins, substances of abuse, and other agents. Based on clinical experience, some cases of TD may worsen over time, others may improve over time, and still others may remain unchanged. Additionally, risk factors may include age and gender and the potency, duration, and dose of the antipsychotic.

Dysfunction of the dopamine transporter has been hypothesized to play a role in the development of TD (Brasic 2018).

References

Brasic JR: Tardive dyskinesia: overview. MedScape, 2018. Available at: https://emedicine.medscape.com/article/1151826-overview?ecd=ppc_google_rlsa-traf_mscp_emed_md_us. Accessed March 31, 2022.

Deutetrabenazine (for Medication-Induced Tardive Dyskinesia)

I. **Mechanism of Action**:

A. Deutetrabenazine and its major metabolites (alpha-dihydrotetrabenazine [HTBZ] and beta-HTBZ) act as reversible inhibitors of the human vesicular monoamine transporter type 2 (VMAT-2). These VMAT-2 proteins decrease the uptake of monoamines (including dopamine, serotonin, norepinephrine, and histamine) into synaptic vesicles and deplete the monoamine stores (TDS Health, n.d.; Teva Pharmaceuticals USA 2020).

II. **Data**:

A. In a randomized double-blind multicenter trial, 117 patients with moderate to severe tardive dyskinesia received deutetrabenazine or placebo. Eligibility criteria included an Abnormal Involuntary Movement Scale (AIMS) score of ≥6. The primary endpoint was the change in AIMS score from baseline to week 12. Deutetrabenazine significantly reduced AIMS scores from baseline to week 12 compared with placebo (least-squares mean [standard error] of –3.0 [0.45] vs. –1.6 [0.46], P=0.019) (Fernandez et al. 2017).

B. A systematic review found that 46% of patients on deutetrabenazine were deemed responders (defined as "much improved" or "very much improved") based on the Clinical Global Impression of change scale rating (pooled dose groups 12 and 18 mg BID) versus 26% of patients taking placebo, yielding a number needed to treat (NNT) of 5 (95% CI 3–19). The percentage of responders (defined by an improvement in AIMS severity score [sum of items 1–7] of 50% or more) was 34% for deutetrabenazine (pooled dosage groups 12 and 18 mg BID) versus 12% for placebo, yielding an NNT of 5 (95% CI 3–11) (Citrome 2017).

C. A 106-week study on the safety and efficacy of deutetrabenazine in patients with tardive dyskinesia analyzed 331 patient-years of exposure. The mean (SE) change in AIMS score was –4.9 (0.4) at week 54 (n=146), –6.3 (0.7) at week 80 (n=66), and –5.1 (2.0) at week 106 (n=8). Long-term treatment with deutetrabenazine was efficacious, safe, and well-tolerated in cohorts of patients with tardive dyskinesia (Fernandez et al. 2019).

III. **Dosing**:

A. Oral: Initial: 6 mg twice daily; may increase the dosage weekly based on response and tolerability in 6 mg/day increments. Administer in two divided doses if the daily dose is ≥12 mg. The maximum recommended dosage is 48 mg/day.

B. For patients who are poor CYP2D6 metabolizers, the maximum recommended dosage is 36 mg/day (i.e., 18 mg twice daily) (Teva Pharmaceuticals USA 2020).

C. If dosing is interrupted for longer than 7 days, re-titration is necessary when resuming.

D. Patients should swallow deutetrabenazine tablets whole; they should not chew, crush, or break them.

E. If adverse reactions such as agitation, akathisia, anxiety, cognitive decline, depression, restlessness, parkinsonism, sedation (intolerable), somnolence, or suicidality occur, dosage decrease or medication discontinuation is recommended.

IV. **Cautions/Monitoring**:

A. Deutetrabenazine is relatively contraindicated in patients with hepatic impairment, Huntington's disease patients with suicidality, or suicidal or very depressed adults.

B. Deutetrabenazine use is contraindicated in patients taking valbenazine or tetrabenazine. Deutetrabenazine should not be coadministered with reserpine or a monoamine oxidase inhibitor (MAOI). Furthermore, deutetrabenazine should not be started within 20 days of discontinuation of reserpine, or within 14 days of discontinuation of an MAOI (Teva Pharmaceuticals USA 2020).

C. There are no guidelines on the frequency of the following assessments during deutetrabenazine treatment: electrolytes; ECG; signs/symptoms of depression or suicidal ideation; signs and/or symptoms of neuroleptic malignant syndrome (NMS), restlessness, and agitation (UpToDate 2024). However, a baseline assessment and repetition of labs after 1 week of treatment seems reasonable.

D. Nasopharyngitis and insomnia are the most common side effects, occurring in more than 4% of treated patients.

E. Deutetrabenazine can cause CNS depression, and patients should be cautioned about operating machinery after taking this medication.

F. Deutetrabenazine is metabolized by CYP2D6, CYP1A2, and CYP3A4. The total daily dosage of deutetrabenazine should not exceed 36 mg when used concomitantly with strong CYP inhibitors (or in individuals who are known phenotypic CYP poor metabolizers at the pathways in question). The maximum single dose of deutetrabenazine should not exceed 18 mg when taken concomitantly with a strong CYP2D6 inhibitor.

G. Patients with a history of depression and/or suicidal ideation should receive a weekly evaluation, particularly at treatment initiation in patients who are CYP2D6 poor metabolizers, because such patients experience increased levels of deutetrabenazine's primary drug metabolites. For these patients, the maximum deutetrabenazine dosage should not exceed 36 mg/day (maximum single dose of 18 mg).

H. Deutetrabenazine may enhance the adverse/toxic effects of antipsychotics; specifically, the risk for akathisia, parkinsonism, or NMS increases. Close observation of physical symptoms is necessary.

I. Deutetrabenazine may cause akathisia severe enough to necessitate dosage reduction. Parkinsonism, including bradykinesia and gait disturbances, has been noted with deutetrabenazine initiation or dosage escalation. These effects may necessitate dosage reduction or discontinuation.

J. Deutetrabenazine enhances the CNS depressant effects of esketamine; of other CNS depressants (e.g., benzodiazepines, buprenorphine, oxycodone); and of hydroxyzine, kava kava, and kratom.

K. Deutetrabenazine can prolong the QTc interval, and QT-prolonging agents may enhance this QTc-prolonging effect of deutetrabenazine. Deutetrabenazine should not be used concomitantly with other drugs that are known to prolong the QTc interval. Deutetrabenazine should be avoided in patients with congenital QT prolongation or a history of cardiac arrhythmias. The risk of QTc prolongation may be increased in patients with bradycardia, hypokalemia, hypomagnesemia, concomitant use of drugs known to cause QT prolongation, or the presence of congenital QTc prolongation.

L. Deutetrabenazine may worsen mood, cognition, rigidity, and functional capacity in patients with Huntington's disease, which can be difficult to differentiate from a progression of Huntington's disease itself.

M. Deutetrabenazine may increase serum prolactin concentrations, which may lead to amenorrhea or impotence.

N. No adverse effect data in pregnancy or lactation in humans are available.

Further Reading

Bashir HH, Jankovic J: Treatment of tardive dyskinesia. Neurol Clin 38(2):379–396, 2020 32279716

DailyMed: Austedo (deutetrabenazine) tablet, coated; Austedo (deutetrabenazine) kit. n.d. Available at: https://dailymed.nlm.nih.gov/dailymed/drugInfo.cfm?setid=7ea3c60a-45c7-44cc-afc2-d87fa53993c0. Accessed February 8, 2022.

Gupta H, Moity AR, Jumonville A, et al: Valbenazine for the treatment of adults with tardive dyskinesia. Health Psychol Res 9(1):24929, 2021 35106396

Khorassani F, Luther K, Talreja O: Valbenazine and deutetrabenazine: vesicular monoamine transporter 2 inhibitors for tardive dyskinesia. Am J Health Syst Pharm 77(3):167–174, 2020 31974564

References

Citrome L: Deutetrabenazine for tardive dyskinesia: a systematic review of the efficacy and safety profile for this newly approved novel medication. Int J Clin Pract 71(11): 2017 29024264

Fernandez HH, Factor SA, Hauser RA, et al: Randomized controlled trial of deutetrabenazine for tardive dyskinesia: the ARM-TD study. Neurology 88(21):2003–2010, 2017 28446646

Fernandez HH, Stamler D, Davis MD, et al: Long-term safety and efficacy of deutetrabenazine for the treatment of tardive dyskinesia. J Neurol Neurosurg Psychiatry 90(12):1317–1323, 2019 31296586

TDS Health: Deutetrabenazine. n.d. StatRef. Available at: https://online.statref.com/document/ad9AfBlts4fvG7lIyZVJUD?searchid=164435929715324063 0andcategoryType=All. February 8, 2022.

UpToDate: Deutetrabenazine: drug information. n.d. Available at: https://pro.uptodatefree.ir/show/112590. Accessed July 31, 2024.

Teva Pharmaceuticals USA: Deutetrabenazine prescribing information. Revised December 2020. Available at: https://www.accessdata.fda.gov/drugsatfda_docs/label/2020/208082s007lbl.pdf. Accessed March 13, 2024.

Tetrabenazine (for Medication-Induced Tardive Dyskinesia) (Off-Label)

I. Mechanism of Action:

A. Tetrabenazine is a reversible inhibitor of the human vesicular monoamine transporter type 2 (VMAT-2), and is not currently approved by the FDA. It decreases the uptake of monoamines (including dopamine, serotonin, norepinephrine, and histamine) into synaptic vesicles and depletes monoamine stores. Hydroxytetrabenazine (HTBZ) also inhibits VMAT-2, with a weak binding affinity for dopamine D_2 receptors (Lundbeck 2017).

II. Data:

A. In a prospective study that included a 6-week treatment period with tetrabenazine started at 50 mg/day, and titration to between 100 mg/day and 150 mg/day, 8 patients (33%) experienced complete resolution of tardive dyskinesia, 6 (25%) experienced marked improvement, another 6 had little or no change, and 4 patients did not complete the study (2 developed severe malaise, 1 withdrew because of an exacerbation of psychosis, and 1 was lost to follow-up). Compared with placebo, tetrabenazine was found to significantly reduce tardive dyskinesia by 64% based on standard rating scales (Kazamatsuri et al. 1972; Lundbeck 2017).

B. Two large retrospective reports of tetrabenazine treatment of hyperkinetic movement disorders supported its beneficial role in tardive dyskinesia. More than 84% of tardive dyskinesia patients (n=242 patients) rated their improvement as either moderate or marked (Bhidayasiri et al. 2013, 2018).

C. Ondo et al. (1999) conducted a prospective single-blind study of 20 patients with tardive dyskinesia (mean duration 43.7 months) treated with tetrabenazine. The average improvement on the Abnormal Involuntary Movement Scale (AIMS) score was 54.2% (from 17.9 to 8.2); after an average treatment period of 20.3 weeks at a mean dosage of 57.9 mg/day, 11 patients rated themselves as markedly, 6 as moderately, and 2 as mildly improved (Ondo et al. 1999).

III. **Dosing**:

A. Tetrabenazine for tardive dyskinesia is started at 50 mg/day in divided doses and is increased as needed by 50 mg every 2 weeks, up to a maximum of 150 mg/day in divided doses (Godwin-Austen and Clark 1971; Kazamatsuri et al. 1972; Ondo et al. 1999; Ricciardi et al. 2019).

B. Alternatively, an initial dosage of 25–37.5 mg/day in 2 or 3 divided doses has been recommended (increasing or decreasing the dosage in 12.5-mg/day increments at weekly intervals). The usual maximum tolerated dosage is 75 mg/day in 3 divided doses; in sporadic cases, dosages up to 200 mg/day have been used (Lundbeck 2017).

IV. **Cautions/Monitoring**:

A. Tetrabenazine is contraindicated in actively suicidal patients or those who have untreated depression. Tetrabenazine also is contraindicated in patients with severe hepatic impairment; those who are taking monoamine oxidase inhibitors (MAOIs; at least a 14-day washout is needed) or reserpine (at least a 20-day washout is needed); and those who are taking deutetrabenazine or valbenazine (Lundbeck 2017).

B. Before prescribing a tetrabenazine dosage greater than 50 mg/day, patients should be genotyped to determine CYP2D6 function. CYP2D6 testing is necessary to determine whether patients are poor metabolizers, extensive metabolizers, or intermediate metabolizers of tetrabenazine (Lundbeck 2017).

C. Tetrabenazine may enhance the adverse/toxic effects of antipsychotic medications and may increase the CNS depressant effects of buprenorphine, hydroxyzine, kava kava, kratom, and zolpidem. Deutetrabenazine, valbenazine, and MAOIs may enhance the adverse/toxic effect of tetrabenazine (Lundbeck 2017).

D. Frequently reported side effects of tetrabenazine include drowsiness (17%–57%), sedation (17%–57%), depression (19%–35%), extrapyramidal symptoms (15%–33%), fatigue (22%), insomnia (22%), akathisia (19%–20%), anxiety (15%), falling (15%), and upper respiratory tract infections (11%) (Lundbeck 2017).

E. It is recommended that clinicians monitor for signs and symptoms of restlessness and agitation. Dosage reduction or discontinuation may be necessary if such symptoms develop or worsen.

F. Tetrabenazine can prolong the QTc interval. Its use should be avoided in patients with congenital QT prolongation, a history of cardiac arrhythmias, or concomitant drugs known to cause QT prolongation.

G. Tetrabenazine carries a risk of developing neuroleptic malignant syndrome or parkinsonian symptoms with disabling orthostatic hypotension, especially during initial dosage titration, which needs close monitoring.

H. Tetrabenazine can increase the risk of depression and suicidal thoughts and behaviors in patients with Huntington's disease. Close observation of patients for the emergence or worsening of depression, suicidality, or notable changes in behavior should accompany treatment. Patients, their caregivers, and their families should be informed of the risk of depression and suicidality. They should be instructed to report behaviors of concern promptly to the treating physician (Lundbeck 2017).

I. Tetrabenazine elevates serum prolactin concentrations in humans. Following administration of 25 mg of tetrabenazine to healthy volunteers, peak plasma prolactin levels increased fourfold to fivefold. Prolactin levels need close monitoring, especially if there is an emergence of sexual side effects (Lundbeck 2017).

J. If treatment is interrupted for more than 5 days, re-titration is recommended. If treatment is interrupted for less than 5 days, resume at the previous maintenance dosage (Lundbeck 2017).

K. Limited information is available about the safety of tetrabenazine during pregnancy or nursing.

Further Reading

Caroff SN: Recent advances in the pharmacology of tardive dyskinesia. Clin Psychopharmacol Neurosci 18(4):493–506, 2020 33124584

Jackson R, Brams MN, Citrome L, et al: Assessment of the impact of tardive dyskinesia in clinical practice: consensus panel recommendations. Neuropsychiatr Dis Treat 17:1589–1597, 2021 34079257

Loonen AJM, Ivanova SA: Neurobiological mechanisms associated with antipsychotic drug-induced dystonia. J Psychopharmacol 35(1):3–14, 2021 32900259

Perju-Dumbrava L, Kempster P: Movement disorders in psychiatric patients. BMJ Neurol Open 2(2):e000057, 2020 33681793

Yahya AS, Khawaja S: Electroconvulsive therapy as a treatment for tardive dyskinesia. Prim Care Companion CNS Disord 23(3):20r02775, 2021 34000170

References

Bhidayasiri R, Fahn S, Weiner WJ, et al; American Academy of Neurology: Evidence-based guideline: treatment of tardive syndromes: report of the Guideline Development Subcommittee of the American Academy of Neurology. Neurology 81(5):463–469, 2013 23897874

Bhidayasiri R, Jitkritsadakul O, Friedman JH, et al: Updating the recommendations for treatment of tardive syndromes: a systematic review of new evidence and practical treatment algorithm. J Neurol Sci 389:67–75, 2018 29454493

Godwin-Austen RB, Clark T: Persistent phenothiazine dyskinesia treated with tetrabenazine. Br Med J 4(5778):25–26, 1971 4938245

Kazamatsuri H, Chien C, Cole JO: Treatment of tardive dyskinesia. I. Clinical efficacy of a dopamine-depleting agent, tetrabenazine. Arch Gen Psychiatry 27(1):95–99, 1972 4555831

Lundbeck: Tetrabenazine prescribing information. Revised September 2017. Available at: https://www.accessdata.fda.gov/drugsatfda_docs/label/2017/021894s013lbl.pdf. Accessed August 4, 2024.

Ondo WG, Hanna PA, Jankovic J: Tetrabenazine treatment for tardive dyskinesia: assessment by randomized videotape protocol. Am J Psychiatry 156(8):1279–1281, 1999 10450276
Ricciardi L, Pringsheim T, Barnes TRE, et al: Treatment recommendations for tardive dyskinesia. Can J Psychiatry 64(6):388–399, 2019 30791698

Valbenazine (for Medication-Induced Tardive Dyskinesia)

I. **Mechanism of Action**:

A. Valbenazine is a vesicular monoamine transporter 2 (VMAT2) inhibitor approved by the FDA to treat adults with tardive dyskinesia (Neurocrine Biosciences 2021). The mechanism of action of valbenazine in the treatment of tardive dyskinesia is unknown but is thought to be mediated through the reversible inhibition of VMAT2, a transporter that regulates monoamine uptake from the cytoplasm to the synaptic vesicle for storage and release.

II. **Data**:

A. A 6-week randomized double-blind, placebo-controlled trial of 205 patients with schizophrenia, schizoaffective disorder, or a mood disorder who had moderate or severe tardive dyskinesia was conducted. Participants were randomly assigned in a 1:1:1 ratio to once-daily placebo, valbenazine 40 mg/day, or valbenazine 80 mg/day. The least-squares mean change from baseline to week 6 in the Abnormal Involuntary Movement Scale (AIMS) dyskinesia score was –3.2 for the 80 mg/day group, a significant difference compared with –0.1 for the placebo group. The AIMS dyskinesia score was also reduced in the 40 mg/day group (–1.9) (Hauser et al. 2017).

B. In the KINECT 3 trial, stable adult patients with schizophrenia or mood disorders with tardive dyskinesia were randomly assigned to receive placebo or valbenazine at 80 mg/day or 40 mg/day. Efficacy assessments included the AIMS (mean score changes, responders) and the Clinical Global Impression of Change–Tardive Dyskinesia (CGI-TD) (mean scores, responders). Of 198 participants, 124 completed treatment (80 mg/day, n=63; 40 mg/day, n=61), and 121 completed follow-up. At week 48, the study showed tardive dyskinesia improvement in both of the valbenazine dosage groups based on AIMS scores. Mean AIMS score changes were as follows for each dosing group: 80 mg/day, –4.8; 40 mg/day, –3.0. The percentage of responders (percentage of subjects with AIMS score reductions ≥50%) was as follows for each dosing group: 52% on 80 mg/day, 28% on 40 mg/day, and. 20% on placebo (Factor et al. 2017).

III. **Dosing**:

A. Valbenazine is dispensed in capsules (40 mg, 60 mg, and 80 mg). The initial dosage is 40 mg once daily (Neurocrine Biosciences 2023). After 1 week, the recommended dosage is 80 mg once daily.

B. Valbenazine can be taken with or without food.

C. The recommended dosage for patients with moderate or severe hepatic impairment is 40 mg once daily. Dosage reduction is suggested based on tolerability in known CYP2D6 poor metabolizers.

D. Continuing therapy at a dosage of 40 mg/day may be considered in some patients (Neurocrine Biosciences 2023). Continued valbenazine therapy is necessary in patients with tardive dyskinesia; symptoms recur following discontinuation of the drug (Factor et al. 2017).

IV. **Cautions/Monitoring**:

A. Valbenazine has been associated with depression and suicidal thoughts/behavior and can cause increased depression and suicidal ideation (McIntyre et al. 2019). Close monitoring for any emergence of severe mood disorder or suicidal ideation is recommended.

B. The AIMS or the Dyskinesia Identification System Condensed User Scale (DISCUS), as well as an ECG for patients at risk of QTc prolongation, are recommended for assessment of progress and to rule out underlying cardiac conditions before initiating valbenazine.

C. Valbenazine should not be combined with monoamine oxidase inhibitors (MAOIs), as valbenazine may enhance the adverse/toxic effects of MAOIs.

D. Valbenazine is also to be avoided in patients taking other strong CYP3A4 inducers (e.g., carbamazepine) or potent CYP3A4 inhibitors (e.g., ketoconazole). Strong CYP2D6 inhibitors (e.g., paroxetine, fluoxetine) may increase exposure to valbenazine's active metabolite. It is suggested that the valbenazine dosage be reduced based on tolerability in patients who are taking a strong CYP2D6 inhibitor or who are known to be CYP2D6 poor metabolizers (Stahl 2020).

E. St. John's wort can decrease the serum concentration of valbenazine, whereas tetrabenazine may worsen the adverse/toxic effects of valbenazine (Neurocrine Biosciences 2021).

F. Valbenazine can cause somnolence; hence, patients should use caution or avoid driving, operating machinery, or any task requiring sustained attention.

G. Valbenazine can cause QTc prolongation.

H. Patients taking valbenazine who develop clinically significant parkinsonian signs or symptoms should have their dosage reduced or the medication discontinued (Neurocrine Biosciences 2021).

I. Valbenazine can increase serum prolactin levels and can elevate hepatic enzymes, including serum alkaline phosphatase, and can also increase serum bilirubin.

J. Valbenazine is available only through a specialty pharmacy (Neurocrine Biosciences 2023). Patients and clinicians should contact the INBRACE Support Program (844-647-3992; https://inbracesupportprogram.com/) for further information (Neurocrine Biosciences 2023).

K. Valbenazine should not be used during pregnancy or nursing (Neurocrine Biosciences 2021).

Further Reading

Gupta H, Moity AR, Jumonville A, et al: Valbenazine for the treatment of adults with tardive dyskinesia. Health Psychol Res 9(1):24929, 2021 35106396

Nikkhah A: A brief review on the role of vesicular monoamine transporter2 inhibitors in hyperkinetic movement disorders. Iran J Child Neurol 15(3):29–33, 2021 34282360

Set KK, Warner JN: Tourette syndrome in children: an update. Curr Probl Pediatr Adolesc Health Care 51(7):101032, 2021 34305006

StatRef: Valbenazine. TDS Health, n.d. Available at: https://online.statref.com/document/nDxp39NByDjIefpOzd6AUt?searchid=1644340372779000790andcategoryType=All. Accessed February 8, 2022.

References

Factor S, Comella C, Correll C, et al: Efficacy of valbenazine (NBI-98854) in subjects with tardive dyskinesia: results of a long-term study (KINECT 3 Extension) (S56.005). Neurology 88(16)(Supplement): 2017

Hauser RA, Factor SA, Marder SR, et al: KINECT 3: A phase 3 randomized, double-blind, placebo-controlled trial of valbenazine for tardive dyskinesia. Am J Psychiatry 174(5):476–484, 2017 28320223

McIntyre RS, Calabrese JR, Nierenberg AA, et al: The effects of valbenazine on tardive dyskinesia in patients with a primary mood disorder. J Affect Disord 246:217–223, 2019 30583148

Neurocrine Biosciences: Ingrezza (valbenazine) US-FDA Package Insert. Neurocrine Biosciences, 2021. Available at: https://www.accessdata.fda.gov/drugsatfda_docs/label/2021/209241s020lbl.pdf. Accessed March 13, 2024.

Neurocrine Biosciences: Ingrezza (valbenazine) capsules prescribing information. Neurocrine Biosciences, 2023. Available at: https://www.neurocrine.com/assets/2023/09/INGREZZA-Full-Prescribing-Information_PPI_Approved-202309.pdf#page24. Accessed March 13, 2024.

Stahl SM: Valbenazine, in Prescriber's Guide: Stahl's Essential Psychopharmacology, 7th Edition. Cambridge, UK, Cambridge University Press, 2020, pp 857–60

Weight Gain

Overview

Weight gain–related side effects are associated with several therapeutic classes, including antidepressants (particularly tricyclic antidepressants), second-generation antipsychotics, and mood stabilizers (Choong et al. 2012). Drug-induced weight gain can be the first step toward the development of obesity and other metabolic complications, which can ultimately reduce life expectancy (Lakka et al. 2002). There is a higher prevalence of metabolic syndrome in mental disorders with psychosis, including schizophrenia and bipolar disorder (Brooks et al. 2007).

An increase in the natural mortality rate of 1.5- to 2-fold in comparison with the general population has been reported for patients with major depressive disorder, bipolar disorder, or schizophrenia (Laursen et al. 2007), which appears to be mainly related to a twofold greater prevalence of cardiovascular risk factors (Birkenaes et al. 2007). However, if left untreated, these diagnoses are also independent risk factors for cardiovascular complications.

A full review of the rapidly changing field of drugs for weight loss, including the glucagon-like peptide-1 (GLP-1) receptor agonists, is beyond the scope of this Handbook.

References

Birkenaes AB, Opjordsmoen S, Brunborg C, et al: The level of cardiovascular risk factors in bipolar disorder equals that of schizophrenia: a comparative study. J Clin Psychiatry 68(6):917–923, 2007 17592917

Brooks NL, Moore KS, Clark RD, et al: Do low levels of circulating adiponectin represent a biomarker or just another risk factor for the metabolic syndrome? Diabetes Obes Metab 9(3):246–258, 2007 17391150

Choong E, Bondolfi G, Etter M, et al: Psychotropic drug-induced weight gain and other metabolic complications in a Swiss psychiatric population. J Psychiatr Res 46(4):540–548, 2012 22316639

Lakka HM, Laaksonen DE, Lakka TA, et al: The metabolic syndrome and total and cardiovascular disease mortality in middle-aged men. JAMA 288(21):2709–2716, 2002 12460094

Laursen TM, Munk-Olsen T, Nordentoft M, et al: Increased mortality among patients admitted with major psychiatric disorders: a register-based study comparing mortality in unipolar depressive disorder, bipolar affective disorder, schizoaffective disorder, and schizophrenia. J Clin Psychiatry 68(6):899–907, 2007 17592915

Metformin (for Medication-Induced Weight Gain)

I. **Mechanism of Action:**

A. Metformin enhances the action of insulin in the liver and decreases the rate of hepatic glucose production (Lee and Morley 1998). Metformin also increases peripheral utilization and suppresses appetite (Hostalek et al. 2015).

B. Metformin is recommended as a first-line treatment in type 2 diabetes mellitus (de Silva et al. 2016). Metformin has been used to treat obesity in nondiabetic individuals, although metformin is not FDA approved for weight loss. Metformin causes weight reduction by reducing insulin resistance and suppressing appetite (Jarskog et al. 2013). The 2016 American Academy of Clinical Endocrinologist guidelines on obesity management recommended the use of metformin in obese patients with evidence of prediabetes or insulin resistance that does not respond to lifestyle modifications or anti-obesity medications (Garvey et al. 2016).

II. **Data:**

A. Use of metformin as an agent for weight loss is off-label, but metformin is frequently used in patients at high risk for metabolic complications who do cannot tolerate or do not respond adequately to other interventions (Yerevanian and Soukas 2019).

B. Metformin effectively decreases weight gain associated with atypical antipsychotics and is well tolerated by children and adolescents with autism spectrum disorder (ASD). One study of metformin in individuals with ASD showed that after 16 weeks, a statistically significantly greater improvement was noted in secondary body composition measures but not in metabolic variables (Anagnostou et al. 2016).

C. Metformin is used off-label to help reduce antipsychotic-induced weight gain and to treat symptoms of polycystic ovary syndrome. It is also used in the treatment of gestational diabetes mellitus and oligomenorrhea secondary to polycystic ovary syndrome (Corcoran and Jacobs 2022).

III. **Dosing:**

A. The oral dosage of immediate-release metformin range from 750 mg to 2 g daily in 2–3 divided doses. Dosages up to 2.55 g/day have been used. To minimize gastrointestinal adverse effects, it is recommended that the patient start with 250 mg or 500 mg twice daily or 850 mg once daily, and increase the dosage gradually based on tolerability (de Silva et al. 2016; Jarskog et al. 2013).

B. The maintenance dosage for extended-release metformin formulations ranges from 1 to 2 g once daily. To minimize gastrointestinal adverse effects, metformin is titrated upward in 500-mg increments every 2–6 weeks based on tolerability (Carrizo et al. 2009; Rado and von Ammon Cavanaugh 2016).

IV. **Cautions/Monitoring**:

A. Metformin is contraindicated in patients with hypersensitivity to metformin or any component of its formulation. Metformin is also contraindicated in patients with severe renal dysfunction (eGFR <30 mL/minute/1.73 m^2) or with acute or chronic metabolic acidosis (including diabetic ketoacidosis) (Bristol-Myers Squibb 2017).

B. Food decreases the extent and slightly delays the absorption of metformin (Bristol-Myers Squibb 2017). Metformin should be administered immediately after a meal to maximize therapeutic benefit. The time to reach maximum plasma metformin concentration is approximately 7–8 hours (Bristol-Myers Squibb 2017). At usual clinical dosages and dosing schedules of metformin, steady-state plasma concentrations of metformin are reached within 24–48 hours and are <1 µg/mL. Metformin is excreted unchanged in the urine and does not undergo hepatic metabolism. Therefore, tubular secretion is the primary route of metformin elimination. Following oral administration, approximately 90% of the absorbed drug is eliminated via the renal route within the first 24 hours, with a plasma elimination half-life of about 6.2 hours.

C. Combining metformin with monoamine oxidase inhibitors (MAOIs) may enhance the hypoglycemic effect. Metformin use with selective serotonin reuptake inhibitors (SSRIs) may also enhance the hypoglycemic effect. On the other hand, combining metformin with a thiazide or thiazide-like diuretics may diminish the therapeutic effect of metformin. In addition, metformin can enhance the adverse/toxic effects of topiramate (UpToDate 2024).

D. Diarrhea is commonly seen with metformin (IR tablet: 53% [placebo: 12%]; ER tablet: 10% [placebo: 3%]). Flatulence (12% [placebo: 6%]) and nausea and vomiting (IR tablet: 26% [placebo 8%]; ER tablet: 7% [placebo: 2%]) are also common (Bonnet and Scheen 2017; Bristol-Myers Squibb 2017).

E. Long-term use of metformin interferes with vitamin B_{12} intrinsic factor absorption in the terminal ileum, potentially leading to anemia and neuropathy (Aroda et al. 2016; Out et al. 2018). Cationic drugs (e.g., amiloride, digoxin, morphine, procainamide, quinidine, quinine, ranitidine, triamterene, trimethoprim, vancomycin) that are eliminated by renal tubular secretion theoretically have the potential to interact with metformin by competing for common renal tubular transport systems (Bristol-Myers Squibb 2017).

F. The use of metformin in patients with hepatic or renal impairment has been associated with lactic acidosis (Bristol-Myers Squibb 2017). Metformin-associated lactic acidosis is characterized by elevated blood lactate levels (>5 mmol/L), anion gap acidosis (without evidence of ketonuria or ketonemia), an increased lactate/pyruvate ratio, and metformin plasma levels >5 mg/mL. In addition to renal or hepatic impairment, other risk factors for metformin-associated lactic acidosis include concomitant use of certain drugs (e.g., carbonic anhydrase inhibitors such as topiramate), age of 65 years or older, having a radiological study with contrast, surgery and other procedures, hypoxic states (e.g., acute congestive heart failure), and excessive alcohol intake, and hepatic impairment.

Further Reading

Campbell JM: Metformin, in Encyclopedia of Biomedical Gerontology. Academic Press, 2019, pp 424–432

Dayabandara M, Hanwella R, Ratnatunga S, et al: Antipsychotic-associated weight gain: management strategies and impact on treatment adherence. Neuropsychiatr Dis Treat 13:2231–2241, 2017 28883731

Handen BL, Anagnostou E, Aman MG, et al: a randomized, placebo-controlled trial of metformin for the treatment of overweight induced by antipsychotic medication in young people with autism spectrum disorder: open-label extension. J Am Acad Child Adolesc Psychiatry 56(10):849–856.e6, 2017 28942807

Inzucchi SE, Lipska KJ, Mayo H, et al: Metformin in patients with type 2 diabetes and kidney disease: a systematic review. JAMA 312(24):2668–2675, 2014 25536258

Walkup JT, Cottingham E: Antipsychotic-induced weight gain and metformin. J Am Acad Child Adolesc Psychiatry 56(10):808–810, 2017a 28942801

References

Anagnostou E, Aman MG, Handen BL, et al: Metformin for treatment of overweight induced by atypical antipsychotic medication in young people with autism spectrum disorder: a randomized clinical trial. JAMA Psychiatry 73(9):928–937, 2016 27556593

Aroda VR, Edelstein SL, Goldberg RB, et al; Diabetes Prevention Program Research Group: Long-term metformin use and vitamin B12 deficiency in the Diabetes Prevention Program Outcomes Study. J Clin Endocrinol Metab 101(4):1754–1761, 2016 26900641

Bonnet F, Scheen A: Understanding and overcoming metformin gastrointestinal intolerance. Diabetes Obes Metab 19(4):473–481, 2017 27987248

Bristol-Myers Squibb: Glucophage XR (metformin hydrochloride) package insert. Revised April 2017. Available at: https://www.accessdata.fda.gov/drugsatfda_docs/label/2017/020357s037s039%2C021202s021s023lbl.pdf. Accessed August 4, 2024.

Carrizo E, Fernández V, Connell L, et al: Extended release metformin for metabolic control assistance during prolonged clozapine administration: a 14 week, double-blind, parallel group, placebo-controlled study. Schizophr Res 113(1):19–26, 2009 19515536

Corcoran C, Jacobs TF: Metformin, in StatPearls. Treasure Island, FL, StatPearls Publishing, 2022. Available at: https://pubmed.ncbi.nlm.nih.gov/30085525/. Accessed March 13, 2024.

de Silva VA, Suraweera C, Suhashini S, et al: Metformin in prevention and treatment of antipsychotic induced weight gain: a systematic review and meta-analysis. BMC Psychiatry 16(1):1–10, 2016 27716110

Garvey WT, Mechanick JI, Brett EM, et al; Reviewers of the AACE/ACE Obesity Clinical Practice Guidelines: American Association of Clinical Endocrinologists and American College of Endocrinology Comprehensive Clinical Practice Guidelines for Medical Care of Patients with Obesity. Endocr Pract 22(Suppl 3):1–203, 2016 27219496

Hostalek U, Gwilt M, Hildemann S: Therapeutic use of metformin in prediabetes and diabetes prevention. Drugs 75(10):1071–1094, 2015 26059289

Jarskog LF, Hamer RM, Catellier DJ, et al; METS Investigators: Metformin for weight loss and metabolic control in overweight outpatients with schizophrenia and schizoaffective disorder. Am J Psychiatry 170(9):1032–1040, 2013 23846733

Lee A, Morley JE: Metformin decreases food consumption and induces weight loss in subjects with obesity with type II non-insulin-dependent diabetes. Obes Res 6(1):47–53, 1998 9526970

Out M, Kooy A, Lehert P, et al: Long-term treatment with metformin in type 2 diabetes and methylmalonic acid: post hoc analysis of a randomized controlled 4.3-year trial. J Diabetes Complications 32(2):171–178, 2018 29174300

Rado J, von Ammon Cavanaugh S: A naturalistic randomized placebo-controlled trial of extended-release metformin to prevent weight gain associated with olanzapine in a US community-dwelling population. J Clin Psychopharmacol 36(2):163–168, 2016 26872112

UpToDate: Metformin: drug information. n.d. Available at: https://pro.uptodatefree.ir/show/9621. Accessed July 31, 2024.

Yerevanian A, Soukas AA: Metformin: mechanisms in human obesity and weight loss. Curr Obes Rep 8(2):156–164, 2019 30874963

Naltrexone-Bupropion (for Medication-Induced Weight Gain)

I. **Mechanism of Action:**

A. Bupropion increases dopamine and norepinephrine by blocking both the dopamine and the norepinephrine transporters. In the hypothalamus, these two neurotransmitters activate proopiomelanocortin neurons, causing the release of proopiomelanocortin. Proopiomelanocortin is then broken down into alpha-melanocyte-stimulating hormone, which binds to melanocortin-4 receptors to suppress appetite. However, stimulation of proopiomelanocortin neurons also activates an endogenous opioid-mediated negative-feedback loop, which mitigates the appetite-suppressing effects (Stahl 2020).

1. Naltrexone can block mu opioid receptors, thus preventing opioid-mediated negative feedback. Such an action would synergize simultaneous activation of the appetite-suppressing pathway by bupropion, resulting in more robust and long-lasting appetite suppression than with either drug alone (Stahl 2020).
2. The combination drug naltrexone-bupropion was approved by the FDA as an adjunct to diet and exercise in patients with a BMI ≥30 kg/m^2 or ≥27 kg/m^2 in the presence of at least one weight-related comorbidity (Takeda Pharmaceuticals America 2014).

II. **Data**:

A. The combination agent naltrexone-bupropion has been shown to reduce weight by approximately 4%–5% (Apovian et al. 2013; Greenway et al. 2010; Wadden et al. 2011).

B. In a randomized double-blind study with 1,742 participants, the mean change in body weight was –1.3% (SE 0.3) in the placebo group, –6.1% (0.3) in the naltrexone 32 mg plus bupropion group (P<0.0001 vs. placebo), and –5.0% (0.3) in the naltrexone 16 mg plus bupropion group (P<0.0001 vs. placebo). Eighty-four (16%) participants assigned to placebo had a decrease in body weight of 5% or more, compared with 226 (48%) assigned to naltrexone 32 mg plus bupropion

(P<0.0001 vs. placebo) and 186 (39%) assigned to naltrexone 16 mg plus bupropion (P<0.0001 vs. placebo) (Greenway et al. 2010).

C. In a double-blind, placebo-controlled study with 1,496 obese (BMI 30–45 kg/m^2) or overweight (27–45 kg/m^2 with dyslipidemia and/or hypertension) participants randomly assigned in a 2:1 ration to combined naltrexone sustained-release (SR) (32 mg/day) plus bupropion SR (360 mg/day) (NB32) or placebo for up to 56 weeks, significantly (P<0.001) greater reductions in body weight were observed with NB32 versus placebo at week 28 (–6.5% vs. –1.9%) and week 56 (–6.4% vs. –1.2%). More NB32-treated participants (P<0.001) experienced ≥5% weight loss versus placebo at week 28 (55.6% vs. 17.5%) and week 56 (50.5% vs. 17.1%) (Apovian et al. 2013).

D. An analysis of three major clinical trials found that the combination of bupropion and naltrexone can produce an average placebo-subtracted weight loss of 4.25% over 56 weeks (Booth and Clements 2016).

E. In a 56-week trial with oral naltrexone extended-release/bupropion extended-release used as an adjunct to a reduced-calorie diet and increased physical activity in adults with an initial BMI of ≥30 kg/m^2 or a BMI of ≥27 kg/m^2 in the presence of at least one body weight–related comorbidity (e.g., type 2 diabetes mellitus, hypertension, dyslipidemia), oral naltrexone ER 32 mg/day with bupropion ER 360 mg/day was significantly more effective than placebo as measured by percentage body weight reductions from baseline and the proportion of patients who achieved body weight reductions of ≥5% and ≥10% (Greig and Keating 2015). Significantly greater improvements in several cardiometabolic risk factors were also observed with naltrexone ER/bupropion ER versus placebo, as well as greater improvements in glycated hemoglobin levels in obese or overweight adults with type 2 diabetes.

III. **Dosing**:

A. The naltrexone-bupropion combination product is an extended-release tablet: 8 mg naltrexone HCl /90 mg bupropion HCl. Naltrexone-bupropion is started with one tablet in the morning for a week and then increased to one tablet twice daily the next week. This is followed by an increase in the dose to two tablets in the morning and a continuation of one tablet in the evening for another week. Finally, from the fourth week onward, two tablets twice daily are continued as tolerated (Takeda Pharmaceuticals America 2014).

IV. **Cautions/Monitoring**:

A. The naltrexone-bupropion combination product is contraindicated when there is known sensitivity to any of its components. Caution is recommended when the naltrexone-bupropion combination product is used by patients with uncontrolled hypertension, seizure disorders (or any condition that can lower the seizure threshold), or anorexia nervosa or bulimia, or by individuals undergoing abrupt discontinuation of alcohol, benzodiazepines, barbiturates, or antiepileptic drugs (Takeda Pharmaceuticals America 2014). Caution is likewise recommended when naltrexone-bupropion is taken with other bupropion-containing products, during long-term opioid use, or within 14 days of taking monoamine oxidase inhibitors (MAOIs) (UpToDate 2024). Bupropion is contraindicated with concurrent use of an MAOI.

B. Prescription of naltrexone-bupropion in adults younger than 24 years requires close monitoring for emergence or worsening of suicidal thoughts and behaviors. The FDA warned of reports of serious neuropsychiatric events in adults taking bupropion for smoking cessation (Takeda Pharmaceuticals America 2014).
C. Measurement of blood glucose levels before and intermittently during treatment is recommended for patients with type 2 diabetes. Measurement of blood pressure and heart rate prior to starting naltrexone-bupropion and intermittently during treatment is also recommended, particularly in patients with cardiac or cerebrovascular disease (Stahl 2020). Cases of hepatitis and clinically significant liver dysfunction have been reported in association with naltrexone exposure in naltrexone clinical trials and in postmarketing studies with patients using naltrexone (Takeda Pharmaceuticals America 2014).
D. Because bupropion is metabolized by CYP2D6 and CYP2B6, bupropion can increase the concentration of SSRIs, tricyclic antidepressants, antipsychotics (haloperidol, risperidone, thioridazine), beta-blockers (metoprolol) and Class 1C antiarrhythmics (propafenone, flecainide) (Takeda Pharmaceuticals America 2014). Concomitant use of CYP2B6 inhibitors (ticlopidine, clopidogrel) can increase bupropion concentration (Takeda Pharmaceuticals America 2014). Similarly, CYP2B6 inducers, including ritonavir, lopinavir, efavirenz, carbamazepine, phenobarbital, and phenytoin, may reduce the efficacy of naltrexone-bupropion by reducing bupropion blood levels; thus, concomitant use should be avoided.
E. The bupropion component of the combination product can lower the seizure threshold, and coadministration of bupropion with other dopaminergic medications can lead to CNS toxicity (Takeda Pharmaceuticals America 2014). Bupropion can cause amphetamine false positives on urine drug tests.
F. The adverse reactions most commonly reported with naltrexone-bupropion include nausea, constipation, headache, vomiting, dizziness, insomnia, dry mouth, and diarrhea (Takeda Pharmaceuticals America 2014).
G. Unlike phentermine-topiramate, naltrexone-bupropion does not have abuse potential. It may be useful in antipsychotic-induced weight gain, especially for nonpsychotic patients taking antipsychotic agents for depression. Naltrexone-bupropion could theoretically exacerbate psychosis in patients with a psychotic disorder; however, there are no controlled trials of this effect (Stahl 2020).
H. A nursing mother should discontinue the naltrexone-bupropion combination (Takeda Pharmaceuticals America 2014). Naltrexone-bupropion has not been studied in pediatric populations.

Further Reading

Gjermeni E, Kirstein AS, Kolbig F, et al: Obesity—an update on the basic pathophysiology and review of recent therapeutic advances. Biomolecules 11(10):1426, 2021 34680059

Laursen TM, Munk-Olsen T, Nordentoft M, et al: Increased mortality among patients admitted with major psychiatric disorders: a register-based study comparing mortality in unipolar depressive disorder, bipolar affective disorder, schizoaffective disorder, and schizophrenia. J Clin Psychiatry 68(6):899–907, 2007 17592915

References

Apovian CM, Aronne L, Rubino D, et al; COR-II Study Group: A randomized, phase 3 trial of naltrexone SR/bupropion SR on weight and obesity-related risk factors (COR-II). Obesity (Silver Spring) 21(5):935–943, 2013 23408728

Booth K, Clements JN: Role of bupropion plus naltrexone for the management of obesity. J Pharm Technol 32(3):125–132, 2016 34860947

Greenway FL, Fujioka K, Plodkowski RA, et al; COR-I Study Group: Effect of naltrexone plus bupropion on weight loss in overweight and obese adults (COR-I): a multicentre, randomised, double-blind, placebo-controlled, phase 3 trial. Lancet 376(9741):595–605, 2010 20673995

Greig SL, Keating GM: Naltrexone ER/bupropion ER: a review in obesity management. Drugs 75(11):1269–1280, 2015 26105116

Stahl SM: Naltrexone-bupropion, in Prescriber's Guide: Stahl's Essential Psychopharmacology, 7th Edition. Cambridge, UK, Cambridge University Press, 2020, pp 557–562

Takeda Pharmaceuticals America: Contrave (naltrexone HCl and bupropion HCl) package insert. Revised September 2014. Available at: https://www.accessdata.fda.gov/drugsatfda_docs/label/2014/200063s000lbl.pdf. Accessed March 13, 2024.

UpToDate: Bupropion and naltrexone. n.d. Available at: https://pro.uptodatefree.ir/Show/97033. Accessed July 31, 2024.

Wadden TA, Foreyt JP, Foster GD, et al: Weight loss with naltrexone SR/bupropion SR combination therapy as an adjunct to behavior modification: the COR-BMOD trial. Obesity (Silver Spring) 19(1):110–120, 2011 20559296

Orlistat (for Medication-Induced Weight Gain)

I. **Mechanism of Action**:

A. Orlistat, a potent natural inhibitor of pancreatic lipase, is isolated from the bacterium *Streptomyces toxytricini*. It is the saturated derivative of lipstatin (Barbier and Schneider 1987). It prevents 25%–30% of ingested fat calories from being absorbed by preventing fat hydrolysis. Orlistat may reduce fat absorption and secondarily increase postprandial secretion of glucagon-like peptide-1 (GLP-1), thus mediating satiety via gut-to-brain signaling. Orlistat facilitates the flow of nonabsorbed fat to the distal gut, with its GLP-1-producing enteroendocrine L-cells (Leblanc et al. 2011).

B. Orlistat has received FDA approval for use in weight management (in combination with a reduced-calorie diet) in obese adolescents age 12 years and older (Aaseth et al. 2021) and in adults. It is also approved to decrease the risk of regaining weight after prior weight loss (U.S. Food and Drug Administration 2015).

II. **Data**:

A. In a double-blind prospective study, 3,305 patients were randomly assigned to lifestyle changes plus either orlistat 120 mg or placebo, taken three times daily. Participants had a BMI ≥30 kg/m^2 and normal (79%) or impaired (21%) glucose tolerance. After 4 years of treatment, the cumulative incidence of diabetes was

9.0% with placebo and 6.2% with orlistat, corresponding to a risk reduction of 37.3% (P=0.0032). Mean weight loss was significantly greater with orlistat (5.8 kg vs. 3.0 kg with placebo; P<0.001) (Torgerson et al. 2004).

B. In a systematic review, orlistat plus behavioral intervention resulted in 3 kg (6.6 lb) more weight loss than placebo after 12 months (Leblanc et al. 2011). A systematic review of randomized controlled trials in adults (mean age ≥18 years, duration ≥6 months) was undertaken to evaluate the effectiveness of orlistat as an anti-obesity treatment. The review found that weight change was between –2.3 kg and –2.8 kg for orlistat (Osei-Assibey et al. 2011).

C. In a study comparing two potent weight loss therapies—1) a low-carbohydrate ketogenic diet (<20 g of carbohydrate daily) and 2) orlistat therapy combined with a low-fat diet (120 mg orally three times daily) plus low-fat diet instruction requiring<30% energy from fat with a 500–1,000 kcal/day deficit, the orlistat therapy group showed an 8.5% body weight reduction with improved low-density lipoprotein cholesterol levels (Yancy et al. 2010).

D. Orlistat improves blood pressure (Siebenhofer et al. 2016) and improves serum lipid values via weight reduction (Davidson et al. 1999).

E. The effects of orlistat on BMI and weight loss were assessed in a 54-week double-blind, placebo-controlled multicenter study in obese adolescents (ages 12–16 years). Following 1 year of treatment with either orlistat 120 mg three times a day or placebo, BMI was found to have decreased by 0.55 kg/m^2 in the orlistat-treated patients and increased by an average of 0.31 kg/m^2 in the placebo-treated patients (P=0.001) (Roche Pharmaceuticals 2009).

F. The use of orlistat for longer than 4 years has not been studied.

III. **Dosing**:

A. Orlistat is available in 120-mg capsules for the long-term treatment of obesity. The recommended dosage is one 120-mg capsule three times a day, with each main meal containing fat (taken during or up to 1 hour after the meal). The patient should be on a nutritionally balanced reduced-calorie diet that contains approximately 30% of calories from fat. The daily intake of fat, carbohydrate, and protein should be distributed over three main meals. If a meal is missed or contains no fat, the orlistat dose can be omitted.

B. Because orlistat has been shown to reduce the absorption of some fat-soluble vitamins and beta-carotene, patients should be counseled to take a multivitamin containing fat-soluble vitamins to ensure adequate nutrition. The vitamin supplement should be taken at least 2 hours before or after administration of orlistat, such as at bedtime (LactMed 2021).

IV. **Cautions/Monitoring**:

A. Orlistat should not be used in patients with chronic malabsorption, cholestasis, or a history of calcium oxalate stones. Substantial weight loss can increase the risk of cholelithiasis. Orlistat-induced fat malabsorption may result in the binding of enteric calcium. When less calcium is available in the intestinal lumen to bind oxalate, intestinal oxalate absorption and urinary oxalate excretion increase. Free oxalate can be deposited in the renal parenchyma, resulting in acute kidney injury, including calcium oxalate stones (Singh et al. 2007; Weir et al. 2011).

B. A multivitamin taken at bedtime is recommended because orlistat may decrease the absorption of fat-soluble vitamins. In a meta-analysis (Padwal et al. 2003), levels of fat-soluble vitamins (A, D, E, K) and beta-carotene were lowered by orlistat therapy, with vitamin D the most frequently affected. A pharmacokinetic interaction study showed a 30% reduction in beta-carotene supplement absorption when it was coadministered with orlistat. Orlistat inhibited absorption of a vitamin E acetate supplement by approximately 60% (Domagała-Rodacka et al. 2016). Use of orlistat by patients taking warfarin can lead to decrease in vitamin K, necessitating a reduction in the warfarin dosage (MacWalter et al. 2003). Hence, close monitoring for the emergence of fat-soluble vitamin deficiency is recommended.

C. Patients treated concomitantly with orlistat and levothyroxine should be monitored for changes in thyroid function (Madhava and Hartley 2005; Roche Pharmaceuticals 2009; Skelin et al. 2017). Orlistat and levothyroxine should be taken at least 4 hours apart.

D. The most common side effects (reported by 15%–30% of patients) of orlistat are gastrointestinal and include intestinal borborygmi and cramps, fecal incontinence, oily spotting, and flatus with discharge (Hollander et al. 1998; Padwal et al. 2003).

E. The incidence of acute liver injury from orlistat use increased (approximately doubled) during the 90 days before and 30 days after the start of treatment compared with background incidence (Douglas et al. 2013).

F. Orlistat inhibits the absorption of cyclosporine. To reduce the chance of a drug-drug interaction, cyclosporine should be taken at least 2 hours before or after orlistat (Roche Pharmaceuticals 2009).

G. The potential exists for misuse of orlistat by patients for whom orlistat is not appropriate (e.g., patients with anorexia nervosa or bulimia).

H. There is no evidence of orlistat causing suppression of ovulation (Roche Pharmaceuticals 2009). Orlistat should not be used during pregnancy. It is not known whether orlistat is secreted in human breast milk. Therefore, nursing women should not take orlistat (Roche Pharmaceuticals 2009).

Further Reading

Ahmad NN, Robinson S, Kennedy-Martin T, et al: Clinical outcomes associated with anti-obesity medications in real-world practice. Obes Rev 22(11):e13326, 2021 34423889

Cignarella A, Busetto L, Vettor R: Pharmacotherapy of obesity: an update. Pharmacol Res 169:105649, 2021 33962014

Hall ME, Cohen JB, Ard JD, et al: Weight-loss strategies for prevention and treatment of hypertension: a scientific statement from the American Heart Association. Hypertension 78(5):e38–e50, 2021 34538096

Hauner H: Obesity treatment—legal and illegal drugs and the future [in German]. Internist (Berl) 62(12):1354–1359, 2021 34591131

Sengupta P, Tiwari N, Bhatt T, et al: Mechanistically acting anti-obesity compositions/formulations of natural origin: a patent review (2010–2021). Exp Opin Ther Patents 32(1):29–46, 2022 34236914

Shi Q, Wang Y, Hao Q, et al: Pharmacotherapy for adults with overweight and obesity: a systematic review and network meta-analysis of randomised controlled trials. Lancet 399(10321):259–269, 2022 34895470

References

Aaseth J, Ellefsen S, Alehagen U, et al: Diets and drugs for weight loss and health in obesity—an update. Biomed Pharmacother 140:111789, 2021 34082399

Barbier P, Schneider F: Syntheses of tetrahydrolipstatin and absolute configuration of tetrahydrolipstatin and lipstatin. Helvetica Chimica Acta 70(1):196–201, 1987

Davidson MH, Hauptman J, DiGirolamo M, et al: Weight control and risk factor reduction in obese subjects treated for 2 years with orlistat: a randomized controlled trial. JAMA 281(3):235–242, 1999 9918478

Domagała-Rodacka R, Cibor D, Szczeklik K, et al: Gastrointestinal tract as a side-effect target of medications. Przegl Lek 73(9):652–658, 2016 29688675

Douglas IJ, Langham J, Bhaskaran K, et al: Orlistat and the risk of acute liver injury: self controlled case series study in UK Clinical Practice Research Datalink. BMJ 346(7906):f1936, 2013 23585064

Hollander PA, Elbein SC, Hirsch IB, et al: Role of orlistat in the treatment of obese patients with type 2 diabetes: a 1-year randomized double-blind study. Diabetes Care 21(8):1288–1294, 1998 9702435

Leblanc ES, O'Connor E, Whitlock EP, et al: Effectiveness of primary care–relevant treatments for obesity in adults: a systematic evidence review for the U.S. Preventive Services Task Force. Ann Intern Med 155(7):434–447, 2011 21969342

MacWalter RS, Fraser HW, Armstrong KM: Orlistat enhances warfarin effect. Ann Pharmacother 37(4):510–512, 2003 12659605

Madhava K, Hartley A: Hypothyroidism in thyroid carcinoma follow-up: orlistat may inhibit the absorption of thyroxine. Clin Oncol (R Coll Radiol) 17(6):492, 2005 16149295

LactMed: Orlistat [updated April 19, 2021]. Bethesda, MD, National Institute of Child Health and Human Development, Drugs and Lactation Database (LactMed). 2006–. Available at: https://www.ncbi.nlm.nih.gov/books/NBK501796/. Accessed July 31, 2024.

Osei-Assibey G, Adi Y, Kyrou I, et al: Pharmacotherapy for overweight/obesity in ethnic minorities and White Caucasians: a systematic review and meta-analysis. Diabetes Obes Metab 13(5):385–393, 2011 21205118

Padwal R, Li SK, Lau DC: Long-term pharmacotherapy for obesity and overweight. Cochrane Database Syst Rev (4):CD004094, 2003 14584004

Roche Pharmaceuticals: Xenical US-FDA package insert. Revised January 2009. Available at: https://www.accessdata.fda.gov/drugsatfda_docs/label/2009/020766s026lbl.pdf. Accessed February 8, 2022.

Siebenhofer A, Jeitler K, Horvath K, et al: Long-term effects of weight-reducing drugs in people with hypertension. Cochrane Database Syst Rev (3):CD007654, 2016 26934640

Singh A, Sarkar SR, Gaber LW, et al: Acute oxalate nephropathy associated with orlistat, a gastrointestinal lipase inhibitor. Am J Kidney Dis 49(1):153–157, 2007 17185156

Skelin M, Lucijani? T,Amidži? Klari? D,et al: Fators affecting gastrointestinal absorption of levothyroxine: a review. Clin Ther 39(2):378–403, 2017 28153426

Torgerson JS, Hauptman J, Boldrin MN, et al: XENical in the prevention of diabetes in obese subjects (XENDOS) study: a randomized study of orlistat as an adjunct to lifestyle changes for the prevention of type 2 diabetes in obese patients. Diabetes Care 27(1):155–161, 2004 14693982

U.S. Food and Drug Administration: Orlistat (marketed as Alli and Xenical) Information. 2015. Available at: https://www.fda.gov/drugs/postmarket-drug-safety-information-patients-and-providers/orlistat-marketed-alli-and-xenical-information. Accessed March 13, 2024.

Weir MA, Beyea MM, Gomes T, et al: Orlistat and acute kidney injury: an analysis of 953 patients. Arch Intern Med 171(7):703–704, 2011 21482850

Yancy WS Jr, Westman EC, McDuffie JR, et al: A randomized trial of a low-carbohydrate diet vs orlistat plus a low-fat diet for weight loss. Arch Intern Med 170(2):136–145, 2010 20101008

Phentermine-Topiramate (for Medication-Induced Weight Gain)

I. **Mechanism of Action:**

A. Phentermine is a sympathomimetic amine with pharmacological properties similar to amphetamines. The mechanism of action in reducing appetite is secondary to stimulation of the hypothalamus and release of norepinephrine (Catalent Pharma Solutions 2012; Rothman and Baumann 2009).

1. Phentermine enhances mainly norepinephrine, but also serotonin and dopamine release in the CNS. Hypothesized sites of phentermine action are the homeostatic-related hypothalamus and reward-related nucleus accumbens (Pilitsi et al. 2019; Srivastava and Apovian 2018; Velazquez and Apovian 2018).
2. Topiramate is a GABA agonist, a glutamate antagonist, and a carbonic anhydrase inhibitor.
3. Phentermine-topiramate (Qsymia) is FDA approved for adults with a body mass index (BMI) ≥30 kg/m^2 or with a BMI ≥27 kg/m^2 with at least one weight-related comorbidity (e.g., hypertension, diabetes, dyslipidemia) (Vivus Inc 2012). Phentermine-topiramate is typically considered for individuals with obesity who do not have comorbid cardiovascular disease (Vivus Inc 2012).

II. **Data:**

A. In a 56-week trial in overweight adults (age 18–70 years) treated with placebo, once-daily phentermine 7.5 mg plus topiramate 46.0 mg, or once-daily phentermine 15.0 mg plus topiramate 92.0 mg, the reported change in body weight was –1.4 kg, –8.1 kg, and –10.2 kg in patients assigned to placebo, those assigned to phentermine 7.5 mg plus topiramate 46.0 mg, and those assigned to phentermine 15.0 mg plus topiramate 92.0 mg, respectively (Gadde et al. 2011).

B. In a double-blind 52-week extension study, 866 volunteers were randomly assigned to treatment (placebo, 7.5 mg phentermine/46 mg controlled-release topiramate [7.5/46], or 15 mg phentermine/92 mg controlled-release topiramate [15/92]) for 108 weeks of the study. The mean percentage changes from baseline in body weight were –1.8%, –9.3%, and –10.5% for placebo, 7.5/46 mg phentermine-topiramate, and 15/92 mg phentermine-topiramate, respectively (Garvey et al. 2012).

C. In a 56-week randomized, placebo-controlled trial, placebo, phentermine-topiramate 3.75/23 mg, or phentermine-topiramate 15/92 mg was added to a reduced-calorie diet. Primary endpoints were percentage body weight reduction and proportion of patients achieving 5% total body weight loss. Secondary endpoints included waist circumference, systolic and diastolic blood pressure, fasting glucose, and lipids. Patients in the placebo, 3.75/23 mg phentermine-topiramate, and 15/92 mg phentermine-topiramate groups lost 1.6%, 5.1%, and 10.9% of baseline body weight, respectively, at 56 weeks (P<0.0001) (Allison et al. 2012).

III. **Dosing**:

A. The initial dose of phentermine-topiramate is 3.75/23 mg for 14 days, followed by 7.5/46 mg after that. If after 12 weeks a 3% loss in baseline body weight is not achieved, the dose can be increased to 11.25/69 mg for 14 days and then to 15/92 mg/day (Two Drugs for Weight Loss 2014).

B. If an individual on phentermine-topiramate does not lose 5% of their body weight after 12 weeks on the highest dose, phentermine-topiramate should be discontinued gradually, as abrupt withdrawal of topiramate can cause seizures (Two Drugs for Weight Loss 2014).

IV. **Cautions/Monitoring**:

A. Phentermine-topiramate is contraindicated in patients with hypersensitivity or idiosyncratic response to phentermine, other sympathomimetic amines, or any component of the formulation. It is likewise contraindicated in patients with a history of cardiovascular disease (e.g., arrhythmias, heart failure, coronary artery disease, stroke, uncontrolled hypertension), hyperthyroidism, glaucoma, agitated states, or substance use disorder. Phentermine-topiramate should not be used during or within 14 days following MAO inhibitor therapy

B. Use of phentermine-topiramate during the first trimester has been associated with cleft palate. Use of phentermine-topiramate is contraindicated during pregnancy and breast-feeding (UpToDate 2024).

C. The phentermine-topiramate combination diminishes the stimulatory effect of amphetamines. It also enhances the hypertensive effect of sympathomimetics such as atomoxetine. The phentermine-topiramate combination may also enhance the tachycardic effect of sympathomimetics.

D. When combined with CYP2D6 inhibitors such as bupropion, phentermine-topiramate may exacerbate neuroexcitatory and/or seizure-potentiating effects. The phentermine-topiramate combination also increases the serum concentration of esketamine. The phentermine-topiramate combination may enhance the hypertensive effect of MAOIs and kratom. Phentermine-topiramate may enhance the serotonergic effect of SSRIs. Tricyclic antidepressants may enhance the adverse/toxic effect of phentermine-topiramate. Tricyclic antidepressants may potentiate the cardiovascular effects of phentermine-topiramate (Catalent Pharma Solutions 2012; UpToDate 2024).

E. The most common adverse effects of phentermine-topiramate are dry mouth (13%–21% on drug vs. 2% on placebo), constipation (15%–17% on drug vs. 6% on placebo), and paresthesia (14%–21% on drug vs. 2% on placebo) (Allison et al. 2012; Gadde et al. 2011). There was a dosage-related increase in the incidence of psychiatric (e.g., depression, anxiety) and cognitive (e.g., disturbance in attention) adverse events in the active treatment group (Catalent Pharma Solutions 2012).

F. Phentermine (alone or in combination) has been associated with acquired valvular heart disease, heart failure, and cardiovascular events (including arrhythmias, acute myocardial infarction, and cardiovascular death) hypothesized to be due to an increase in 5-HT and subsequent vascular remodeling (Gorelik et al. 2020; Page et al. 2016).

G. Phentermine (alone and in combination) has been associated with CNS effects, including delirium, mania, and psychosis, related to the release of norepinephrine and dopamine (Homola and Hieber 2018; Jo et al. 2019).

H. The literature has reported insomnia, irritability, and anxiety in 24%–27% of users (Brauer et al. 1996; Jo et al. 2019).

I. Primary pulmonary hypertension (PPH) has been reported in patients receiving a combination of phentermine and fenfluramine or dexfenfluramine (Gorelik et al. 2020).

J. Phentermine is a Schedule IV controlled substance. Clinicians who prescribe phentermine-topiramate should enroll in a Risk Evaluation and Mitigation Strategy (REMS) program, which includes an online or print formal training module detailing safety information.

Further Reading

Ahmad NN, Robinson S, Kennedy-Martin T, et al: Clinical outcomes associated with anti-obesity medications in real-world practice: a systematic literature review. Obes Rev 22(11):e13326, 2021 34423889

Cignarella A, Busetto L, Vettor R: Pharmacotherapy of obesity: an update. Pharmacol Res 169(July):105649, 2021 33962014

Hall ME, Cohen JB, Ard JD, et al: Weight-loss strategies for prevention and treatment of hypertension: a scientific statement from the American Heart Association. Hypertension 78(5):e38–e50, 2021 34538096

National Center for Biotechnology Information: PubChem compound summary for CID 4771, phentermine. National Center for Biotechnology Information, n.d. Available at: https://pubchem.ncbi.nlm.nih.gov/compound/Phentermine. Accessed February 7, 2022.

References

Allison DB, Gadde KM, Garvey WT, et al: Controlled-release phentermine/topiramate in severely obese adults: a randomized controlled trial (EQUIP). Obesity (Silver Spring) 20(2):330–342, 2012 22051941

Brauer LH, Johanson CE, Schuster CR, et al: Evaluation of phentermine and fenfluramine, alone and in combination, in normal, healthy volunteers. Neuropsychopharmacology 14(4):233–241, 1996 8924191

Catalent Pharma Solutions: QSYMIA (phentermine and topiramate extended-release) package insert. Catalent Pharma Solutions, 2012. Available at: https://www.accessdata.fda.gov/drugsatfda_docs/label/2012/022580s000lbl.pdf. Accessed March 13, 2024.

Gadde KM, Allison DB, Ryan DH, et al: Effects of low-dose, controlled-release, phentermine plus topiramate combination on weight and associated comorbidities in overweight and obese adults (CONQUER): a randomised, placebo-controlled, phase 3 trial. Lancet 377(9774):1341–1352, 2011 21481449

Garvey WT, Ryan DH, Look M, et al: Two-year sustained weight loss and metabolic benefits with controlled-release phentermine/topiramate in obese and overweight adults (SEQUEL): a randomized, placebo-controlled, phase 3 extension study. Am J Clin Nutr 95(2):297–308, 2012 22158731

Gorelik E, Gorelik B, Masarwa R, et al: The cardiovascular safety of antiobesity drugs—analysis of signals in the FDA Adverse Event Report System Database. Int J Obes (Lond) 44(5):1021–1027, 2020 32152496

Homola J, Hieber R: Combination of venlafaxine and phentermine/topiramate induced psychosis: a case report. Ment Health Clin 8(2):95–99, 2018 29955552

Jo HS, Wang SM, Kim JJ: Recurrent psychosis after phentermine administration in a young female: a case report. Clin Psychopharmacol Neurosci 17(1):130–133, 2019 30690949

Page RL 2nd, O'Bryant CL, Cheng D, et al: Drugs that may cause or exacerbate heart failure: a scientific statement from the American Heart Association. Circulation 134(6):e32–e69, 2016 27400984

Pilitsi E, Farr OM, Polyzos SA, et al: Pharmacotherapy of obesity: available medications and drugs under investigation. Metabolism 92:170–192, 2019 30391259

Rothman RB, Baumann MH: Appetite suppressants, cardiac valve disease and combination pharmacotherapy. Am J Ther 16(4):354–364, 2009 19092640

Srivastava G, Apovian CM: Current pharmacotherapy for obesity. Nat Rev Endocrinol 14(1):12–24, 2018 29027993

Two drugs for weight loss. JAMA 312(9):955–957, 2014 25182105

UpToDate: Phentermine. n.d. Available at: https://pro.uptodatefree.ir/Show/9765. Accessed July 31, 2024.

Velazquez A, Apovian CM: Updates on obesity pharmacotherapy. Ann N Y Acad Sci 1411(1):106–119, 2018 29377198

Vivus Inc: Qsymia (phentermine and topiramate extended-release) capsules. Vivus, 2012. Available at: https://www.accessdata.fda.gov/drugsatfda_docs/nda/2012/022580orig1s000_qsymia_toc.cfm. Accessed March 13, 2024.

Topiramate (for Medication-Induced Weight Gain)

I. **Mechanism of Action**:

A. Although the weight-loss effect of topiramate is based on the selective inhibition of mitochondrial carbonic anhydrase isoforms (Khalil et al. 2019), topiramate is not FDA approved as monotherapy for weight loss.

B. Topiramate enhances the activity of the inhibitory neurotransmitter GABA at a nonbenzodiazepine site on $GABA_A$ receptors (Johnson et al. 2004, 2007; Upsher-Smith Laboratories 2023). Topiramate blocks voltage-dependent sodium channels; augments the activity of GABA in some subtypes of the $GABA_A$ receptor; antagonizes the AMPA/kainate subtype of the glutamate receptor; and inhibits carbonic anhydrase (particularly the CA-II and CA-IV isoenzymes) (Edmonds et al. 1996; White 1997).

C. Topiramate is used as initial monotherapy in the management of partial-onset seizures or primary generalized tonic-clonic seizures in adults and pediatric patients age 2 years or older (Arroyo et al. 2005; Janssen Pharmaceuticals 2023). Topiramate is used as adjunctive therapy (i.e., in combination with other anticonvulsants) in managing primary generalized tonic-clonic seizures in adults and pediatric patients age 2 years or older (Langtry et al. 1997; Sachdeo 1998). Topiramate is used as adjunctive therapy (i.e., in combination with other anticonvulsants) in the management of seizures associated with Lennox-Gastaut syndrome in adults and pediatric patients age 2 years or older (Janssen Pharmaceuticals 2023). Topiramate has been recommended as a second-line anticonvulsant option in patients with Dravet syndrome (Wirrell and Nabbout 2019; Wirrell et al. 2017).

D. Topiramate is used for the prevention of migraine headaches in adults and adolescents age 12 years or older (Brandes et al. 2004; Silberstein et al. 2004; Wirrell and Nabbout 2019; Wirrell et al. 2017). Anecdotally and with limited supporting evidence, topiramate has been used successfully in adults for the off-label management of alcohol dependence (Johnson 2004; Johnson et al. 2007).

II. **Data**:

A. Topiramate at an average dosage of 200–600 mg/day caused a mean weight loss of 7.75 kg (SD=6.9 kg, $P<0.001$), and at 12 months, 9 patients had lost a mean of 9.61 kg (SD=6.7 kg, $P=0.003$) (Kirov and Tredget 2005). Other studies have shown that topiramate can cause up to 5% or more body weight loss over 52 weeks of topiramate treatment (Khera et al. 2016).

B. A meta-analysis of randomized controlled trials (RCTs) examining use of topiramate in patients with schizophrenia for weight reduction included 10 double-blind RCTs and 7 open-label RCTs. Topiramate was significantly superior to the control condition in mitigating weight gain and psychopathology in antipsychotic-treated patients with schizophrenia (Goh et al. 2019).

C. Another systematic review and meta-analysis of 257 randomized trials (54 different drugs; 84,696 patients enrolled) found that topiramate caused an average 3.8-kg weight loss (Domecq et al. 2015).

D. Another review found that topiramate induced weight loss, especially in patients with a high baseline BMI, and that the amount of weight lost was not strictly dependent on daily dosage and was not influenced by gender (Verrotti et al. 2011).

III. **Dosing**:

A. Topiramate is started at 50 mg/day and increased in 25- to 50-mg increments at weekly intervals based on response and tolerability up to a recommended dose of 200 mg/day (Hasan et al. 2013; Ko et al. 2005).

B. Because of the bitter taste, immediate-release topiramate tablets should be swallowed intact and not broken or chewed. If the tablets are broken, they should be used immediately, because the stability of the exposed drug beyond a brief period cannot be ensured; any unused portion should be discarded. For patients experiencing difficulty in swallowing the tablets, contents of the capsule/sprinkle formulation may be sprinkled on a small amount of food (Ortho-McNeil 1997).

IV. **Cautions/Monitoring**:

A. If untreated, topiramate-induced chronic metabolic acidosis may have potentially serious sequelae (e.g., increased risk of nephrolithiasis or nephrocalcinosis, development of osteomalacia and/or osteoporosis with an increased risk for fractures, reduced growth rates in pediatric patients). Hence, serum bicarbonate concentrations should be measured at baseline and periodically during treatment (Upsher-Smith Laboratories 2023).

B. All patients receiving or beginning therapy with any anticonvulsant for any indication should be closely monitored for the emergence or worsening of depression, suicidal thoughts or behavior (suicidality), and/or unusual changes in mood or behavior.

C. When topiramate therapy is started in patients receiving pioglitazone or vice versa, careful attention should be given to the routine monitoring of patients for adequate glycemic control (Janssen Pharmaceuticals 2023).

D. Topiramate, when combined with amitriptyline, may increase blood levels of the antidepressant by up to 12% and can precipitate toxicity (Janssen Pharmaceuticals 2023).

E. Concomitant use of topiramate and valproic acid has been associated with hyperammonemia with or without encephalopathy in patients who have previously tolerated either drug alone (Janssen Pharmaceuticals 2023).

F. Plasma concentrations of phenytoin were increased by 25% in some patients also taking topiramate.

G. Carbamazepine can decrease the plasma levels of topiramate by up to 40% (Janssen Pharmaceuticals 2023).

H. Concomitant use of topiramate with other carbonic anhydrase inhibitors (e.g., acetazolamide, dichlorphenamide, zonisamide) may increase the risk or severity of metabolic acidosis and may also increase the risk of kidney stone formation (Janssen Pharmaceuticals 2023).

I. The peak concentrations and area under the concentration-time curve (AUC) of lithium increased by 27% and 26%, respectively, during concurrent administration of topiramate at dosages up to 600 mg. Therefore, serum lithium concentrations should be monitored in patients receiving concurrent lithium and high-dose topiramate therapy.

J. Use of topiramate by patients taking combination oral contraceptives can increase the risk of contraceptive failure and breakthrough bleeding, and contraceptive efficacy can be reduced even in the absence of breakthrough bleeding (Janssen Pharmaceuticals 2023). For this reason, additional barrier methods should be discussed with women of reproductive age.

K. Cognitive and related difficulties include confusion, psychomotor slowing, difficulty with concentration or attention, difficulty with memory, and speech or language problems, particularly word-finding difficulties.

L. Psychiatric or behavior difficulties include depression and mood problems (Collins et al. 2006; Janssen Pharmaceuticals 2023; Johnson et al. 2003, 2008).

M. A syndrome consisting of acute myopia associated with secondary angle-closure glaucoma has been reported in some adult and pediatric patients receiving topiramate (Janssen Pharmaceuticals 2023; Johnson et al. 2008).

N. Because of the risk of acute myopia associated with secondary angle-closure glaucoma and other visual defects, patients receiving topiramate should be advised to seek immediate medical attention if they experience blurred vision, visual disturbances, or periorbital pain during therapy with the drug (Janssen Pharmaceuticals 2023).

O. Bleeding (e.g., epistaxis, ecchymosis, increased menstrual bleeding, life-threatening hemorrhage) was reported in about 4.5% of adults and pediatric patients (Janssen Pharmaceuticals 2023).

P. Decreased sweating and elevated body temperature above normal (hyperthermia) can be seen (Janssen Pharmaceuticals 2023).

Q. Topiramate does not appear to be superior to other mood stabilizers in the long-term treatment of patients with treatment-resistant mood disorders.

Further Reading

Ahmad NN, Robinson S, Kennedy-Martin T, et al: Clinical outcomes associated with anti-obesity medications in real-world practice: a systematic literature review. Obes Rev 22(11):e13326, 2021 34423889

Shi Q, Wang Y, Hao Q, et al: Pharmacotherapy for adults with overweight and obesity: a systematic review and network meta-analysis of randomised controlled trials. Lancet 399(10321):259–269, 2022 34895470

Wang Y, Wang D, Cheng J, et al: Efficacy and tolerability of pharmacological interventions on metabolic disturbance induced by atypical antipsychotics in adults: a systematic review and network meta-analysis. J Psychopharmacol 35(9):1111–1119, 2021 34311625

References

Arroyo S, Dodson WE, Privitera MD, et al; EPMN-106/INT-28 Investigators: Randomized dose-controlled study of topiramate as first-line therapy in epilepsy. Acta Neurol Scand 112(4):214–222, 2005 16146489

Brandes JL, Saper JR, Diamond M, et al; MIGR-002 Study Group: Topiramate for migraine prevention: a randomized controlled trial. JAMA 291(8):965–973, 2004 14982912

Collins GB, McAllister MS, Adury K: Drug adjuncts for treating alcohol dependence. Cleve Clin J Med 73(7):641–656, 2006 16845975

Domecq JP, Prutsky G, Leppin A, et al: Clinical review: drugs commonly associated with weight change: a systematic review and meta-analysis. J Clin Endocrinol Metab 100(2):363–370, 2015 25590213

Edmonds HL Jr, Jiang YD, Zhang PY, et al: Anticonvulsant activity of topiramate and phenytoin in a rat model of ischemia-induced epilepsy. Life Sci 59(10):PL127–PL131, 1996 8761322

Goh KK, Chen CH, Lu ML: Topiramate mitigates weight gain in antipsychotic-treated patients with schizophrenia: meta-analysis of randomised controlled trials. Int J Psychiatry Clin Pract 23(1):14–32, 2019 29557263

Hasan A, Falkai P, Wobrock T, et al; WFSBP Task force on Treatment Guidelines for Schizophrenia: World Federation of Societies of Biological Psychiatry (WFSBP) guidelines for biological treatment of schizophrenia, part 2: update 2012 on the long-term treatment of schizophrenia and management of antipsychotic-induced side effects. World J Biol Psychiatry 14(1):2–44, 2013 23216388

Janssen Pharmaceuticals: Topamax (topiramate) tablets and sprinkle capsules prescribing information. Janssen Pharmaceuticals, revised May 2023. Available at: https://www.janssenlabels.com/package-insert/product-monograph/prescribing-information/TOPAMAX-pi.pdf. Accessed July 31, 2024.

Johnson BA: Uses of topiramate in the treatment of alcohol dependence. Expert Rev Neurother 4(5):751–758, 2004 15853502

Johnson BA, Ait-Daoud N, Bowden CL, et al: Oral topiramate for treatment of alcohol dependence: a randomised controlled trial. Lancet 361(9370):1677–1685, 2003 12767733

Johnson BA, Ait-Daoud N, Akhtar FZ, et al: Oral topiramate reduces the consequences of drinking and improves the quality of life of alcohol-dependent individuals: a randomized controlled trial. Arch Gen Psychiatry 61(9):905–912, 2004 15351769

Johnson BA, Rosenthal N, Capece JA, et al; Topiramate for Alcoholism Advisory Board; Topiramate for Alcoholism Study Group: Topiramate for treating alcohol dependence: a randomized controlled trial. JAMA 298(14):1641–1651, 2007 17925516

Johnson BA, Rosenthal N, Capece JA, et al; Topiramate for Alcoholism Advisory Board; Topiramate for Alcoholism Study Group: Improvement of physical health and quality of life of alcohol-dependent individuals with topiramate treatment: US multisite randomized controlled trial. Arch Intern Med 168(11):1188–1199, 2008 18541827

Khalil NY, AlRabiah HK, Al Rashoud SS, et al: Topiramate: comprehensive profile. Profiles Drug Subst Excip Relat Methodol 44:333–378, 2019 31029222

Khera R, Murad MH, Chandar AK, et al: Association of pharmacological treatments for obesity with weight loss and adverse events: a systematic review and meta-analysis. JAMA 315(22):2424–2434, 2016 27299618

Kirov G, Tredget J: Add-on topiramate reduces weight in overweight patients with affective disorders: a clinical case series. BMC Psychiatry 5(1):19, 2005 15817130

Ko YH, Joe SH, Jung IK, et al: Topiramate as an adjuvant treatment with atypical antipsychotics in schizophrenic patients experiencing weight gain. Clin Neuropharmacol 28(4):169–175, 2005 16062095

Langtry HD, Gillis JC, Davis R: Topiramate: a review of its pharmacodynamic and pharmacokinetic properties and clinical efficacy in the management of epilepsy. Drugs 54(5):752–773, 1997 9360061

Ortho-McNeil: Topamax (topiramate) tablets product information reference source. 1997. Available at: https://www.accessdata.fda.gov/drugsatfda_docs/nda/99/20505S3_Topamax_admindocs_corres.pdf. Accessed July 31, 2024.

Sachdeo RC: Topiramate: clinical profile in epilepsy. Clin Pharmacokinet 34(5):335–346, 1998 9592618

Silberstein SD, Neto W, Schmitt J, et al; MIGR-001 Study Group: Topiramate in migraine prevention: results of a large controlled trial. Arch Neurol 61(4):490–495, 2004 15096395

Upsher-Smith Laboratories: Topiramate capsule, extended release [prescribing information]. Revised February 2023. Available at: https://dailymed.nlm.nih.gov/dailymed/fda/fdaDrugXsl.cfm?setid=691d276c-9cc1-4d39-828f-0f44d7ef6328&type=display. Accessed July 31, 2024.

Verrotti A, Scaparrotta A, Agostinelli S, et al: Topiramate-induced weight loss: a review. Epilepsy Res 95(3):189–199, 2011 21684121

White HS. Clinical significance of animal seizure models and mechanism of action studies of potential antiepileptic drugs. Epilepsia 38(Suppl 1):S9–S17, 1997 9092952

Wirrell EC, Laux L, Donner E, et al: Optimizing the diagnosis and management of Dravet syndrome: recommendations from a North American consensus panel. Pediatr Neurol 68(March):18–34.e3, 2017 28284397

Wirrell EC, Nabbout R: Recent advances in the drug treatment of Dravet syndrome. CNS Drugs 33(9):867–881, 2019 31549357

Xerostomia

Overview

Psychotropic medications can affect the amount of saliva secreted and may alter the composition of saliva via their receptor effects on the dual sympathetic and parasympathetic innervation of the salivary glands (Szabadi and Tavernor 2012). A 50% reduction in saliva flow may occur before patients become aware of the problem (Guggenheimer and Moore 2003).

Failure to recognize xerostomia caused by psychotropic medications may increase cavities, periodontal disease, and chronic systemic inflammatory conditions that can shorten a patient's life span.

A simple in-office assessment of the oral cavity can be achieved by visual inspection and by placing a dry tongue blade against the inside of the cheek mucosa. If the blade sticks to the mucosa and a gentle tug is needed to lift it away, xerostomia may be present (Navazesh and ADA Council on Scientific Affairs and Division of Science 2003).

References

Guggenheimer J, Moore PA: Xerostomia: etiology, recognition and treatment. J Am Dent Assoc 134(1):61–69, quiz 118–119, 2003 12555958

Navazesh M; ADA Council on Scientific Affairs and Division of Science: How can oral health care providers determine if patients have dry mouth? J Am Dent Assoc 134(5):613–620, 2003 12785497

Szabadi, E, Tavernor S. Hypo- and hypersalivation induced by psychoactive drugs. CNS Drugs 11:(6):449–466, 2012

Bethanechol (for Medication-Induced Xerostomia)

I. **Mechanism of Action**:

A. Bethanechol is a centrally acting parasympathomimetic drug. Bethanechol is a carbamate ester that is resistant to the action of cholinesterase, and most of its action is linked to activity at the M_3 muscarinic receptor (Clinical Key 2022).

II. **Data**:

A. The most frequent cause of hyposalivation is the use of certain medications (e.g., anticoagulants, antidepressants, antihypertensives, antiretrovirals, hypoglycemics, levothyroxine, multivitamins and supplements, nonsteroidal anti-inflammatory drugs, steroid inhalers) (Villa et al. 2014).

B. Nonpharmacological interventions include proper hydration; increase in humidity at nighttime; avoidance of irritating dentifrices and crunchy/hard foods; and use of sugar-free chewing gums/candy (Visvanathan and Nix 2010).

C. A total of 58 publications were identified (46 addressing preventive interventions and 12 addressing therapeutic interventions). A majority of the evidence focused on the setting of radiation therapy for head and neck cancer. For the management of salivary gland hypofunction and/or xerostomia, intermediate-quality evidence supports the use of topical mucosal lubricants, saliva substitutes, and agents that stimulate the salivary reflex. Other risk-reducing interventions that may be offered during radiation therapy for head and neck cancer include bethanechol and acupuncture (Mercadante et al. 2021). A number of clinical studies of patients with multiple causes of dry mouth report a clinical response to orally administered pilocarpine with an improvement of mouth wetting in up to 90% of patients.

D. In a randomized clinical trial, Jham et al. (2007) evaluated the effect of bethanechol on salivary flow when used concomitantly with head and neck radiotherapy in 43 participants. One group received 25 mg oral bethanechol three times daily, and the other received artificial saliva. The drug was used during and after the radiotherapy treatment. Samples of stimulated and unstimulated saliva were collected in four moments: at the beginning, between the 15th and 19th sessions of radiotherapy, immediately after the final radiotherapy treatment and 2 months after the end of radiotherapy. The use of bethanechol was associated with significantly higher whole resting (unstimulated) saliva flow rates immediately after radiotherapy.

E. The effect of bethanechol on the salivary flow was investigated by Jaguar et al. (2015) in 97 participants with oropharyngeal and nasopharyngeal carcinoma. They took a 25-mg bethanechol tablet twice a day from the beginning of radiotherapy to 1 month after the end of radiotherapy. Participants in the placebo group had significantly higher degrees of xerostomia in comparison with those receiving bethanechol. In irradiated participants, bethanechol preserved both unstimulated and stimulated salivary flow compared with placebo. Hence, the use of bethanechol during radiotherapy may increase salivary flow and reduce the damage to the salivary glands. However, it was also noted that after bethanechol therapy was stopped in the study, the number of participants with xerostomia increased (Jaguar et al. 2015).

III. **Dosing**:

A. The recommended oral dosage range for bethanechol is 25–200 mg/day (Jaguar et al. 2015). The usual adult oral dosage range is 10–50 mg three or four times a day. The minimum effective dose is determined by giving 5–10 mg initially and repeating the same amount at hourly intervals until a satisfactory response occurs or a maximum of 50 mg (total daily dosage) has been given/reached.

B. The effects of the drug sometimes appear within 30 minutes and are usually maximal within 60–90 minutes. The drug effects persist for about 1 hour (Drugs.com 2024).

C. The dosage must be individualized, based on the type and severity of the condition to be treated. It is helpful to give the drug when the stomach is empty. If taken soon after eating, nausea and vomiting may occur.

IV. **Cautions/Monitoring**:

A. Bethanechol is contraindicated in asthma and chronic obstructive pulmonary disease (COPD) patients because cholinergic stimulation constricts the airways. Bethanechol is also contraindicated in patients with hypersensitivity to bethanechol or any component of the formulation.

B. Caution is recommended in patients with hyperthyroidism, peptic ulcer disease, epilepsy, asthma, pronounced bradycardia or hypotension, vasomotor instability, coronary artery disease, or parkinsonism.
C. Caution is also warranted in situations involving mechanical obstruction of the gastrointestinal or genitourinary tract; when the increased muscular activity of the gastrointestinal tract or bladder might prove harmful; and in patients with bladder neck obstruction, spastic gastrointestinal disturbances, acute inflammatory lesions of the gastrointestinal tract, peritonitis, or marked vagotonia (Clinical Key 2022; UpToDate/Lexicomp 2024).
D. Laboratory monitoring is not necessary (Clinical Key 2022).
E. Acetylcholinesterase inhibitors may enhance the adverse/toxic effects of bethanechol chloride. Specifically, cholinergic effects may be improved or increased (it is recommended that patients be monitored throughout the treatment).
F. Beta-blockers may enhance the adverse/toxic effects of bethanechol. Of particular concern is the potential for cardiac conduction abnormalities and bronchoconstriction (close monitoring is recommended) (UpToDate/Lexicomp 2024).
G. Bethanechol can cause flushing, hypotension, and tachycardia. It can also cause colic, headache, malaise, and seizures.
H. Diaphoresis is a significant side effect that can produce several gastrointestinal side effects, including abdominal cramps, borborygmi, diarrhea, eructation, nausea, salivation, and vomiting.
I. Bethanechol can increase urinary urgency. Ophthalmic complications include lacrimation miosis. Bethanechol can also precipitate asthma and bronchoconstriction.

Further Reading

American Society of Health-System Pharmacists: Bethanecol. 2021. Available at: https://online.statref.com/document/tjcvuox9IdRsQtjT0b-8yD?searchid=1644607080512029110 categoryType=All. Accessed March 13, 2024.

Riley P, Glenny AM, Hua F, et al: Pharmacological interventions for preventing dry mouth and salivary gland dysfunction following radiotherapy. Cochrane Database Syst Rev (7):CD012744, 2017 28759701

Salum FG, Medella-Junior FAC, Figueiredo MAZ, et al: Salivary hypofunction: an update on therapeutic strategies. Gerodontology 35(4):305–316, 2018 29956369

References

Clinical Key: Bethanechol. Elsevier, n.d. Available at: https://www.clinicalkey.com/#!/content/drug_monograph/6-s2.0–66. Accessed February 11, 2022.

Drugs.com: Urecholine (bethanechol chloride) prescribing information. Last updated June 17, 2024. Available at: https://www.drugs.com/pro/urecholine.html. Accessed July 31, 2024.

Jaguar GC, Lima EN, Kowalski LP, et al: Double blind randomized prospective trial of bethanechol in the prevention of radiation-induced salivary gland dysfunction in head and neck cancer patients. Radiother Oncol 115(2):253–256, 2015 25890572

Jham BC, Teixeira IV, Aboud CG, et al: A randomized phase III prospective trial of bethanechol to prevent radiotherapy-induced salivary gland damage in patients with head and neck cancer. Oral Oncol 43(2):137–142, 2007 16798061

Mercadante V, Jensen SB, Smith DK, et al: Salivary gland hypofunction and/or xerostomia induced by nonsurgical cancer therapies: ISOO/MASCC/ASCO Guideline. J Clin Oncol 39(25):2825–2843, 2021 34283635
UpToDate/Lexicomp: Bethanechol: drug information. n.d. Available at: https://pro.uptodatefree.ir/show/9153. Accessed July 31, 2024.
Villa A, Connell CL, Abati S: Diagnosis and management of xerostomia and hyposalivation. Ther Clin Risk Manag 11:45–51, 2014 25653532
Visvanathan V, Nix P: Managing the patient presenting with xerostomia: a review. Int J Clin Pract 64(3):404–407, 2010 19817913

Pilocarpine (for Medication-Induced Xerostomia)

I. Mechanism of Action:

A. The agonist action of pilocarpine on the cholinergic receptors causes increased secretion from exocrine glands, including sweat, salivary, lacrimal, gastric, pancreatic and intestinal glands, as well as increased tone and motility of the smooth muscle cells in the eye and in the respiratory and gastrointestinal tracts (Pilocarpine 2020).

1. Oral pilocarpine stimulates salivary flow within 15 minutes and peak flow rates are maintained for at least 1–2 hours after dosing in patients with xerostomia. The mean salivary flow rate with oral pilocarpine is 2- to 10-fold higher after pilocarpine treatment than after placebo (Wiseman et al. 2012).
2. Oral pilocarpine is recommended for the treatment of symptoms of dry mouth from salivary gland hypofunction caused by radiotherapy for cancer of the head and neck.
3. Oral pilocarpine is also used to treat the symptoms of dry mouth in patients with Sjögren syndrome (U.S. Food and Drug Administration 2022).

II. Data:

A. In a prospective randomized, double-blind, placebo-controlled trial, patients received either placebo or pilocarpine (5 mg or 10 mg orally three times a day) for 12 weeks and were evaluated at baseline and every 4 weeks thereafter. There was an overall improvement in 54% of the 5-mg group, as compared with 25% of the placebo group (P=0.003). Thirty-one percent of the 5-mg group had improved comfort of the mouth and tongue, compared with 10% of the placebo group (P=0.002). Speaking ability improved in 33% of the 5-mg group, compared with 18% of the placebo group (P=0.037). There were comparable improvements in the group receiving the 10-mg dose (Johnson et al. 1993).

B. In another study, 162 patients who had received radiation with clinically significant xerostomia were enrolled in a randomized, double-blind, placebo-controlled multicenter clinical investigation. Patients received 2.5-mg tablets for the first 4 weeks, 5.0-mg tablets for the second 4 weeks, and 10.0-mg tablets for the last 4 weeks of the 12-week study. There were statistically more significant postdose improvements in parotid salivary flow in the pilocarpine-treated groups versus placebo. All pilocarpine dosages tested were safe. The study concluded that pilocarpine produces clinically substantial benefits for xerostomia. Best results were obtained with continuous treatment for 8–12 weeks with dosages greater than 2.5 mg three times per day (LeVeque et al. 1993).

C. Another study involved patients with autoimmune conditions and related clinically significant dry mouth who were randomly assigned to receive 2.5 mg pilocarpine, 5 mg pilocarpine, or placebo tablets four times daily for 12 weeks. A significantly greater proportion of the patients in the 5-mg pilocarpine group than in the placebo group showed improvement in global assessments of dry mouth. The salivary flow was significantly increased 2- to 3-fold after administration of the first dose and was maintained throughout the 12-week study. The most common adverse effect was sweating (Vivino et al. 1999).

III. **Dosing**:

A. The recommended dosage for the initiation of treatment of xerostomia is 5 mg taken three times daily (Hawthorne and Sullivan 2000). This dosage may be titrated up to 10 mg three times daily in patients who do not respond adequately to, but can tolerate, the lower dosage. The lowest dosage that is effective and tolerable should be used for maintenance therapy.

IV. **Cautions/Monitoring**:

A. Hypersensitivity to pilocarpine or any component of the formulation; uncontrolled asthma; when miosis is undesirable (e.g., acute iritis, angle-closure glaucoma).

B. Pilocarpine can cause flushing (8%–13% of patients), chills (3%–15%), nausea (6%–15%) dizziness (5%–12%), and headache (11%). Other adverse effects include urinary frequency (9%–12%), neuromuscular and skeletal weakness (2%–12%), and diaphoresis (29%–68%) (Lexicomp/UpToDate 2024; U.S. Food and Drug Administration 2022).

C. Fatal overdose with pilocarpine has been reported in the scientific literature at doses presumed to be greater than 100 mg. Overdose should be treated with atropine titration (0.5–1.0 mg given subcutaneously or intravenously) and supportive measures to maintain respiration and circulation. Epinephrine (0.3 mg–1.0 mg, subcutaneously or intramuscularly) may also be of value in the presence of severe cardiovascular depression or bronchoconstriction.

D. Use of pilocarpine by patients with severe hepatic impairment (Child-Pugh score 10–15) is not recommended. In patients with mild to moderate hepatic impairment, a single 5-mg dose administration results in a 30% decrease in total plasma clearance and a doubling of exposure. Peak plasma levels increase by about 30%, and half-life increases to 2.1 hours in hepatically impaired patients (U.S. Food and Drug Administration 2022).

E. Acetylcholinesterase inhibitors may enhance the adverse/toxic effect of pilocarpine. Specifically, cholinergic effects may be enhanced or increased. Therefore, close monitoring is recommended throughout treatment.

F. Beta-blockers may enhance the adverse/toxic effect of pilocarpine. Of particular concern is the potential for cardiac conduction abnormalities and bronchoconstriction.

G. Pilocarpine was previously classified as FDA Category C in pregnancy; therefore, close monitoring is recommended throughout treatment (Lexicomp/UpToDate 2024).

Further Reading

Marchand DK, McCormack S: Pilocarpine for radiotherapy-induced dry mouth and dry eyes: a review of clinical effectiveness, cost-effectiveness, and guidelines. Ottawa, ON, Canadian Agency for Drugs and Technologies in Health, 2020

Thakkar JP, Lane CJ: Hyposalivation and xerostomia and burning mouth syndrome: medical management. Oral Maxillofac Surg Clin North Am 34(1):135–146, 2020 31685347

References

Hawthorne M, Sullivan K: Pilocarpine for radiation-induced xerostomia in head and neck cancer. Int J Palliat Nurs 6(5):228–232, 2000 12419994

Johnson JT, Ferretti GA, Nethery WJ, et al: Oral pilocarpine for post-irradiation xerostomia in patients with head and neck cancer. N Engl J Med 329(6):390–395, 1993 8326972

LeVeque FGM, Montgomery M, Potter D, et al: A multicenter, randomized, double-blind, placebo-controlled, dose-titration study of oral pilocarpine for treatment of radiation-induced xerostomia in head and neck cancer patients. J Clin Oncol 11(6):1124–1131, 1993 8501499

Lexicomp/UpToDate: Pilocarpine (systemic): drug information. n.d. Available at: https://pro.uptodatefree.ir/Show/9905. Accessed July 31, 2024.

Pilocarpine [updated June 15, 2020], in LiverTox: Clinical and Research Information on Drug-Induced Liver Injury [Internet]. Bethesda, MD, National Institute of Diabetes and Digestive and Kidney Diseases, 2012–. Available at: https://www.ncbi.nlm.nih.gov/books/NBK548815/. Accessed March 13, 2024.

U.S. Food and Drug Administration: Pilocarpine Prescribing Information. Available at: https://www.accessdata.fda.gov/drugsatfda_docs/label/2010/200890s001lbl.pdf. Accessed February 11, 2022.

Vivino FB, Al-Hashimi I, Khan Z, et al: Pilocarpine tablets for the treatment of dry mouth and dry eye symptoms in patients with Sjögren syndrome: a randomized, placebo-controlled, fixed-dose, multicenter trial. P92–01 Study Group. Arch Intern Med 159(2):174–181, 1999 9927101

Wiseman LR, Faulds D, Bowen WB, et al: Oral pilocarpine: a review of its pharmacological properties and clinical potential in xerostomia. Drugs 49(1):143–155, 2012

PART IV
Other Agents/Treatments

13

Nutraceuticals and Phytoceuticals

Erick Calvario-Sanchez, M.D.
Patricia Aguayo, M.D., M.P.H.
Becky Kinkead, Ph.D.
Mark H. Rapaport, M.D.

***Nutraceuticals* are products** derived from food sources that offer health benefits beyond basic nutrition. The word *nutraceutical* is a portmanteau, blending the words *nutrition* and *pharmaceutical*, indicating that these products intersect food and medicine. *Phytoceuticals* are bioactive compounds from plants that provide health benefits beyond basic nutrition. These substances are often used for their medicinal and/or therapeutic properties and can include a wide range of phytochemicals, such as flavonoids, carotenoids, polyphenols, and alkaloids. The term *phytoceutical* originates from the Greek words *phyto*, meaning "plant," and *ceutical*, meaning "pharmaceutical." Therefore, because vitamins are essential for maintaining health, help to prevent and treat deficiencies, and fall under the classification of nutraceuticals, we included B vitamins in this chapter.

Acetyl-L-Carnitine

I. **Generic Names**: Acetyl-L-carnitine, carnitine

II. **Brand Names**: None

III. **Scientific Name**: L-3-hydroxytrimethylaminobutanoate

IV. **Class**: Common nutraceutical

V. **Mechanism of Action**

A. Acetyl-L-carnitine (ALC) facilitates the uptake of acetyl coenzyme A (acetyl-CoA) in the mitochondria during fatty acid oxidation, enhances acetylcholine production, and stimulates the synthesis of proteins and membrane phospholipids (Traina 2016).

B. ALC may increase the release of dopamine (Goodison et al. 2017). ALC also influences functional aspects of serotonergic, noradrenergic, and GABAergic neurotransmission (Traina 2016).

VI. **Evidence-Based Uses**

A. Major depressive disorder (MDD) (Ravindran et al. 2018; Veronese et al. 2018).

VII. **Common/Other Uses**

A. Antioxidant; treatment of cachexia, cardiovascular disease, diabetes, dyslipidemias, fatigue, hematological disorders, infertility, renal disease; enhancement of exercise performance (Lexicomp 2022)

VIII. **Major Contraindications and When to Use Caution**

A. None

IX. **Dosage Ranges and Guidelines**

A. The Canadian Network for Mood and Anxiety Treatments (CANMAT) clinical guidelines for the management of major depressive disorder in adults recommend acetyl-L-carnitine as a third-line monotherapy for mild to moderate MDD (level 2) (Ravindran et al. 2018).

B. Only two studies have demonstrated pharmacokinetic profiles in humans. One study administered a dose of 500 mg (Kwon and Chung 2004), while the other used a dose of 590 mg (Baek et al. 2015). In both studies, ALC was well tolerated by the subjects. Given that most commercially available formulations contain 500 mg of ALC, it is reasonable to recommend a daily dose of 500 mg.

X. **Monitoring**: Not applicable

XI. **Relevant Pharmacokinetics/Pharmacodynamics**

A. In healthy adult males given a one-time dose of a commercially available ALC product containing 500 mg of ALC, the C_{max} was approximately 1.7 μg/mL. Plasma levels returned to baseline roughly 4 hours postdose, and bioavailability was approximately 20%. Rather than being metabolized, excess ALC is excreted in the urine as needed to maintain stable blood concentrations (Baek et al. 2015).

XII. **Clinically Relevant Drug Interactions**

A. Carbamazepine, phenobarbital, phenytoin, and valproic acid may decrease blood concentrations of ALC.

B. Pivampicillin and other pivalate-conjugated antibiotics may decrease blood concentrations of ALC (Office of Dietary Supplements 2023).

XIII. **Adverse Effects**

A. **Common**: Nausea, vomiting, abdominal cramps, diarrhea, and a "fishy" body odor (Office of Dietary Supplements 2023)

B. **Rare**: Mania (Goodison et al. 2017); headache and insomnia (Martinotti et al. 2011).

C. **Risks in pregnancy and lactation**: Insufficient reliable information is available on ALC's safety in pregnancy and lactation; avoid use.

XIV. **Clinical Pearls/Guidelines**

A. As an over-the-counter product, ALC is regulated differently from prescription drugs, and the quality and content of available preparations may vary. Consider consultation with a pharmacist.

References

Baek S-M, Zheng R, Seo E-J, et al: Pharmacokinetic comparisons of two acetyl-L-carnitine formulations in healthy Korean volunteers. Int J Clin Pharmacol Ther 53(11):980–986, 2015 26396135

Goodison G, Overeem K, de Monte V, et al: Mania associated with self-prescribed acetyl-l-carnitine in a man with bipolar I disorder. Australas Psychiatry 25(1):13–14, 2017 27406927

Kwon OS, Chung YB: HPLC determination and pharmacokinetics of endogenous acetyl-L-carnitine (ALC) in human volunteers orally administered a single dose of ALC. Arch Pharm Res 27(6):676–681, 2004 15283472

Lexicomp. Acetyl-L-carnitine. n.d. Available (but accessible only by subscribers) at: https://online.lexi.com/lco/action/doc/retrieve/docid/fc_rnp2/6032226?cesid=8B5FEl9eHlMandsearchUrl=/lco/action/search%3Fq%3Dacetyl-L-carnitine%26t%3Dname%26va%3Dacetyl-L-carnitine#. Accessed May 4, 2022.

Martinotti G, Andreoli S, Reina D, et al: Acetyl-L-carnitine in the treatment of anhedonia, melancholic and negative symptoms in alcohol dependent subjects. Prog Neuropsychopharmacol Biol Psychiatry 35(4):953–958, 2011

Office of Dietary Supplements: Carnitine: fact sheet for health professionals. National Institutes of Health, Office of Dietary Supplements. Updated April 17, 2023. Available at: https://ods.od.nih.gov/factsheets/Carnitine-HealthProfessional/. Accessed March 13, 2024.

Ravindran AV, Balneaves LG, Faulkner G, et al; CANMAT Depression Work Group: Canadian Network for Mood and Anxiety Treatments (CANMAT) 2016 Clinical Guidelines for the Management of Adults with Major Depressive Disorder: Section 5: Complementary and alternative medicine treatments. Focus (Am Psychiatr Publ) 16(1):85–94, 2018 32015703

Traina G: The neurobiology of acetyl-L-carnitine. Front Biosci (Landmark Ed) 21(7):1314–1329, 2016 27100509

Veronese N, Stubbs B, Solmi M, et al: Acetyl-l-carnitine supplementation and the treatment of depressive symptoms: a systematic review and meta-analysis. Psychosom Med 80(2):154–159, 2018 29076953

Alpha-Lipoic Acid

I. **Generic Names**: Alpha-lipoic acid, thioctic acid, thioctacid (thioctic acid), lipoic acid

II. **Brand Names**: None

III. **Scientific Name**: 1,2-dithiolane-3-pentanoic acid

IV. **Class**: Common nutraceutical

V. **Mechanism of Action**

A. Alpha-lipoic acid (ALA) is a compound commonly found in mitochondria; it is a necessary cofactor for mitochondrial α-ketoacid dehydrogenases and thus serves a critical role in energy metabolism. ALA is also involved in glucose and lipid metabolism, manages gene transcription, and works as an antioxidant (Salehi et al. 2019; Shay et al. 2009).

VI. **Evidence-Based Uses**

A. Alzheimer's disease (Holmquist et al. 2007; Shinto et al. 2014)

VII. **Common/Other Uses**

A. Antioxidant; treatment of diabetic neuropathy, HIV/AIDS, liver disease; chelation of transition and heavy metals; promotion of weight loss (Nguyen et al. 2024)

VIII. **Major Contraindications and When to Use Caution**

A. Use with caution in patients with liver disease, patients who consume large amounts of alcohol, and patients with diabetes, thyroid disorders, or thiamine deficiency (Nguyen et al. 2024).

IX. **Dosage Ranges and Guidelines**

A. ALA at 600 mg/day slowed the progression rate of dementia dramatically, in comparison with the rate in untreated patients or patients receiving cholinesterase inhibitors (Hager et al. 2007; Holmquist et al. 2007).

X. **Monitoring**: Not applicable

XI. **Relevant Pharmacokinetics/Pharmacodynamics**

A. ALA is rapidly absorbed after oral ingestion of 50–600 mg thioctic acid, with a time to peak plasma concentration of approximately 0.5–1 hour (Salehi et al. 2019). It is extensively metabolized in the liver and rapidly conjugated (Teichert et al. 2003), and its half-life is about 0.5 hour (Breithaupt-Grögler et al. 1999).

XII. **Clinically Relevant Drug Interactions**

A. Antidiabetic drugs: ALA may enhance the hypoglycemic effect of antidiabetic drugs (Porasuphatana et al. 2012).

XIII. **Adverse Effects**

A. **Common**: Headache, heartburn, nausea, vomiting (Gilron et al. 2021)

B. **Rare**: Delayed hypersensitivity (Rizzi et al. 2015); insulin autoimmune syndrome (Gullo et al. 2014; Moffa et al. 2019); strong odor of the urine (Bobe et al. 2020)

C. **Risks in pregnancy and lactation**: Insufficient reliable information is available on ALA's safety in pregnancy and lactation; avoid use.

XIV. Clinical Pearls/Guidelines

A. A dosage of 200–2,400 mg/day of ALA is deemed safe and free of side effects (Nguyen et al. 2024).

B. In addition to its potential benefits for dementia, ALA has demonstrated clear benefit in peripheral neuropathy, likely related to its activity as a lipophilic free-radical scavenger of peripheral nerves, stimulation of nerve growth factor, and promotion of fiber regeneration (Vallianou et al. 2009; Ziegler et al. 2002).

C. As an over-the-counter product, ALA is regulated differently from prescription drugs, and the quality and content of available preparations may vary. Consider consultation with a pharmacist.

References

Bobe G, Michels AJ, Zhang W-J, et al: A randomized controlled trial of long-term (R)-alpha-lipoic acid supplementation promotes weight loss in overweight or obese adults without altering baseline elevated plasma triglyceride concentrations. J Nutr 150(9):2336–2345, 2020 32692358

Breithaupt-Grögler K, Niebch G, Schneider E, et al: Dose-proportionality of oral thioctic acid—coincidence of assessments via pooled plasma and individual data. Eur J Pharm Sci 8(1):57–65, 1999 10072479

Gilron I, Robb S, Tu D, et al: Double-blind, randomized, placebo-controlled crossover trial of alpha-lipoic acid for the treatment of fibromyalgia pain: the IMPALA trial. Pain 162(2):561–568, 2021 32773602

Gullo D, Evans JL, Sortino G, et al: Insulin autoimmune syndrome (Hirata disease) in European Caucasians taking alpha-lipoic acid. Clin Endocrinol (Oxf) 81(2):204–209, 2014 24111525

Hager K, Kenklies M, McAfoose J, et al: Alpha-lipoic acid as a new treatment option for Alzheimer's disease—a 48 months follow-up analysis. J Neural Transm Suppl 72(72):189–193, 2007 17982894

Holmquist L, Stuchbury G, Berbaum K, et al: Lipoic acid as a novel treatment for Alzheimer's disease and related dementias. Pharmacol Ther 113(1):154–164, 2007 16989905

Moffa S, Improta I, Rocchetti S, et al: Potential cause-effect relationship between insulin autoimmune syndrome and alpha lipoic acid: two case reports. Nutrition 57:1–4, 2019 30086435

Nguyen H, Pellegrini MV, Gupta V: Alpha-Lipoic Acid, in StatPearls. Treasure Island, FL, StatPearls Publishing, last update January 26, 2024. Available at: https://www.ncbi.nlm.nih.gov/books/NBK564301/. Accessed March 13, 2024.

Porasuphatana S, Suddee S, Nartnampong A, et al: Glycemic and oxidative status of patients with type 2 diabetes mellitus following oral administration of alpha-lipoic acid: a randomized double-blinded placebo-controlled study. Asia Pac J Clin Nutr 21(1):12–21, 2012 22374556

Rizzi A, Nucera E, Buonomo A, et al: Delayed hypersensitivity to alpha-lipoic acid: look at dietary supplements. Contact Dermatitis 73(1):62–63, 2015 25864490

Salehi B, Berkay Yılmaz Y, Antika G, et al: Insights on the use of alpha-lipoic acid for therapeutic purposes. Biomolecules 9(8):356, 2019 31405030

Shay KP, Moreau RF, Smith EJ, et al: Alpha-lipoic acid as a dietary supplement: molecular mechanisms and therapeutic potential. Biochim Biophys Acta 1790(10):1149–1160, 2009 19664690

Shinto L, Quinn J, Montine T, et al: A randomized placebo-controlled pilot trial of omega-3 fatty acids and alpha lipoic acid in Alzheimer's disease. J Alzheimers Dis 38(1):111–120, 2014 24077434

Teichert J, Hermann R, Ruus P, et al: Plasma kinetics, metabolism, and urinary excretion of alpha-lipoic acid following oral administration in healthy volunteers. J Clin Pharmacol 43(11):1257–1267, 2003 14551180

Vallianou N, Evangelopoulos A, Koutalas P: Alpha-lipoic acid and diabetic neuropathy. Rev Diabet Stud 6(4):230–236, 2009 20043035

Ziegler G, Ploch M, Miettinen-Baumann A, et al: Efficacy and tolerability of valerian extract LI 156 compared with oxazepam in the treatment of non-organic insomnia—a randomized, double-blind, comparative clinical study. Eur J Med Res 7(11):480–486, 2002 12568976

B Vitamins[1]

I. **Generic Names**: Cobalamine (B_{12}), folate (B_9), pyridoxine (B_6)

II. **Brand Names**: None

III. **Scientific Names**: As in "Generic Names"

IV. **Class**: Water-soluble vitamin

V. **Mechanism of Action**

A. The B vitamins comprise a group of eight water-soluble vitamins that perform essential, closely interrelated roles in cellular functioning, acting as coenzymes in a vast array of catabolic and anabolic enzymatic reactions. They play an important role in numerous aspects of brain function, including energy production, DNA/RNA synthesis/repair, genomic and nongenomic methylation, and the synthesis of several neurochemicals and signaling molecules (Kennedy 2016).

VI. **Evidence-Based Uses**

A. Dementia (Gil Martínez et al. 2022).

B. Depression (Almeida et al. 2014, 2015).

VII. **Common/Other Uses**

A. B_{12}: Treatment of cancer, cardiovascular disease, stroke; enhancement of cognitive function, energy, and endurance (Office of Dietary Supplements 2024).

B. B_6: Treatment of cardiovascular disease, cancer, premenstrual syndrome, nausea and vomiting in pregnancy; enhancement of cognitive function (Office of Dietary Supplements 2023).

VIII. **Major Contraindications and When to Use Caution**

A. Patients with sensitivity to the cobalt moiety or the cobalamin molecule should abstain from using vitamin B_{12} (Al Amin and Gupta 2023).

B. Use with caution in patients with Leber hereditary optic neuropathy and also in those with renal failure (Al Amin and Gupta 2023).

IX. **Dosage Ranges and Guidelines**

A. A recent meta-analysis and systematic review suggested that supplementation of B vitamins (especially with folic acid supplementation) may have a positive effect on delaying and preventing the risk of cognitive decline, particularly in populations who received early and long-duration intervention (Gil Martínez et al. 2022).

---

[1]For information on folic acid (vitamin B_9), see the Folic Acid section in this chapter.

B. Several studies have shown that treatment with folate and vitamin B_{12} does not reduce depressive symptoms over a short period of time but may be helpful in the long-term management of depression in certain populations (Almeida et al. 2015). A randomized double-blind, placebo-controlled trial showed that taking citalopram plus B_{12} (0.5 mg), folic acid (2 mg), and B_6 (25 mg) did not increase the 12-week efficacy of antidepressant treatment but did enhance and sustain the antidepressant response over 1 year (Almeida et al. 2014).

X. Monitoring

A. Folic acid can aggravate vitamin B_{12} deficiency; first correct the B_{12} deficiency, and then use folate supplementation, unless the patient has a concomitant folate deficiency (Al Amin and Gupta 2023).

XI. Relevant Pharmacokinetics/Pharmacodynamics

A. Dietary vitamin B_{12} is primarily absorbed by binding with intrinsic factor (IF) to be actively transported in the terminal ileum. Vitamin B_{12} has a C_{max} of 7 hours and a half-life of ~25 hours (Alpers 2016).

B. Vitamin B_6 is absorbed in the upper small intestine by simple diffusion and is transported to the liver for biotransformation into the active coenzyme pyridoxal phosphate ("Vitamin B6 [pyridoxine and pyridoxal 5'-phosphate]—monograph" 2001).

XII. Clinically Relevant Drug Interactions

A. Pyridoxin may increase the metabolism of phenytoin and fosphenytoin and may decrease the serum concentrations of the active metabolites of primidone (UpToDate 2024).

XIII. Adverse Effects

A. Vitamin B_{12}

1. **Common**: Fever, itching or rash, tingling or numbness of joints, shortness of breath, rapid weight gain, polycythemia, hypokalemia, congestive heart failure, pulmonary edema, vascular thrombosis
2. **Rare**: Allergic reactions, especially with hydroxocobalamin injections (Al Amin and Gupta 2023)

B. Vitamin B_6

1. **Common**: Sensory neuropathy (this effect rarely occurs below toxic doses [i.e., ≥1 g/day for adults]); indigestion, nausea, breast tenderness, photosensitivity
2. **Rare**: Vesicular dermatosis (with higher doses below levels of toxicity) (Abosamak and Gupta 2023)

XIV. Clinical Pearls/Guidelines

A. The evidence base supporting B vitamin use in each of the conditions noted is mixed (Abosamak and Gupta 2023; Al Amin and Gupta 2023).

References

Abosamak NR, Gupta V: Vitamin B6 (pyridoxine), in StatPearls. Treasure Island, FL, StatPearls Publishing, last update August 17, 2023. Available at: https://www.ncbi.nlm.nih.gov/books/NBK557436/. Accessed March 13, 2024.

Al Amin ASM, Gupta V: Vitamin B12 (cobalamin), in StatPearls. Treasure Island, FL, StatPearls Publishing, last update July 16, 2023. Available at: https://www.ncbi.nlm.nih.gov/books/NBK559132/. Accessed March 13, 2024.

Almeida OP, Ford AH, Hirani V, et al: B vitamins to enhance treatment response to antidepressants in middle-aged and older adults: results from the B-VITAGE randomised, double-blind, placebo-controlled trial. Br J Psychiatry 205(6):450–457, 2014 25257064

Almeida OP, Ford AH, Flicker L: Systematic review and meta-analysis of randomized placebo-controlled trials of folate and vitamin B12 for depression. Int Psychogeriatr 27(5):727–737, 2015 25644193

Alpers DH: Absorption and blood/cellular transport of folate and cobalamin: pharmacokinetic and physiological considerations. Biochimie 126:52–56, 2016 26586110

Gil Martínez V, Avedillo Salas A, Santander Ballestín S: Vitamin supplementation and dementia: a systematic review. Nutrients 14(5):1033, 2022 35268010

Kennedy DO: B vitamins and the brain: mechanisms, dose and efficacy—a review. Nutrients 8(2):68, 2016 26828517

Office of Dietary Supplements: Vitamin B6: Fact Sheet for Health Professionals. National Institutes of Health, Office of Dietary Supplements. Updated June 16, 2023. Available at: https://ods.od.nih.gov/factsheets/VitaminB6-HealthProfessional/. Accessed March 13, 2024.

Office of Dietary Supplements: Vitamin B12: fact sheet for health professionals. National Institutes of Health, Office of Dietary Supplements, updated March 26, 2024. Available at: https://ods.od.nih.gov/factsheets/VitaminB12-HealthProfessional/. Accessed April 21, 2024.

UpToDate: Vitamin B6 (pyridoxine): drug information. n.d. Available at: https://pro.uptodate-free.ir/Show/9839. Accessed August 4, 2024.

Vitamin B6 (pyridoxine and pyridoxal 5'-phosphate)—monograph. Altern Med Rev 6(1):87–92, 2001 11207460

Folic Acid

I. **Generic Names**: folic acid, folate, folacin, methylfolate, vitamin B_9

II. **Brand Names**: Deplin, Metafolin

III. **Scientific Name**: pteroylglutamic acid

IV. **Class**: Water-soluble vitamin

V. **Mechanism of Action**

A. Folic acid is necessary for the formation of several coenzymes in many metabolic systems, particularly for purine and pyrimidine synthesis. It is also required for nucleoprotein synthesis and maintenance in erythropoiesis (Merrell and McMurry 2023).

B. Folic acid is required for the remethylation of homocysteine to methionine and S-adenosylmethionine (SAM) conversion (Bottiglieri 2013).

C. Folic acid also participates in the methylation of tetrahydrobiopterin, an essential cofactor for the hydroxylase enzymes involved in the production of neurotransmitters such as serotonin (Taylor et al. 2003).

VI. **Evidence-Based Uses**

A. Major depressive disorder (MDD) (Sarris et al. 2022).

VII. **Common/Other Uses**

A. Neural tube defects, cancer, heart disease, stroke, anemias due to folate deficiency, dementia, Alzheimer's disease, congenital heart defects, autism spectrum disorder (Office of Dietary Supplements 2022).

VIII. **Major Contraindications and When to Use Caution**

A. Folic acid supplementation is not recommended for patients with hypersensitivity to folic acid or to any constituent of the formulation (Merrell and McMurry 2023).

IX. **Dosage Ranges and Guidelines**

A. Methylfolate (15 mg/day) is provisionally recommended for adjunctive use in MDD. Folic acid, however, is not recommended for this use (Sarris et al. 2022).

X. **Monitoring**: Not applicable

XI. **Relevant Pharmacokinetics/Pharmacodynamics**

A. Folate absorption occurs by both passive and carrier-mediated mechanisms in the proximal intestine. Intestinal folate transport is a saturable process with an optimal pH between 5.5 and 6.0, which explains why antacids reduce its absorption (Scaglione and Panzavolta 2014).

B. Several studies have reported a higher relative bioavailability of supplemental folic acid compared with food folates (Scaglione and Panzavolta 2014). The range of folate bioavailability from the diet is widely variable (44%–80%) (Alpers 2016).

C. Folate is both filtered and secreted; most of the secreted folate is reabsorbed. Biliary excretion of folate has been estimated to be as high as 100 μg/day (Institute of Medicine 1998).

XII. **Clinically Relevant Drug Interactions**

A. Folic acid may enhance the adverse/toxic effects of fluorouracil products (Mainwaring and Grygiel 1995).

B. Folate supplements could interfere with methotrexate's anticancer effects (Office of Dietary Supplements 2022).

C. Taking folate supplements could reduce blood levels of phenytoin, carbamazepine, and valproate. Also, these drugs could reduce blood levels of folate (Office of Dietary Supplements 2022).

D. Green tea (Navarro-Perán et al. 2005) and sulfasalazine (Jansen et al. 2004) may decrease the serum concentration of folic acid.

E. Folic acid may have antagonistic effects on phenobarbital (Fröscher et al. 1995).

F. Folic acid may decrease serum concentrations of phenytoin (Lewis et al. 1995) and of primidone and its active metabolites (e.g., phenobarbital) (Fröscher et al. 1995).

XIII. **Adverse Effects**

A. **Common**: None; folic acid is relatively nontoxic.

B. **Rare**: Erythema, rash, itching, general malaise, bronchospastic respiratory difficulty, anaphylaxis (UpToDate 2024)

XIV. **Clinical Pearls/Guidelines**

A. Deplin is a pharmaceutical-grade form of L-methylfolate that is available by prescription.

B. Post hoc analyses found that depressed patients with inflammation and/or obesity responded better to adjunctive L-methylfolate than did those without inflammation or obesity who participated in the same clinical trials (Macaluso 2022).

References

Alpers DH: Absorption and blood/cellular transport of folate and cobalamin: pharmacokinetic and physiological considerations. Biochimie 126:52–56, 2016 26586110

Bottiglieri T: Folate, vitamin B12, and S-adenosylmethionine. Psychiatr Clin North Am 36(1):1–13, 2013 23538072

Fröscher W, Maier V, Laage M, et al: Folate deficiency, anticonvulsant drugs, and psychiatric morbidity. Clin Neuropharmacol 18(2):165–182, 1995 8635176

Institute of Medicine: Dietary Reference Intakes for Thiamin, Riboflavin, Niacin, Vitamin B6, Folate, Vitamin B12, Pantothenic Acid, Biotin, and Choline. Standing Committee on the Scientific Evaluation of Dietary Reference Intakes and its Panel on Folate, Other B Vitamins, and Choline. Washington, DC, National Academies Press, 1998

Jansen G, van der Heijden J, Oerlemans R, et al: Sulfasalazine is a potent inhibitor of the reduced folate carrier: implications for combination therapies with methotrexate in rheumatoid arthritis. Arthritis Rheum 50(7):2130–2139, 2004 15248210

Lewis DP, Van Dyke DC, Willhite LA, et al: Phenytoin-folic acid interaction. Ann Pharmacother 29(7–8):726–735, 1995 8520091

Macaluso M: L-Methylfolate in antidepressant non-responders: the impact of body weight and inflammation. Front Psychiatry 13:840116, 2022 35370812

Mainwaring P, Grygiel JJ: Interaction of 5-fluorouracil with folates. Aust NZ J Med 25(1):60–60, 1995 7786254

Merrell BJ, McMurry JP: Folic Acid, in StatPearls. Treasure Island, FL, StatPearls Publishing, last update August 8, 2023. Available at: https://www.ncbi.nlm.nih.gov/books/NBK554487/. Accessed March 13, 2024.

Navarro-Perán E, Cabezas-Herrera J, García-Cánovas F, et al: The antifolate activity of tea catechins. Cancer Res 65(6):2059–2064, 2005 15781612

Office of Dietary Supplements: Folate: fact sheet for health professionals. National Institutes of Health, Office of Dietary Supplements. Updated November 30, 2022. Available at: https://ods.od.nih.gov/factsheets/Folate-HealthProfessional/. Accessed March 13, 2024.

Sarris J, Ravindran A, Yatham LN, et al: Clinician guidelines for the treatment of psychiatric disorders with nutraceuticals and phytoceuticals: the World Federation of Societies of Biological Psychiatry (WFSBP) and Canadian Network for Mood and Anxiety Treatments (CANMAT) Taskforce. World J Biol Psychiatry 23(6):424–455, 2022 35311615

Scaglione F, Panzavolta G: Folate, folic acid and 5-methyltetrahydrofolate are not the same thing. Xenobiotica 44(5):480–488, 2014 24494987

Taylor MJ, Carney S, Geddes J, et al: Folate for depressive disorders. Cochrane Database Syst Rev (2):CD003390, 2003 12804463

UpToDate. Folic acid: drug information. n.d. Available at: https://pro.uptodatefree.ir/show/8475. Accessed August 4, 2024.

Ginkgo

I. **Generic Names**: Ginkgo, ginkgo biloba, fossil tree, maidenhair tree, Japanese silver apricot, baiguo, yinhsing

II. **Brand Names**: None

III. **Scientific Name**: *Ginkgo biloba*

IV. **Class**: Phytoceutical

V. **Mechanism of Action**

A. Ginkgo leaf and its extracts contain a variety of components, such as flavonoids, terpenoids, and organic acids (Liu et al. 2021).

B. Ginkgo enhances the body's ability to scavenge free radicals by increasing glutathione levels (Suter et al. 2011).

C. Many possible mechanisms of action have been proposed for ginkgo leaf and its extracts, including antioxidant effects; anti-inflammatory effects; anti-apoptosis effects; defense against mitochondrial dysfunction, amyloidogenesis, and Aβ aggregation; and modulation of phosphorylation of tau protein (Lu et al. 2021; Singh et al. 2019).

VI. **Evidence-Based Uses**

A. Schizophrenia (as adjunct to antipsychotic treatment) (Sarris et al. 2022).

VII. **Common/Other Uses**

A. Anxiety (Woelk et al. 2007), allergies, dementia, diabetic retinopathy, glaucoma, peripheral artery disease, tinnitus, premenstrual syndrome, vertigo (National Center for Complementary and Integrative Health 2020). The evidence base supporting ginkgo's use in each of these conditions varies; for further information, readers are referred to comprehensive sources in the literature (e.g., Nguyen and Alzahrani 2023).

VIII. **Major Contraindications and When to Use Caution**

A. Ginkgo is contraindicated in patients who are hypersensitive to ginkgo preparations.

B. The typical recommended dosage range for Ginkgo biloba extract (EGb 761) is 120–240 mg/day, taken in divided doses (Nguyen and Alzahrani 2023).

C. Consuming more than 10 roasted seeds per day can cause difficulty breathing, weak pulse, seizures, loss of consciousness, and shock (Kajiyama et al. 2002; Miwa et al. 2001).

D. Caution is warranted for patients who have bleeding disorders or who are on anticoagulant drugs, as well as for patients with seizure disorders (Granger 2001; Gregory 2001; Kupiec and Raj 2005).

IX. **Dosage Ranges and Guidelines**

A. Ginkgo extracts at doses of 120–360 mg (50:1 standardized extract) are weakly recommended for adjunctive use in schizophrenia (primarily for negative symptoms) (Sarris et al. 2022).

B. A clinical study (N= 107) showed that 4 weeks of treatment with a ginkgo extract or placebo reduced anxiety rating scores by at least 50% in 44% of patients treated with ginkgo at 480 mg/day, 39% of patients treated with 240 mg/day, and 22% of patients treated with placebo (Woelk et al. 2007).

X. **Monitoring**

A. Close monitoring is needed for people at risk of bleeding, including those who are taking anticoagulants (Tan and Lee 2021).

XI. **Relevant Pharmacokinetics/Pharmacodynamics**

A. After oral administration of a ginkgo extract at 120 mg or 240 mg per person, bilobalide (79%), ginkgolide A (80%), and ginkgolide B (88%) demonstrated high oral bioavailability, with rapid absorption (T_{max} <2 hours) and half-lives ranging from 2.08 to 6.04 hours. Bilobalide is mainly excreted from the body through renal transport, mediated by organic anion transporter 1/3 (OAT1 or OAT3?). It may undergo an unknown metabolic process, but there is no enterohepatic circulation (Lu et al. 2021).

XII. **Clinically Relevant Drug Interactions**

A. Weak inhibition of cytochrome P450 (CYP) 3A4 and CYP2C19 at higher-than-recommended doses (Naccarato et al. 2012; Unger 2013).

B. Ginkgo may decrease the serum concentration of efavirenz (Naccarato et al. 2012) and antiseizure agents (Kupiec and Raj 2005).

C. Ginkgo may increase the risk of bleeding if used with blood thinners (Sarris et al. 2022; Stanger et al. 2012; Tan and Lee 2021).

D. Ginkgo may enhance the anticoagulant effect of salicylates (Gardner et al. 2007; Wolf 2006).

XIII. **Adverse Effects**

A. **Common**: Dizziness, gastrointestinal symptoms, headache

B. **Rare**: Bleeding (Bent et al. 2005), allergic skin reactions (Pennisi 2006), mood dysregulation (Rho et al. 2018)

C. **Risks in pregnancy and lactation**: Avoid use of ginkgo during pregnancy and lactation (Dugoua et al. 2006).

XIV. **Clinical Pearls/Guidelines**

A. As an over-the-counter product, ginkgo is regulated differently from prescription drugs, and the quality and content of available preparations may vary. Consider consultation with a pharmacist.

References

Bent S, Goldberg H, Padula A, et al: Spontaneous bleeding associated with ginkgo biloba: a case report and systematic review of the literature: a case report and systematic review of the literature. J Gen Intern Med 20(7):657–661, 2005 16050865

Dugoua, J.-J., Mills, E., Perri, D., et al: Safety and efficacy of ginkgo (Ginkgo biloba) during pregnancy and lactation. Can J Clin Pharmacol 13(3):e277–e284, 2006

Gardner CD, Zehnder JL, Rigby AJ, et al: Effect of Ginkgo biloba (EGb 761) and aspirin on platelet aggregation and platelet function analysis among older adults at risk of cardiovascular disease: a randomized clinical trial. Blood Coagul Fibrinolysis 18(8):787–793, 2007 17982321

Granger AS: Ginkgo biloba precipitating epileptic seizures. Age Ageing 30(6):523–525, 2001 11742783
Gregory PJ: Seizure associated with Ginkgo biloba? Ann Intern Med 134(4):344, 2001 11182853
Kajiyama Y, Fujii K, Takeuchi H, et al: Ginkgo seed poisoning. Pediatrics 109(2):325–327, 2002 11826216
Kupiec T, Raj V: Fatal seizures due to potential herb-drug interactions with Ginkgo biloba. J Anal Toxicol 29(7):755–758, 2005 16419414
Liu L, Wang Y, Zhang J, et al: Advances in the chemical constituents and chemical analysis of Ginkgo biloba leaf, extract, and phytopharmaceuticals. J Pharm Biomed Anal 193:113704, 2021 33157480
Lu J, Xie L, Liu K, et al: Bilobalide: a review of its pharmacology, pharmacokinetics, toxicity, and safety. Phytother Res 35(11):6114–6130, 2021 34342079
Miwa H, Iijima M, Tanaka S, et al: Generalized convulsions after consuming a large amount of gingko nuts. Epilepsia 42(2):280–281, 2001 11240603
Naccarato M, Yoong D, Gough K: A potential drug-herbal interaction between Ginkgo biloba and efavirenz. J Int Assoc Physicians AIDS Care (Chic) 11(2):98–100, 2012 22323244
National Center for Complementary and Integrative Health. Ginkgo. Last updated August 2020. Available at: https://www.nccih.nih.gov/health/ginkgo. Accessed May 3, 2022.
Nguyen T, Alzahrani T: Ginkgo Biloba, in StatPearls. Treasure Island, FL, StatPearls Publishing, last update July 3, 2023. Available at: https://www.ncbi.nlm.nih.gov/books/NBK541024/. Accessed August 4, 2024.
Pennisi RS: Acute generalised exanthematous pustulosis induced by the herbal remedy Ginkgo biloba. Med J Aust 184(11):583–584, 2006 16768668
Rho SS, Woo YS, Bahk W-M: Ginkgo biloba induced mood dysregulation: a case report. BMC Complement Altern Med 18(1):14, 2018 29334964
Sarris J, Ravindran A, Yatham LN, et al: Clinician guidelines for the treatment of psychiatric disorders with nutraceuticals and phytoceuticals: the World Federation of Societies of Biological Psychiatry (WFSBP) and Canadian Network for Mood and Anxiety Treatments (CANMAT) Taskforce. World J Biol Psychiatry 23(6):424–455, 2022 35311615
Singh SK, Srivastav S, Castellani RJ, et al: Neuroprotective and antioxidant effect of Ginkgo biloba extract against AD and other neurological disorders. Neurotherapeutics 16(3):666–674, 2019 31376068
Stanger MJ, Thompson LA, Young AJ, et al: Anticoagulant activity of select dietary supplements. Nutr Rev 70(2):107–117, 2012 22300597
Suter A, Niemer W, Klopp R: A new ginkgo fresh plant extract increases microcirculation and radical scavenging activity in elderly patients. Adv Ther 28(12):1078–1088, 2011 22120894
Tan CSS, Lee SWH: Warfarin and food, herbal or dietary supplement interactions: a systematic review. Br J Clin Pharmacol 87(2):352–374, 2021 32478963
Unger M: Pharmacokinetic drug interactions involving Ginkgo biloba. Drug Metab Rev 45(3):353–385, 2013 23865865
Woelk H, Arnoldt KH, Kieser M, et al: Ginkgo biloba special extract EGb 761 in generalized anxiety disorder and adjustment disorder with anxious mood: a randomized, double-blind, placebo-controlled trial. J Psychiatr Res 41(6):472–480, 2007 16808927
Wolf HRD: Does Ginkgo biloba special extract EGb 761 provide additional effects on coagulation and bleeding when added to acetylsalicylic acid 500 mg daily? Drugs R D 7(3):163–172, 2006 16752942

Inositol

I. **Generic Name**: Inositol

II. **Brand Names**: None

III. **Scientific Name**: Hexahydroxycyclohexane

IV. **Class**: Common nutraceutical

V. **Mechanism of Action**

A. Inositol is a constituent of the intracellular phosphatidylinositol second-messenger system, which is linked to several neurotransmitters, including α_1-noradrenergic, serotonin, dopamine, norepinephrine, glutamate, and cholinergic receptors (Wozniak et al. 2015).

B. Inositol may play a role in the interactions between G protein–coupled receptors and their ligands, particularly in the serotonergic pathway (Wozniak et al. 2015).

C. Inositol may reverse the desensitization of serotonin receptors (Levine 1997).

VI. **Evidence-Based Uses**

A. Panic disorder (Benjamin et al. 1995; Palatnik et al. 2001)

B. Obsessive-compulsive disorder (Fux et al. 1996)

VII. **Common/Other Uses**

A. Metabolic syndrome, bipolar depression, polycystic ovary syndrome (PCOS), anxiety, major depressive disorder, bipolar disorder, diabetes, dyslipidemia (Natural Medicines—Professional 2022; Sarris et al. 2022)

VIII. **Major Contraindications and When to Use Caution**

A. None

IX. **Dosage Ranges and Guidelines**

A. Panic disorder: A small clinical study found that taking inositol 18 g/day for 1 month may be as effective as fluvoxamine 150 mg/day (Palatnik et al. 2001). However, further studies are needed to properly establish efficacy.

B. OCD: One preliminary clinical study found that taking inositol 18 g/day for 6 weeks improved Yale-Brown Obsessive-Compulsive Scale (Y-BOCS) scores when compared with placebo (Fux et al. 1996). However, further studies are needed to properly establish efficacy.

X. **Monitoring**: Not applicable

XI. **Relevant Pharmacokinetics/Pharmacodynamics**

A. Inositol is metabolized by myoinositol oxidase, which is located in the renal cortex. However, metabolism is complex; it appears to change in utero and at birth and is affected by enteral intake and endogenous production (Phelps et al. 2013). Further studies are needed for accurate information.

XII. **Clinically Relevant Drug Interactions**

A. Theoretically, concomitant use of inositol with antidiabetic drugs may increase the risk of hypoglycemia by lowering blood glucose levels and glycated hemoglobin A1c (HbA1c) levels (Crawford et al. 2015).

XIII. **Adverse effects**

A. **Common**: Diarrhea, gas, nausea
B. **Rare**: Dizziness, tiredness, insomnia, agitation, headache (Wozniak et al. 2015)

XIV. **Clinical Pearls/Guidelines**

A. As an over-the-counter product, inositol is regulated differently from prescription drugs, and the quality and content of available preparations may vary. Consider consultation with a pharmacist.
B. Inositol is also found naturally in certain foods, such as citrus fruits and fiber-rich whole grains (e.g., brown rice, corn).

References

Benjamin J, Agam G, Levine J, et al: Inositol treatment in psychiatry. Psychopharmacol Bull 31(1):167–175, 1995 7675981

Crawford TJ, Crowther CA, Alsweiler J, et al: Antenatal dietary supplementation with myo-inositol in women during pregnancy for preventing gestational diabetes. Cochrane Database Syst Rev 2015(12):CD011507, 2015 26678256

Fux M, Levine J, Aviv A, et al: Inositol treatment of obsessive-compulsive disorder. Am J Psychiatry 153(9):1219–1221, 1996 8780431

Levine J: Controlled trials of inositol in psychiatry. Eur Neuropsychopharmacol 7(2):147–155, 1997 9169302

Natural Medicines—Professional: Inositol. n.d. Available (but accessible only by subscribers) at: https://naturalmedicines-therapeuticresearch-com.ezproxy.lib.utah.edu/databases/food,-herbs-supplements/professional.aspx?productid=299#effectiveness. Accessed May 3, 2022.

Palatnik A, Frolov K, Fux M, et al: Double-blind, controlled, crossover trial of inositol versus fluvoxamine for the treatment of panic disorder. J Clin Psychopharmacol 21(3):335–339, 2001 11386498

Phelps DL, Ward RM, Williams RL, et al: Pharmacokinetics and safety of a single intravenous dose of myo-inositol in preterm infants of 23–29 wk. Pediatr Res 74(6):721–729, 2013 24067395

Sarris J, Ravindran A, Yatham LN, et al: Clinician guidelines for the treatment of psychiatric disorders with nutraceuticals and phytoceuticals: the World Federation of Societies of Biological Psychiatry (WFSBP) and Canadian Network for Mood and Anxiety Treatments (CANMAT) Taskforce. World J Biol Psychiatry 23(6):424–455, 2022 35311615

Wozniak J, Faraone SV, Chan J, et al: A randomized clinical trial of high eicosapentaenoic acid omega-3 fatty acids and inositol as monotherapy and in combination in the treatment of pediatric bipolar spectrum disorders: a pilot study. J Clin Psychiatry 76(11):1548–1555, 2015 26646031

Kava

I. **Generic Names**: Kava, kava kava, ava pepper, ava root, kawa
II. **Brand Names**: None
III. **Scientific Name**: *Piper methysticum*
IV. **Class**: Phytoceutical

V. **Mechanism of Action**

A. Kava derives its pharmacological effects from the kavapyrones (also known as kavalactones), which are concentrated in the rhizomes and roots (Bilia et al. 2002; He et al. 1997).

B. Kava enhances ligand binding to $GABA_A$ receptors (Jussofie et al. 1994).

C. Kava reduces neuronal reuptake of norepinephrine and dopamine (Baum et al. 1998).

VI. **Evidence-Based Uses**

A. Generalized anxiety disorder (GAD) (Sarris et al. 2022; Smith and Leiras 2018)

VII. **Common/Other Uses**

A. Treatment of anxiety, epilepsy, insomnia, menopausal symptoms, myalgia, premenstrual syndrome, stress; enhancement of sexual arousal (Natural Medicines—Professional 2022)

VIII. **Major Contraindications and When to Use Caution**

A. Kava should be used with caution in individuals with preexisting liver disease (FDA advisory).

IX. **Dosage Ranges and Guidelines**

A. The Australian Therapeutic Goods Administration recommends a maximum daily dose of kavalactone of 250 mg (Teschke and Lebot 2011).

B. Kava rootstock extracts standardized to kavalactones at 60–250 mg are not recommended for adjunctive or monotherapy use for GAD (Sarris et al. 2022).

X. **Monitoring**

A. Because long-term studies are lacking, use of kava for more than 8 weeks is not recommended (Smith and Leiras 2018).

B. Kava should be used cautiously in patients with renal or liver disease, blood disorders, Parkinson's disease, or depression. Regular/frequent liver function tests may be warranted (Fetrow and Avila 2003).

XI. **Relevant Pharmacokinetics/Pharmacodynamics**

A. Studies of kava have not been conducted in humans, only in rats, and findings vary widely according to the kind of kavalactone (or active substance from kava) used (Mathews et al. 2005).

XII. **Clinically Relevant Drug Interactions**

A. Kava may enhance the adverse/toxic effects of paroxetine (Izzo and Ernst 2009), benzodiazepines, and CNS depressants (Almeida and Grimsley 1996; Izzo and Ernst 2009; Sarris et al. 2011).

B. Kava may diminish the therapeutic effects of antiparkinsonian agents (dopamine agonists) (Schelosky et al. 1995).

C. Theoretically, kava can be a moderate inhibitor of cytochrome P450 (CYP) 2C19 and CYP2C9 (Mathews et al. 2002).

D. Combining kava with alcohol may increase the risk of sedation and/or hepatotoxicity (Li and Ramzan 2010).

XIII. **Adverse Effects**

A. **Common**: Drowsiness, dry mouth, dizziness, gastrointestinal upset, headache, memory problems, tremors

B. **Rare**: Hepatotoxicity (European Association for the Study of the Liver 2019; Navarro et al. 2014), kava dermopathy (scale-like lesions on the palms of hands, soles of the feet, and back) (Fetrow and Avila 2003), rhabdomyolysis (Bodkin et al. 2012), parkinsonian-like symptoms (Meseguer et al. 2002)

C. **Risks in pregnancy and lactation**: Use of kava during pregnancy/lactation should be avoided (Ernst 2002; Pearl et al. 2011).

XIV. **Clinical Pearls/Guidelines**

A. As an over-the-counter product, kava is regulated differently from prescription drugs, and the quality and content of available preparations may vary. Consider consultation with a pharmacist.

References

Almeida JC, Grimsley EW: Coma from the health food store: interaction between kava and alprazolam. Ann Intern Med 125(11):940–941, 1996 8967683

Baum SS, Hill R, Rommelspacher H: Effect of kava extract and individual kavapyrones on neurotransmitter levels in the nucleus accumbens of rats. Prog Neuropsychopharmacol Biol Psychiatry 22(7):1105–1120, 1998 9829291

Bilia AR, Gallon S, Vincieri FF: Kava-kava and anxiety: growing knowledge about the efficacy and safety. Life Sci 70(22):2581–2597, 2002 12269386

Bodkin R, Schneider S, Rekkerth D, et al: Rhabdomyolysis associated with kava ingestion. Am J Emerg Med 30(4):635.e1–635.e3, 2012 21458945

EASL Clinical Practice Guidelines: Drug-induced liver injury. Elsevier Enhanced Reader. n.d.

European Association for the Study of the Liver: EASL Clinical Practice Guidelines: Drug-induced liver injury. J Hepatol 70(6):1222–1261, 2019 30926241

Ernst E: Herbal medicinal products during pregnancy: are they safe? BJOG 109(3):227–235, 2002 11950176

Fetrow CH, Avila JR: Professional's Handbook of Complementary and Alternative Medicines. Philadelphia, Wolters Kluwer Health, 2003

He XG, Lin LZ, Lian LZ: Electrospray high performance liquid chromatography-mass spectrometry in phytochemical analysis of kava (Piper methysticum) extract. Planta Med 63(1):70–74, 1997 17252331

Izzo AA, Ernst E: Interactions between herbal medicines and prescribed drugs: an updated systematic review. Drugs 69(13):1777–1798, 2009

Jussofie A, Schmiz A, Hiemke C: Kavapyrone enriched extract from Piper methysticum as modulator of the GABA binding site in different regions of rat brain. Psychopharmacology (Berl) 116(4):469–474, 1994 7701051

Li XZ, Ramzan I: Role of ethanol in kava hepatotoxicity. Phytother Res 24(4):475–480, 2010 19943335

Mathews JM, Etheridge AS, Black SR: Inhibition of human cytochrome P450 activities by kava extract and kavalactones. Drug Metab Dispos 30(11):1153–1157, 2002 12386118

Mathews JM, Etheridge AS, Valentine JL, et al: Pharmacokinetics and disposition of the kavalactone kawain: interaction with kava extract and kavalactones in vivo and in vitro. Drug Metab Dispos 33(10):1555–1563, 2005 16033948

Meseguer E, Taboada R, Sánchez V, et al: Life-threatening parkinsonism induced by kava-kava. Mov Disord 17(1):195–196, 2002 11835463
Natural Medicines—Professional: Kava. n.d. Available (but accessible only by subscribers) at: https://naturalmedicines-therapeuticresearch-com.ezproxy.lib.utah.edu/databases/food,-herbs-supplements/professional.aspx?productid=872#effectiveness. Accessed May 3, 2022.
Navarro VJ, Barnhart H, Bonkovsky HL, et al: Liver injury from herbals and dietary supplements in the U.S. Drug-Induced Liver Injury Network. Hepatology 60(4):1399–1408, 2014 25043597
Pearl PL, Drillings IM, Conry JA: Herbs in epilepsy: evidence for efficacy, toxicity, and interactions. Semin Pediatr Neurol 18(3):203–208, 2011 22062945
Sarris J, LaPorte E, Schweitzer I: Kava: a comprehensive review of efficacy, safety, and psychopharmacology. Aust N Z J Psychiatry 45(1):27–35, 2011 21073405
Sarris J, Ravindran A, Yatham LN, et al: Clinician guidelines for the treatment of psychiatric disorders with nutraceuticals and phytoceuticals: the World Federation of Societies of Biological Psychiatry (WFSBP) and Canadian Network for Mood and Anxiety Treatments (CANMAT) Taskforce. World J Biol Psychiatry 23(6):424–455, 2022 35311615
Schelosky L, Raffauf C, Jendroska K, et al: Kava and dopamine antagonism. J Neurol Neurosurg Psychiatry 58(5):639–640, 1995 7745421
Smith K, Leiras C: The effectiveness and safety of Kava kava for treating anxiety symptoms: a systematic review and analysis of randomized clinical trials. Complement Ther Clin Pract 33:107–117, 2018 30396607
Teschke R, Lebot V: Proposal for a kava quality standardization code. Food Chem Toxicol 49(10):2503–2516, 2011 21756963

Lavender

I. **Generic Names**: Lavender, English lavender, common lavender, French lavender
II. **Brand Names**: Silexan
III. **Scientific Names**: *Lavandula angustifolia*; *Lavandula officinalis*
IV. **Class**: Phytoceutical
V. **Mechanism of Action**

A. The applicable parts of lavender are the flowers, leaves, and oil. Several pharmacological and biological tests have reported that lavender has CNS depressant, anticonvulsive, sedative, spasmolytic, local anesthetic, antioxidant, antibacterial, and mast cell degranulation inhibitory effects (Hajhashemi et al. 2003).

B. Lavender may exert some activity at the $GABA_A$ receptor; it also inhibits the presynaptic calcium channels (Generoso et al. 2017), as well as modulating the *N*-methyl-D-aspartate (NMDA) receptor and inhibiting the serotonin transporter (SERT) (López et al. 2017).

VI. **Evidence-Based Uses**

A. Major depressive disorder (MDD) (Sarris et al. 2022).

B. Generalized anxiety disorder (GAD) (Sarris et al. 2022).

VII. **Common/Other Uses**

A. Antimicrobial, anticonvulsant, spasmolytic, anti-inflammatory, and insect repellent effects; treatment of cancer, dementia, fatigue, insomnia, dysmenorrhea (Lexicomp 2022)

VIII. **Major Contraindications and When to Use Caution**

A. Lavender should be used with caution in patients taking sedatives (Donelli et al. 2019).

IX. **Dosage Ranges and Guidelines**

A. Lavender at dosages of 80–160 mg per day of essential oil (in the form of soft gels)—or 500 mg to 1.5 g twice per day of dried flower (preferably in the form of standardized formulations)—is weakly recommended for monotherapy or adjunctive use in MDD. Lavender at the same dosages used for the essential oil (80–160 mg/day) but in the form of a specialized oil (in capsule form) is provisionally recommended for monotherapy or adjunctive use in GAD (Sarris et al. 2022).

X. **Monitoring**: Not applicable

XI. **Relevant Pharmacokinetics/Pharmacodynamics**

A. The linalool constituent of lavender is absorbed and eliminated quickly, with a half-life of 4 hours after a single dose and of approximately 9 hours after 14 days of treatment (Doroshyenko et al. 2013).

XII. **Clinically Relevant Drug Interactions**

A. The narcotic and sedative effects of CNS depressants and anticonvulsants may be increased if these agents are used concomitantly with lavender-containing products.

B. Anticoagulants may convey an increased risk of bleeding when given concomitantly with lavender (Denner 2009).

XIII. **Adverse Effects**

A. **Common**: Constipation, nausea, vomiting (Fetrow and Avila 2003)

B. **Rare**: Topical products containing lavender oil may cause allergic contact dermatitis, eczema (Bingham et al. 2019), or prepubertal gynecomastia/thelarche (Diaz et al. 2016; Henley et al. 2007).

C. **Risks in pregnancy and lactation**: Avoid use of lavender during pregnancy and lactation.

XIV. **Clinical Pearls/Guidelines**

A. A controlled study that compared Silexan (a lavender oil preparation) and lorazepam in adults with GAD found comparable decreases in Hamilton Anxiety Rating Scale scores (decreases of ~45%–46%) for the two agents (Woelk and Schläfke 2010). In addition to its benefits for anxiety, Silexan was also shown to have some benefit in comorbid depression, impaired sleep, somatic complaints, and quality-of-life measures, without causing significant sedation, withdrawal, or major adverse effects (Kasper et al. 2018).

B. The evidence base supporting lavender's use in each of the conditions noted varies; for further information, readers are referred to comprehensive sources in the literature (e.g., Kasper et al. 2018).

References

Bingham LJ, Tam MM, Palmer AM, et al: Contact allergy and allergic contact dermatitis caused by lavender: a retrospective study from an Australian clinic. Contact Dermatitis 81(1):37–42, 2019 30779160

Denner SS: Lavandula angustifolia Miller: English lavender. Holist Nurs Pract 23(1):57–64, 2009 19104276

Diaz A, Luque L, Badar Z, et al: Prepubertal gynecomastia and chronic lavender exposure: report of three cases. J Pediatr Endocrinol Metab 29(1):103–107, 2016 26353172

Donelli D, Antonelli M, Bellinazzi C, et al: Effects of lavender on anxiety: a systematic review and meta-analysis. Phytomedicine 65:153099, 2019 31655395

Doroshyenko O, Rokitta D, Zadoyan G, et al: Drug cocktail interaction study on the effect of the orally administered lavender oil preparation silexan on cytochrome P450 enzymes in healthy volunteers. Drug Metab Dispos 41(5):987–993, 2013 23401474

Fetrow CH, Avila JR: Professional's Handbook of Complementary and Alternative Medicines. Philadelphia, Wolters Kluwer Health, 2003

Generoso MB, Soares A, Taiar IT, et al: Lavender oil preparation (silexan) for treating anxiety: an updated meta-analysis. J Clin Psychopharmacol 37(1):115–117, 2017 27861196

Hajhashemi V, Ghannadi A, Sharif B: Anti-inflammatory and analgesic properties of the leaf extracts and essential oil of Lavandula angustifolia Mill. J Ethnopharmacol 89(1):67–71, 2003 14522434

Henley DV, Lipson N, Korach KS, et al: Prepubertal gynecomastia linked to lavender and tea tree oils. N Engl J Med 356(5):479–485, 2007 17267908

Kasper S, Müller WE, Volz H-P, et al: Silexan in anxiety disorders: clinical data and pharmacological background. World J Biol Psychiatry 19(6):412–420, 2018 28511598

Lexicomp: Lavender. n.d. Available (but accessible only by subscribers) at: https://online.lexi.com/lco/action/doc/retrieve/docid/fc_rnp2/3750228?cesid=2D55mEnrmhkandsearchUrl=/lco/action/search%3Fq%3Dlavender%26t%3Dname%26va%3Dlavender. Accessed May 4, 2022.

López V, Nielsen B, Solas M, et al: Exploring pharmacological mechanisms of lavender (Lavandula angustifolia) essential oil on central nervous system targets. Front Pharmacol 8:280, 2017 28579958

Sarris J, Ravindran A, Yatham LN, et al: Clinician guidelines for the treatment of psychiatric disorders with nutraceuticals and phytoceuticals: the World Federation of Societies of Biological Psychiatry (WFSBP) and Canadian Network for Mood and Anxiety Treatments (CANMAT) Taskforce. World J Biol Psychiatry 23(6):424–455, 2022 35311615

Woelk H, Schläfke S: A multi-center, double-blind, randomised study of the lavender oil preparation silexan in comparison to lorazepam for generalized anxiety disorder. Phytomedicine 17(2):94–99, 2010 19962288

N-Acetylcysteine

I. **Generic Names**: *N*-acetylcysteine, acetyl cysteine, *N*-acetyl-L-cysteine

II. **Brand Names**: Cetylev

III. **Scientific Name**: As in "Generic Names"

IV. **Class**: Antidote to acetaminophen toxicity, mucolytic agent, nutraceutical

V. **Mechanism of Action**

A. *N*-acetylcysteine (NAC) acts as a hepatoprotective agent; its sulfhydryl groups serve as a substrate for the toxic acetaminophen metabolite in place of glutathione in the liver (ClinicalKey 2022.

B. NAC stimulates glutamate efflux by activating the cysteine/glutamate antiporter (system x_c^- [Sx_c^-]), thereby enhancing the endogenous activation of metabotropic glutamate receptors. In addition, NAC enhances the clearance of synaptic glutamate by inducing the glutamate transporter 1 (Raghu et al. 2021).
C. NAC also has antioxidant properties and can modulate neurotransmitters such as glutamate and dopamine (Raghu et al. 2021).

VI. **Evidence-Based Uses**

A. Obsessive-compulsive disorder (OCD) (Sarris et al. 2022)
B. Schizophrenia (Sarris et al. 2022)

VII. **Common/Other Uses**

A. Mucolytic; treatment of acetaminophen toxicity, bipolar disorder, depression, *Helicobacter pylori* infections, necrotizing enterocolitis (Ershad et al. 2023)

VIII. **Major Contraindications and When to Use Caution**

A. Use is contraindicated in patients with hypersensitivity to acetylcysteine or any component of the formulation (Ershad et al. 2023).
B. NAC has antiplatelet effects; its use should be stopped at least 2 weeks before any surgical procedure (Niemi et al. 2006).

IX. **Dosage Ranges and Guidelines**

A. NAC at dosages of 2–3 g/day is weakly recommended for adjunctive use in OCD (Sarris et al. 2022).
B. NAC at dosages of 1–3 g/day is provisionally recommended for adjunctive use in schizophrenia (primarily for negative symptoms) (Sarris et al. 2022).

X. **Monitoring**: Not applicable

XI. **Relevant Pharmacokinetics/Pharmacodynamics**

A. Protein binding: 66%–87%
B. **Metabolism**: NAC is deacetylated by the liver and intracellularly in most tissues to cysteine and disulfides.
C. **Half-life**: Intravenous solution: 5.6 hours; effervescent tablets: 18.1 hours
D. **Excretion**: Urine (renal clearance accounts for roughly 30% of total clearance) (ClinicalKey 2022)

XII. **Clinically Relevant Drug Interactions**

A. Activated charcoal may inhibit the oral absorption of acetylcysteine (Watson and McKinney 1991).
B. Nitroglycerin: NAC can increase the risk for hypotension (Horowitz et al. 1988) and headaches (Iversen 1992) when taken with intravenous or transdermal nitroglycerin.
C. NAC may increase the risk of bleeding when taken with anticoagulant or antiplatelet drugs (Niemi et al. 2006; Wijeysundera et al. 2009).
D. NAC may increase the risk of hypotension when taken with antihypertensive drugs (Ruiz et al. 1994).
E. NAC may reduce the antimalarial effects of chloroquine by increasing cellular levels of glutathione (Deharo et al. 2003).

XIII. **Adverse Effects**

A. **Common**: Diarrhea, dry mouth, dyspepsia, heartburn, loss of appetite, nausea, vomiting

B. **Rare**: Anaphylaxis (Perry and Shannon 1998), chest tightness, palpitations (Hansen et al. 1994)

C. **Risks in pregnancy and lactation**: Advise mothers to consider waiting 30 hours after NAC administration before re-initiating breastfeeding (ClinicalKey 2022).

XIV. **Clinical Pearls/Guidelines**

A. As an over-the-counter product, NAC is regulated differently from prescription drugs, and the quality and content of available preparations may vary. Consider consultation with a pharmacist.

B. NAC has been studied—and has shown some promise—in a variety of psychiatric disorders, including bipolar depression, OCD, trichotillomania, substance use disorders, schizophrenia (Bradlow et al. 2022; Ooi et al. 2018). The evidence base supporting NAC use in each of the conditions noted varies; for further information, readers are referred to comprehensive sources in the literature (e.g., Ershad et al. 2023).

References

Bradlow RCJ, Berk M, Kalivas PW, et al: The potential of N-acetyl-L-cysteine (NAC) in the treatment of psychiatric disorders. CNS Drugs 36(5):451–482, 2022 35316513

ClinicalKey: Acetylcysteine. n.d. Available (but accessible only by subscribers) at: https://www-clinicalkey-com.ezproxy.lib.utah.edu/#!/content/drug_monograph/6-s2.0–7?scrollTo=%23Administration. Accessed April 6, 2022.

Deharo E, Barkan D, Krugliak M, et al: Potentiation of the antimalarial action of chloroquine in rodent malaria by drugs known to reduce cellular glutathione levels. Biochem Pharmacol 66(5):809–817, 2003 12948862

Ershad M, Naji A, Vearrier D: NAcetylcysteine, in StatPearls. Treasure Island, FL, StatPearls Publishing, last update February 19, 2023. Available at: https://www.ncbi.nlm.nih.gov/books/NBK537183/. Accessed March 13, 2024.

Hansen NC, Skriver A, Brorsen-Riis L, et al: Orally administered N-acetylcysteine may improve general well-being in patients with mild chronic bronchitis. Respir Med 88(7):531–535, 1994 7972979

Horowitz JD, Henry CA, Syrjanen ML, et al: Nitroglycerine/N-acetylcysteine in the management of unstable angina pectoris. Eur Heart J 9(Suppl A):95–100, 1988

Iversen HK: N-acetylcysteine enhances nitroglycerin-induced headache and cranial arterial responses. Clin Pharmacol Ther 52(2):125–133, 1992 1505148

Niemi TT, Munsterhjelm E, Pöyhiä R, et al: The effect of N-acetylcysteine on blood coagulation and platelet function in patients undergoing open repair of abdominal aortic aneurysm. Blood Coagul Fibrinolysis 17(1):29–34, 2006 16607076

Ooi SL, Green R, Pak SC: N-acetylcysteine for the treatment of psychiatric disorders: a review of current evidence. BioMed Res Int 2018:2469486, 2018 30426004

Perry HE, Shannon MW: Efficacy of oral versus intravenous N-acetylcysteine in acetaminophen overdose: results of an open-label, clinical trial. J Pediatr 132(1):149–152, 1998 9470017

Raghu G, Berk M, Campochiaro PA, et al: The multifaceted therapeutic role of N-acetylcysteine (NAC) in disorders characterized by oxidative stress. Curr Neuropharmacol 19(8):1202–1224, 2021 33380301

Ruiz FJ, Salom MG, Inglés AC, et al: N-acetyl-L-cysteine potentiates depressor response to captopril and enalaprilat in SHRs. Am J Physiol 267(3 Pt 2):R767–R772, 1994 8092321

Sarris J, Ravindran A, Yatham LN, et al: Clinician guidelines for the treatment of psychiatric disorders with nutraceuticals and phytoceuticals: the World Federation of Societies of Biological Psychiatry (WFSBP) and Canadian Network for Mood and Anxiety Treatments (CANMAT) Taskforce. World J Biol Psychiatry 23(6):424–455, 2022 35311615

Watson WA, McKinney PE: Activated charcoal and acetylcysteine absorption: issues in interpreting pharmacokinetic data. DICP 25(10):1081–1084, 1991 1803797

Wijeysundera DN, Karkouti K, Rao V, et al: N-acetylcysteine is associated with increased blood loss and blood product utilization during cardiac surgery. Crit Care Med 37(6):1929–1934, 2009 19384218

Omega-3 Fatty Acids

I. **Generic Names**: Omega-3 fatty acids

II. **Brand Names**: Lovaza, Epanova, Omacor

III. **Scientific Names**: eicosapentaenoic acid (EPA), docosahexaenoic acid (DHA), alpha-linolenic acid (ALA)

IV. **Class**: Common nutraceutical

V. **Mechanism of Action**

A. There are three omega-3 fatty acids (O3FAs): eicosapentaenoic acid (EPA), docosahexaenoic acid (DHA), and alpha-linolenic acid (ALA) (Cholewski et al. 2018).

B. Inhibition of diacylglycerol acyltransferase-2 (DGAT2), increased mitochondrial and hepatic peroxisomal beta-oxidation, decreased hepatic lipogenesis, and increased plasma lipoprotein lipase activity are potential mechanisms of action (Bays et al. 2008; Kris-Etherton et al. 2002).

C. The exact role of fatty acids in psychiatric disorders is unknown. EPA seems to act through inhibition of phospholipase A2 (Bennett and Horrobin 2000) or protein kinase C (Seung Kim et al. 2001), or as an anti-inflammatory (Gaughran 2002).

VI. **Evidence-Based Uses**

A. Major depressive disorder (MDD) (Sarris et al. 2022)

B. Schizophrenia (adjunctive) (Çakici et al. 2019; Qiao et al. 2020)

VII. **Common/Other Uses**

A. Heart disease, stroke, hypertriglyceridemia, ADHD, Alzheimer's disease, age-related macular degeneration, dry eye disease, retinitis pigmentosa, rheumatoid arthritis (GlaxoSmithKline 2020). The evidence base supporting use of omega-3 fatty acids in each of these conditions varies; for further information, readers are referred to comprehensive sources in the literature (e.g., Krupa et al. 2024).

VIII. Major Contraindications and When to Use Caution

A. Omega-3 fatty acids should be used with caution in patients with coagulopathy; the risk of bleeding may increase with concomitant anticoagulant/antiplatelet use (Kris-Etherton et al. 2002).

B. Omega-3 fatty acids should be used with caution in patients with a known fish allergy or a history of atrial fibrillation/atrial flutter (GlaxoSmithKline 2020).

C. Because of the effects of omega-3 fatty acids on platelet function, it is recommended that they be discontinued before any elective surgical procedure (Ang-Lee et al. 2001; Sarris et al. 2022).

IX. Dosage Ranges and Guidelines

A. Omega-3 fatty acids at doses standardized to 1–2 g of EPA are recommended for adjunctive use in MDD (Sarris et al. 2022).

B. Omega-3 fatty acids at doses standardized to 1–2 g of EPA or mixed EPA/DHA are recommended for adjunctive use in schizophrenia (Çakici et al. 2019; Qiao et al. 2020).

C. Lovaza brand capsule: Each 1-g capsule contains a combination of EPA (~465 mg) and DHA (~375 mg) ethyl esters (GlaxoSmithKline 2020).

X. Monitoring

A. In patients with hepatic impairment who are taking omega-3 fatty acids, low-density lipoprotein (LDL) levels and hepatic transaminases should be periodically monitored (GlaxoSmithKline 2020).

XI. Relevant Pharmacokinetics/Pharmacodynamics

A. **Absorption**: Directly in the small intestine

B. **Protein binding**: EPA: >99%

C. **Metabolism**: EPA and DHA are mainly oxidized in the liver, similar to other fatty acids derived from dietary sources.

D. **Half-life** (elimination): EPA: ~37 hours; DHA: ~46 hours

E. **Time to peak plasma concentration**: Following repeated dosing with low-fat meals for ~2 weeks (steady-state): EPA: 5–8 hours; DHA: 5–9 hours (GlaxoSmithKline 2020)

XII. Clinically Relevant Drug Interactions

A. Omega-3 fatty acids may enhance the effect of warfarin (Tan and Lee 2021), antiplatelet drugs (Larson et al. 2008), and anticoagulant drugs (Vanschoonbeek et al. 2004).

B. Omega-3 fatty acids may enhance the antiplatelet effect of ibrutinib (GlaxoSmithKline 2020).

XIII. Adverse Effects

A. Cardiovascular: Atrial fibrillation, atrial flutter

B. Gastrointestinal: Dysgeusia, dyspepsia, eructation

C. Dermatological: Pruritus, skin rash

D. Endocrine and metabolic: Increased low-density lipoprotein cholesterol

E. Hepatic: Increased serum alanine aminotransferase (ALT) and aspartate transaminase (AST)

F. **Risks in pregnancy and lactation**: Until further information is available, omega-3 fatty acids should be used with caution in pregnancy and lactation (Kris-Etherton et al. 2002).

XIV. **Clinical Pearls/Guidelines**

A. Omega-3 fatty acids are available in prescription and over-the-counter (OTC) formulations. When using OTC products, it is important to remember that these products are regulated differently from prescription drugs and that the quality and content of available preparations may vary. Consider consultation with a pharmacist.

Further Reading

National Center for Complementary and Integrative Health: Omega-3 supplements: in depth. Last Updated: May 2018. Available at: https://www.nccih.nih.gov/health/omega3-supplements-in-depth. Accessed May 3, 2022.

References

Ang-Lee MK, Moss J, Yuan C-S: Herbal medicines and perioperative care. JAMA 286(2):208–216, 2001 11448284

Bays HE, Tighe AP, Sadovsky R, et al: Prescription omega-3 fatty acids and their lipid effects: physiologic mechanisms of action and clinical implications. Expert Rev Cardiovasc Ther 6(3):391–409, 2008 18327998

Bennett CN, Horrobin DF: Gene targets related to phospholipid and fatty acid metabolism in schizophrenia and other psychiatric disorders: an update. Prostaglandins Leukot Essent Fatty Acids 63(1–2):47–59, 2000 10970713

Çakici N, van Beveren NJM, Judge-Hundal G, et al: An update on efficacy of anti-inflammatory agents for patients with schizophrenia: a meta-analysis. Psychol Med 49(14):2307–2319, 2019 31439071

Cholewski M, Tomczykowa M, Tomczyk M: A comprehensive review of chemistry, sources and bioavailability of omega-3 fatty acids. Nutrients 10(11):E1662, 2018 30400360

Gaughran F: Immunity and schizophrenia: autoimmunity, cytokines, and immune responses. Int Rev Neurobiol 52:275–302, 2002 12498108

GlaxoSmithKline: Lovaza (omega-3-acid ethyl esters) capsules prescribing information. Revised September 2020. Available at: https://www.accessdata.fda.gov/drugsatfda_docs/label/2020/021654s044lbl.pdf. Accessed August 4, 2024.

Kris-Etherton PM, Harris WS, Appel LJ; American Heart Association, Nutrition Committee: Fish consumption, fish oil, omega-3 fatty acids, and cardiovascular disease. Circulation 106(21):2747–2757, 2002 12438303

Krupa KN, Fritz K, Parmar M: Omega-3 Fatty Acids, in StatPearls. Treasure Island, FL, StatPearls Publishing, last update February 28, 2024. Available at: https://www.ncbi.nlm.nih.gov/books/NBK564314/. Accessed August 4, 2024.

Larson MK, Ashmore JH, Harris KA, et al: Effects of omega-3 acid ethyl esters and aspirin, alone and in combination, on platelet function in healthy subjects. Thromb Haemost 100(4):634–641, 2008 18841286

Qiao Y, Liu CP, Han HQ, et al: No impact of omega-3 fatty acid supplementation on symptoms or hostility among patients with schizophrenia. Front Psychiatry 11:312, 2020 32372988

Sarris J, Ravindran A, Yatham LN, et al: Clinician guidelines for the treatment of psychiatric disorders with nutraceuticals and phytoceuticals: the World Federation of Societies of Biological Psychiatry (WFSBP) and Canadian Network for Mood and Anxiety Treatments (CANMAT) Taskforce. World J Biol Psychiatry 23(6):424–455, 2022 35311615

Seung Kim HF, Weeber EJ, Sweatt JD, et al: Inhibitory effects of omega-3 fatty acids on protein kinase C activity in vitro. Mol Psychiatry 6(2):246–248, 2001 11317232

Tan CSS, Lee SWH: Warfarin and food, herbal or dietary supplement interactions: a systematic review. Br J Clin Pharmacol 87(2):352–374, 2021 32478963

Vanschoonbeek K, Feijge MAH, Paquay M, et al: Variable hypocoagulant effect of fish oil intake in humans: modulation of fibrinogen level and thrombin generation. Arterioscler Thromb Vasc Biol 24(9):1734–1740, 2004 15217806

Rhodiola

I. **Generic Names**: Rhodiola, arctic root, golden root, rose root, king's crown

II. **Brand Names**: None

III. **Scientific Name**: *Rhodiola rosea*

IV. **Class**: Phytoceutical

V. **Mechanism of Action**

A. *R. rosea* has been recognized as a botanical adaptogen with antifatigue, antistress, and antidepressant properties (Tao et al. 2019).

B. Animal research suggests that Rhodiola may improve mood by regulating the activity of serotonin, dopamine, acetylcholine, and norepinephrine (Chen et al. 2009; Kelly 2001).

C. Compounds isolated from Rhodiola roots appear to inhibit monoamine oxidase A in vitro (van Diermen et al. 2009).

D. The active compounds rhodioloside, salidroside, and tyrosol have been associated with antidepressant effects (Tao et al. 2019).

VI. **Evidence-Based Uses**

A. Major depressive disorder (MDD) (Sarris et al. 2022)

VII. **Common/Other Uses**

A. Rhodiola is promoted as increasing energy, stamina, strength, and mental capacity; improving athletic performance; protecting against the effects of stress; and helping to manage anxiety and other symptoms (National Center for Complementary and Integrative Health 2020).

VIII. **Major Contraindications and When to Use Caution**

A. None

IX. **Dosage Ranges and Guidelines**

A. No dosage recommendations are available for Rhodiola; however, recent guidelines state that Rhodiola root at a dosage of 340–680 mg (once daily to three times daily, depending on extract) is *not recommended* for monotherapy or adjunctive use in MDD (Sarris et al. 2022).

X. **Monitoring**: Not applicable

XI. **Relevant Pharmacokinetics/Pharmacodynamics**

A. In animal studies, salidroside was rapidly absorbed, reaching C_{max} in approximately 0.5 hour after orally dosing. The bioavailability varied from 32% to 98% owing to diversified administration routes and doses. Salidroside metabolism is mainly hepatic; its half-life is 0.5–2 hours, and it is primarily excreted in the urine (Fan et al. 2020).

XII. **Clinically Relevant Drug Interactions**

A. Inhibitor of cytochrome P450 (CYP) 2C9 (Thu et al. 2016)

XIII. **Adverse Effects**

A. Possible side effects of Rhodiola include dizziness and either dry mouth or excessive saliva production (National Center for Complementary and Integrative Health 2020).

B. **Risks in pregnancy and lactation**: Insufficient reliable information is available on Rhodiola's safety in pregnancy and lactation; avoid use.

XIV. **Clinical Pearls/Guidelines**

A. As an over-the-counter product, Rhodiola is regulated differently from prescription drugs, and the quality and content of available preparations may vary. Consider consultation with a pharmacist.

B. The evidence base supporting use of Rhodiola in each of the conditions noted varies; for further information, readers are referred to comprehensive sources in the literature (e.g., National Center for Complementary and Integrative Health 2020).

References

Chen QG, Zeng YS, Qu ZQ, et al: The effects of Rhodiola rosea extract on 5-HT level, cell proliferation and quantity of neurons at cerebral hippocampus of depressive rats. Phytomedicine 16(9):830–838, 2009 19403286

Fan F, Yang L, Li R, et al: Salidroside as a potential neuroprotective agent for ischemic stroke: a review of sources, pharmacokinetics, mechanism and safety. Biomed Pharmacother 129:110458, 2020 32603893

Kelly GS: Rhodiola rosea: a possible plant adaptogen. Altern Med Rev 6(3):293–302, 2001

National Center for Complementary and Integrative Health: Rhodiola. Last updated October 2020. Available at: https://www.nccih.nih.gov/health/rhodiola. Accessed May 4, 2022.

Sarris J, Ravindran A, Yatham LN, et al: Clinician guidelines for the treatment of psychiatric disorders with nutraceuticals and phytoceuticals: the World Federation of Societies of Biological Psychiatry (WFSBP) and Canadian Network for Mood and Anxiety Treatments (CANMAT) Taskforce. World J Biol Psychiatry 23(6):424–455, 2022 35311615

Tao H, Wu X, Cao J, et al: Rhodiola species: a comprehensive review of traditional use, phytochemistry, pharmacology, toxicity, and clinical study. Med Res Rev 39(5):1779–1850, 2019 30652331

Thu OK, Spigset O, Nilsen OG, et al: Effect of commercial Rhodiola rosea on CYP enzyme activity in humans. Eur J Clin Pharmacol 72(3):295–300, 2016 26613955

van Diermen D, Marston A, Bravo J, et al: Monoamine oxidase inhibition by Rhodiola rosea L. roots. J Ethnopharmacol 122(2):397–401, 2009 19168123

S-Adenosyl Methionine (SAM)

I. **Generic Names**: *S*-adenosyl methionine, SAM, ademetionine, *S*-adenosyl-L-methionine

II. **Brand Names**: SAMe, SAM-e, AdoMet

III. **Scientific Name**: As in "Generic Names"

IV. **Class**: Common nutraceutical

V. **Mechanism of Action**

A. SAM is made in the body from methionine, an amino acid found in foods (National Center for Complementary and Integrative Health 2017). Its synthesis is closely linked to vitamin B_{12} and folate metabolism; deficiencies of these vitamins can result in decreased SAM concentrations in the CNS.

B. SAM may enhance monoamine systems and is involved in the production of monoaminergic neurotransmitters; it is also associated with increased serotonin turnover and elevated dopamine and norepinephrine levels (Bottiglieri 2013).

VI. **Evidence-Based Uses**

A. Major depressive disorder (MDD)

VII. **Common/Other Uses**

A. Osteoarthritis, liver diseases, fibromyalgia, migraine, schizophrenia, Alzheimer's disease, attention-deficit hyperactivity disorder (ADHD). The evidence base supporting SAM's use in each of these conditions varies; for further information, readers are referred to comprehensive sources in the literature (e.g., National Center for Complementary and Integrative Health 2017).

VIII. **Major Contraindications and When to Use Caution**

A. Avoid use in patients with bipolar disorder. SAM has been reported to cause a switch from a depressed state to a hypomanic or manic state (Gören et al. 2004).

B. SAM may worsen the symptoms of Lesch-Nyhan syndrome (Dolcetta et al. 2013).

C. SAM methylates levodopa, which could theoretically worsen parkinsonian symptoms. However, this effect has not been reported in humans (Charlton and Crowell 1992).

D. SAM may cause serotonin syndrome when used in conjunction with clomipramine, and it could theoretically increase the effects and adverse effects of herbs and supplements that increase serotonin levels (Iruela et al. 1993).

E. There is theoretical reason to believe that taking SAM may promote *Pneumocystis* infection in people who are immunocompromised (National Center for Complementary and Integrative Health 2017).

IX. **Dosage Ranges and Guidelines**

A. SAM at 800–3,200 mg is weakly recommended for adjunctive use in MDD (Sarris et al. 2022).

B. Ideally, SAM should be taken earlier in the day (i.e., before 4 P.M.) to prevent insomnia (Bottiglieri 2013).

X. **Monitoring**

A. Toxicological studies have concluded that SAM is safe even at high doses. However, data on long-term use of SAM are lacking.

XI. **Relevant Pharmacokinetics/Pharmacodynamics**

A. SAM should be taken on an empty stomach 30–60 minutes before meals or 2 hours after meals.

B. SAM tosylate disulfate salt reaches peak plasma levels in about 5 hours, and the half-life is about 6 hours (Yang et al. 2009).

C. SAM crosses the blood-brain barrier and also enters the synovial fluid (Giulidori et al. 1984).

D. SAM is excreted in the urine and feces (Friedel et al. 1989).

XII. **Clinically Relevant Drug Interactions**

A. SAM may reduce the effectiveness of levodopa (Charlton and Crowell 1992).

B. In combination with serotonergic drugs, SAM may increase the risk of serotonin syndrome and other serotonergic side effects (Iruela et al. 1993).

XIII. **Adverse Effects**

A. **Common**: Anorexia, constipation, diarrhea, dizziness, dry mouth, flatulence, headache, insomnia, nausea, nervousness, sweating, vomiting

B. **Rare**: Rash, itching, increased urinary frequency, blurred vision, anxiety, tiredness

C. **Risks in pregnancy and lactation**: Insufficient information available.

XIV. **Clinical Pearls/Guidelines**

A. As an over-the-counter product, SAM is regulated differently from prescription drugs, and the quality and content of available preparations may vary. Consider consultation with a pharmacist.

References

Bottiglieri T: Folate, vitamin B12, and S-adenosylmethionine. Psychiatr Clin North Am 36(1):1–13, 2013 23538072

Charlton CG, Crowell B Jr: Parkinson's disease-like effects of S-adenosyl-L-methionine: effects of L-dopa. Pharmacol Biochem Behav 43(2):423–431, 1992 1359575

Dolcetta D, Parmigiani P, Salmaso L, et al: Quantitative evaluation of the clinical effects of S-adenosylmethionine on mood and behavior in Lesch-Nyhan patients. Nucleosides Nucleotides Nucleic Acids 32(4):174–188, 2013 24001191

Friedel HA, Goa KL, Benfield P: S-adenosyl-L-methionine: a review of its pharmacological properties and therapeutic potential in liver dysfunction and affective disorders in relation to its physiological role in cell metabolism. Drugs 38(3):389–416, 1989 2680435

Giulidori P, Cortellaro M, Moreo G, et al: Pharmacokinetics of S-adenosyl-L-methionine in healthy volunteeers. Eur J Clin Pharmacol 27(1):119–121, 1984 6489422

Gören JL, Stoll AL, Damico KE, et al: Bioavailability and lack of toxicity of S-adenosyl-L-methionine (SAMe) in humans. Pharmacotherapy 24(11):1501–1507, 2004 15537554

Iruela LM, Minguez L, Merino J, et al: Toxic interaction of S-adenosylmethionine and clomipramine. Am J Psychiatry 150(3):522, 1993 8434674

National Center for Complementary and Integrative Health: S-adenosyl-L-methionine (SAMe): in depth. Last updated January 2017. Available at: https://www.nccih.nih.gov/health/sadenosyllmethionine-same-in-depth. Accessed April 27, 2022.

Sarris J, Ravindran A, Yatham LN, et al: Clinician guidelines for the treatment of psychiatric disorders with nutraceuticals and phytoceuticals: the World Federation of Societies of Biological Psychiatry (WFSBP) and Canadian Network for Mood and Anxiety Treatments (CANMAT) Taskforce. World J Biol Psychiatry 23(6):424–455, 2022 35311615

Yang J, He Y, Du Y-X, et al: Pharmacokinetic properties of S-adenosylmethionine after oral and intravenous administration of its tosylate disulfate salt: a multiple-dose, open-label, parallel-group study in healthy Chinese volunteers. Clin Ther 31(2):311–320, 2009 19302903

St. John's Wort

I. **Generic Name**: St. John's wort
II. **Brand Names**: None
III. **Scientific Name**: *Hypericum perforatum*
IV. **Class**: Phytoceutical
V. **Mechanism of Action**

A. Several compounds isolated from St. John's wort possess pharmacological activity, including naphthodianthrones, xanthones, flavonoids, phloroglucinols (e.g. hyperforin), and hypericin (Russo et al. 2014; UpToDate 2022).
B. Hyperforin has been shown to inhibit monoamine oxidase type A (MAO-A) and MAO-B as well as the reuptake of norepinephrine, dopamine, and serotonin (Müller et al. 1998; Singer et al. 1999; Thiede and Walper 1994).
C. Hyperforin has a strong affinity for GABA, glutamate, and adenosine receptors (Sood et al. 2010). Downregulation of beta-adrenergic receptors has also been documented (Müller et al. 1998).

VI. **Evidence-Based Uses**

A. Mild to moderate depression (Sarris et al. 2022)

VII. **Common/Other Uses**

A. Menopausal symptoms, ADHD, somatic symptom disorder, obsessive-compulsive disorder, and other conditions. Topical use of St. John's wort is promoted for various skin conditions, including wounds, bruises, and muscle pain (National Center for Complementary and Integrative Health 2020). The evidence base supporting use of St. John's wort in each of these conditions varies; for further information, readers are referred to comprehensive sources in the literature (e.g., Peterson and Nguyen 2023).

VIII. **Major Contraindications and When to Use Caution**

A. St. John's wort can weaken the effects of many medicines (see "Clinically Relevant Drug Interactions" below).
B. Taking St. John's wort with serotonergic antidepressants or other drugs that affect serotonin may lead to increased serotonin-related side effects (National Center for Complementary and Integrative Health 2020).
C. St. John's wort may interfere with surgical procedures via its serotonergic CNS effects and/or its serotonergic effects on the vascular system (Ang-Lee et al. 2001). Its use should be discontinued preoperatively, because it can increase the metabolism of some drugs used in anesthesia.
D. St. John's wort can induce hypomania or mania when used in patients with bipolar disorder or in depressed patients with occult bipolar disorder (Nierenberg et al. 1999).

E. St. John's wort may induce psychosis in patients with schizophrenia (Lal and Iskandar 2000).

IX. **Dosage Ranges and Guidelines**

A. Preparations vary greatly in chemical content and quality but may be standardized regarding hyperforin (commonly 2%–5%) or hypericin (commonly 0.12%–0.3%) content (Asher et al. 2017).

B. Clinical trials evaluating the efficacy of St. John's wort in depression have commonly used 900 mg of extract daily in 3 divided doses for periods of up to 12 weeks (range: 200–1,800 mg/day) (Kasper et al. 2008).

C. St. John's wort flowers at dosages of 600–1,800 mg/day standardized to a dose of approximately 0.2%–0.3% hypericin and/or 5%–6% hyperforin (1–3 times a day, depending on extract) are recommended for monotherapy use in mild to moderate depression (Sarris et al. 2022).

X. **Monitoring**

A. Not applicable

XI. **Relevant Pharmacokinetics/Pharmacodynamics**

A. St. John's wort has low penetration of the blood-brain barrier, with only about 5% of hypericin likely to reach the brain; hypericin's half-life in the brain appears to be several weeks (Russo et al. 2014).

B. Time to peak plasma concentration (C_{max}) was reported to range from about 2.8 to 3.6 hours for hyperforin after a single dose of St. John's wort (300–1,800 mg) (Russo et al. 2014).

C. A distribution half-life of 3 hours was noted for hyperforin (Biber et al. 1998).

D. In animal research, hyperforin was metabolized in the liver by the hydroxylation pathway. Four major phase I metabolites (19-hydroxyhyperforin, 24-hydroxyhyperforin, 29-hydroxyhyperforin, and 34-hydroxyhyperforin) were isolated (Cui et al. 2004). Hyperforin's elimination half-life is 9–20 hours (Biber et al. 1998; Schulz et al. 2005).

E. When taken orally, St. John's wort is generally well tolerated.

XII. **Clinically Relevant Drug Interactions**:

A. Because of the complex interactions among Hypericum constituents in any particular St. John's wort product or dose form, drug interactions with St. John's wort are highly variable and are often difficult to predict based solely on the St. John's wort dosage (Chrubasik-Hausmann et al. 2019, p. 129).

B. St. John's wort induces cytochrome P450 (CYP) 1A2, CYP2C19, CYP2C9, and CYP3A4 and intestinal P-glycoprotein/multidrug efflux pump (MDR)-1 drug transporters.

C. St. John's wort can weaken the effects of many medicines, including antidepressants, hormonal contraceptives, cyclosporine, digoxin, ivabradine, indinavir, nevirapine, irinotecan, imatinib, warfarin, and simvastatin (National Center for Complementary and Integrative Health 2020).

D. Concomitant use of St. John's wort can reduce peak plasma levels of the antiretroviral protease inhibitor indinavir by more than 50% (Piscitelli et al. 2000).

E. St. John's wort increases the clearance of hormonal contraceptives (presumably by lowering the concentrations of ethinylestradiol), thereby reducing their clinical effects Pfrunder et al. 2003).

F. St. John's wort increases the clearance of alprazolam, reducing its clinical effects (Markowitz et al. 2003).

G. St. John's wort reduces the levels and clinical effects of digoxin (Chrubasik-Hausmann et al. 2019), docetaxel (Goey et al. 2014), and ketamine (Peltoniemi et al. 2012).

H. St. John's wort increases the clearance of imatinib, reducing its clinical effects (Frye et al. 2004).

I. St. John's wort increases the metabolism of phenytoin, reducing its plasma concentrations and consequently its clinical effects (Henderson et al. 2002).

XIII. **Adverse Effects**

A. **Common**: Agitation, anxiety, dizziness, diarrhea, constipation, stomach discomfort, dry mouth (Mayo Clinic 2022)

B. **Other**: Fatigue, insomnia, headache, and photosensitivity (Mayo Clinic 2022)

C. **Risks in pregnancy and lactation**: Use of St. John's wort is contraindicated in pregnancy and lactation.

XIV. **Clinical Pearls/Guidelines**

A. As an over-the-counter product, St. John's wort is regulated differently from prescription drugs, and the quality and content of available preparations may vary. Consider consultation with a pharmacist.

References

Ang-Lee MK, Moss J, Yuan C-S: Herbal medicines and perioperative care. JAMA 286(2):208–216, 2001 11448284

Asher GN, Gartlehner G, Gaynes BN, et al: Comparative benefits and harms of complementary and alternative medicine therapies for initial treatment of major depressive disorder: systematic review and meta-analysis. J Altern Complement Med 23(12):907–919, 2017 28700248

Biber A, Fischer H, Römer A, et al: Oral bioavailability of hyperforin from hypericum extracts in rats and human volunteers. Pharmacopsychiatry 31(S 1):36–43, 1998

Chrubasik-Hausmann S, Vlachojannis J, McLachlan AJ: Understanding drug interactions with St John's wort (Hypericum perforatum L.): impact of hyperforin content. J Pharm Pharmacol 71(1):129–138, 2019 29411879

Cui Y, Ang CYW, Beger RD, et al: In vitro metabolism of hyperforin in rat liver microsomal systems. Drug Metab Dispos 32(1):28–34, 2004 14709617

Frye RF, Fitzgerald SM, Lagattuta TF, et al: Effect of St John's wort on imatinib mesylate pharmacokinetics. Clin Pharmacol Ther 76(4):323–329, 2004 15470331

Goey AKL, Meijerman I, Rosing H, et al: The effect of St John's wort on the pharmacokinetics of docetaxel. Clin Pharmacokinet 53(1):103–110, 2014 24068654

Henderson L, Yue QY, Bergquist C, et al: St John's wort (Hypericum perforatum): drug interactions and clinical outcomes. Br J Clin Pharmacol 54(4):349–356, 2002 12392581

Kasper S, Gastpar M, Müller WE, et al: Efficacy of St. John's wort extract WS 5570 in acute treatment of mild depression: a reanalysis of data from controlled clinical trials. Eur Arch Psychiatry Clin Neurosci 258(1):59–63, 2008 18084790

Lal S, Iskandar H: St. John's wort and schizophrenia. CMAJ 163(3):262–263, 2000 10951721

Markowitz JS, Donovan JL, DeVane CL, et al: Effect of St John's wort on drug metabolism by induction of cytochrome P450 3A4 enzyme. JAMA 290(11):1500–1504, 2003 13129991
Mayo Clinic. St. John's wort. n.d. Available at: https://www.mayoclinic.org/drugs-supplements-st-johns-wort/art-20362212. Accessed May 2, 2022.
Müller W, Singer A, Wonnemann M, et al: Hyperforin represents the neurotransmitter reuptake inhibiting constituent of hypericum extract. Pharmacopsychiatry 31(S 1):16–21, 1998
National Center for Complementary and Integrative Health: St John's wort. Last updated October 2020. Available at: https://www.nccih.nih.gov/health/st-johns-wort. Accessed May 2, 2022.
Nierenberg AA, Burt T, Matthews J, et al: Mania associated with St. John's wort. Biol Psychiatry 46(12):1707–1708, 1999 10624554
Peltoniemi MA, Saari TI, Hagelberg NM, et al: St John's wort greatly decreases the plasma concentrations of oral S-ketamine. Fundam Clin Pharmacol 26(6):743–750, 2012 21635359
Peterson B, Nguyen H: St. John's Wort, in StatPearls. Treasure Island, FL, StatPearls Publishing, last update May 16, 2023. Available at: https://www.ncbi.nlm.nih.gov/books/NBK557465/. Accessed August 4, 2024.
Pfrunder A, Schiesser M, Gerber S, et al: Interaction of St John's wort with low-dose oral contraceptive therapy: a randomized controlled trial. Br J Clin Pharmacol 56(6):683–690, 2003 14616430
Piscitelli SC, Burstein AH, Chaitt D, et al: Indinavir concentrations and St John's wort. Lancet 355(9203):547–548, 2000 10683007
Russo E, Scicchitano F, Whalley BJ, et al: Hypericum perforatum: pharmacokinetic, mechanism of action, tolerability, and clinical drug-drug interactions. Phytother Res 28(5):643–655, 2014 23897801
Sarris J, Ravindran A, Yatham LN, et al: Clinician guidelines for the treatment of psychiatric disorders with nutraceuticals and phytoceuticals: the World Federation of Societies of Biological Psychiatry (WFSBP) and Canadian Network for Mood and Anxiety Treatments (CANMAT) Taskforce. World J Biol Psychiatry 23(6):424–455, 2022 35311615
Schulz H-U, Schürer M, Bässler D, et al: Investigation of the bioavailability of hypericin, pseudohypericin, hyperforin and the flavonoids quercetin and isorhamnetin following single and multiple oral dosing of a hypericum extract containing tablet. Arzneimittelforschung 55(1):15–22, 2005 15727160
Singer A, Wonnemann M, Müller WE: Hyperforin, a major antidepressant constituent of St. John's Wort, inhibits serotonin uptake by elevating free intracellular Na+1. J Pharmacol Exp Ther 290(3):1363–1368, 1999 10454515
Sood A, Ebbert JO, Prasad K, et al: A randomized clinical trial of St. John's wort for smoking cessation. J Altern Complement Med 16(7):761–767, 2010 20590478
Thiede H-M, Walper A: Inhibition of MAO and COMT by hypericum extracts and hypericin. J Geriatr Psychiatry Neurol 7(1)(Suppl 1):S54–S56, 1994 7857510
UpToDate. Clinical use of St. John's wort. Literature review current through December 2022. Available at: https://pro.uptodatefree.ir/show/1391. Accessed August 4, 2024.

Valerian

I. **Generic Names**: Valerian, all-heal, garden heliotrope
II. **Brand Names**: None
III. **Scientific Name**: *Valeriana officinalis*
IV. **Class**: Phytoceutical, sedative-hypnotic agent

V. **Mechanism of Action**

A. Valerenic acid and other constituents of valerian are GABA agonists.

B. Valerian may inhibit the enzyme system responsible for the catabolism of GABA. It may also bind directly to $GABA_A$ receptors and stimulate the release and reuptake of GABA (Komori et al. 2006; Yuan et al. 2004).

C. Valerian may affect sleep regulation via its activity at adenosine (A_1) and serotonin ($5\text{-}HT_1$) receptors (Yuan et al. 2004).

VI. **Evidence-Based Uses**

A. Insomnia (Shinjyo et al. 2020)

1. A fixed valerian hops extract combination (Ze 91019) taken daily for 4 weeks was found to be superior to placebo in patients with ICD-10 nonorganic insomnia and without any safety concerns (Koetter et al. 2007). Another clinical study showed that 600 mg/day of valerian extract LI 156 (Sedonium) had efficacy comparable to 10 mg/day of oxazepam in the treatment of ICD-10 nonorganic insomnia (Ziegler et al. 2002). A systematic review and meta-analysis found that the primary therapeutic benefits of valerian were its sleep-promoting and anxiolytic effects (Shinjyo et al. 2020).

VII. **Common/Other Uses**

A. Anxiety, depression, premenstrual syndrome (PMS), menopause symptoms, headaches (National Center for Complementary and Integrative Health 2020)

VIII. **Major Contraindications and When to Use Caution**

A. **Perioperative**: Valerian has sedative effects that may cause additive CNS depression when combined with anesthesia and other medications used perioperatively (Houghton 1999).

IX. **Dosage Ranges and Guidelines**

A. Valerian has most often been used at dosages of 300–600 mg/day for up to 6 weeks (Shinjyo et al. 2020).

X. **Monitoring**: Not applicable

XI. **Relevant Pharmacokinetics/Pharmacodynamics**

A. Following a 600-mg oral dose of a specific valerian extract in healthy volunteers, maximum valerenic acid serum concentrations of 0.9–2.3 ng/mL were reached within 1–2 hours, and the elimination half-life was about 1.1 hours (Anderson et al. 2005).

XII. **Clinically Relevant Drug Interactions**

A. Valerian may enhance the adverse/toxic effects of benzodiazepines (Carrasco et al. 2009; Yuan et al. 2004).

B. Concomitant use of valerian with barbiturates or CNS depressants can induce additive sedative effects (Carrasco et al. 2009; Yuan et al. 2004).

C. Valerian may interact with other herbs and supplements that have sedative effects (Houghton 1999) and may also interact with alcohol (Office of Dietary Supplements 2013).

XIII. **Adverse Effects**

A. **Common**: Diarrhea and gastrointestinal problems, dizziness, headaches, fatigue, sleepiness, mental dullness, restlessness, excitability, uneasiness, agitation, vivid dreams (Cuellar and Ratcliffe 2009)
B. **Rare**: Tachycardia, high-output cardiac failure with withdrawal after long-term use (Garges et al. 1998)
C. **Risks in pregnancy and lactation**: Insufficient reliable information is available on valerian's safety in pregnancy and lactation; avoid use.

XIV. **Clinical Pearls/Guidelines**

A. Advise patients to taper dosages slowly when discontinuing valerian after extended use.
B. Valerian is usually taken 2 hours before bedtime.
C. As an over-the-counter product, valerian is regulated differently from prescription drugs, and the quality and content of available preparations may vary. Consider consultation with a pharmacist.

References

Anderson GD, Elmer GW, Kantor ED, et al: Pharmacokinetics of valerenic acid after administration of valerian in healthy subjects. Phytother Res 19(9):801–803, 2005 16220575

Carrasco MC, Vallejo JR, Pardo-de-Santayana M, et al: Interactions of Valeriana officinalis L. and Passiflora incarnata L. in a patient treated with lorazepam. Phytother Res 23(12):1795–1796, 2009 19441067

Cuellar NG, Ratcliffe SJ: Does valerian improve sleepiness and symptom severity in people with restless legs syndrome? Altern Ther Health Med 15(2):22–28, 2009

Garges HP, Varia I, Doraiswamy PM: Cardiac complications and delirium associated with valerian root withdrawal. JAMA 280(18):1566–1567, 1998 9820254

Houghton PJ: The scientific basis for the reputed activity of valerian. J Pharm Pharmacol 51(5):505–512, 1999 10411208

Koetter U, Schrader E, Käufeler R, et al: A randomized, double blind, placebo-controlled, prospective clinical study to demonstrate clinical efficacy of a fixed valerian hops extract combination (Ze 91019) in patients suffering from non-organic sleep disorder. Phytother Res 21(9):847–851, 2007 17486686

Komori T, Matsumoto T, Motomura E, et al: The sleep-enhancing effect of valerian inhalation and sleep-shortening effect of lemon inhalation. Chem Senses 31(8):731–737, 2006 16857858

National Center for Complementary and Integrative Health: Valerian. Last updated October 2020. Available at: https://www.nccih.nih.gov/health/valerian. Accessed May 3, 2022.

Office of Dietary Supplements: Valerian. Updated March 15, 2013. Available at: https://ods.od.nih.gov/factsheets/Valerian-HealthProfessional/. Accessed May 3, 2022.

Shinjyo N, Waddell G, Green J: Valerian root in treating sleep problems and associated disorders—a systematic review and meta-analysis. J Evid Based Integr Med 25:2515690X2096732, 2020

Yuan C-S, Mehendale S, Xiao Y, et al: The gamma-aminobutyric acidergic effects of valerian and valerenic acid on rat brainstem neuronal activity. Anesth Analg 98(2):353–358, 2004 14742369

Ziegler G, Ploch M, Miettinen-Baumann A, et al: Efficacy and tolerability of valerian extract LI 156 compared with oxazepam in the treatment of non-organic insomnia—a randomized, double-blind, comparative clinical study. Eur J Med Res 7(11):480–486, 2002 12568976

14

Interventional Psychiatry

Sahand Babapoor-Farrokhran, M.D., Ph.D.
Joan A. Camprodon, M.D., M.P.H., Ph.D.

Interventional psychiatry is an emerging subspecialty that uses procedural interventions, primarily device neuromodulation therapies, to treat patients with brain disorders associated with mood, behavioral, and/or cognitive disturbances. This therapeutic field has developed thanks to advances in neuroscience that have revealed the brain circuit mechanisms of neuropsychiatric disorders. Device neuromodulation interventions are generally categorized into three main groups: surgical or invasive, convulsive, and noninvasive. Therapeutic protocols using techniques such as deep brain stimulation (DBS), vagal nerve stimulation (VNS [both surgical and invasive]), electroconvulsive therapy (ECT [convulsive]), and transcranial magnetic stimulation (TMS [noninvasive]) exist to treat patients with a wide variety of conditions, such as mood disorders, obsessive-compulsive disorder, tobacco use disorder, psychosis, and catatonia. The same technologies, with different disease-specific protocols, are used to treat diverse psychiatric and also neurological conditions, such as movement disorders and epilepsy, or to support poststroke motor rehabilitation, highlighting the relevance of an integrated clinical neuroscience approach focused on a clinical understanding of brain circuitry. It is important to emphasize that DBS, VNS, TMS, ECT, and all other modalities are technologies, not treatments; the specific combination of stimulation parameters in a concrete protocol is what defines a treatment. In this chapter we focus on the most relevant surgical, convulsive, and noninvasive modalities with approved indications, but readers should note that this is a rapidly evolving field with new indications, new protocols, and new technologies being developed and entering clinical practice at an unprecedented rate.

Deep Brain Stimulation

I. **Class**: Invasive surgical neuromodulation

II. **Indications**

A. The first FDA-cleared indication for deep brain stimulation (DBS) was chronic pain, but this was eventually revoked due to inconsistent efficacy evidence.

B. The most common indications are movement disorders: Parkinson's disease, essential tremor, and dystonia.

C. Psychiatrically, DBS was cleared by the FDA for treatment-resistant OCD in 2009 under a humanitarian device exception.

D. While significant research has taken place in major depressive disorder (MDD), DBS is not currently approved for this indication. Other experimental applications have been described for Tourette's syndrome, schizophrenia, eating disorders, substance use disorder, obesity, bipolar disorder, PTSD, and Alzheimer's dementia.

III. **Mechanism of Action**

A. DBS at typical frequencies (which are high and nonphysiological) is thought to inhibit neurons locally around the electrodes, producing circuit-wide transsynaptic effects.

IV. **Contraindications**

A. **Relative contraindications**: Acute psychosis, substance use disorder in the past 6 months, antisocial personality disorder, pregnancy, pacemaker/defibrillator

B. Any condition that would contraindicate general anesthesia

V. **Medical Clearance**

A. Regular preoperative assessment, including anesthesia clearance

VI. **Process**

A. Under general or local anesthesia, a stereotactic frame is affixed and a magnetic resonance imaging (MRI) or a computed tomography (CT) scan is obtained. Thereafter, a route to the target area is planned in a way that the implanted electrodes do not damage vessels or vital structures on their course. Then a burr hole is drilled and an electrode is moved to the target through the predetermined route, using the stereotactic apparatus.

B. Anatomic targets for OCD include the ventral capsule/ventral striatum (VC/VS [FDA cleared in 2009]) and also the anterior limb of the internal capsule, the subthalamic nucleus, the nucleus accumbens, and the inferior thalamic peduncle.

C. Targets for other conditions include the subgenual cingulate (depression); the anterior limb of the internal capsule (depression, anorexia); the nucleus accumbens (depression, addiction, Lesch-Nyhan syndrome, OCD, Tourette's syndrome); the inferior thalamic peduncle (depression); the dorsomedial ventro-anterior, ventrolateral, and infralaminar thalamus (Tourette's syndrome); the centromedian-parafascicular complex (Tourette's syndrome); the internal globus pallidus (Tourette's syndrome, Lesch-Nyhan syndrome); the lateral habenula (depression); the medial forebrain bundle (depression); the ventromedial hypothalamus (obesity); the posterior hypothalamus (obesity); the mammillothalamic and mammillotegmental tracts (dementia), and the basolateral amygdala (PTSD).

D. After device implantation, the parameters of the stimulator are adjusted with a wireless device on an outpatient basis.
E. Newer "closed loop" stimulation dynamically reads and adapts to the real-time intrinsic brain rhythms.

VII. **Side Effects**

A. Potential surgical complications include intracerebral hematoma, seizure, delirium, electrode displacement, and infection.
B. Stimulation-related side effects include recurrence of depression and suicidality, hypomania, anxiety, hypersexuality and disinhibition (including gambling), psychosis, paralalia, flushing, and nausea/vomiting.
C. Glial scars around electrodes may affect efficacy.

VIII. **Clinical Pearls/Treatment Guidelines**

A. The stimulation parameters are voltage (0–10 V), pulse width (typically 60–450 microseconds), frequency (typically 70–220 Hz), selection of active and inactive electrodes and their polarity, and duty cycle (i.e., the duration the stimulator is on and off [however, the stimulator usually is continuously on]).
B. In DBS studies in OCD, the response rate was about 60% regardless of the target (Gadot et al. 2022). In MDD, DBS led to a >50% response rate in open-label trials (Holtzheimer et al. 2012), but a large randomized, placebo-controlled trial (Dougherty et al. 2015) was not positive. In Tourette's syndrome, DBS led to a >50% decrease in tic severity (Baldermann et al. 2016).

Further Reading

Arulpragasam AR, Chou T, Kaur N, et al: Future directions of deep brain stimulation: current disorders, new technologies. Psychiatr Ann 43:366–373, 2013

Corse D, Chou T, Arulpragasam AR, et al: Deep brain stimulation for obsessive-compulsive disorder. Psychiatr Ann 43:351–357, 2013

Kaur N, Chou T, Corse AK, et al: Deep brain stimulation for treatment-resistant depression. Psychiatr Ann 43:358–365, 2013

Schwalb JM, Hamani C: The history and future of deep brain stimulation. Neurotherapeutics 5(1):3–13, 2008 18164479

Yu H, Neimat JS: The treatment of movement disorders by deep brain stimulation. Neurotherapeutics 5(1):26–36, 2008 18164481

References

Baldermann JC, Schüller T, Huys D, et al: Deep brain stimulation for Tourette syndrome: a systematic review and meta-analysis. Brain Stimul 9(2):296–304, 2016 26827109

Dougherty DD, Rezai AR, Carpenter LL, et al: A randomized sham-controlled trial of deep brain stimulation of the ventral capsule/ventral striatum for chronic treatment-resistant depression. Biol Psychiatry 78(4):240-248, 2015 25726497

Gadot R, Najera R, Hirani S, et al: Efficacy of deep brain stimulation for treatment-resistant obsessive-compulsive disorder: systematic review and meta-analysis. J Neurol Neurosurg Psychiatry jnnp-2021-328738 [Online ahead of print], 2022 36127157

Holtzheimer PE, Kelley ME, Gross RE, et al: Subcallosal cingulate deep brain stimulation for treatment-resistant unipolar and bipolar depression. Arch Gen Psychiatry 69(2):150–158, 2012 22213770

Electroconvulsive Therapy

I. **Class**: Convulsive neuromodulation technique

II. **Indications**

A. Primary

1. Major depressive episode, with or without psychotic features
2. Psychotic disorders (e.g., schizophrenia, schizoaffective disorder)
3. Mania
4. Catatonia (secondary to psychiatric, medical, or neurological etiologies), malignant catatonia, and neuroleptic malignant syndrome

B. Also consider

1. Acute suicidal ideation
2. Severe self-injurious behavior and aggression in autism spectrum disorder (Park et al. 2021)
3. Status epilepticus
4. Parkinson's disease
5. When a rapid response is desired (e.g., for patients without adequate oral intake, who have significant agitation, or who are experiencing acute severe exacerbation of their psychiatric symptoms)
6. When symptoms fail to respond to pharmacotherapy, psychotherapy, or other interventions
7. Patient preference

III. **Mechanism of Action**

A. ECT differentially affects the noradrenergic, serotonergic, dopaminergic, and GABAergic systems (e.g., increased D_1 and D_3 activity).

B. ECT could increase growth factors such as brain-derived neurotrophic factor (BDNF) and nerve growth factor (NGF).

C. ECT causes volumetric increases in limbic midtemporal structures (e.g., hippocampus, amygdala) and anterior cingulate cortex.

D. ECT causes increased cerebral blood flow (CBF) during the induced seizure and decreased CBF during the postictal period. There is slowing of the EEG signal during the postictal period as well. The decreased CBF correlates with the clinical response in depression.

IV. **Contraindications**

A. There are no absolute contraindications to ECT.

B. Patients with an intracranial mass, increased intracranial pressure, cerebrovascular disease, or aneurysms are at increased risk of complications such as herniation and bleeding. However, close monitoring of blood pressure and pretreatment with dexamethasone (for space-occupying lesions) could minimize the risks.

C. Patients with recent myocardial infarction are at increased risk, although the risk is greatly diminished 2 weeks after the infarction.

D. Epilepsy is not a contraindication; in fact, ECT has been used effectively in the treatment of status epilepticus.

V. **Medical Clearance**

A. Standard history, physical exam (including neurological exam), preanesthesia clearance, complete blood count and chemistry (including liver, kidney, and thyroid function tests), and electrocardiogram
B. Further tests, such as chest, spine, or limb X ray, for any suspicion of abnormalities in corresponding areas
C. Brain MRI if there is any suspicion of intracranial pathology
D. Cardiology investigation if there is any suspicion of ischemia, abnormal rhythm, or other cardiac pathologies

VI. **Process**

A. Informed consent by patient if capable, and in cases of impaired capacity, consent by health care proxy (substitute decision maker), legal guardian, or court order
B. It is advisable to gradually decrease and discontinue lithium, antiepileptics, benzodiazepines, or other medications with seizure threshold–increasing properties. If discontinuation is not feasible, hold these medications before 5 P.M. the evening before ECT treatments.
C. Patients should receive nothing by mouth from the midnight prior to the procedure. On the day of the procedure, patients receive a general anesthetic and muscle relaxant, and after confirmation of full muscle relaxation, the electrical stimulus is delivered.
D. Treatment parameters include electrode placement (right unilateral, bitemporal, or bifrontal), pulse width (0.3 millisecond, or *ultrabrief*; 0.5–1.0 millisecond, or *brief*), stimulus duration (in seconds), stimulus amplitude (in milliamps), and total dose (in millicoulombs). Frequency of stimulation is generally 20–120 Hz.
   1. Right unilateral electrode position and ultrabrief pulse width have fewer cognitive side effects but take longer to achieve therapeutic effects.
   2. A switch from right unilateral to bilateral ECT may be necessary if right unilateral ECT is insufficient to improve symptoms.
E. The acute course starts with three treatments per week (two per week in some countries [e.g., the UK]) for 3 weeks or until response or remission is reached. The frequency of treatments can be reduced depending on response, tolerability, and side effects. Most patients respond in 6–20 sessions.
F. After the initial acute course, some patients require long-term maintenance treatments, the frequency of which is gradually decreased to biweekly, monthly, or longer intervals. Some patients require indefinite maintenance treatments.

VII. **Side Effects**

A. The most common side effects of ECT are headaches, muscle pain, and jaw pain (which can be treated with acetaminophen, ibuprofen, or.similar agents). Nausea and vomiting can also occur after the procedure.
B. Memory impairment (most commonly anterograde amnesia) can occur. Permanent memory loss is extremely rare; almost all patients return to their cognitive baseline within 6 months.
C. Confusion and delirium may occur acutely after ECT, but these effects are usually short-lived.

D. ECT may cause a switch from depression to mania in patients with underlying bipolar disorder, although this occurs only rarely. At the same time, ECT is also a treatment of mania.

E. A rare adverse effect of ECT involves bone or tooth fractures and ligament injuries, likely associated with insufficient pharmacological paralysis.

VIII. **Clinical Pearls/Treatment Guidelines**

A. The duration of the induced seizure should be at least 20 seconds for treatment to be effective.

B. The most commonly used anesthetics are methohexital, propofol, ketamine, and etomidate. The most frequently used muscle relaxants are succinylcholine and rocuronium.

Further Reading

American Psychiatric Association Committee on Electroconvulsive Therapy: The Practice of Electroconvulsive Therapy: Recommendations for Treatment, Training, and Privileging, 2nd Edition. Washington, DC, American Psychiatric Association, 2001

Camprodon JA, Rauch SL, Greenberg BD, et al: Psychiatric Neurotherapeutics: Contemporary Surgical and Device-Based Treatments in Psychiatry. New York, NY, Humana Press (Springer), 2016

Espinoza RT, Kellner CH: Electroconvulsive therapy. N Engl J Med 386(7):667–672, 2022 35172057

Ousdal OT, Brancati GE, Kessler U, et al: The neurobiological effects of electroconvulsive therapy studied through magnetic resonance: what have we learned, and where do we go? Biol Psychiatry 91(6):540–549, 2022 34274106

UK ECT Review Group: Efficacy and safety of electroconvulsive therapy in depressive disorders: a systematic review and meta-analysis. Lancet 361(9360):799–808, 2003 12642045

References

Park SE, Grados M, Wachtel L, et al: Use of electroconvulsive therapy in autism. Psychiatr Clin North Am 44(1):23–33, 2021 33526235

Ketamine/Esketamine

I. **Brand Name**: Ketalar (ketamine); Spravato (esketamine nasal spray)

II. **Therapeutic Class**: Anesthetic

III. **Mechanism-Based Class**: Noncompetitive *N*-methyl-D-aspartate (NMDA) glutamate receptor antagonist

IV. **Mechanism(s) of Action**

A. Esketamine is the *S*-enantiomer of ketamine and is FDA approved for treatment-resistant major depressive disorder (MDD) and depressive symptoms in adults with MDD and acute suicidal ideation or behavior (also called major depressive disorder with suicidal ideation [MDSI]).

B. Although it is a pharmacological intervention, ketamine/esketamine is generally considered to fall within the space of interventional neuropsychiatry, as it requires IV infusions (or intranasal administration in the case of esketamine) and monitoring in specialized interventional settings.

V. **Indications**

A. Esketamine was approved by the FDA in 2019 to treat adults (in conjunction with oral antidepressants) with treatment-resistant depression.

B. Esketamine was approved by the FDA in 2020 to treat adults (in conjunction with oral antidepressants) with major depressive disorder with suicidal ideation (MDSI).

C. The use of IV ketamine to treat mood disorders remains an off-label indication.

VI. **Mechanism of Action**

A. Ketamine is a glutamatergic (NMDA) antagonist, and its metabolite activates α-amino-3-hydroxy-5-methyl-4-isoxazolepropionic acid (AMPA) receptors. In addition, ketamine's antidepressant action is exerted through modulation of GABA-ergic, opioidergic, brain-derived neurotrophic factor (BDNF), and downstream second-messenger systems affecting neural plasticity and neurogenesis.

VII. **Contraindications**

A. Active psychosis or mania, history of psychosis, recent manic episode, lifetime history of ketamine or phencyclidine use disorder, ongoing active substance use disorder

B. Medical contraindications include predisposition to laryngospasm or apnea; severe uncontrolled cardiovascular disease such as heart failure or angina; uncontrolled or malignant hypertension; recent myocardial infarction; recent cerebrovascular accident; cerebrospinal fluid obstruction (as in head injury, intracranial mass, similar conditions); intracranial aneurysmal vascular disease or arteriovenous malformation; history of intracerebral hemorrhage; intraocular pressure pathology (e.g., glaucoma, acute globe injury); uncontrolled hyperthyroidism; and porphyria.

C. Ketamine treatment is not recommended during pregnancy or breastfeeding.

VIII. **Medical Clearance**

A. An anesthesia consult could be requested in cases where there is any doubt about the safety of esketamine/ketamine treatments.

IX. **Process**

A. Informed consent should be obtained after the clinician explains the benefits, risks, and alternative treatments.

B. Naltrexone has been shown to negatively affect the efficacy of ketamine treatment. Consider reducing the dose or discontinuing medications with GABAergic activity (e.g., benzodiazepines, lamotrigine, gabapentin), or consider skipping these medications on the day of ketamine treatment.

C. Esketamine (FDA approved) is administered twice a week for weeks 1–4, once a week for weeks 5–8, and weekly or biweekly thereafter according to the package label of the product used. For detailed information, refer to the esketamine monograph (manufacturer's full prescribing information [Janssen Pharmaceuticals 2023]).

   1. Starting dose for esketamine is 56 mg, and subsequent doses could be 56 mg or 84 mg, depending on response and tolerability. Blood pressure should be monitored before, during, and at the end of esketamine administration.

D. Ketamine infusions are administered twice a week for 3 weeks. The frequency is then gradually decreased to once a month or even longer intervals, depending on the response and tolerability; however, there is variability in scheduling across centers.

   1. Ketamine infusions start with a subanesthetic 0.5 mg/kg infusion over 40 minutes. (*Note*: An infusion of 0.2 mg/kg has been tried in some studies [Domany et al. 2020], with less benefit but fewer side effects. Doses up to 2 mg/kg for infusions have been tried.) Blood pressure should be monitored before, during, and at the end of ketamine administration.

E. Patients should not engage in potentially dangerous activities, such as driving or operating machinery, until the next day, following a night of refreshing sleep. Patients should be accompanied by a chaperone after ketamine or esketamine treatments.

F. As mentioned earlier, maintenance treatment can be administered at weekly, biweekly, or at even longer intervals, depending on response and tolerability.

X. Side Effects

A. Sedation, somnolence, anxiety, dissociation, hallucinations and perceptual disturbances, dizziness, vertigo

B. Nausea and vomiting, hypertension, ulcerative or interstitial cystitis, respiratory suppression

XI. Clinical Pearls/Treatment Guidelines

A. Ketamine (and esketamine) has potential for dependence and diversion. Therefore, it is prudent to assess the risk of diversion and developing (or relapsing into) a substance use disorder during treatment. Consider consultation with an addiction specialist. That said, such risk should not be an absolute contraindication for treatment.

Further Reading

Sanacora G, Katz R: Ketamine: a review for clinicians. Focus Am Psychiatr Publ 16(3):243–250, 2018 31975918

Yavi M, Lee H, Henter ID, et al: Ketamine treatment for depression: a review. Discov Ment Health 2(1):9, 2022 35509843

Zanos P, Gould TD: Mechanisms of ketamine action as an antidepressant. Mol Psychiatry 23(4):801–811, 2018 29532791

References

Domany Y, Shelton RC, McCullumsmith CB: Ketamine for acute suicidal ideation. An emergency department intervention: a randomized, double-blind, placebo-controlled, proof-of-concept trial. Depress Anxiety 37(3):224–233, 2020 31733088

Janssen Pharmaceuticals: Spravato (esketamine) nasal spray [package insert]. Revised October 2023. Available at: https://www.janssenlabels.com/package-insert/product-monograph/prescribing-information/SPRAVATO-pi.pdf. Accessed July 4, 2024.

Transcranial Magnetic Stimulation

I. **Class**: Noninvasive neuromodulation technique

II. **Indications**

A. Different therapeutic TMS protocols have been cleared by the FDA for use in treatment-resistant major depressive disorder (MDD, which was the first approved indication, in 2008), acute migraine headaches with aura (in 2013), OCD (in 2017), and smoking cessation (in 2020).

B. In addition to its therapeutic clinical applications, TMS also has diagnostic applications in clinical neurophysiology for the assessment of pathologies affecting the corticospinal motor tract and for noninvasive presurgical cortical mapping of motor (FDA cleared in 2009) and language (FDA cleared in 2012) areas.

III. **Mechanism of Action**

A. TMS exerts its effects by increasing or decreasing the activity of brain regions, leading to neuroplastic changes in brain circuit dynamics.

B. These neuromodulatory effects are accomplished by engaging neurophysiological mechanisms similar to long-term potentiation (LTP) and long-term depression (LTD) but at the level of populations of neurons, not single synapses.

IV. **Contraindications**

A. Presence of implanted metallic devices in the head and neck, including cochlear implants (absolute contraindication), deep brain stimulators, aneurysmal clips, metal plates, and medication pumps.

B. Extra caution should be exercised in patients with cardiac pacemakers and vagal nerve stimulators.

C. Comorbid epilepsy is considered a partial contraindication, and many clinics will not treat patients with a history of seizures.

D. Medications that modulate the seizure threshold are not contraindicated and can be continued (with caution) during treatment.

V. **Medical Clearance**

A. No specific workup is necessary for TMS clearance, other than a detailed history and examination to identify absolute and relative contraindications.

VI. **Process**

A. **Informed consent** should be obtained after the clinician explains the benefits, risks, and alternative treatments.

B. **Assessment of cortical excitability**: In the first session, the patient's cortical excitability is assessed by measuring the resting motor threshold (MT). The MT defines the minimum amount of energy required to activate cortical neurons. This procedure involves application of single pulses of TMS at varying intensities over the primary motor cortex representation of a hand muscle (upper extremity) or the anterior tibialis (lower extremity). After each pulse, clinicians assess the evoked response in the muscle by visually observing a contraction or measuring an evoked neurophysiological response with an electromyogram (EMG). The MT is defined as the TMS pulse intensity capable of eliciting an evoked peripheral response 50% of the time (i.e., 5 out of 10 pulses).

C. **Dose definition**: The TMS dose is individualized for every patient as a function of their cortical excitability or MT. Typical doses range from 90% to 120% of the MT, depending on the indication and protocol.

D. **Target definition**: The TMS target is then defined using standardized scalp measurements or stereotactic MRI-guided neuronavigation. Protocols for MDD generally target the left (or right) dorsolateral prefrontal cortex (DLPFC), those for OCD the dorsomedial prefrontal cortex/anterior cingulate cortex (DMPFC/ACC) or the pre-supplementary motor area (pre-SMA), those for smoking cessation the ventrolateral prefrontal cortex/anterior insula (VLPFC/AI) bilaterally, and those for migraines the occipital pole.

E. **Protocol selection**: Once cortical excitability is defined, the dose determined, and the target identified, clinicians should select the appropriate protocol. This involves choosing the type of coil, frequency of stimulation, number of pulses, and number of sessions in the course of treatment. Each indication is associated with a different protocol with distinct biological, behavioral, and clinical effects.

F. **Common therapeutic protocols**:

1. MDD: For the left DLPFC target, 10 Hz repetitive TMS (rTMS) with ≥3,000 pulses per session or intermittent theta burst stimulation (iTBS) with ≥600 pulses per session at 120% of the MT (accelerated protocols use iTBS at 90% of the MT, 1,800 pulses per session, 10 sessions per day, for 5 sequential days). For the right DLPFC target, 1 Hz rTMS or cTBS. Some patients may benefit from sequential bilateral (both right and left DLPFC targets) TMS using the above protocols. Other targets and protocols exist but are experimental.
2. OCD: For the DMPFC/ACC target, 20 Hz rTMS with ≥2,000 pulses per session at 100% of the MT using a deep coil. Other experimental targets include the pre-SMA, which requires 1 Hz rTMS or cTBS at 110%–120% of the MT.
3. Smoking cessation: For the bilateral VLPFC/AI target, 10 Hz rTMS with ≥1,800 pulses per session at 120% of the MT using a deep coil.
4. Migraines: Single pulses of TMS over the occipital pole with a home-based device.

G. **Frequency of treatments**:

1. Generally, patients receive TMS daily (except for weekends) for 5–6 weeks (acute period), followed by a gradual tapering down over a few weeks.
2. In accelerated protocols, patients receive up to 50 treatments over 5 consecutive days (up to 10 treatments per day).
3. The treatment of migraines is an exception to the requirement of multiple repeated days of treatment. For migraines, TMS is applied as needed when a migraine is starting in order to abort it.
4. No maintenance protocol is uniformly accepted. Suggested protocols include clustered protocols (monthly 5–10 sessions over 3–5 days) or continuation at a lower frequency (e.g., once a week, biweekly).

H. There are no particular aftercare guidelines for TMS. Patients can resume their usual activities following the treatment.

VII. **Side Effects**

A. Adverse effects are rare and usually mild. TMS is generally well tolerated.

B. The most common adverse effects are discomfort or pain at the stimulation site and headaches. These are mild and can be treated by over-the-counter analgesics.

C. Twitching of the jaw and forehead muscles due to direct peripheral stimulation of the corresponding muscles may occur. If this causes discomfort, it could be alleviated by repositioning the coil.

D. Uncommonly, patients may experience presyncope or syncope. This is generally vasovagal, most common during the first visit, and more common in individuals with phobias in the blood-needle spectrum.

E. Hearing loss is a potential side effect, and ear plugs are used during treatment.

F. Seizure is a rare (1/35,000 treatments) adverse effect. TMS does not increase the risk of epilepsy.

VIII. **Clinical Pearls/Treatment Guidelines**

A. The frequency of stimulation defines the physiological effects of TMS; thus, high-frequency repetitive TMS (rTMS) (≥5 Hz, although generally 10–20 Hz) and intermittent theta burst stimulation (iTBS) are excitatory, while low-frequency rTMS (1 Hz) and continuous theta burst stimulation (cTBS) are inhibitory.

B. The right DLPFC target for MDD can be considered in patients with anxious depression or a comorbid anxiety disorder.

C. Resting-state fMRI-based treatment targeting has been cleared by the FDA in the context of accelerated protocols. This technology has shown some promise in improving outcomes while reducing treatment durations.

Further Reading

Camprodon JA: Transcranial magnetic stimulation, in Psychiatric Neurotherapeutics: Contemporary Surgical and Device-Based Treatments in Psychiatry. Edited by Camprodon JA, Rauch SL, Greenberg BD, Dougherty DD. New York, Humana Press, 2016, pp 165–186

Carmi L, Tendler A, Bystritsky A, et al: Efficacy and safety of deep transcranial magnetic stimulation for obsessive-compulsive disorder: a prospective multicenter randomized double-blind placebo-controlled trial. Am J Psychiatry 176(11):931–938, 2019 31109199

Cole EJ, Phillips AL, Bentzley BS, et al: Stanford Neuromodulation Therapy (SNT): a double-blind randomized controlled trial. Am J Psychiatry 179(2):132–141, 2022 34711062

O'Reardon JP, Solvason HB, Janicak PG, et al: Efficacy and safety of transcranial magnetic stimulation in the acute treatment of major depression: a multisite randomized controlled trial. Biol Psychiatry 62(11):1208–1216, 2007 17573044

Zangen A, Moshe H, Martinez D, et al: Repetitive transcranial magnetic stimulation for smoking cessation: a pivotal multicenter double-blind randomized controlled trial. World Psychiatry 20(3):397–404, 2021 34505368

Vagus Nerve Stimulation

I. **Class**: Invasive surgical neuromodulation

II. **Indications**

A. Vagus nerve stimulation (VNS) is FDA cleared for epilepsy (1997) and as an add-on treatment for treatment-resistant major depressive disorder (MDD) (2005).

III. **Mechanism of Action**

A. Although the mechanism of action of VNS is not fully understood, brain imaging has been helpful in elucidating underlying processes.

B. Afferent fibers of the left vagus nerve project to the nucleus tractus solitarius, which relays signals to the locus coeruleus and dorsal raphe, which contain noradrenergic and serotonergic neurons projecting across the CNS. Therefore, stimulation of the left vagus nerve modulates the neurophysiological activity of these neurotransmitter systems in the brain.

IV. **Contraindications**

A. Absolute contraindication: Left vagotomy (resected left vagus nerve)

B. Relative contraindications: MDD with psychotic features, paranoid delusions, history of manic episodes, schizoaffective disorder, unstable personality disorders such as borderline personality disorder

C. Any condition that would contraindicate general anesthesia

V. **Medical Clearance**

A. Regular preoperative assessment, including anesthesia clearance

VI. **Process**

A. The procedure is carried out under general anesthesia. One incision is made halfway between the mandible and the sternal notch to place the helical electrodes. The second incision is made 1 cm below the clavicle to make a pocket for the pulse generator.

B. Note that VNS electrodes are placed on the left vagus nerve because a predominance (up to 80%) of its fibers are afferent (i.e., go to the brain), whereas the right vagus nerve has many more efferent fibers (i.e., going to the end organs), and thus its stimulation has a higher risk of side effects (e.g., bradycardia) (Giordano et al. 2017; Ohemeng and Parham 2020).

C. VNS stimulation parameters are monitored and adjusted by a clinician in the outpatient setting using a wireless device. Patients generally have a simpler device that allows them to turn the device on and off, but not adjust the full range of parameters.

VII. **Side Effects**

A. Surgical complications (e.g., infection, bleeding); complications from anesthesia

B. Voice alteration (most common; reported in 54%–60%), neck pain, cough, dyspnea, paresthesias. These stimulation-related side effects commonly improve with time and can also be managed by changing treatment parameters.

VIII. **Clinical Pearls/Treatment Guidelines**

A. The stimulation parameters are current charge, pulse width, frequency, and duty cycle (note that VNS devices are usually not stimulating continuously; instead, they alternate periods of stimulation with off-periods).

B. A longitudinal follow-up of pilot studies of VNS in patients with severe treatment-resistant depression (Nahas et al. 2005) found that at 2-year follow-up, the response rate was 42% and the remission rate was 22%. Response and remission rates improved at 1-year follow-up compared with the first 10 weeks.

Further Reading

Cristancho MA, Cristancho P, Altinay M, et al: Vagus nerve stimulation (VNS), in Psychiatric Neurotherapeutics: Contemporary Surgical and Device-Based Treatments in Psychiatry. Edited by Camprodon JA, Rauch SL, Greenberg BD, et al. New York, Humana Press, 2016, pp 99–11

Rush AJ, Marangell LB, Sackeim HA, et al: Vagus nerve stimulation for treatment-resistant depression: a randomized, controlled acute phase trial. Biol Psychiatry 58(5):347–354, 2005 16139580

Thompson SL, O'Leary GH, Austelle CW, et al: A review of parameter settings for invasive and non-invasive vagus nerve stimulation (VNS) applied in neurological and psychiatric disorders. Front Neurosci 15:709436, 2021 34326720

References

Giordano F, Zicca A, Barba C, et al: Vagus nerve stimulation: surgical technique of implantation and revision and related morbidity. Epilepsia 58(Suppl 1):85–90, 2017 28386925

Nahas Z, Marangell LB, Husain MM, et al: Two-year outcome of vagus nerve stimulation (VNS) for treatment of major depressive episodes. J Clin Psychiatry 66(9):1097–1104, 2005 16187765

Ohemeng KK, Parham K: Vagal nerve stimulation: indications, implantation, and outcomes. Otolaryngol Clin North Am 53(1):127–143, 2020 31685239

PART V
Treatment of Special Populations

15

Women: Pregnancy, Postpartum, and Breastfeeding

Laura Kenkel, M.D.
Shanon Astley, M.D.
Linda Kang, M.D.

Importance of Psychiatric Treatment During Pregnancy and Lactation

- Risks of exposure to medications in utero must be balanced with risks of untreated mental illness, which include possible increased risk of preterm birth, low birthweight, poor involvement in prenatal care, and engagement in high-risk behaviors (ACOG Committee on Practice Bulletins—Obstetrics 2008; Betcher and Wisner 2020).
- Although some studies have suggested that pregnancy is protective against mental disorders, others have found high rates of relapse during pregnancy in women with major depressive disorder (26% of women still taking medication, 68% of women who discontinued medication [Cohen et al. 2006]) or bipolar disorder (71% overall risk of at least one mood episode recurrence during pregnancy; women who discontinued mood stabilizers had a twofold greater risk of relapse and a five times greater proportion of weeks ill [40%, versus 9% among women who continued mood stabilizer treatment] during pregnancy [Viguera et al. 2007]).
- Untreated ADHD can have a significant negative impact on social, occupational, and academic functioning in addition to increasing the risk of substance use and car/other accidents (Freeman 2014; Ornoy 2018).
- Pregnant women with severe mental illness also have an increased rate of "near miss" obstetric complications (i.e., conditions from which the woman almost dies) during pregnancy or childbirth, with rates being highest for acute renal failure; cardiac arrest, failure, or infarction; and obstetric embolism. Easter et al. (2021) posited that "diagnostic overshadowing" (in this context, the misattribution of symptoms of a serious medical illness to an already diagnosed comorbid mental illness) was one of several possible factors contributing to this increased risk.

Challenges of Accurate Risk Assessment

- Because few randomized double-blind, placebo-controlled pharmacological studies include pregnant women as participants, very limited data are available on a drug's pregnancy-specific pharmacokinetics, pharmacodynamics, efficacy, and safety (Payne 2019).
- The involvement of pregnant women in randomized controlled trials raises complex ethical concerns, both about the risk the research may pose to the woman and fetus and about the risks to the woman and fetus posed by a lack of reliable data to guide clinical care (Kaye 2019).
- Animal models used to investigate drug safety in pregnancy provide important information but cannot be relied on to determine safety in human pregnancy. Interspecies differences (animal-to-animal and animal-to-human) cause variability in teratogenic dose levels and malformations caused by pharmaceuticals. For example, interspecies differences in placental anatomy limit the translatability of animal model findings on placental drug transfer to humans (Nau 1986; Schmidt et al. 2021).
- Risk determination is hampered by studies that often have small numbers of subjects and lack statistical power. Not all cohort studies utilize reference groups of unexposed pregnancies. The number of exposed infants reported in many studies is too low for many drugs to accurately gauge teratogenicity (van Gelder et al. 2014).
- Research studies investigating psychotropic use and negative infant outcomes have not consistently controlled for underlying psychiatric illnesses; studies that have controlled for underlying psychiatric illness have generally found that the risk of adverse outcomes associated with psychotropic medication is significantly less than previously estimated (or is nonexistent) (Payne 2019).
- Given the above factors, the authors of this chapter have, to the best of their ability, based the information presented here on human data from larger studies that controlled for confounders.

Physiological Changes During Pregnancy and Postpartum

- Multiple physiological changes occur during pregnancy, including alterations in apparent volume of distribution, weight gain, and increased renal clearance as well as hormone-driven alterations in metabolic activity of enzymes within the cytochrome P450 (CYP) family (increased CYP2D6 and CYP3A activity and decreased CYP1A2 activity, among others) and the uridine diphosphate glucuronosyltransferase (UGT) family (upregulated UGT1A4 and UGT2B7). An individual woman's metabolic phenotype (poor, intermediate, extensive, or ultrarapid metabolizer) also affects metabolic rate (Betcher and Wisner 2020; Ke et al. 2014; Kokras et al. 2019; Tracy et al. 2005).
- Hemodynamic changes result in an increase in plasma volume and a decrease in plasma protein binding; in late pregnancy, serum albumin decreases by as much as 31% and alpha-1 acid glycoprotein (α_1-AGP) decreases by as much as 19%. The unbound plasma fraction of drugs that are highly protein bound can change as much as 30% (Ke et al. 2014).

- During the postpartum period, maternal physiology undergoes several changes over a short period of time: renal blood flow and glomerular filtration rate decrease back to their normal range, plasma volume normalizes, sex hormone levels decrease rapidly, and hepatic enzyme activity returns to baseline. These changes may lead to high maternal drug plasma concentrations, which require close monitoring (Kokras et al. 2019).

Breastfeeding

- The benefits of breastfeeding are widely recognized, and breast milk is considered to be the gold standard for newborn and infant nutrition (Newton and Hale 2015).
- Studies examining the safety of drugs in breastfeeding use various calculations to gauge a drug's impact on the breastfeeding infant. This chapter includes the range (across available studies) of the measured relative infant dosages (RIDs) for medications, which is the same as the weight-adjusted maternal dosage.

  - The RID is the mg/kg infant dosage divided by the mg/kg maternal dosage, multiplied by 100 (Newton and Hale 2015).
  - RIDs less than or equal to 10% are considered relatively safe, caution is necessary for RIDS between 10%–25%, and RIDs greater than 25% should be avoided (Drugs and Lactation Database (LactMed) 2006–). It should be noted that the RID does not account for variable dosage ranges that may be prescribed to mothers, postnatal age, and variability in toxicity between drugs. Additionally, studies estimating RID do not always consider active metabolites (Anderson and Sauberan 2016).

Overarching Treatment Principles

- Assume that all women of childbearing age will become pregnant, and counsel them about the potential risk of their medications and what to do in the event of unexpected pregnancy (Payne 2019).
- Engage patients who want to become pregnant in prepregnancy planning 6–12 months before they attempt conception to allow time to achieve stability after any necessary medication changes (Payne 2019).
- In the event of an unexpected pregnancy, abrupt cessation of all psychiatric medications is not recommended, because it causes stress and anxiety in the patient, may produce withdrawal or discontinuation symptoms, and may lead to a relapse of the psychiatric illness. Consider stopping medications with known teratogenicity. Taper when possible if discontinuing medications (Payne 2019).
- Strive to minimize both the number of exposures to different medications AND the number of episodes of psychiatric illness (Payne 2019).
- Use monotherapy and lowest effective dosages whenever possible. Because of the physiological changes associated with pregnancy, **consider monitoring serum drug levels** rather than focusing on a specific dosage,. If possible, obtain serum drug levels prior to pregnancy when the patient is stable to establish a baseline level (Raffi et al. 2019; Westin et al. 2018).

Medication Classes

Antidepressants

Impact of Pregnancy-Related Physiological Changes

- Serum levels of most antidepressants decline as pregnancy progresses. Dosages may have to be increased during the second and third trimesters and subsequently decreased postpartum. *Sertraline may be an exception*, in that one systematic review found increased dosage-adjusted levels of sertraline in the third trimester (Schoretsanitis et al. 2020). Therapeutic drug monitoring can help augment clinical assessment regarding dosage changes (Betcher and Wisner 2020).

Malformations

- The increased risk of malformations (specifically cardiac) associated with **SSRIs** and **SNRIs** is often diminished or no longer significant after adjustment for confounders (Betcher and Wisner 2020). Some reports have associated **paroxetine** with an increased risk of cardiac malformations, although this association has not been substantiated by more recent evidence. Consider fetal echocardiography if there is first-trimester exposure to paroxetine (ACOG Committee on Practice Bulletins—Obstetrics 2008; Gao et al. 2018; Huybrechts et al. 2014; Ornoy and Koren 2019; Yonkers et al. 2009).
- **Bupropion** has been associated with risk of cardiovascular malformations, with a projected absolute risk of approximately 2/1,000 births (Hendrick et al. 2017).
- Based on limited data, consistent evidence of teratogenicity is lacking for the following: TCAs, trazodone, nefazodone, and mirtazapine (Gentile 2014; Yonkers et al. 2009).
- Very limited or no teratogenicity data are available for the following: levomilnacipran, milnacipran, desvenlafaxine, vilazodone, vortioxetine, and MAOIs (Carvalho et al. 2016; Einarson et al. 2003; Hendrick et al. 2017; Yonkers et al. 2009).

Maternal Effects

- End-of-pregnancy exposure to **all antidepressants** has been associated with a 1.3-fold higher risk of postpartum hemorrhage (PPH), although findings are limited by imprecise assessments of PPH and inconsistent exposure windows (Jiang et al. 2016).
- Late-pregnancy exposure to **SSRIs, SNRIs, or TCAs** has been associated with preeclampsia and gestational hypertension (Carvalho et al. 2016; Gadot and Koren 2015; Gentile 2014; Palmsten et al. 2013; Raffi et al. 2019).

- Studies reporting associations between **SSRIs** and early miscarriages are likely confounded by underlying disease and/or early gestational age at first contact (most miscarriages occur early in pregnancy) (Bellantuono et al. 2015; Ornoy and Koren 2019).
- **MAOIs and atypical antidepressant** have limited to no data regarding maternal adverse effects.

Infant Effects

- **SSRI** exposure late in pregnancy (>20 weeks) is associated with a <1% absolute risk of persistent pulmonary hypertension of the newborn (PPHN), with an increase in baseline incidence from approximately 2/1,000 to 4/1,000. Note the FDA warning and Category D rating for paroxetine (Bérard et al. 2017; Ornoy and Koren 2019; 't Jong et al. 2012; Yonkers et al. 2009).
- Neonatal abstinence syndrome (NAS) occurs in up to 30% of infants with SSRI exposure late in pregnancy. Symptoms include tremulousness, jitteriness, and tachypnea and are usually mild and transient, self-resolving within the first few days after birth. NAS is more common with **paroxetine, venlafaxine, and fluoxetine** than with other SSRIs. Concurrent benzodiazepine exposure increases NAS risk (Betcher and Wisner 2020; Ornoy and Koren 2019; Yonkers et al. 2009).
- Studies that have reported an association between intrauterine growth restriction (IUGR) or prematurity and use of SSRIs are likely confounded by underlying maternal disease (Bellantuono et al. 2015; Ornoy and Koren 2019).
- There are no consistent associations between adverse neurodevelopmental outcomes and in utero exposure to SSRIs/SNRIs when studies adjust for confounders (Andrade 2022; Ornoy and Koren 2019; Rommel et al. 2020).
- Exposure to **TCAs, particularly clomipramine**, in late pregnancy is associated with an increased risk of withdrawal symptoms similar to those seen in NAS (Gentile 2014).
- **MAOIs and atypical antidepressants** have limited to no data regarding infant adverse effects.

Breastfeeding

- Table 15–1 provides breastfeeding guidelines for commonly prescribed antidepressant medications based on the most recently available data from LactMed, the majority of which are from case reports. Safety ratings are determined via a combination of RID, infant serum levels, active metabolites, and reported adverse effects.

Table 15–1. Antidepressants: guidelines for breastfeeding

Medication	RID	Safety rating[a]	Notes
SSRIs			
Citalopram	2.5%–18.4%	AM	Monitor infant for excessive drowsiness, restlessness, agitation, poor feeding, poor weight gain.
Escitalopram	0.8%–11.3%	AM	Monitor infant for excessive drowsiness, restlessness, agitation, poor feeding, poor weight gain.
Fluoxetine	0.54%–20%	AM	Monitor infant for colic, agitation, irritability, poor feeding, poor weight gain.
Fluvoxamine	0.8%–1.38%	S	Monitor infant for diarrhea, vomiting, decreased sleep, agitation.
Paroxetine	1.1%–3.2%	S	
Sertraline	0.5%–2.4%	S	
SNRIs			
Desvenlafaxine	6.8%–7.8%	AM	Monitor infant for sedation, adequate weight gain.
Duloxetine	0.14%–0.82%	LI	Monitor infant for drowsiness, adequate feeding, weight gain, developmental milestones.
Levomilnacipran	N/A	LI	
Milnacipran	2.8%	LI	
Venlafaxine	3%–11.8%	AM	Monitor infant for sedation, adequate weight gain.
TCAs			
Amitriptyline	0.9%–1.8%	S	Monitor infant for sedation.
Desipramine	N/A; infant levels undetectable	S	
Doxepin	2.2%	X	If used, monitor for infant sedation, hypotonia, vomiting, weight loss
Imipramine	2.9%	S	
Nortriptyline	1.3%	S	
MAOIs			
Isocarboxazid	N/A	LI	
Phenelzine	N/A	LI	
Selegiline	N/A	LI	Do not breastfeed until 7 days after final dose when using the transdermal patch.
Tranylcypromine	N/A	LI	

Table 15–1. Antidepressants: guidelines for breastfeeding *(continued)*

Medication	RID	Safety rating[a]	Notes
Others			
Bupropion	1.4%–10.6%	AM	Monitor infant for vomiting, diarrhea, jitteriness, sedation.
Mirtazapine	0.6%–2.8%	S	If exclusively breastfed, monitor infant for adequate growth and behavioral side effects.
Trazodone	0.65%	S	

Note. MAOIs=monoamine oxidase inhibitors; N/A=not available; RID=relative infant dose; SNRIs=serotonin-norepinephrine reuptake inhibitors; SSRIs=selective serotonin reuptake inhibitors; TCAs=tricyclic antidepressants.

[a]**Safety ratings**:

- AM—Additional monitoring required if used while breastfeeding, because of high breast milk levels, higher infant plasma levels, and/or associated adverse effects.
- LI—Limited or no information available; use of alternative medications is recommended (especially in preterm infant or newborn).
- S—Considered to be safe for breastfeeding because of low breast milk levels, low infant plasma levels, short half-life, and/or low toxicity.
- X—Avoid breastfeeding while taking.

Source. Drugs and Lactation Database (LactMed) 2006–.

Antianxiety Medications

Impact of Pregnancy-Related Physiological Changes

- Several anxiolytic medications are metabolized via the CYP enzymes, which may be induced or inhibited by hormones in pregnancy. Substrates of CYP3A4 (increased activity in pregnancy) include midazolam, diazepam, buspirone, and propranolol. Substrates of CYP2C19 (decreased activity) include diazepam and propranolol. Propranolol is additionally a substrate of CYP1A2 (decreased activity) and CYP2D6 (increased activity) (Flockhart et al. 2021; Ke et al. 2014).

Malformations

- **Chlordiazepoxide** and **diazepam** are the drugs of choice for first-trimester use if benzodiazepine treatment is needed (Bellantuono et al. 2013).
- **Clonazepam** and **lorazepam** should be used cautiously in the first trimester in light of reports of higher risks of major malformations, although the absolute risk is low (<1%) (Bellantuono et al. 2013).

- Current data are insufficient to gauge the risk of major malformations with first-trimester use of **alprazolam** (Bellantuono et al. 2013).
- **Gabapentin** has been associated with increased risk of cardiac defects (relative risk [RR] 1.40) but not major malformations (Patorno et al. 2020).
- **Propranolol** has not been associated with malformations (Briggs et al. 2021).
- Data in humans are too limited to accurately gauge the risk of major malformations associate with the following drugs: buspirone (Bristol Myers Squibb 2010), midazolam, oxazepam, and temazepam (McElhatton 1994).

Maternal Effects

- **Alprazolam and buspirone** have been found to increase prolactin levels, although this is not expected to adversely affect a mother's ability to breastfeed (Drugs and Lactation Database [LactMed] 2006–; Zemishlany et al. 1990–1991).

Infant Effects

- **Benzodiazepine** use in later pregnancy has been associated with neonatal abstinence syndrome (also called "opiate-like withdrawal syndrome") and floppy infant syndrome (Convertino et al. 2016).
- Infants exposed to benzodiazepines at any point in pregnancy may have a higher likelihood of neonatal intensive care unit (NICU) hospitalization and small head circumference (Freeman et al. 2018)
- Early- and late-pregnancy **gabapentin** exposure has been associated with an increased risk of preterm labor (RR 1.22–1.28), small size for gestational age (RR 1.17–1.39), and NICU admission (RR 1.35) (Patorno et al. 2020).
- **Propranolol** has been associated with increased risk of intrauterine growth restriction (especially with treatment beginning in the early second trimester) and reduced placental weight. Infants of mothers taking propranolol near delivery should be monitored for symptoms of beta blockade (bradycardia, hypoglycemia) for 24–48 hours after birth (Briggs et al. 2021).

Breastfeeding

- Table 15–2 provides breastfeeding guidelines for commonly prescribed anxiolytics based on the most recently available data from LactMed, the majority of which are from case reports. Safety ratings are determined via a combination of RID, infant serum levels, active metabolites, and reported adverse effects.

Table 15–2. Antianxiety medications: guidelines for breastfeeding

Medication	Relative infant dose	Safety rating[a]	Notes
Benzodiazepines			
Alprazolam	3%	X	If used repeatedly while nursing, monitor infants for sedation; possible withdrawal symptoms if breastfeeding is discontinued.
Chlordiazepoxide	N/A	LI	
Clonazepam	2.5%	AM	Monitor for infant drowsiness, weight gain, and developmental milestones; monitor infant serum levels if excessive persistent sedation.
Diazepam	3%	X	Long half-life leads to accumulation in the newborn. If used, monitor for lethargy and weight loss. After a single dose, wait 6 to 8 hours before feeding a preterm or newborn infant.
Lorazepam	8.5%	S	
Midazolam	0.06%	S	Delay breastfeeding for 4 hours following dose (6–8 hours for newborn or preterm infant).
Oxazepam	0.7%	S	
Temazepam	N/A	S	Take bedtime dose after last feeding.
Other agents			
Buspirone	N/A	LI	
Gabapentin	1.3%–3.8%	S	
Pregabalin	7%	S	
Propranolol	<0.1%–0.9%	S	

Note. N/A=not available.
[a]**Safety ratings**:
- AM—Additional monitoring required if used while breastfeeding, because of high breast milk levels, higher infant plasma levels, and/or associated adverse effects.
- LI—Limited or no information available; use of alternative medications is recommended (especially in preterm infant or newborn).
- S—Considered to be safe for breastfeeding because of low breast milk levels, low infant plasma levels, short half-life, and/or low toxicity.
- X—Avoid breastfeeding while taking.

Source. Briggs et al. 2021; Drugs and Lactation Database (LactMed) 2006–.

Mood Stabilizers

Impact of Pregnancy-Related Physiological Changes

- **Lithium**—Changes in total body water, plasma volume, and glomerular filtration rate (GFR) may cause lithium levels to decrease in the second trimester and increase the risk of toxic lithium levels in the third trimester. Monitor levels every 4 weeks until 34–36 weeks gestation. Dose should be held with initiation of labor. Lower the dosage after delivery, then monitor with twice-weekly serum levels until 2 weeks postpartum (Chokhawala et al. 2022; Poels et al. 2018; Wesseloo et al. 2017).
- **Lamotrigine**—Increased renal clearance in the first trimester and increased estrogen-induced liver metabolism in the third trimester necessitate lamotrigine dosage adjustments. If possible, obtain a baseline serum level at the patient's optimal dose prior to conception. Anticipate increasing dosage by 20%–25% during pregnancy to maintain prepregnancy levels. Check serum levels every 4–5 weeks during pregnancy and every 1–2 weeks postpartum. Clearance and metabolism return to normal after 1 month postpartum (Payne 2021; Stahl 2017).
- **Valproic acid**—Total valproic acid concentration may decrease during pregnancy, and unbound valproic acid concentration may increase (due to a decrease in serum albumin). Monitor total and unbound valproic acid concentrations before conception, monthly during pregnancy, and weekly for 3 weeks after delivery (Arfman et al. 2020).
- **Carbamazepine**—Carbamazepine concentration and clearance undergo minimal changes during pregnancy. Obtain a prepregnancy level; clinical changes should prompt a recheck of the level and comparison to the baseline prepregnancy value (Arfman et al. 2020).
- **Oxcarbazepine**—Increased oxcarbazepine clearance in the second trimester may require dosage adjustments (Iqbal et al. 2001; Stahl 2017).

Malformations

- **Lithium** has been associated with an increased risk of cardiovascular malformations, including Ebstein's anomaly (RR 1.9% vs. RR 1.15% for general population) (Patorno et al. 2017). If lithium is used during the first trimester, offer fetal anomaly scanning at 20 weeks gestation (Poels et al. 2018).
- **Lithium** is also associated with an increased risk of other major malformations (adjusted risk [AR] 7.4% vs. AR 4.3% for general population); the risk of malformation may increase with higher dosages (Fornaro et al. 2020).
- **Lamotrigine** has not been associated with an increased risk of major malformations in recent large studies (Payne 2021).

- **Valproic acid, carbamazepine, and oxcarbazepine** are associated with several major malformations and should be discontinued or transitioned to an alternative medication prior to pregnancy (Iqbal et al. 2001; Jentink et al. 2010; Payne 2021; Stahl 2017). If valproic acid, carbamazepine, or oxcarbazepine must be continued in pregnancy, use the lowest effective dosage or serum level; obtaining an alpha-fetoprotein level and fetal anatomy scan at 16–18 weeks is recommended (Matlow and Koren 2012).

Maternal Effects

- **Lithium** is associated with increased risk of euthyroid/hypothyroid goiter, weight gain, and nephrogenic diabetes insipidus. Monitor thyroid-stimulating hormone (TSH) and basic metabolic panel (BMP) frequently (Poels et al. 2018; Wesseloo et al. 2017).
- **Carbamazepine** is associated with increased risk of transient hepatic dysfunction and preeclampsia. Monitor the comprehensive metabolic panel (CMP) and protein-to-creatinine ratio in the third trimester (Iqbal et al. 2001).

Infant Effects

- Infants of mothers who receive **lithium** during labor should be monitored postpartum for floppy infant syndrome (Yonkers et al. 2004).
- Routine maternal folate supplementation of 0.4–0.8 mg/day has not been found to prevent neural tube defects (NTDs) associated with **antiepileptic drugs (AEDs)** (Hill et al. 2010). Some guidelines recommend that women at high risk for NTDs should be prescribed high-dosage folate supplementation (4–5 mg/day) (Tomson et al. 2020). To date, it is unclear whether high-dosage folate prevents AED-associated NTDs (Patel et al. 2018; Tomson et al. 2019; Wilson and O'Connor 2021).
- Some guidelines recommend oral vitamin K supplementation (10–20 mg/day) in the last month of pregnancy for mothers taking enzyme-inducing AEDs, such as **carbamazepine**, to reduce the risk of maternal postpartum hemorrhage and neonatal hemorrhage (Borgelt et al. 2016). The American Academy of Pediatrics recommends that all infants receive a single dose of intramuscular vitamin K to prevent vitamin K deficiency bleeding (Hand et al. 2022).

Breastfeeding

- Table 15–3 provides breastfeeding guidelines for commonly prescribed mood stabilizers based on the most recently available data from LactMed, the majority of which are from case reports. Safety ratings are determined via a combination of RID, infant serum levels, active metabolites, and reported adverse effects.}

Table 15–3. Mood stabilizers: guidelines for breastfeeding

Medication	Relative infant dose	Safety rating[a]	Notes
Carbamazepine	<10%[b]	AM	High levels in breast milk; infant serum levels are sometimes measurable but often below anticonvulsant therapeutic range. Monitor infant for signs of hepatic dysfunction/jaundice, drowsiness, adequate weight gain, developmental milestones.
Lamotrigine	2%–31%	AM	High levels in breast milk. Monitor infant for apnea, rash, sedation, poor suckling.
Lithium	0%–42%	AM	Monitor infant for hypotonia, dehydration, impaired thyroid function. Check infant lithium level, creatinine, blood urea nitrogen, and TSH 2–10 days after birth, then periodically or if concerned for toxicity.
Oxcarbazepine	1.5%–1.7%	S	Monitor for drowsiness, adequate weight gain, and developmental milestones.
Valproic acid/ divalproex	<10%[b]	S	Monitor for bruising, bleeding, or jaundice (theoretical risk for hepatotoxicity).

Note. TSH=thyroid-stimulating hormone.
[a]**Safety ratings:**
- AM—Additional monitoring required if used while breastfeeding, because of high breast milk levels, higher infant plasma levels, and/or associated adverse effects.
- S—Considered to be safe for breastfeeding because of low breast milk levels, low infant plasma levels, short half-life, and/or low toxicity.

[b]Tomson et al. 2022.
Source. Drugs and Lactation Database (LactMed) 2006–; .

Antipsychotics

Impact of Pregnancy-Related Physiological Changes

- Serum concentrations of **aripiprazole and quetiapine** decrease by 50% or more as pregnancy progresses. **Olanzapine and clozapine** concentrations do not appear to decrease during pregnancy. Concentrations of **haloperidol and perphenazine** may also decrease over the course of pregnancy, although additional data are needed to confirm this (Westin et al. 2018).

Malformations

- A large 2016 study found that use of first- or second-generation antipsychotics in early pregnancy does not increase the risk of overall congenital malformations and cardiac malformations, with the exception being use of **risperidone**, which has been associated with a small increased risk of overall malformations (RR 1.26) and cardiac malformations (RR 1.26) (Huybrechts et al. 2016).

Maternal Effects

- Exposure to **second-generation antipsychotics** during pregnancy is associated with an increased risk of gestational diabetes (OR 1.43), cesarean section (OR 1.35), large-for-gestational-age newborn (OR 1.57), and preterm birth (OR 1.29) compared with nonexposure to second-generation antipsychotics. Second-generation antipsychotics are associated with an increased risk of cesarean section and large-for-gestational-age newborns compared with first-generation antipsychotics (Ellfolk et al. 2020).
- Monitor maternal complete blood count (CBC), CMP, and hemoglobin A1c (HbA1c) and consider an early glucose challenge test. Offer routine ultrasound monitoring of fetal size in late pregnancy (Payne 2017; Stahl 2017).
- **Aripiprazole** may lower serum prolactin, with resultant cessation of lactation in some cases (Drugs and Lactation Database [LactMed] 2006–).

Infant Effects

- Exposure to **first- or second-generation antipsychotics** is associated with lower Apgar scores, a greater need for neonatal or NICU treatment, and more frequent hospitalization at 7 days postpartum compared with infants not exposed to either first- or second-generation antipsychotics (Ellfolk et al. 2020).
- Use of **first- or second-generation antipsychotics** late in pregnancy has been associated with neonatal withdrawal syndrome and/or extrapyramidal symptoms, which are noted more prominently with **haloperidol**. Use of more than one psychotropic drug increases the risk of withdrawal symptoms. Timing of onset of withdrawal symptoms ranges from delivery to 1 month postpartum. Infants who are exclusively breastfed may have less risk of withdrawal or reduced symptoms of withdrawal (Convertino et al. 2016; Kanemura et al. 2020; Payne 2017; Stahl 2017; U.S. Food and Drug Administration 2011).
- **Clozapine** has been associated with floppy infant syndrome and neonatal seizures in case reports (Mehta and Van Lieshout 2017).
- Some authors recommend monitoring infants exposed to **clozapine** for agranulocytosis with routine CBCs for up to 6 months after delivery (Kulkarni et al. 2015; Payne 2017). This recommendation appears to be based on case report data from the 1990s (Dev and Krupp 1995). A more recent case series did not find any instances of agranulocytosis; however, more information is needed to accurately gauge this risk (Imaz et al. 2018).

- A large birth cohort study found a possible association between exposure to **aripiprazole** during the first and/or second half of pregnancy and increased risk of neurodevelopmental disorders (e.g., autism spectrum disorder [ASD], ADHD, speech or language disorder, behavioral disorder); there was no increased risk of neurodevelopmental disorder associated with any of the other antipsychotics examined in the study (Straub et al. 2022). Another large population-based cohort study did not find convincing evidence to support an increased risk of ADHD or ASD in infants exposed to antipsychotics during gestation (Hálfdánarson et al. 2022).

Breastfeeding

- Table 15–4 provides breastfeeding guidelines for commonly prescribed antipsychotic medications based on the most recently available data from LactMed, the majority of which are from case reports. Safety ratings are determined via a combination of RID, infant serum levels, active metabolites, and reported adverse effects.

Table 15–4. Antipsychotics: guidelines for breastfeeding

Medication	Relative infant dose	Safety rating[a]	Notes
FGAs			
Chlorpromazine	—[a]	AM	Monitor for infant drowsiness.
Fluphenazine	LND	LI	
Haloperidol	—[a]	AM	Daily doses up to 10 mg do not usually affect breastfed infant. Hindmilk drug levels greater than foremilk drug levels.
Loxapine	LND	LI	
Perphenazine	0.1%	AM	Monitor for excessive drowsiness and for developmental milestones.
Prochlorperazine	LND	LI	Intermittent use for nausea likely safe.
SGAs			
Aripiprazole	0.7%–12.7%	LI	
Asenapine	LND	S	
Brexpiprazole	LND	LI	
Cariprazine	LND	LI	
Clozapine	LND	X	If used, monitor for excessive sedation and periodically monitor infant's WBC.

Table 15–4. Antipsychotics: guidelines for breastfeeding *(continued)*

Medication	Relative infant dose	Safety rating[a]	Notes
Lurasidone	—[d]	LI	
Olanzapine	0.13%–1.6%	S	
Paliperidone	<1%	LI	
Quetiapine	0.005%–0.43%	S	
Risperidone	2.2%–4.7%	LI	
Ziprasidone	—[e]	S	

Note. FGAs=first-generation antipsychotics; LND=limited to no data; N/A=not available; SGAs=second-generation antipsychotics; WBC=white blood count.

[a]**Safety ratings**:

- AM—Additional monitoring required if used while breastfeeding, because of high breast milk levels, higher infant plasma levels, and/or associated adverse effects.
- LI—Limited or no information available; use of alternative medications is recommended (especially in preterm infant or newborn).
- S—Considered to be safe for breastfeeding because of low breast milk levels, low infant plasma levels, short half-life, and/or low toxicity.
- X—Avoid breastfeeding while taking.

[b]Chlorpromazine shows no clear or consistent relationship for RID; some transmission but limited data.

[c]Haloperidol is excreted in breast milk, but RID not known or limited data.

[d]Lurasidone likely excretes no drug in breast milk, given that 99% of drug is plasma-bound proteins (Lurasidone 2023).

[e]Ziprasidone RID may be <10% (Schlotterbeck et al. 2009).

Source. Drugs and Lactation Database (LactMed) 2006–.

Stimulants

Impact of Pregnancy-Related Physiological Changes

- **Amphetamine, atomoxetine, and clonidine** are substrates of CYP2D6, which has increased activity in pregnancy. **Atomoxetine** is also a substrate of CYP2C19, which has decreased activity in pregnancy (Flockhart et al. 2021; Ke et al. 2014).

Malformations

- In utero exposure to prescribed **amphetamines** has not been associated with an increased risk of malformation (Huybrechts et al. 2018; Kittel-Schneider et al. 2021).
- Maternal use of **methylphenidate** in the first trimester has been associated with increased risk of cardiac malformations in the newborn, although absolute risk remains small (adjusted relative risk [aRR] 1.28) (Huybrechts et al. 2018).

- First-trimester exposure to **modafinil or armodafinil** has been associated with increased risk of major malformations, with an absolute risk of 12% (adjusted OR 2.7) compared with unexposed pregnancies (Damkier and Broe 2020; Kaplan et al. 2021; Kittel-Schneider et al. 2021).
- Data on use of **atomoxetine or guanfacine** in pregnancy are very limited; consider discontinuation (Kittel-Schneider et al. 2021; Ornoy 2018).
- Studies examining use of **clonidine** as an antihypertensive during pregnancy have found no evidence of teratogenicity (Ornoy 2018).

Maternal Effects

- **Amphetamines and methylphenidate** have been associated with a minor increased risk of preeclampsia (Cohen et al. 2017; Kittel-Schneider et al. 2021).
- **Methylphenidate and atomoxetine** have been associated with increased risk of miscarriage, although similar adjusted relative risks for treated (aRR 1.55) and untreated (aRR 1.56) ADHD indicated that the underlying disorder may contribute to the association (Bro et al. 2015).
- **Guanfacine, methylphenidate, and high doses of amphetamines** may interfere with milk production via serum prolactin reduction (Drugs and Lactation Database [LactMed] 2006–).

Infant Effects

- The long-term impact of in utero exposure to stimulant medication is unknown (Ornoy 2018).
- In utero exposure to ADHD medications (not specific to any one medication) is associated with an increased risk (RR 1.88) of NICU admission (Jiang et al. 2019).
- **Stimulant monotherapy (amphetamines or methylphenidate)** during the second half of pregnancy has been associated with increased risk (aRR 1.30) of preterm birth (Cohen et al. 2017).
- Methylphenidate and atomoxetine have been associated with a risk (aRR 2.06) of Apgar scores less than 10 (Bro et al. 2015).

Breastfeeding

- Table 15–5 provides breastfeeding guidelines for commonly prescribed ADHD medications based on the most recently available data from LactMed, the majority of which are from case reports. Safety ratings are determined via a combination of RID, infant serum levels, active metabolites, and reported adverse effects.

Table 15–5. Stimulants: guidelines for breastfeeding

Medication	Relative infant dose	Safety rating[a]	Notes
Amphetamines	1.9%–2.1%	X	No definitive evidence of adverse infant effects, but high transfer into breast milk occurs even at lower maternal dosages. Use lowest effective dosage if unable to discontinue.
Atomoxetine	N/A	LI	
Clonidine	4.1%–8.4%	X	High transfer to breast milk and infant serum. Monitor infant for hypotonia, drowsiness, apnea, seizure-like episodes.
Guanfacine	N/A	LI	
Methylphenidate	0.16%–0.7%	S	
Modafinil/armodafinil	5.3%	LI	

Note. N/A=not available.
[a]**Safety ratings**:
- LI—Limited or no information available; use of alternative medications is recommended (especially in preterm infant or newborn).
- S—Considered to be safe for breastfeeding because of low breast milk levels, low infant plasma levels, short half-life, and/or low toxicity.
- X—Avoid breastfeeding while taking.

Source. Drugs and Lactation Database (LactMed) 2006–; Kittel-Schneider et al. 2021; Ornoy 2018.

Hypnotics

Impact of Pregnancy-Related Physiological Changes

- **Zolpidem, zaleplon, and suvorexant** are substrates of CYP3A4, which has increased activity in pregnancy. **Suvorexant** is also a substrate of CYP2C19, which has decreased activity in pregnancy (Flockhart et al. 2021).

Malformations

- Data on first-trimester use of **zopiclone, zolpidem, or zaleplon** indicate that these agents carry no increased risk for congenital malformations (Juric et al. 2009; Wikner and Källén 2011).

- Data on the effects of eszopiclone, suvorexant, lemborexant, or ramelteon in human pregnancy are very limited (Drugs and Lactation Database [LactMed] 2006–; Esai Inc 2019; Merck Sharp and Dohme Corp 2020; Takeda Pharmaceuticals America 2010).
- Very limited data are available on use of **exogenous melatonin** in human pregnancy—specifically, how such use may affect the development of the fetal neuroendocrine reproductive axis. Occasional low doses (<10 mg) during pregnancy may be safe, but high and/or frequent doses should be avoided (Briggs et al. 2021).
- A systematic review and meta-analysis found that offspring exposed to **H_1 antihistamines (e.g., diphenhydramine, hydroxyzine)** did not have a higher risk of major malformations compared with the unexposed control population (Etwel et al. 2017).

Maternal Effects

- **Ramelteon** can increase prolactin levels; one study found an increase of 34% in nonbreastfeeding women who took 16 mg every night for 6 months, but there was no report of hyperprolactinemia symptoms (Richardson and Wang-Weigand 2009).
- A systematic review and meta-analysis found that women who took **H1 antihistamines (e.g., diphenhydramine, hydroxyzine)** during pregnancy did not have a higher risk of spontaneous abortion or premature birth (Etwel et al. 2017).

Infant Effects

- A study comparing 45 women who received **zolpidem** during pregnancy and 45 matched pregnant women without zolpidem exposure found an increased rate of preterm delivery and low birthweight in the zolpidem cohort, but this increase was not statistically significant. Also increased, but not reaching statistical significance, were symptoms of respiratory difficulty, lethargy, and hypotonia in the zolpidem-exposed neonates (Juric et al. 2009).
- If **zopiclone** is used during the last weeks of pregnancy, monitor for reduced fetal movement and fetal heart rate variability and for neonatal hypothermia, hypotonia, and feeding difficulties. Infants should also be monitored for withdrawal symptoms in the postnatal period (Sanofi-Aventis Canada 2018).

Breastfeeding

- Table 15–6 provides breastfeeding guidelines for commonly prescribed hypnotic drugs based on the most recently available data from LactMed, the majority of which are from case reports. Safety ratings are determined via a combination of RID, infant serum levels, active metabolites, and reported adverse effects.

Table 15–6. Hypnotics: guidelines for breastfeeding

Medication	Relative infant dose	Safety rating[a]	Notes
Diphenhydramine	N/A	LI	If used, consider bedtime doses after last feeding of the day.
Eszopiclone	N/A	LI	If used, monitor infant for excessive sedation.
Hydroxyzine	N/A	LI	Small occasional doses unlikely to cause adverse effects; avoid larger doses/prolonged use.
Lemborexant	N/A	LI	
Melatonin	N/A	LI	
Ramelteon	0.24%	LI	If used, monitor for infant somnolence and feeding problems. Consider interrupting breastfeeding and pumping/discarding milk during treatment and for 25 hours after mother's last ingestion.
Suvorexant	N/A	LI	If used, monitor infant for somnolence.
Zaleplon	1.4%	LI	
Zolpidem	0.004%–0.019%	S	Avoid nighttime feeding after taking dose. Monitor infant for sedation, hypotonia, respiratory depression.
Zopiclone	1.2%–3.2%	LI	

Note. N/A=not available.

[a]**Safety ratings**:

- LI—Limited or no information available; use of alternative medications is recommended (especially in preterm infant or newborn).
- S—Considered to be safe for breastfeeding because of low breast milk levels, low infant plasma levels, short half-life, and/or low toxicity.

Source. Briggs et al. 2021; Drugs and Lactation Database (LactMed) 2006–; Saito et al. 2022; Takeda Pharmaceuticals America 2010.

Medications Used in Substance Use Disorders

Impact of Pregnancy-Related Physiological Changes

- **Methadone** dosing in pregnant women usually starts at 20–30 mg/day; the dosage is increased in 5- to 10-mg increments with a goal of reaching a dosage that mitigates withdrawal symptoms and cravings with minimum sedation. Physiological changes associated with pregnancy may necessitate split dosing (12-hour intervals) (Rodriguez and Klie 2019).
- **Methadone** is a substrate of CYP3A4 and CYP2B6, both of which have increased activity in pregnancy (Flockhart et al. 2021; Ke et al. 2014).

Malformations

- A 2019 study found that neonates exposed to **acamprosate** did not have significant differences in birthweight or congenital abnormalities (including fetal alcohol syndrome) in comparison with an alcohol-exposed group and a community control group (Kelty et al. 2019).
- Limited data are available on **varenicline** in pregnancy. A 2013 prospective cohort study examined 23 women with varying durations (1 day to 16 weeks) of varenicline use during pregnancy (Harrison-Woolrych et al. 2013). Out of 17 live births, 5 had adverse outcomes (1 with birth asphyxia and recurrent chest infections, 1 with gastroesophageal reflux, 1 with ankyloglossia, and 2 with feeding difficulties).
- A 2020 study examining **naltrexone** exposure found no differences in obstetric outcomes or birth anomalies between mothers taking naltrexone and mothers taking buprenorphine or methadone (Towers et al. 2020).
- A 2016 population-based study found that infants born to women treated with **methadone** during pregnancy were two times more likely than infants of mothers taking buprenorphine to have any congenital malformations or major malformations when compared with the general population. However, the authors noted that the increased risk with methadone could be related to confounders as well as to the higher proportion of women older than 35 years on methadone compared with the younger population on buprenorphine (Wurst et al. 2016).
- The same 2016 population-based study found no statistical difference in the frequency of congenital malformations or major malformations in the infants of women treated with **buprenorphine** during pregnancy when compared with the general population (Wurst et al. 2016).
- Although **nicotine replacement therapy** (NRT) has not been adequately studied in pregnancy, impaired fetal growth is a concern due to the possibility of related decreases in uterine blood flow and increases in uterine vascular resistance. NRT use during pregnancy may be reasonable if other nonpharmacological approaches to smoking cessation have failed. Women should be counseled that continuing to smoke while using NRT may pose a higher risk to the fetus than either smoking or NRT use alone (Briggs et al. 2021).

- Insufficient human data are available to estimate the risk of major birth defects or miscarriage associated with **naloxone** use in pregnancy. The fetus should be evaluated for signs of opioid withdrawal distress if naloxone is administered to the mother (Adapt Pharma 2020).

Maternal Effects

- A 2019 study found that rates of hospital admission during pregnancy among women treated with **acamprosate** during pregnancy and during the first 42 days postpartum were not significantly different from rates among women in the community control group but were significantly lower than rates among women with a recent history of problematic alcohol use (alcohol comparison group) (Kelty et al. 2019).
- A 2016 population study found higher frequencies of cesarean section and preterm birth for women treated with **methadone or buprenorphine** compared with the general population, but these findings did not reach the level of statistical significance (Wurst et al. 2016).
- Treatment with **methadone or buprenorphine** during pregnancy has been associated with a decreased probability of maternal overdose; the probability steadily declines as treatment duration increases. In one study, women with opioid use disorders who were treated with methadone or buprenorphine during pregnancy had a decreased probability of low-birthweight and preterm birth in comparison with those who did not receive treatment during pregnancy (Krans et al. 2021).

Infant Effects

- A 2020 study examining **naltrexone** exposure found that neonates of mothers with opioid use disorder who took naltrexone during pregnancy had a significantly lower rate of neonatal abstinence syndrome compared with neonates of mothers who took buprenorphine or methadone (Towers et al. 2020).
- A 2016 population study found higher frequencies of low-birthweight, small-for-gestational-age infants and lower Apgar scores for infants whose mothers received **methadone** compared with the general population, but these findings did not reach the level of statistical significance (Wurst et al. 2016).

Breastfeeding

- Table 15–7 provides breastfeeding guidelines for drugs commonly prescribed for treatment of substance use disorders based on the most recently available data from LactMed, the majority of which are from case reports. Safety ratings are determined via a combination of RID, infant serum levels, active metabolites, and reported adverse effects.

Table 15–7. Medications used to treat substance use disorders: guidelines for breastfeeding

Medication	Relative infant dose	Safety rating[a]	Notes
Acamprosate	N/A	LI	Benefits of taking acamprosate may outweigh unknown risks if it successfully helps mother to abstain from alcohol.
Buprenorphine	0.18%–2.4%	S	Enters breast milk but is poorly absorbed by infant. Monitor infant for drowsiness, respiratory depression, adequate weight gain, and developmental milestones.
Methadone	0.6%–6%	AM	Breastfeeding is encouraged for stable women who took methadone during pregnancy for opioid use disorder; it may decrease neonatal withdrawal symptoms in infants. Monitor infant for increased sleepiness, limpness, and difficulty breathing.
Naloxone	N/A	S	Should not affect infant because it is not orally bioavailable.
Naltrexone	0.86%	S	
Nicotine replacement therapy (NRT)	1.9%–7.8%	X	Nicotine reduces infant's ability to auto-resuscitate in hypoxic episodes (risk factor for sudden infant death syndrome [SIDS]). Nicotine from a 21-mg transdermal patch passes into breast milk at an equivalence of smoking 17 cigarettes/day. Concentrations in breast milk vary, depending on method of NRT.
Varenicline	N/A	LI	Benefits of taking varenicline may outweigh unknown risks if it successfully helps mother to abstain from smoking.

Note. N/A=not available.

[a]**Safety ratings**:

- AM—Additional monitoring required if used while breastfeeding, because of high breast milk levels, higher infant plasma levels, and/or associated adverse effects.
- LI—Limited or no information available; use of alternative medications is recommended (especially in preterm infant or newborn).
- S—Considered to be safe for breastfeeding because of low breast milk levels, low infant plasma levels, short half-life, and/or low toxicity.
- X—Avoid breastfeeding while taking.

Source. Briggs et al. 2021; Drugs and Lactation Database (LactMed) 2006–.

Neuroactive Steroids for Treatment of Postpartum Depression

- Brexanolone (Zulresso) and zuranolone (Zurzuvae) are positive allosteric modulators of $GABA_A$ receptors that are FDA approved for the treatment of postpartum depression (PPD) (Cornett et al. 2021; Deligiannidis et al. 2023). Brexanolone is approved for people age 15 years and older (Sage Therapeutics 2022), and zuranolone is approved for adults (Sage Therapeutics and Biogen 2023).

Brexanolone

Administration and Safety

- Brexanolone is administered intravenously over a 60-hour period in the presence of a health care professional, with continuous pulse-oximetry monitoring ti mitigate the risk of excess sedation or sudden loss of consciousness (Reddy et al. 2023; Sage Therapeutics 2022). Excess sedation has been most commonly linked to concomitant use of benzodiazepines (Patterson et al. 2024). Brexanolone is available only through a Risk Evaluation and Mitigation Strategies (REMS) program (Reddy et al. 2023).

Maternal/Infant Effects

- Insufficient data on brexanolone use in pregnant people are available to determine risk of birth defects or adverse maternal or fetal outcomes in humans; however, serious adverse outcomes have been identified in animal studies (Reddy et al. 2023).

Breastfeeding

- A study of 12 women receiving brexanolone calculated a maximum relative infant dose (RID) of 1.3% via breast milk (Wald et al. 2022). Although no data are available on the effects of brexanolone in breast-fed infants, Wald et al. (2022) estimated the risk of adverse effects to infants to be low because of the low RID and brexanolone's low oral bioavailability (less than 5% in adults).

Zuranolone

Administration and Safety

- Zuranolone is administered orally once daily in the evening for 14 days and requires administration with fat-containing food (Deligiannidis et al. 2023; Sage Therapeutics and Biogen 2023). Zuranolone can be used alone or as an adjunctive treatment with oral antidepressants (Sage Therapeutics and Biogen 2023).

Maternal/Infant Effects

- As with brexanolone, there are no available data on the effects of zuranolone in pregnant people, but data from animal studies suggest that zuranolone may cause adverse fetal effects (Sage Therapeutics and Biogen 2023).

Breastfeeding

- Lactation data are limited to one study with 14 women who were administered 30 mg zuranolone daily for 5 days; he daily RID was estimated to be 0.357% (Sage Therapeutics and Biogen 2023). There are no available data on zuranolone's effects in breastfed infants.

Neuromodulation Therapies

Electroconvulsive Therapy

Impact of Pregnancy-Related Physiological Changes

- The care team for pregnant women receiving electroconvulsive therapy (**ECT**) should include an anesthesiologist who has experience with pregnant patients and can adjust medications as necessary (Rose et al. 2020).
- The patient's physical positioning during ECT must take into account the aortocaval compression that occurs in advanced pregnancy (Rose et al. 2020).

Malformations

- The estimated safety of **ECT** in pregnancy is based on case series of ECT in pregnancy. Although data are limited, it does not appear that ECT increases the risk of malformations (Rose et al. 2020).

Maternal Effects

- Pregnant women have a higher risk of aspiration and intubation challenges that must be considered by the **ECT** anesthesiologist.

Infant Effects

- Care must be taken during **ECT** to ensure adequate oxygenation and perfusion, given that ECT-induced seizures increase oxygen demand and cardiac work, which may decrease uterine and placental perfusion (Rose et al. 2020).
- Continuous fetal monitoring during ECT or pre-/postprocedure nonstress tests to ensure fetal well-being should be conducted for **ECT** treatments administered after 23 weeks gestation, and the ECT treatment setting should be able to accommodate emergent delivery (Rose et al. 2020).

Breastfeeding

- Available data, although limited, indicate that **ECT** does not adversely affect lactation and does not adversely affect the breastfeeding infant. The risks associated with anesthetic agents are minimal and can be further mitigated by delaying breastfeeding until a few hours posttreatment. Alternatively, breast milk can be collected and stored on the day prior to ECT (Babu et al. 2013; Gressier et al. 2015).

Transcranial Magnetic Stimulation

Malformations

- Repetitive transcranial magnetic stimulation (**rTMS**) has not been associated with an increased risk for malformations, although data are extremely limited (Lee et al. 2021).

Maternal Effects

- Pregnant women undergoing **rTMS** may experience minor side effects, including headaches, discomfort, and pain in the stimulation area. These side effects should remit by the end of the treatment. Supine hypotension has been noted in some pregnant women receiving rTMS, but this effect may be prevented through postural correction (Lee et al. 2021).

Infant Effects

- None of the 23 studies in a 2023 systematic review examining TMS for peripartum depression reported major side effects for newborns (Miuli et al. 2023).

Breastfeeding

- **rTMS** has not been shown to adversely affect lactation or breastfeeding (Cox et al. 2020).

References

ACOG Committee on Practice Bulletins—Obstetrics: ACOG Practice Bulletin: clinical management guidelines for obstetrician-gynecologists number 92, April 2008 (replaces practice bulletin number 87, November 2007). Use of psychiatric medications during pregnancy and lactation. Obstet Gynecol 111(4):1001–1020, 2008 18378767

Adapt Pharma: Narcan (naloxone) package insert. Plymouth Meeting, PA, Adapt Pharma, revised August 2020. Available at: https://www.accessdata.fda.gov/drugsatfda_docs/label/2020/208411Orig1s004lbl.pdf. Accessed March 13, 2024.

Anderson PO, Sauberan JB: Modeling drug passage into human milk. Clin Pharmacol Ther 100(1):42–52, 2016 27060684

Andrade C: Gestational exposure to antidepressant drugs and neurodevelopment: an examination of language, mathematics, intelligence, and other cognitive outcomes. J Clin Psychiatry 83(1):22f14388, 2022 35081278

Arfman IJ, Wammes-van der Heijden EA, Ter Horst PGJ, et al: Therapeutic drug monitoring of antiepileptic drugs in women with epilepsy before, during, and after pregnancy. Clin Pharmacokinet 59(4):427–445, 2020 31912315

Babu GN, Thippeswamy H, Chandra PS: Use of electroconvulsive therapy (ECT) in postpartum psychosis—a naturalistic prospective study. Arch Womens Ment Health 16(3):247–251, 2013 23568390

Bellantuono C, Tofani S, Di Sciascio G, et al: Benzodiazepine exposure in pregnancy and risk of major malformations: a critical overview. Gen Hosp Psychiatry 35(1):3–8, 2013 23044244
Bellantuono C, Vargas M, Mandarelli G, et al: The safety of serotonin-noradrenaline reuptake inhibitors (SNRIs) in pregnancy and breastfeeding: a comprehensive review. Hum Psychopharmacol 30(3):143–151, 2015 25784291
Bérard A, Sheehy O, Zhao J-P, et al: SSRI and SNRI use during pregnancy and the risk of persistent pulmonary hypertension of the newborn. Br J Clin Pharmacol 83(5):1126–1133, 2017 27874994
Betcher HK, Wisner KL: Psychotropic treatment during pregnancy: research synthesis and clinical care principles. J Womens Health (Larchmt) 29(3):310–318, 2020 31800350
Borgelt LM, Hart FM, Bainbridge JL: Epilepsy during pregnancy: focus on management strategies. Int J Womens Health 8:505–517, 2016 27703396
Briggs GG, Freeman RK, Towers CV, et al: Drugs in Pregnancy and Lactation: A Reference Guide to Fetal and Neonatal Risk, 12th Edition. Philadelphia, Lippincott Williams & Wilkins, 2021, p 1775
Bristol Myers Squibb: Buspar (buspirone) package insert, Princeton, NJ, Bristol Myers Squibb, 2010. Available at: https://www.accessdata.fda.gov/drugsatfda_docs/label/2010/018731s051lbl.pdf. Accessed March 13, 2024.
Bro SP, Kjaersgaard MIS, Parner ET, et al: Adverse pregnancy outcomes after exposure to methylphenidate or atomoxetine during pregnancy. Clin Epidemiol 7:139–147, 2015 25657597
Carvalho AF, Sharma MS, Brunoni AR, et al: The safety, tolerability and risks associated with the use of newer generation antidepressant drugs: a critical review of the literature. Psychother Psychosom 85(5):270–288, 2016 27508501
Chokhawala K, Lee S, Saadabadi A: Lithium, in StatPearls. Treasure Island, FL, StatPearls Publishing, 2022. Available at: https://www.ncbi.nlm.nih.gov/books/NBK519062/. Accessed March 13, 2024.
Cohen JM, Hernández-Díaz S, Bateman BT, et al: Placental complications associated with psychostimulant use in pregnancy. Obstet Gynecol 130(6):1192–1201, 2017 29112657
Cohen LS, Altshuler LL, Harlow BL, et al: Relapse of major depression during pregnancy in women who maintain or discontinue antidepressant treatment. JAMA 295(5):499–507, 2006 16449615
Convertino I, Sansone AC, Marino A, et al: Neonatal adaptation issues after maternal exposure to prescription drugs: withdrawal syndromes and residual pharmacological effects. Drug Saf 39(10):903–924, 2016 27289228
Cornett EM, Rando L, Labbé AM, et al: Brexanolone to treat postpartum depression in adult women. Psychopharmacol Bull 51(2):115–130, 2021 34092826
Cox EQ, Killenberg S, Frische R, et al: Repetitive transcranial magnetic stimulation for the treatment of postpartum depression. J Affect Disord 264:193–200, 2020 32056750
Damkier P, Broe A: First-trimester pregnancy exposure to modafinil and risk of congenital malformations. JAMA 323(4):374–376, 2020 31990303
Deligiannidis KM, Meltzer-Brody S, Maximos B, et al: Zuranolone for the treatment of postpartum depression. Am J Psychiatry 180(9):668–675, 2023 37491938
Dev V, Krupp P: The side effects and safety of clozapine. Rev Contemp Pharmacother 6(2):197–208, 1995
Drugs and Lactation Database (LactMed) [Internet]. Bethesda, MD, National Institute of Child Health and Human Development, 2006–. Available at: https://www.ncbi.nlm.nih.gov/books/NBK501922/. Accessed March 13, 2024.
Easter A, Sandall J, Howard LM: Obstetric near misses among women with serious mental illness: data linkage cohort study. Br J Psychiatry 219(3):494–500, 2021 33427147
Einarson A, Bonari L, Voyer-Lavigne S, et al: A multicentre prospective controlled study to determine the safety of trazodone and nefazodone use during pregnancy. Can J Psychiatry 48(2):106–110, 2003 12655908
Eisai Inc: Dayvigo (lemborexant) package insert. Woodcliff Lake, NJ, Eisai, 2019. Available at: https://www.accessdata.fda.gov/drugsatfda_docs/label/2019/212028s000lbl.pdf. Accessed March 13, 2024.

Ellfolk M, Leinonen MK, Gissler M, et al: Second-generation antipsychotics and pregnancy complications. Eur J Clin Pharmacol 76(1):107–115, 2020 31680189

Etwel F, Faught LH, Rieder MJ, et al: The risk of adverse pregnancy outcome after first trimester exposure to H1 antihistamines: a systematic review and meta-analysis. Drug Saf 40(2):121–132, 2017 27878468

Flockhart DA, Thacker D, McDonald C, et al: The Flockhart Cytochrome P450 Drug-Drug Interaction Table. Bloomington, IN, Division of Clinical Pharmacology, Indiana University School of Medicine, 2021. Available at: https://drug-interactions.medicine.iu.edu. Accessed March 13, 2024.

Fornaro M, Maritan E, Ferranti R, et al: Lithium exposure during pregnancy and the postpartum period: a systematic review and meta-analysis of safety and efficacy outcomes. Am J Psychiatry 177(1):76–92, 2020 31623458

Freeman MP: ADHD and pregnancy. Am J Psychiatry 171(7):723–728, 2014 24980168

Freeman MP, Góez-Mogollón L, McInerney KA, et al: Obstetrical and neonatal outcomes after benzodiazepine exposure during pregnancy: results from a prospective registry of women with psychiatric disorders. Gen Hosp Psychiatry 53:73–79, 2018 29958100

Gadot Y, Koren G: The use of antidepressants in pregnancy: focus on maternal risks. J Obstet Gynaecol Can 37(1):56–63, 2015 25764038

Gao S-Y, Wu Q-J, Sun C, et al: Selective serotonin reuptake inhibitor use during early pregnancy and congenital malformations: a systematic review and meta-analysis of cohort studies of more than 9 million births. BMC Med 16(1):205, 2018 30415641

Gentile S: Tricyclic antidepressants in pregnancy and puerperium. Expert Opin Drug Saf 13(2):207–225, 2014 24383525

Gressier F, Rotenberg S, Cazas O, et al: Postpartum electroconvulsive therapy: a systematic review and case report. Gen Hosp Psychiatry 37(4):310–314, 2015 25929986

Hálfdánarson Ó, Cohen JM, Karlstad Ø, et al: Antipsychotic use in pregnancy and risk of attention/deficit-hyperactivity disorder and autism spectrum disorder: a Nordic cohort study. Evid Based Ment Health 25(2):54–62, 2022 34810174

Hand I, Noble L, Abrams SA: Vitamin K and the newborn infant. Pediatrics 149(3):e2021056036, 2022 35190810

Harrison-Woolrych M, Paterson H, Tan M: Exposure to the smoking cessation medicine varenicline during pregnancy: a prospective nationwide cohort study. Pharmacoepidemiol Drug Saf 22(10):1086–1092, 2013 23926076

Hendrick V, Suri R, Gitlin MJ, et al: Bupropion use during pregnancy: a systematic review. Prim Care Companion CNS Disord 19(5):17r02160, 2017 28973846

Hill DS, Wlodarczyk BJ, Palacios AM, et al: Teratogenic effects of antiepileptic drugs. Expert Rev Neurother 10(6):943–959, 2010 20518610

Huybrechts KF, Palmsten K, Avorn J, et al: Antidepressant use in pregnancy and the risk of cardiac defects. N Engl J Med 370(25):2397–2407, 2014 24941178

Huybrechts KF, Hernández-Díaz S, Patorno E, et al: Antipsychotic use in pregnancy and the risk for congenital malformations. JAMA Psychiatry 73(9):938–946, 2016 27540849

Huybrechts KF, Bröms G, Christensen LB, et al: Association between methylphenidate and amphetamine use in pregnancy and risk of congenital malformations: a cohort study from the international pregnancy safety study consortium. JAMA Psychiatry 75(2):167–175, 2018 29238795

Imaz ML, Oriolo G, Torra M, et al: Clozapine use during pregnancy and lactation: a case-series report. Front Pharmacol 9:264, 2018 29636684

Iqbal MM, Sohhan T, Mahmud SZ: The effects of lithium, valproic acid, and carbamazepine during pregnancy and lactation. J Toxicol Clin Toxicol 39(4):381–392, 2001 11527233

Jentink J, Loane MA, Dolk H, et al; EUROCAT Antiepileptic Study Working Group: Valproic acid monotherapy in pregnancy and major congenital malformations. N Engl J Med 362(23):2185–2193, 2010 20558369

Jiang H-Y, Xu L-L, Li Y-C, et al: Antidepressant use during pregnancy and risk of postpartum hemorrhage: a systematic review and meta-analysis. J Psychiatr Res 83:160–167, 2016 27637098
Jiang H-Y, Zhang X, Jiang C-M, et al: Maternal and neonatal outcomes after exposure to ADHD medication during pregnancy: a systematic review and meta-analysis. Pharmacoepidemiol Drug Saf 28(3):288–295, 2019 30585374
Juric S, Newport DJ, Ritchie JC, et al: Zolpidem (Ambien) in pregnancy: placental passage and outcome. Arch Womens Ment Health 12(6):441–446, 2009 19657707
Kanemura A, Masamoto H, Kinjo T, et al: Evaluation of neonatal withdrawal syndrome in neonates delivered by women taking psychotropic or anticonvulsant drugs: a retrospective chart review of the effects of multiple medications and breastfeeding. Eur J Obstet Gynecol Reprod Biol 254:226–230, 2020 33011505
Kaplan S, Braverman DL, Frishman I, et al: Pregnancy and fetal outcomes following exposure to modafinil and armodafinil during pregnancy. JAMA Intern Med 181(2):275–277, 2021 33074297
Kaye DK: The moral imperative to approve pregnant women's participation in randomized clinical trials for pregnancy and newborn complications. Philos Ethics Humanit Med 14(1):11, 2019 31492178
Ke AB, Rostami-Hodjegan A, Zhao P, et al: Pharmacometrics in pregnancy: an unmet need. Annu Rev Pharmacol Toxicol 54:53–69, 2014 24392692
Kelty E, Tran D, Lavin T, et al: Prevalence and safety of acamprosate use in pregnant alcohol-dependent women in New South Wales, Australia. Addiction 114(2):206–215, 2019 30152012
Kittel-Schneider S, Quednow BB, Leutritz AL, et al: Parental ADHD in pregnancy and the postpartum period—a systematic review. Neurosci Biobehav Rev 124:63–77, 2021 33516734
Kokras N, Sotiropoulos MG, Poulogiannopoulou E, et al: Maternal and infant pharmacokinetics of psychotropic medications during pregnancy and lactation, in Perinatal Psychopharmacology. Edited by Uguz F, Orsolini L. New York, Springer International, 2019, pp 17–35
Krans EE, Kim JY, Chen Q, et al: Outcomes associated with the use of medications for opioid use disorder during pregnancy. Addiction 116(12):3504–3514, 2021 34033170
Kulkarni J, Storch A, Baraniuk A, et al: Antipsychotic use in pregnancy. Expert Opin Pharmacother 16(9):1335–1345, 2015 26001182
Lee HJ, Kim SM, Kwon JY: Repetitive transcranial magnetic stimulation treatment for peripartum depression: systematic review and meta-analysis. BMC Pregnancy Childbirth 21(1):118, 2021 33563220
Lurasidone [Updated January 15, 2023], in Drugs and Lactation Database (LactMed) [Internet]. Bethesda, MD, National Institute of Child Health and Human Development, 2006-. Available at: https://www.ncbi.nlm.nih.gov/books/NBK501728/. Accessed August 7, 2024.
Matlow J, Koren G: Is carbamazepine safe to take during pregnancy? Can Fam Physician 58(2):163–164, 2012 22337738
McElhatton PR: The effects of benzodiazepine use during pregnancy and lactation. Reprod Toxicol 8(6):461–475, 1994 7881198
Mehta TM, Van Lieshout RJ: A review of the safety of clozapine during pregnancy and lactation. Arch Womens Ment Health 20(1):1–9, 2017 27704220
Merck Sharp and Dohme Corp: Belsomra (suvorexant) package insert. Whitehouse Station, NJ, Merck Sharp and Dohme, 2020. Available at: https://www.accessdata.fda.gov/drugsatfda_docs/label/2020/204569s006lbl.pdf. Accessed March 13, 2024.
Miuli A, Pettorruso M, Stefanelli G, et al: Beyond the efficacy of transcranial magnetic stimulation in peripartum depression: a systematic review exploring perinatal safety for newborns. Psychiatry Res 326:115251, 2023 37270864
Nau H: Species differences in pharmacokinetics and drug teratogenesis. Environ Health Perspect 70:113–129, 1986 3104022
Newton ER, Hale TW: Drugs in breast milk. Clin Obstet Gynecol 58(4):868–884, 2015 26457856

Ornoy A: Pharmacological treatment of attention deficit hyperactivity disorder during pregnancy and lactation. Pharm Res 35(3):46, 2018 29411149

Ornoy A, Koren G: SSRIs and SNRIs (SRI) in pregnancy: effects on the course of pregnancy and the offspring: how far are we from having all the answers? Int J Mol Sci 20(10):2370, 2019 31091646

Palmsten K, Huybrechts KF, Michels KB, et al: Antidepressant use and risk for preeclampsia. Epidemiology 24(5):682–691, 2013 23873072

Patel N, Viguera AC, Baldessarini RJ: Mood-stabilizing anticonvulsants, spina bifida, and folate supplementation: commentary. J Clin Psychopharmacol 38(1):7–10, 2018 29215383

Patorno E, Huybrechts KF, Bateman BT, et al: Lithium use in pregnancy and the risk of cardiac malformations. N Engl J Med 376(23):2245–2254, 2017 28591541

Patorno E, Hernandez-Diaz S, Huybrechts KF, et al: Gabapentin in pregnancy and the risk of adverse neonatal and maternal outcomes: a population-based cohort study nested in the US Medicaid Analytic eXtract dataset. PLoS Med 17(9):e1003322, 2020 32870921

Patterson R, Balan I, Morrow AL, et al: Novel neurosteroid therapeutics for post-partum depression: perspectives on clinical trials, program development, active research, and future directions. Neuropsychopharmacology 49(1):67–72, 2024 37715106

Payne JL: Psychopharmacology in pregnancy and breastfeeding. Psychiatr Clin North Am 40(2):217–238, 2017 28477649

Payne JL: Psychopharmacology in pregnancy and breastfeeding. Med Clin North Am 103(4):629–650, 2019 31078197

Payne JL: Psychiatric medication use in pregnancy and breastfeeding. Obstet Gynecol Clin North Am 48(1):131–149, 2021 33573783

Poels EMP, Bijma HH, Galbally M, et al: Lithium during pregnancy and after delivery: a review. Int J Bipolar Disord 6(1):26, 2018 30506447

Raffi ER, Nonacs R, Cohen LS: Safety of psychotropic medications during pregnancy. Clin Perinatol 46(2):215–234, 2019 31010557

Reddy DS, Mbilinyi RH, Estes E: Preclinical and clinical pharmacology of brexanolone (allopregnanolone) for postpartum depression: a landmark journey from concept to clinic in neurosteroid replacement therapy. Psychopharmacology (Berl) 240(9):1841–1863, 2023 37566239

Richardson G, Wang-Weigand S: Effects of long-term exposure to ramelteon, a melatonin receptor agonist, on endocrine function in adults with chronic insomnia. Hum Psychopharmacol 24(2):103–111, 2009 19090503

Rodriguez CE, Klie KA: Pharmacological treatment of opioid use disorder in pregnancy. Semin Perinatol 43(3):141–148, 2019 30755340

Rommel A-S, Bergink V, Liu X, et al: Long-term effects of intrauterine exposure to antidepressants on physical, neurodevelopmental, and psychiatric outcomes: a systematic review. J Clin Psychiatry 81(3):19r12965, 2020 32412703

Rose S, Dotters-Katz SK, Kuller JA: Electroconvulsive therapy in pregnancy: safety, best practices, and barriers to care. Obstet Gynecol Surv 75(3):199–203, 2020 32232498

Sage Therapeutics: Zulresso (brexanolone) injection, for intravenous use; prescribing information. Revised June 2022. Available at: https://assets.sagerx.com/zulresso/prescribing-information.pdf. Accessed June 9, 2024.

Sage Therapeutics and Biogen: Zurzuvae (zuranolone) capsules, for oral use; prescribing information. Revised November 2023. Available at: https://documents.sage-biogen.com/us/zurzuvae/pi.pdf. Accessed June 8, 2024.

Saito J, Tachibana Y, Sano Wada Y, et al: Presence of hypnotics in the cord blood and breast milk, with no adverse effects in the infant: a case report. Breastfeed Med 17(4):349–352, 2022 34935466

Sanofi-Aventis Canada: Imovane (zopiclone) package insert. Laval, QC, Canada, Sanofi-Aventis Canada, 2018. Available at: https://pdf.hres.ca/dpd_pm/00047597.PDF. Accessed March 13, 2024.

Schmidt A, Schmidt A, Markert UR: The road (not) taken—placental transfer and interspecies differences. Placenta 115:70–77, 2021 34562829

Schoretsanitis G, Spigset O, Stingl JC, et al: The impact of pregnancy on the pharmacokinetics of antidepressants: a systematic critical review and meta-analysis. Expert Opin Drug Metab Toxicol 16(5):431–440, 2020 32238008

Schlotterbeck P, Saur R, Hiemke C, et al: Low concentration of ziprasidone in human milk: a case report. Int J Neuropsychopharmacol 12(3):437–438, 2009 19203410

Stahl SM: Prescriber's Guide: Stahl's Essential Psychopharmacology, 6th Edition. Cambridge, UK, Cambridge University Press, 2017

Straub L, Hernández-Díaz S, Bateman BT, et al: Association of antipsychotic drug exposure in pregnancy with risk of neurodevelopmental disorders: a national birth cohort study. JAMA Intern Med 182(5):522–533, 2022 35343998

Takeda Pharmaceuticals America: Rozerem (ramelteon) package insert. Deerfield, IL, Takeda Pharmaceuticals America, 2010. Available at: https://www.accessdata.fda.gov/drugsatfda_docs/label/2010/021782s011lbl.pdf. Accessed March 13, 2024.

'tJong GW, Einarson T, Koren G, et al: Antidepressant use in pregnancy and persistent pulmonary hypertension of the newborn (PPHN): a systematic review. Reprod Toxicol 34(3):293–297, 2012 22564982

Tomson T, Battino D, Bromley R, et al: Management of epilepsy in pregnancy: a report from the International League Against Epilepsy Task Force on Women and Pregnancy. Epileptic Disord 21(6):497–517, 2019 31782407

Tomson T, Battino D, Bromley R, et al: Global survey of guidelines for the management of epilepsy in pregnancy: a report from the International League Against Epilepsy Task Force on Women and Pregnancy. Epilepsia Open 5(3):366–370, 2020 32913945

Tomson T, Battino D, Bromley R, et al: Breastfeeding while on treatment with antiseizure medications: a systematic review from the ILAE Women Task Force. Epileptic Disord 24(6):1020–1032, 2022 36193017

Towers CV, Katz E, Weitz B, et al: Use of naltrexone in treating opioid use disorder in pregnancy. Am J Obstet Gynecol 222(1):83.e1–83.e8, 2020 31376396

Tracy TS, Venkataramanan R, Glover DD, et al; National Institute for Child Health and Human Development Network of Maternal-Fetal-Medicine Units: Temporal changes in drug metabolism (CYP1A2, CYP2D6 and CYP3A activity) during pregnancy. Am J Obstet Gynecol 192(2):633–639, 2005 15696014

U.S. Food and Drug Administration: Antipsychotic drug labels updated on use during pregnancy and risk of abnormal muscle movements and withdrawal symptoms in newborns. FDA Drug Safety Communication, 2011. Available at: https://www.fda.gov/drugs/drug-safety-and-availability/fda-drug-safety-communication-antipsychotic-drug-labels-updated-use-during-pregnancy-and-risk. Accessed March 13, 2024.

van Gelder MMHJ, de Jong-van den Berg LTW, Roeleveld N: Drugs associated with teratogenic mechanisms, part II: a literature review of the evidence on human risks. Hum Reprod 29(1):168–183, 2014 24108217

Viguera AC, Whitfield T, Baldessarini RJ, et al: Risk of recurrence in women with bipolar disorder during pregnancy: prospective study of mood stabilizer discontinuation. Am J Psychiatry 164(12):1817–1824, quiz 1923, 2007 18056236

Wald J, Henningsson A, Hanze E, et al: Allopregnanolone concentrations in breast milk and plasma from healthy volunteers receiving brexanolone injection, with population pharmacokinetic modeling of potential relative infant dose. Clin Pharmacokinet 61(9):1307–1319, 2022 35869362

Wesseloo R, Wierdsma AI, van Kamp IL, et al: Lithium dosing strategies during pregnancy and the postpartum period. Br J Psychiatry 211(1):31–36, 2017 28673946

Westin AA, Brekke M, Molden E, et al: Treatment with antipsychotics in pregnancy: changes in drug disposition. Clin Pharmacol Ther 103(3):477–484, 2018 28643331

Wikner BN, Källén B: Are hypnotic benzodiazepine receptor agonists teratogenic in humans? J Clin Psychopharmacol 31(3):356–359, 2011 21508851

Wilson RD, O'Connor DL: Maternal folic acid and multivitamin supplementation: international clinical evidence with considerations for the prevention of folate-sensitive birth defects. Prev Med Rep 24:101617, 2021 34976673

Wurst KE, Zedler BK, Joyce AR, et al: A Swedish population-based study of adverse birth outcomes among pregnant women treated with buprenorphine or methadone: preliminary findings. Subst Abuse 10:89–97, 2016 27679504

Yonkers KA, Wisner KL, Stowe Z, et al: Management of bipolar disorder during pregnancy and the postpartum period. Am J Psychiatry 161(4):608–620, 2004 15056503

Yonkers KA, Wisner KL, Stewart DE, et al: The management of depression during pregnancy: a report from the American Psychiatric Association and the American College of Obstetricians and Gynecologists. Gen Hosp Psychiatry 31(5):403–413, 2009 19703633

Zemishlany Z, McQueeney R, Gabriel SM, et al: Neuroendocrine and monoaminergic responses to acute administration of alprazolam in normal subjects. Neuropsychobiology 23(3):124–128, 1990–1991 2098668

16

Children and Adolescents

Austin Campbell, Pharm.D., BCPP
Laine Young-Walker, M.D.

Pharmacokinetic and Pharmacodynamic Differences in Children Versus Adults

- Children have relatively more body water and less fat than adults, which can lead to variations in drug concentrations.
- Despite having plasma protein levels similar to those in adults, children frequently have higher free fractions of medications in circulation because of lower concentrations of albumin (van den Anker et al. 2018).
- Drug metabolism via cytochrome P450 (CYP) in children is normal/unchanged relative to metabolism in adults for major enzymes, such as CYP2D6 and CYP3A4/5, but is slower than metabolism in adults for CYP1A2.
- Renal elimination of weight-corrected medications appears to be very similar for adults, adolescents, and children.
- Some medications (e.g., first-generation antihistamines such as diphenhydramine [Benadryl]) have greater CNS penetration in children than in adults, potentially contributing to increased side effects.
- Children and adolescents appear to be more susceptible than adults to a number of psychotropic medication–induced side effects, including sedation, gastrointestinal disturbances, metabolic changes, and prolactin elevation (Birmaher et al. 2007; Liu et al. 2019).
- Compared with adults, children have a greater likelihood of experiencing paradoxical reactions (i.e., the opposite of the intended effect) to medications such as benzodiazepines and first-generation antihistamines (Mancuso et al. 2004).
- For most psychiatric medications, safety and tolerability data in pediatric and adolescent populations are much more sparse than data in adult populations, and far fewer long-term safety studies have been conducted in children than in adults to evaluate the distal risks/benefits of these medications.

Antidepressants

- Selective serotonin reuptake inhibitors (SSRIs) are considered to be the first-line treatment option for moderate to severe depression in children and adolescents (National Institute for Health and Care Excellence 2019).
- Fluoxetine and escitalopram are the preferred agents, both having FDA approvals, with sertraline and citalopram considered reasonable alternatives (Cheung et al. 2018).
- Serotonin-norepinephrine reuptake inhibitors (SNRIs) and bupropion may be less well tolerated than first-line treatments and should be considered after SSRIs for depression in children and adolescents (Boaden et al. 2020).
- Desvenlafaxine, mirtazapine, paroxetine, vilazodone, and vortioxetine are not recommended for the treatment of depression in children and adolescents because there is insufficient evidence demonstrating their efficacy in this age group (Findling et al. 2020; Hetrick et al. 2021; National Institute for Health and Care Excellence 2019).
- Tricyclic antidepressants (TCAs) are no longer recommended for the treatment of depression in children and adolescents because of side effects and safety concerns (Birmaher et al. 2007; National Institute for Health and Care Excellence 2019). Furthermore, TCAs have not been shown to be superior to placebo in treating depression in children (Hazell et al. 2013).
- The side effects most commonly reported with SSRI and SNRI medications in children and adolescents are gastrointestinal symptoms, sleep changes (i.e., insomnia or somnolence), restlessness, diaphoresis, headaches, changes in appetite (increase or decrease), and sexual dysfunction.
- Behavioral activation is much more common in children and adolescents than in adults and has been reported in as many as 20%–50% of individuals treated with an antidepressant (Patel et al. 2018).
  - Behavioral activation is more common during the first few days after starting or increasing the dosage of a medication.
- Starting medications at the lowest dosage and increasing the dosage gradually may help mitigate many adverse effects, reduce the risk for behavioral activation, and improve overall tolerability (Walter et al. 2020).
- Table 16–1 presents information on dosing and FDA-approved indications for antidepressants used in children and adolescents.

Boxed Warning for Suicidal Ideation and Behavior

- An FDA class warning was issued in 2004 for all antidepressants and/or medications with similar mechanisms of action. For detailed information, the reader is referred to comprehensive sources in the literature (e.g., Fergusson et al. 2005).
- The warning was based on a large review of clinical trials involving nine antidepressants for MDD, OCD, or anxiety that showed that children and adolescents taking antidepressant medications spontaneously reported more suicidal thoughts or attempts (4%) than did those receiving placebo (2%) (Cheung et al. 2018; Spielmans et al. 2020).

Table 16–1. Antidepressant indications (both FDA and off-label) and dosage guidelines for pediatric patients

Medication	FDA-approved pediatric indications (age)	Starting daily dosage	Maximum recommended daily dosage	Off-label uses in pediatric patients (age)*	Starting daily dosage*	Maximum recommended daily dosage*
SSRIs						
Citalopram	N/A			AD (≥7 years) MDD (≥7 years) OCD (≥7 years)	7–11 years: 2.5–10 mg ≥12 years: 10 mg	40 mg
Escitalopram	MDD (≥12 years)	5–10 mg	20 mg	AD (≥10 years)		
Fluoxetine	OCD (≥7 years) MDD (≥8 years)	7–11 years: 5 mg ≥12 years: 10 mg	60 mg	AD/GAD (≥6 years) Anorexia/bulimia nervosa (≥12 years)		
Fluvoxamine	OCD (≥8 years)	8–11 years: 12.5–25 mg ≥12 years: 25–50 mg	8–11 years: 200 mg ≥12 years: 300 mg	MDD (≥13 years)		
Paroxetine	N/A			SocAD (≥8 years) OCD (≥7 years)	10 mg	60 mg
Sertraline	OCD (≥6 years)	25 mg	200 mg	AD (≥6 years) MDD (≥6 years)		

Table 16–1. Antidepressant indications (both FDA and off-label) and dosage guidelines for pediatric patients *(continued)*

Medication	FDA-approved pediatric indications (age)	Starting daily dosage	Maximum recommended daily dosage	Off-label uses in pediatric patients (age)*	Starting daily dosage*	Maximum recommended daily dosage*
SNRIs						
Duloxetine	GAD (≥7 years) Fibromyalgia (≥13 years)	30 mg 30 mg	120 mg 60 mg	MDD (≥7 years)		
Venlafaxine	N/A			GAD (≥6 years) MDD (≥12 years)	37.5 mg	150 mg
TCAs[a]						
Amitriptyline	N/A			MDD (≥9 years) Migraine prophylaxis (≥12 years)	Varies[a]	200 mg
Clomipramine	OCD (≥10 years)	25 mg	3 mg/kg or 200 mg	AD (≥10 years)		
Desipramine	N/A			ADHD (≥7 years) MDD (≥6 years)	Varies[a]	6–12 years: 3 mg/kg or 100 mg ≥13 years: 150 mg
Doxepin	N/A			AD (≥7 years) MDD (≥7 years)	Varies[a]	7–11 years: 3 mg/kg ≥12 years: 300 mg
Imipramine	Enuresis (≥6 years)	10–25 mg	6–11 years: 50 mg ≥12 years: 75 mg	ADHD MDD		Dosages up to 200 mg/day
Protriptyline	N/A			MDD (≥13 years)	Varies[a]	60 mg

Table 16–1. Antidepressant indications (both FDA and off-label) and dosage guidelines for pediatric patients *(continued)*

Medication	FDA-approved pediatric indications (age)	Starting daily dosage	Maximum recommended daily dosage	Off-label uses in pediatric patients (age)*	Starting daily dosage*	Maximum recommended daily dosage*
Other						
Bupropion[b]	N/A			ADHD (≥6 years) MDD (≥8 years) (IR) Smoking cessation (≥14 years) (IR)	1.5–3.0 mg/kg divided	6 mg/kg/day or 400 mg
Mirtazapine	N/A			Insomnia	7.5 mg	30 mg

Note. AD=anxiety disorder; ADHD=attention-deficit/hyperactivity disorder; GAD=generalized anxiety disorder; IR=immediate release; MDD=major depressive disorder; OCD=obsessive-compulsive disorder; SNRIs=serotonin-norepinephrine reuptake inhibitors; SocAD=social anxiety disorder; SSRIs=selective serotonin reuptake inhibitors; TCAs=tricyclic antidepressants.

*N/A= not approved (off-label). Dosing for off-label uses of medications may vary from dosing for FDA-approved indications.

[a]TCA dosing can vary greatly, depending on indication, age, and size/weight of child. Recommend consulting individual product information for safe dosing when using off-label.

[b]Bupropion may be initiated with the immediate-release product and then transitioned to the 12-hour or 24-hour formulation once titrated to a corresponding dosage.

Source. Drugs@FDA 2024; Missouri Department of Social Services 2022.

- No suicides occurred in any of these trials, and overall rates of suicidal ideation decreased from baseline in all treatment groups (Cheung et al. 2018; Emslie et al. 2006). By contrast, a large correlational study conducted in 2014 demonstrated that reductions in antidepressant prescriptions (likely related in part to the boxed warning) were associated with an increase in suicide attempts (Lu et al. 2014).
- In subsequent research, evidence did not suggest an increased risk for worsening of suicidality or an increased emergence of suicidality in individuals who did not have it at baseline (Emslie et al. 2006; Hammad et al. 2006).
- Suicidal ideation and behavior are unpredictable and are associated with uncertainty. This uncertainty should be acknowledged by clinicians and discussed openly with patients, parents, and guardians. All children and adolescents experiencing suicidal thoughts should be monitored closely, especially after treatment initiation (Boaden et al. 2020).
- Informed consent regarding the FDA boxed warning and psychoeducation regarding suicidality and crisis planning for the same are critical.

Antianxiety Medications

Antidepressants

- SSRIs are the treatment of choice for most children and adolescents with generalized anxiety disorder, panic disorder, separation anxiety disorder, or social anxiety disorder. SNRIs may also be a reasonable alternative for some patients (Walter et al. 2020).
- The SSRIs fluoxetine, escitalopram, and sertraline and the SNRI duloxetine have the largest amount of evidence supporting their use in pediatric anxiety disorders (Hetrick et al. 2021; Walter et al. 2020).
- TCAs are not recommended as first- or second-line treatment options for anxiety disorders in children and adolescents because of their limited supporting evidence, increased side effects, and less-favorable safety profile (Hetrick et al. 2021; Walter et al. 2020).
- Refer to Table 16–1 for information on FDA-approved indications as well as recommended starting and maximum dosages for antidepressants in children and adolescents.
- SSRI and SNRI medications can cause behavioral activation and/or agitation. This adverse effect is more common in younger children than in older children and occurs more frequently in patients with anxiety disorders than in those with depression (Walter et al. 2020).
- See earlier subsection "Boxed Warning for Suicidal Ideation and Behavior" under "Antidepressants."

Other Medications for Anxiety

- There is insufficient evidence to support the use of benzodiazepines in the treatment of anxiety disorders in children and adolescents. Because of these agents' significant risk for abuse, diversion, and adverse effects, use of benzodiazepines should be limited to special circumstances and for limited durations of time (Patel et al. 2018; Walter et al. 2020).
- Buspirone has limited evidence supporting its use in children and adolescents but is generally safe and well tolerated (Patel et al. 2018). Buspirone has shown benefit in some patients as adjunctive treatment or monotherapy.
- Hydroxyzine is not recommended for use in the treatment of anxiety disorders in children and adolescents (Patel et al. 2018). It may have acute benefit in some patients for short-term use.
- Propranolol has insufficient evidence to support its use in managing anxiety disorders in children and adolescents (Patel et al. 2018). It may have a small role in specific situations (i.e., performance anxiety). Use caution in patients with bradycardia, heart disease, diabetes mellitus, asthma, or depression.
- Table 16–2 presents information on dosing for off-label uses of other anxiolytic medications in children and adolescents.

Table 16–2. Off-label uses of other anxiolytic medications in pediatric patients

Medication	Off-label uses in pediatric patients*	Starting dosage*	Maximum recommended daily dosage*
Buspirone	AD (≥6 years)	5 mg	60 mg divided
Hydroxyzine	AD	0.5 mg/kg/dose every 6 hours	Age <6 years: 50 mg Age ≥6 years: 100 mg)
Propranolol	Disruptive behavior	10 mg	60 mg

AD=anxiety disorders.
*Dosing for off-label uses of medications may vary from dosing for FDA-approved indications.
Source. Drugs@FDA 2024; Missouri Department of Social Services 2022.

Mood Stabilizers

- Lithium or second-generation antipsychotics (SGAs) are considered the first-line treatment options in the management of bipolar disorder (mania and maintenance) for children and adolescents (McClellan et al. 2007; Yatham et al. 2018).
- Antiepileptic medications used as mood stabilizers have lower-quality evidence supporting their efficacy in children and adolescents and should be considered second-line options for bipolar disorder (mania and maintenance) (Davico et al. 2018; Yatham et al. 2018). Because of the teratogenic risks associated with these medications, caution should be used when prescribing mood stabilizers for girls/women of childbearing age.
- Although monotherapy is encouraged, the combination of two traditional mood stabilizers or of a mood stabilizer plus an SGA may be necessary acutely when there is only partial response and/or when mixed or psychotic features are present (McClellan et al. 2007; Yatham et al. 2018).
- Carbamazepine is no longer recommended as a treatment option for bipolar disorder (mania) for most children and adolescents, given that alternative agents with better safety and efficacy data are available.
- Acute mania has been the focus of most research for child and adolescent bipolar disorder (Davico et al. 2018; McClellan et al. 2007; Yatham et al. 2018).
  - Lithium, aripiprazole, asenapine, quetiapine, and risperidone are the preferred medication options for acute mania in this population.
  - Because of safety concerns, tolerability issues, and/or lower-quality evidence, divalproex, olanzapine, and ziprasidone are considered to be second-line options.
- Limited data are available regarding treatment options for bipolar depression in children and adolescents (DelBello et al. 2022; Yatham et al. 2018).
  - Lurasidone is considered the preferred medication option for bipolar depression by many experts.
  - Lithium and lamotrigine are reasonable alternatives to lurasidone as treatment options for pediatric bipolar depression.
  - The combination of olanzapine + fluoxetine (marketed as Symbyax) may also be effective but is not recommended as a first- or second-line choice because olanzapine carries a significant risk of metabolic side effects.
  - Quetiapine has conflicting data supporting its use in pediatric bipolar depression and may be considered a third-line choice.
  - Evidence supporting the benefit of combining antidepressants is very limited. Antidepressants should not be used in suspected bipolar depression without a mood stabilizer or an SGA because of the risk of cycle acceleration and worsening of long-term prognosis.

- Evidence supporting the efficacy of specific medications in the maintenance treatment of pediatric bipolar disorder is also very limited (Yatham et al. 2018; Yee et al. 2019).
  - Aripiprazole, lithium, and divalproex monotherapy and adjunctive lamotrigine have longer-term data in child and adolescent patients available/published.
  - Some evidence suggests that patients who respond well to initial treatment with asenapine, quetiapine, risperidone, or ziprasidone may be continued on the same agent for maintenance treatment.
- Common and serious side effects of mood stabilizers reported in children and adolescents typically mirror those reported in adults.
- The risk of Stevens-Johnson syndrome with lamotrigine is greater in children and adolescents than in adults.
- Table 16–3 presents information on dosing and FDA-approved indications for mood stabilizers used to treat bipolar disorder in children and adolescents.

Table 16–3. Indications and dosage guidelines for lithium and antiepileptic medications used to treat pediatric bipolar disorder

Medication	FDA-approved pediatric indications (age)	Common off-label uses for pediatric bipolar disorder*	Starting daily dosage*	Maximum recommended daily dosage*
Lithium	Acute mania and maintenance (≥12 years)	Acute mania Depression Maintenance	300 mg twice daily	<22 kg: 600 mg 22–41 kg: 900 mg >41 kg: 1,200 mg
Divalproex/ valproic acid	N/A[a]	Acute mania Mixed features Maintenance	10 mg/kg/day (ER form only for ≥10 years)	1,000 mg
Carbamazepine	N/A[a]	Acute mania Mixed features	≥6 years: 100 mg twice daily	6–15 years: 1,000 mg ≥16 years: 1,200 mg
Lamotrigine	N/A[a]	Depression Maintenance	25 mg	200 mg

Note. ER=extended release.
*Dosing for off-label uses of medications may vary from dosing for FDA-approved indications.
[a]N/A: Not approved for use in bipolar disorder in patients ≤18 years but frequently used and guideline recommended in younger age groups.
Source. Drugs@FDA 2024; Missouri Department of Social Services 2022.

Antipsychotics

- Second-generation antipsychotics (SGAs) are considered to be the treatments of choice for schizophrenia spectrum and other psychotic disorders in children and adolescents (McClellan et al. 2013; National Institute for Health and Care Excellence 2013).
- Aripiprazole, olanzapine, quetiapine, and risperidone have the greatest amount of supportive evidence for use in pediatric populations, but brexpiprazole, lurasidone, and paliperidone are also FDA approved for use in children and adolescents (Krause et al. 2018; McClellan et al. 2013).
- Olanzapine is not typically recommended as a first-line treatment because of its relatively higher risk of significant weight gain and other metabolic side effects (Krause et al. 2018; McClellan et al. 2013).
- Ziprasidone has one of the most benign metabolic risk profiles in children and adolescents; however, it is not recommended as a first-line agent because of its less favorable efficacy data and lack of approved indications in this population (Krause et al. 2018; McClellan et al. 2013).
- Currently, cariprazine, iloperidone, and lumateperone lack sufficient evidence/information to recommend their use or to provide guidance on dosing in children and adolescents (Drugs@FDA 2024).
- First-generation antipsychotics (FGAs) are no longer recommended for routine use in children and adolescents because of insufficient supporting evidence and increased safety concerns. For further information, readers are referred to the published literature on the potential neurotoxic effects of FGAs in general (e.g., Nasrallah and Chen 2017).
- Antipsychotic medications are typically not recommended for off-label use in children and adolescents in the absence of approved or evidence-based indications. However, usage data suggest that the majority of antipsychotics are not prescribed for FDA-approved indications (American Psychiatric Association 2018; Dinnissen et al. 2020; Hoekstra and Dietrich 2022; Penfold et al. 2013).
  - In children and adolescents, antipsychotics are currently approved only for use in bipolar disorder, schizophrenia, Tourette syndrome, and irritability associated with autism spectrum disorder.
  - The symptom for which antipsychotics are most often used off-label is disruptive behavior or irritability, and the most common co-occurring diagnoses are ADHD, anxiety disorders, autism spectrum disorder, and other mood disorders.
- For further information on SGA use in bipolar disorder, see Chapter 6, "Antipsychotics," in this Handbook.
- Patterns of antipsychotic efficacy, tolerability, and adverse effects in children and adolescents are very similar to those in adults. However, a dearth of pediatric studies makes drawing firm conclusions difficult (Krause et al. 2018).

- Children and adolescents are more susceptible than adults to some SGA adverse effects, including metabolic side effects, extrapyramidal symptoms, and prolactin elevation (Birmaher et al. 2007; Liu et al. 2019; Vitiello et al. 2009).
- The adverse effects most commonly experienced by children and adolescents taking SGAs are sedation, nausea, age-inappropriate weight gain, changes in blood pressure or heart rate, and headache.
- Table 16–4 presents information on dosing and FDA-approved indications for SGAs used to treat bipolar disorder in children and adolescents.

Table 16–4. Indications and dosage guidelines for antipsychotics used to treat pediatric bipolar disorder

Medication	FDA-approved pediatric indications (age)	Starting daily dosage	Maximum recommended daily dosage
Aripiprazole	Acute/mixed mania (≥10 years)	10 mg	30 mg
	Autism-associated irritability (≥6 years)	5–10 mg	15 mg
	Schizophrenia (≥13 years)	10 mg	30 mg
	Tourette syndrome (≥6 years)	≥6 years and <50 kg: 5 mg ≥6 years and ≥50 kg: 10 mg	≥6 years and <50 kg: 10 mg ≥6 years and ≥50 kg: 20 mg
Asenapine	Acute/mixed mania (≥10 years)	2.5 mg twice daily	10 mg twice daily
Brexpiprazole	Schizophrenia (≥13 years)	0.5 mg	4 mg
Clozapine*	N/A	12.5–25 mg	400 mg
Lurasidone	Bipolar depression (≥10 years) Schizophrenia (≥13 years)	20 mg	80 mg
Olanzapine	Acute/mixed mania (≥13 years) Schizophrenia (≥13 years)	2.5–5 mg	20 mg
Paliperidone	Schizophrenia (12+)	3 mg	12 mg
Quetiapine	Acute/mixed mania (≥10 years) Schizophrenia (≥13 years)	25 mg twice daily (IR) 50 mg (XR)	800 mg
Risperidone	Acute mania (≥10 years) Autism-associated irritability (≥5 years) Schizophrenia (≥13 years)	0.25–0.5 mg	5–10 years: 3 mg ≥11 years: 6 mg
Ziprasidone*	N/A	20 mg	160 mg

Note. IR=immediate release; N/A=not approved (off-label); XR=extended release.
*Shaded rows indicate off-label use.
Source. Drugs@FDA 2024; Missouri Department of Social Services 2022.

Medications Used for ADHD

Psychostimulants

- Stimulant medications (methylphenidate and mixed amphetamine salt products) have multiple dosage and release mechanisms, such as short-acting, long-acting, transdermal, delayed-onset, and prodrug formulations. For further information on the advantages and disadvantages of these individual products, as well as detailed dosing tables and guidelines for their use, readers are referred to Chapter 7, "Stimulants," in this Handbook.
- Use of stimulant medications for management of ADHD in children and adolescents is strongly supported by the literature, and these agents are considered to be the first-line therapies (National Institute for Health and Care Excellence 2018; Wolraich et al. 2019).
- All methylphenidate and most amphetamine formulations are FDA approved for use in children ages 6 years and older; however, immediate-release amphetamine salts and dextroamphetamine are approved for children as young as 3 years, while one extended-release product using a three-bead system is approved for adolescents ages 13 years and older (Drugs@FDA 2024).
- Although not FDA approved for use in this age group, methylphenidate is the recommended treatment for children younger than 6 years with severe ADHD because the evidence base supporting safety and efficacy in this population is larger for methylphenidate than for mixed amphetamine salt products (Wolraich et al. 2019). Methylphenidate products are generally considered to be less potent than mixed amphetamine salts.
- Some evidence suggests methylphenidate products may have better efficacy and tolerability in children and adolescents, whereas amphetamine products may be preferred in adults (Cortese et al. 2018).
- Methylphenidate and amphetamine products have similar rates of most adverse effects; however, amphetamine salts may be associated with a greater risk of irritability (Stuckelman et al. 2017).
- Common adverse effects of stimulants in children and adolescents include anorexia, poor growth or weight loss during childhood, sleep disturbance, jitteriness, and emotional lability.

Nonstimulant Medications

- Because of their delayed onset of action and less-robust therapeutic effects, nonstimulant medications are usually reserved for individuals who have contraindications, intolerances, or inadequate responses to psychostimulants (National Institute for Health and Care Excellence 2018; Wolraich et al. 2019).
- The greatest amount of supportive evidence (from larger to smaller) exists for atomoxetine, extended-release guanfacine, and extended-release clonidine (Wolraich et al. 2019).
- For both guanfacine and clonidine, the extended-release and immediate-release products are NOT interchangeable on a milligram-per-milligram basis.

- Viloxazine is the newest FDA-approved nonstimulant medication and may play a role similar to that of atomoxetine in the treatment algorithm for ADHD. However, current evidence supporting viloxazine use is limited (Nasser et al. 2020).
- Atomoxetine and viloxazine carry warnings for suicidal thinking and behavior. Although these symptoms are very rare, all children and adolescents initiating treatment for ADHD should be monitored closely for suicidality (Chen et al. 2014; Man et al. 2017).
- Table 16–5 presents information on dosing and the use of nonstimulant medications in ADHD. For detailed tables with dosing guidelines for the use of stimulant medication in ADHD, see Chapter 7, "Stimulants," in this *Handbook*.
- Bupropion (off-label) appears to be well tolerated in pediatric ADHD and has shown some efficacy in treating this disorder. It may be considered as a third-line treatment option after failure of other medications (Biederman and Spencer 2000; Cortese et al. 2018)
- TCAs, particularly desipramine, have also demonstrated benefit in treating ADHD. However, TCA use is typically not recommended because of safety concerns (Otasowie et al. 2014).

Table 16–5. Dosage guidelines for nonstimulant medications used to treat ADHD in pediatric patients

Medication	FDA-approved uses in ADHD (age)	Starting daily dosage	Maximum recommended daily dosage
Norepinephrine reuptake inhibitors			
Atomoxetine	Monotherapy (≥6 years)	≤70 kg: 0.5 mg/kg >70 kg: 40 mg	≤70 kg: 1.4 mg/kg >70 mg: 100 mg
Viloxazine	Monotherapy (≥6 years)	6–11 years: 100 mg ≥12 years: 200 mg	400 mg
Alpha2-adrenergic agonists			
Clonidine ER	Monotherapy or adjunctive (≥6 years)	0.1 mg	0.4 mg
Clonidine IR*	N/A	≤45 kg: 0.05 mg >45 kg: 0.1 mg	27–40.5 kg: 0.2 mg 40.5–45 kg: 0.3 mg >45 kg: 0.4 mg
Guanfacine ER	Monotherapy or adjunctive (≥6 years)	1 mg	Monotherapy: 6–12 years: 4 mg ≥13 years: 7 mg Adjunctive: 4 mg
Guanfacine IR*	N/A	≤45 kg: 0.5 mg >45 kg: 1 mg	27–40.5 kg: 2 mg 40.5–45 kg: 3 mg >45 kg: 4 mg

Note. ER=extended release; IR=immediate release; N/A=not approved (off-label).
*Shaded rows indicate off-label use.
Source. Drugs@FDA 2024; Missouri Department of Social Services 2022.

Medications Used in Substance Use Disorders

- There is an absence of clinical trial data supporting the efficacy of pharmacotherapy in adolescents with substance use disorders (SUDs). Currently, no medications used to treat SUDs in adults have FDA approved indications in children and adolescents (Drugs@FDA 2024).

Alcohol Use Disorder

- Naltrexone has shown preliminary evidence of tolerability, safety, and efficacy in adolescents with alcohol use disorder; however, controlled trials are lacking (Hammond and Gray 2016).
- Disulfiram demonstrated some benefit and was well tolerated in a small study of adolescents with alcohol use disorder (Niederhofer and Staffen 2003).

Opioid Use Disorder

- Among medications for adolescents with opioid use disorder, only buprenorphine has been tested in clinical trials and is FDA approved for young people ages 16 years and older (Drugs@FDA 2024; Hammond and Gray 2016).
  - A clinical trial comparing buprenorphine and clonidine in adolescents with opioid use disorder found buprenorphine to be more effective than clonidine in retaining patients in treatment and increasing the number of opiate-free urine tests (Marsch et al. 2005).
- Limited uncontrolled data suggest that naltrexone is well tolerated and is a feasible treatment option for adolescents with opioid use disorder (Fishman et al. 2010).
- The safety and effectiveness of methadone has not been established in adolescents; methadone's use is largely restricted to individuals older than 18 years (Hammond and Gray 2016; Moolchan et al. 2005). Readers are referred to the methadone prescribing regulations (e.g., Substance Abuse and Mental Health Services Administration 2024).

Tobacco Use Disorder

- Nicotine replacement therapy (NRT) is the most studied and preferred treatment option for smoking cessation in adolescents. The nicotine patch is most commonly used and may offer adherence advantages over other NRT formulations (Hammond and Gray 2016).
- Although bupropion appears to be a safe option, its sustained efficacy in adolescents has not been demonstrated (Hammond and Gray 2016; Yan and Goldman 2021).
- In controlled trials, varenicline did not demonstrate efficacy for smoking cessation in adolescents but was well tolerated and may hasten abstinence (Gray et al. 2019). Readers are referred to Chapter 10, "Treatment of Substance Use Disorders," for further information on varenicline, including the risks of prescribing this medication for individuals with mental disorders.

References

American Psychiatric Association (APA): Five things physician and patients should question. Choosing Wisely; last reviewed 2018. Available at: https://www.choosingwisely.org/societies/american-psychiatric-association/. Accessed May 24, 2022.

Biederman J, Spencer T: Non-stimulant treatments for ADHD. Eur Child Adolesc Psychiatry 9(Suppl 1):I51–I59, 2000 11140780

Birmaher B, Brent D, Bernet W, et al: Practice parameter for the assessment and treatment of children and adolescents with depressive disorders. J Am Acad Child Adolesc Psychiatry 46(11):1503–1526, 2007 18049300

Boaden K, Tomlinson A, Cortese S, et al: Antidepressants in children and adolescents: meta-review of efficacy, tolerability, and suicidality in acute treatment. Front Psychiatry 11:717, 2020 32982805

Chen Q, Sjölander A, Runeson B, et al: Drug treatment for attention-deficit/hyperactivity disorder and suicidal behaviour: register based study. BMJ 348:g3769, 2014 24942388

Cheung AH, Zuckerbrot RA, Jensen PS, et al: Guidelines for adolescent depression in primary care (GLAD-PC): part II. Treatment and ongoing management. Pediatrics 141(3):e20174082, 2018 29483201

Cortese S, Adamo N, Del Giovane C, et al: Comparative efficacy and tolerability of medications for attention-deficit hyperactivity disorder in children, adolescents, and adults: a systematic review and network meta-analysis. Lancet Psychiatry 5(9):727–738, 2018 30097390

Davico C, Canavese C, Vittorini R, et al: Anticonvulsants for psychiatric disorders in children and adolescents: a systematic review of their efficacy. Front Psychiatry 9:270, 2018 29988399

DelBello MP, Kadakia A, Heller V, et al: Systematic review and network meta-analysis: Efficacy and safety of second-generation antipsychotics in youth with bipolar depression. J Am Acad Child Adolesc Psychiatry 61(2):243–254, 2022 34420839

Dinnissen M, Dietrich A, van der Molen JH, et al: Prescribing antipsychotics in child and adolescent psychiatry: guideline adherence. Eur Child Adolesc Psychiatry 29(12):1717–1727, 2020 32052173

Drugs@FDA. FDA-Approved Drugs (Database for information about drugs approved for human use in the United States). Available at: https://www.accessdata.fda.gov/scripts/cder/daf/index.cfm. Accessed August 5, 2024..

Emslie G, Kratochvil C, Vitiello B, et al: Treatment for adolescents with depression study (TADS): safety results. J Am Acad Child Adolesc Psychiatry 45(12):1440–1455, 2006

Fergusson D, Doucette S, Glass KC, et al: Association between suicide attempts and selective serotonin reuptake inhibitors: systematic review of randomised controlled trials. BMJ 330(7488):396, 2005 15718539

Findling RL, McCusker E, Strawn JRA: A randomized, double-blind, placebo-controlled trial of vilazodone in children and adolescents with major depressive disorder with twenty-six-week open-label follow-up. J Child Adolesc Psychopharmacol 30(6):355–365, 2020 32460523

Fishman MJ, Winstanley EL, Curran E, et al: Treatment of opioid dependence in adolescents and young adults with extended release naltrexone: preliminary case-series and feasibility. Addiction 105(9):1669–1676, 2010 20626723

Gray KM, Baker NL, McClure EA, et al: Efficacy and safety of varenicline for adolescent smoking cessation: a randomized clinical trial. JAMA Pediatr 173(12):1146–1153, 2019 31609433

Hammad TA, Laughren T, Racoosin J: Suicidality in pediatric patients treated with antidepressant drugs. Arch Gen Psychiatry 63(3):332–339, 2006 16520440

Hammond CJ, Gray KM: Pharmacotherapy for substance use disorders in youths. J Child Adolesc Subst Abuse 25(4):292–316, 2016 28082828

Hazell P, Mirzaie M: Tricyclic drugs for depression in children and adolescents. Cochrane Database Syst Rev (6):CD002317, 2013 23780719

Hetrick SE, McKenzie JE, Bailey AP, et al: New generation antidepressants for depression in children and adolescents: a network meta-analysis. Cochrane Database Syst Rev (5):CD013674, 2021 34029378

Hoekstra PJ, Dietrich A: First do no harm: use off-label antipsychotic medication in children and adolescents with great caution. Eur Child Adolesc Psychiatry 31(1):1–3, 2022 35064827

Krause M, Zhu Y, Huhn M, et al: Efficacy, acceptability, and tolerability of antipsychotics in children and adolescents with schizophrenia: a network meta-analysis. Eur Neuropsychopharmacol 28(6):659–674, 2018 29802039

Liu XI, Schuette P, Burckart GJ, et al: A comparison of pediatric and adult safety studies for antipsychotic and antidepressant drugs submitted to the United States Food and Drug Administration. J Pediatr 208:236–242.e3, 2019 30679050

Lu CY, Zhang F, Lakoma MD, et al: Changes in antidepressant use by young people and suicidal behavior after FDA warnings and media coverage: quasi-experimental study. BMJ 348:g3596, 2014 24942789

Man KKC, Coghill D, Chan EW, et al: Association of risk of suicide attempts with methylphenidate treatment. JAMA Psychiatry 74(10):1048–1055, 2017 28746699

Mancuso CE, Tanzi MG, Gabay M: Paradoxical reactions to benzodiazepines: literature review and treatment options. Pharmacotherapy 24(9):1177–1185, 2004 15460178

Marsch LA, Bickel WK, Badger GJ, et al: Comparison of pharmacological treatments for opioid-dependent adolescents: a randomized controlled trial. Arch Gen Psychiatry 62(10):1157–1164, 2005 16203961

McClellan J, Kowatch R, Findling RL; Work Group on Quality Issues: Practice parameter for the assessment and treatment of children and adolescents with bipolar disorder. J Am Acad Child Adolesc Psychiatry 46(1):107–125, 2007 17195735

McClellan J, Stock S; American Academy of Child and Adolescent Psychiatry (AACAP) Committee on Quality Issues (CQI): Practice parameter for the assessment and treatment of children and adolescents with schizophrenia. J Am Acad Child Adolesc Psychiatry 52(9):976–990, 2013 23972700

Missouri Department of Social Services: Psychotropic Medication Settlement, Excessive Dosage Guide. Last updated and approved July 25, 2022. Available at: https://dss.mo.gov/docs/settlment-2019/excessive-dosage-guidelines.xlsx. Accessed May 24, 2022.

Moolchan ET, Robinson ML, Ernst M, et al: Safety and efficacy of the nicotine patch and gum for the treatment of adolescent tobacco addiction. Pediatrics 115(4):e407–e414, 2005 15805342

Nasrallah HA, Chen AT: Multiple neurotoxic effects of haloperidol resulting in neuronal death. Ann Clin Psychiatry 29(3):195–202, 2017 28738100

Nasser A, Liranso T, Adewole T, et al: A Phase III, randomized, placebo-controlled trial to assess the efficacy and safety of once-daily SPN-812 (viloxazine extended-release) in the treatment of attention-deficit/hyperactivity disorder in school-age children. Clin Ther 42(8):1452–1466, 2020 32723670

National Institute for Health and Care Excellence: Guideline: Psychosis and schizophrenia in children and young people: recognition and management. Clinical guideline [CG155]. Published January 23, 2013. London, National Institute for Health and Care Excellence, 2013. Available at: https://www.nice.org.uk/guidance/cg155. Accessed January 29, 2024.

National Institute for Health and Care Excellence: Guideline: Attention deficit hyperactivity disorder: diagnosis and management. NICE guideline [NG87]. Published March 14, 2018. London, National Institute for Health and Care Excellence, 2018. Available at: https://www.nice.org.uk/guidance/ng87. Accessed January 29, 2024.

National Institute for Health and Care Excellence: Guideline: Depression in children and young people. NICE guideline [NG134]. Published June 25, 2019. London, National Institute for Health and Care Excellence, 2019. Available at: https://www.nice.org.uk/guidance/ng134. Accessed January 29, 2024.

Niederhofer H, Staffen W: Comparison of disulfiram and placebo in treatment of alcohol dependence of adolescents. Drug Alcohol Rev 22(3):295–297, 2003 15385223

Otasowie J, Castells X, Ehimare UP, et al: Tricyclic antidepressants for attention deficit hyperactivity disorder (ADHD) in children and adolescents. Cochrane Database Syst Rev (9):CD006997, 2014 25238582

Patel DR, Feucht C, Brown K, et al: Pharmacological treatment of anxiety disorders in children and adolescents: a review for practitioners. Transl Pediatr 7(1):23–35, 2018 29441280

Penfold RB, Stewart C, Hunkeler EM, et al: Use of antipsychotic medications in pediatric populations: what do the data say? Curr Psychiatry Rep 15(12):426, 2013 24258527

Substance Abuse and Mental Health Services Administration: Methadone Take-Home Flexibilities Extension Guidance. Last updated 01/23/2024. Available at: https://www.samhsa.gov/medications-substance-use-disorders/statutes-regulations-guidelines/methadone-guidance. Accessed July 31, 2024.

Spielmans GI, Spence-Sing T, Parry P: Duty to warn: antidepressant black box suicidality warning is empirically justified. Front Psychiatry 11:18, 2020 32116839

Stuckelman ZD, Mulqueen JM, Ferracioli-Oda E, et al: Risk of irritability with psychostimulant treatment in children with ADHD: a meta-analysis. J Clin Psychiatry 78(6):e648–e655, 2017 28682529

van den Anker J, Reed MD, Allegaert K, et al: Developmental changes in pharmacokinetics and pharmacodynamics. J Clin Pharmacol 58(Suppl 10):S10–S25, 2018 30248190

Vitiello B, Correll C, van Zwieten-Boot B, et al: Antipsychotics in children and adolescents: increasing use, evidence for efficacy and safety concerns. Eur Neuropsychopharmacol 19(9):629–635, 2009 19467582

Walter HJ, Bukstein OG, Abright AR, et al: Clinical practice guideline for the assessment and treatment of children and adolescents with anxiety disorders. J Am Acad Child Adolesc Psychiatry 59(10):1107–1124, 2020 32439401

Wolraich ML, Hagan JF Jr, Allan C, et al: Clinical Practice Guideline for the Diagnosis, Evaluation, and Treatment of Attention-Deficit/Hyperactivity Disorder in Children and Adolescents. Pediatrics 144(4):e20192528, 2019 31570648

Yan T, Goldman RD: Bupropion for smoking cessation in adolescents. Can Fam Physician 67(10):743–745, 2021 34649897

Yatham LN, Kennedy SH, Parikh SV, et al: Canadian Network for Mood and Anxiety Treatments (CANMAT) and International Society for Bipolar Disorders (ISBD) 2018 guidelines for the management of patients with bipolar disorder. Bipolar Disord 20(2):97–170, 2018 29536616

Yee CS, Hawken ER, Baldessarini RJ, et al: Maintenance pharmacological treatment of juvenile bipolar disorder: review and meta-analysis. Int J Neuropsychopharmacol 22(8):531, 2019 31211354

17

Older Adults

Tammy Duong, M.D.
J. Craig Nelson, M.D.

Overview of Physiological Changes in Older Adults

- Selection of psychopharmacological agents for older adults requires careful consideration. Age-related changes in pharmacokinetics, pharmacodynamics, comorbid disease, and polypharmacy should be considered.
- Older adults may require lower dosages than those used in younger adults. In addition, the time required for an adequate medication trial may be longer for older versus younger patients.
- Absorption affects how quickly a drug can take effect and occurs in the stomach or small intestine. Factors affecting absorption include delayed gastric emptying and changes in pH due either to decreased acid production or to medications (i.e., proton pump inhibitors or antacids) (Patel et al. 2020).
- P-glycoproteins (Pgps) are efflux pumps that move drugs back into the lumen. Pgps line the intestines, liver, kidneys, and blood-brain barrier. Pgps can be less functional in older patients, resulting in higher end-organ drug concentrations (van Assema et al. 2012).
- First-pass metabolism can be reduced as a result of decreased hepatic blood flow and hepatic mass. Therefore, drugs with extensive first-pass metabolism, such as propranolol, can have greater bioavailability in older adults (Mangoni and Jackson 2004).
- Older adults lose lean muscle mass and total body water, whereas fat composition increases. As a result, lipophilic drugs (e.g., diazepam, chlordiazepoxide) will have an increased volume of distribution, leading to an increased half-life. Hydrophilic drugs (e.g., lithium, ethanol, digoxin) will have a reduced volume of distribution, leading to higher serum concentrations (Mangoni and Jackson 2004).

- Drug metabolism occurs via phase I oxidation by cytochrome P450 (CYP) enzymes or Phase II glucuronidation. The rate of phase I metabolism can decline as much as 30% in older adults (Klotz 2009).
- Elimination is mediated by the kidneys. Kidney mass starts to decline in an individual's 30s, but up to one-third of individuals have preserved renal function in older age (Klotz 2009).
- Glomerular filtration rate (GFR) is a proxy used to quantify renal function. Equations such as the Cockcroft-Gault or the modification of diet in renal disease (MDRD) can be used to approximate GFR and help determine whether a medication's dosage should be adjusted based on the patient's renal function.
- Dopaminergic D_1 and D_2, serotonergic 5-HT_{1A} and 5-HT_{2A}, and muscarinic M_1 receptor densities are reduced with aging. Patients may become more sensitive to the effects of medications affecting these receptors, leading to a higher risk of experiencing adverse effects (Pollock 1998).
- Recommended starting dosages for older adults are one-half or less of the normal starting dosage for younger adults. Dosages should be increased gradually, at intervals no less than 1 or 2 weeks, to the lowest effective dosage.

Medication Classes

Antidepressants

Pharmacokinetic/Pharmacodynamic Considerations

- The half-life of antidepressants may be prolonged in older adults as a result of age-related larger volume of distribution, reduced metabolism by CYP enzymes, reduced P-glycoprotein activity, and decreased elimination via the kidneys.
- Antidepressants commonly have significant CYP enzyme interactions, which may lead to drug-drug interactions.

Dosing

- In general, start with half or less of the normal starting dosage used in younger adults to minimize initial side effects.
- Maximum dosages of tricyclic antidepressants (TCAs), monoamine oxidase inhibitors (MAOIs), citalopram, and escitalopram should be reduced in older adults.

Selected Side Effects

Central Nervous System/Neuropsychiatric

- The 2004 FDA Boxed Warning regarding antidepressants and increased risk of suicidality applied only to young adults, and there is no evidence of increased suicidality risk in adults older than 24 years. In fact, in older adults (age 65 years and older), antidepressants have been shown to be protective against the development of suicidal ideation and behavior (Fornaro et al. 2019).
- Older adults can be more susceptible to extrapyramidal side effects (EPS) from all antidepressants. These effects may include tremor, akathisia, and parkinsonian symptoms (Hawthorne and Caley 2015).
- Dream enactment and restless legs syndrome can be exacerbated by antidepressants. Among the antidepressants, mirtazapine may confer the greatest risk for restless legs syndrome (Rottach et al. 2008).

Cardiovascular

- α_1-Receptor blockade is associated with orthostasis and reflex tachycardia, leading to an increased risk of falls. TCAs, MAOIs, trazodone, and mirtazapine are all associated with orthostasis. Concomitant use of diuretics can exacerbate these side effects.
- Risk factors for prolongation of the corrected QT interval include older age, history of long QTc, female sex, cardiovascular disease, and hypokalemia. TCAs and citalopram are associated with QTc prolongation (Drew et al. 2010).

Endocrinological

- Selective serotonin reuptake inhibitors (SSRIs) are associated with the syndrome of inappropriate antidiuretic hormone secretion (SIADH), which can result in hyponatremia. Other risk factors for SIADH include older age, female sex, body mass index (BMI) less than 18.5 kg/m^2, malignancy, infections, and CNS pathology (Pinkhasov et al. 2021).

Hematological

- SSRIs and serotonin-norepinephrine reuptake inhibitors (SNRIs) are associated with platelet dysfunction (Halpern and Reber 2007). The bleeding risk increases significantly if an SSRI is used in combination with a nonsteroidal anti-inflammatory drug.

Genitourinary

- TCAs and SNRIs can be associated with urinary retention because of their antimuscarinic properties.

Antianxiety Medications

Pharmacokinetic/Pharmacodynamic Considerations

- Because they are lipophilic, benzodiazepines have a large volume of distribution in older adults.
- Intramuscular delivery of benzodiazepines can lead to erratic absorption for older adults.
- Benzodiazepines that are metabolized oxidatively, such as clorazepate, diazepam, and flurazepam, have active metabolites and decreased clearance and are long acting. These drugs are generally not recommended for use in older adults because they produce more sedation and psychomotor impairment (Greenblatt et al. 1991).
- Benzodiazepines that are metabolized via conjugation (glucuronidation), such as lorazepam, oxazepam, and temazepam, have no active metabolites and in general are more often recommended for use in older adults (Greenblatt et al. 1991).

Dosing

- Consider using one-quarter to one-half of the benzodiazepine dosage typically used in younger adults.
- Benzodiazepines that are short- to intermediate-acting, such as lorazepam, are preferred over long-acting agents.

Selected Side Effects

Central Nervous System/Neuropsychiatric

- Older adults may be more sensitive to the amnestic effects of high-dose benzodiazepines (American Geriatrics Society 2019).
- Benzodiazepines may impair motor coordination and increase reaction times, leading to falls and fractures (Markota et al. 2016).
- In medically complicated older adult patients, benzodiazepines may precipitate confusion, delirium, irritability, and/or hyperactivity and may impair cognition (Markota et al. 2016).

Cardiovascular

- Benzodiazepines are associated with lowered heart rate and blood pressure (Jacobson 2014).

Respiratory

- Benzodiazepines may worsen obstructive sleep apnea by relaxing the oropharyngeal muscles (Jacobson 2014).
- Respiratory depression can occur with use of high doses of benzodiazepines and use of benzodiazepines in combination with other respiratory depressant drugs.

Mood Stabilizers

Pharmacokinetic/Pharmacodynamic Considerations

- Clearance of carbamazepine, divalproex, lamotrigine, levetiracetam, and lithium may be reduced in older patients.
- In older patients, dehydration, kidney disease, concomitant use of nonsteroidal anti-inflammatory drugs (NSAIDs) and certain other medications, and changes in salt intake can significantly affect lithium's renal clearance and lead to toxicity.
- Lithium has a decreased volume of distribution in older adults as a result of reductions in total body water.

- Divalproex has increased free drug (i.e., protein unbound) levels in older adults, meaning that there is more available active drug. Checking bound versus unbound (free) plasma levels may at times be helpful clinically, as this ratio correlates better with side effects.

Dosing

- For older adults, consider using one-half the typical dosage used in younger adults.
- Lamotrigine may require a slower titration to the target dosage. The titration regimen provided in the manufacturer's package insert should be employed. See Table 5–1 in Chapter 5, "Mood Stabilizers," for detailed information on prescribing and dosage escalation of lamotrigine.
- The target lithium level for older adults is 0.4–0.8 mEq/L. CNS levels may be higher than reflected by serum levels (De Fazio et al. 2017).
- The target divalproex level for older adults is 65–90 µg/mL (Jacobson 2014).

Selected Side Effects

Central Nervous System/Neuropsychiatric

- Dizziness, somnolence, confusion, and cognitive changes are common side effects associated with mood stabilizers.
- Older adults can be more sensitive than younger patients to the motor effects (e.g., tremor, ataxia) of mood stabilizers.

Endocrinological

- Older adults may be more susceptible to SIADH, which is associated with carbamazepine and divalproex (Chan 1997).

Musculoskeletal

- Skeletal muscle weakness can occur with divalproex use and can lead to difficulty with standing and ambulation in older adults (Jacobson 2014).

Renal

- Lithium use in older adults can lead to polyuria and urinary incontinence secondary to lithium's impairment of the kidneys' ability to concentrate urine (Jacobson 2014).
- In rare cases, lithium use can cause diabetes insipidus.

Antipsychotics

Pharmacokinetic/Pharmacodynamic Considerations

- Antipsychotics are lipophilic and have a larger volume of distribution in older adults than in younger adults.
- Antipsychotics are metabolized via CYP enzymes and glucuronidation. CYP1A2, which metabolizes clozapine, haloperidol, and olanzapine, becomes less efficient with age (Jacobson 2014).
- Long-acting injectable antipsychotics can be used in older adults, but injections may be more painful in individuals with reduced muscle mass.

Dosing

- Consider using one-half the typical dosage used in younger adults.
- In older adults, low-potency antipsychotics (e.g., quetiapine) have a larger and less predictable therapeutic range compared with high-potency antipsychotics (e.g., risperidone, olanzapine, brexpiprazole).

Selected Side Effects

Central Nervous System/Neuropsychiatric

- **Boxed warning**: Increased mortality in elderly patients with dementia-related psychosis taking antipsychotics. The initial warning was for second-generation antipsychotics only and cautioned clinicians regarding the potential for increased risk of death—particularly death related to cardiovascular (e.g., heart failure, sudden death) or infectious (e.g., pneumonia) causes. In 2008, the warning was expanded to apply to all antipsychotics after further studies indicated that first-generation antipsychotics carried similar (and in fact greater) risk (Schneeweiss et al. 2007; Wang et al. 2005).
  - A 2005 meta-analysis of 15 randomized controlled trials demonstrated an increased risk of mortality (3.5% vs. 2.3% for placebo; odds ratio [OR] = 1.5) in patients with Alzheimer's disease or dementia who were treated with second-generation antipsychotics (Schneider et al. 2005; U.S. Food and Drug Administration 2005).
- Older adults may be more susceptible to the anticholinergic side effects of chlorpromazine, clozapine, thioridazine, and olanzapine, which can lead to confusion, worsening cognition, and delirium.
- Older adults tend to be more susceptible to EPS such as parkinsonism, whereas akathisia and dystonia occur slightly less frequently in older compared with younger adults (Jacobson 2014).

- Prophylactic use of anticholinergic drugs to prevent EPS is generally not recommended in older adults. Instead, use a lower dosage of the antipsychotic to address/ameliorate EPS.
- Antipsychotics can exacerbate motor symptoms in patients with Parkinson's disease or Lewy body disease. If an antipsychotic is required, use of a dopamine-sparing drug (e.g., clozapine, pimavanserin, quetiapine) should be considered.
- Older adults are at an increased risk of tardive dyskinesia (Savitt and Jankovic 2018).
- Seizure risk in association with antipsychotics is highest for patients taking clozapine or chlorpromazine. Individuals with structural brain disease or prior seizures are at greater risk (Hedges et al. 2003).

Cardiovascular

- All antipsychotics confer an increased risk for cerebrovascular accidents (e.g., strokes, transient ischemic attacks) when used to treat dementia-related psychosis in older adults (Wang et al. 2012). The FDA issued a boxed warning for all antipsychotics regarding this usage.
- Older adults are more susceptible to the orthostatic side effects of antipsychotics (mediated by α_1-adrenergic receptor antagonism), which can contribute to falls and fractures.

Hematological

- The risk of agranulocytosis associated with clozapine use is less than 1%, but it may be slightly higher for older adults (Bishara and Taylor 2014).

Stimulants

Pharmacokinetic/Pharmacodynamic Considerations

- Use of stimulants for the treatment of apathy, depression, catatonia, or Parkinson's disease or for prevention of falls is considered to be off-label. Heterogeneous studies of methylphenidate or amphetamines have demonstrated limited positive outcomes in older adults with these conditions (Sassi et al. 2020).
- Stimulants such as dextroamphetamine have decreased clearance in older adults (Ermer et al. 2013).

Dosing

- There are no established dosing guidelines for off-label uses of stimulants.
- For older adults, consider starting with one-quarter to one-half of the dosage typically used for younger adults.

Selected Side Effects

Central Nervous System/Neuropsychiatric

- Insomnia is a common side effect of stimulants.
- Less frequently, stimulants can induce or exacerbate anxiety, restlessness, headache, delirium, and hallucinations.

Ophthalmological

- Stimulants can exacerbate narrow-angle glaucoma (Lu et al. 2006).

Cardiovascular

- Stimulants are associated with an increased risk of myocardial infarction, stroke, and sudden death in individuals with preexisting cardiovascular disease (Franzen et al. 2012).
- Stimulants can increase the heart rate and blood pressure and can induce palpitations, all of which should be monitored throughout treatment (Franzen et al. 2012).

Gastrointestinal

- Decreased appetite is a common side effect of stimulants.

Hypnotics

Pharmacokinetic/Pharmacodynamic Considerations

- Hypnotic medications are indicated for short-term use in older adults. Long-term use may require regular/frequent evaluation for side effects.
- Hypnotics are largely metabolized via CYP3A4. Coadministration of hypnotics with CYP3A4 inhibitors will lead to an increased risk of side effects such as hallucinations or falls.

Dosing

- Maximum dosages in older adults: Eszopiclone 2 mg/day; zaleplon 5 mg/day; zolpidem 5 mg/day

Selected Side Effects

Central Nervous System/Neuropsychiatric

- Common side effects of hypnotic medications include somnolence, dizziness, headache, confusion, and amnesia. Side effects are more prominent at higher doses of medications with longer half-lives (Jacobson 2014).
- Hypnotics' sedative effects are associated with falls (Ryba and Rainess 2020).
- Hypnotics can be associated with hallucinations.
- Less-common side effects include irritability, emotional lability, apathy, and agitation.

Medications Used in Substance Use Disorders

Considerations

- Older adults are more likely to misuse alcohol, nicotine, and benzodiazepines compared with other drugs (Seim et al. 2020), although medicinal and recreational cannabis use in older adults is also on the rise (Han and Palamar 2020; Solomon et al. 2021).
- Because medications for substance use disorders are generally understudied in geriatric populations, their safety is not well established in this age group (Tampi et al. 2019).
- Nicotine replacement therapy (NRT) has not been rigorously studied in geriatric populations. Transdermal nicotine patches, which release nicotine slowly, are the preferred replacement delivery system for older adults.
- Methadone is lipophilic and has a large volume of distribution, which can be problematic in older adults.

Dosing

- Target dosages for naltrexone, acamprosate, and NRT in older adults are typically one-half the dosages normally used in younger adults.
- Use caution with disulfiram dosages higher than 250 mg/day.
- Target dosages of buprenorphine for older adults have not been established, but lower dosages are generally recommended.

Selected Side Effects

Central Nervous System/Neuropsychiatric

- Buprenorphine, disulfiram, and long-acting benzodiazepines can lead to dizziness, confusion, and oversedation.
- Topiramate can lead to cognitive slowing, and its use is often avoided in older adults (Sommer and Fenn 2010).
- Varenicline can exacerbate depression and suicidal thinking. See Chapter 10, "Treatment of Substance Use Disorders," for further information on varenicline, including the risks of prescribing this medication for individuals with mental disorders.

Cardiovascular

- Disulfiram can induce flushing, palpitations, tachycardia, and hypotension, which can lead to cardiovascular collapse in older adults. Use of disulfiram is often avoided in older adults (Bourcier et al. 2013).
- Clonidine can be used for symptomatic treatment of opioid withdrawal, but side effects include orthostasis, bradycardia, atrioventricular block, and syncope.
- Methadone has the potential to prolong the QTc interval.

Neuromodulation Therapies

Electroconvulsive Therapy

Considerations

- Electroconvulsive therapy (ECT) remains the gold standard for treatment-refractory mood disorders.
- ECT is well tolerated in older adults who are frail, have difficulty tolerating medications, or are acutely suffering from catatonia or suicidality.
- Patients with medical comorbidities are not excluded from receiving ECT treatment. Clinicians should use evidence-based screening and medical clearance criteria.
- Patients without medial temporal lobe atrophy are three times more likely to respond to ECT than are those with mild or moderate atrophy (Geduldig and Kellner 2016).

Dosing

- Bifrontal and right unilateral ECT have equal response rates in depressed older adults (Geduldig and Kellner 2016).
- ECT adjustments for older adults may include reducing the frequency (e.g., from 3 times a week to 2 times a week) and changing from bilateral to unilateral electrode placement (Geduldig and Kellner 2016).

Selected Side Effects

Central Nervous System/Neuropsychiatric

- ECT can cause short-term anterograde amnesia that improves with time, even in patients with cognitive impairment (Geduldig and Kellner 2016).
- Some older adults with cognitive impairment may be more susceptible to developing transient delirium during ECT treatments (Geduldig and Kellner 2016).

Transcranial Magnetic Stimulation

Considerations

- Varying levels of brain atrophy may decrease the efficacy of repetitive transcranial magnetic stimulation (rTMS) in older adults (Cappon et al. 2022).

Dosing

- rTMS intensity may need to be adjusted to compensate for increased scalp-to-cortex distance in patients with brain atrophy (Cappon et al. 2022).
- Older adults may require longer treatment durations and a higher total number of pulses for optimal response to rTMS (Yip et al. 2017).

Selected Side Effects

Central Nervous System/Neuropsychiatric

- Headaches, pain at the procedure site, and toothache are the most common side effects associated with rTMS (Valiengo et al. 2022).
- rTMS is associated with a rare increased risk of generalized tonic-clonic seizures (Cappon et al. 2022).

References

American Geriatrics Society Beers Criteria Update Expert Panel: Updated AGS Beers Criteria for Potentially Inappropriate Medication Use in Older Adults. J Am Geriatr Soc 67(4):674–694, 2019 30693946

Bishara D, Taylor D: Adverse effects of clozapine in older patients: epidemiology, prevention and management. Drugs Aging 31(1):11–20, 2014 24338220

Bourcier S, Mongardon N, Daviaud F, et al: Disulfiram ethanol reaction mimicking anaphylactic, cardiogenic, and septic shock. Am J Emerg Med 31(1):270.e1–270.e3, 2013 22809767

Cappon D, den Boer T, Jordan C, et al: Transcranial magnetic stimulation (TMS) for geriatric depression. Ageing Res Rev 74:101531, 2022 34839043

Chan TY: Drug-induced syndrome of inappropriate antidiuretic hormone secretion: causes, diagnosis and management. Drugs Aging 11(1):27–44, 1997 9237039

De Fazio P, Gaetano R, Caroleo M, et al: Lithium in late-life mania: a systematic review. Neuropsychiatr Dis Treat 13:755–766, 2017 28331326

Drew BJ, Ackerman MJ, Funk M, et al: Prevention of torsade de pointes in hospital settings: a scientific statement from the American Heart Association and the American College of Cardiology Foundation. Circulation 121(8):1047–1060, 2010 20185054

Ermer J, Haffey MB, Richards C, et al: Double-blind, placebo-controlled, two-period, crossover trial to examine the pharmacokinetics of lisdexamfetamine dimesylate in healthy older adults. Neuropsychiatr Dis Treat 9:219–229, 2013 23431065

Fornaro M, Anastasia A, Valchera A, et al: The FDA "black box" warning on antidepressant suicide risk in young adults: more harm than benefits? Front Psychiatry 10:294, 2019 31130881

Franzen JD, Wetzel MW, Padala PR, et al: Psychostimulants for older adults. Curr Psychiatr 11(1):23–32, 2012

Geduldig ET, Kellner CH: Electroconvulsive therapy in the elderly: new findings in geriatric depression. Curr Psychiatry Rep 18(4):40, 2016 26909702

Greenblatt DJ, Harmatz JS, Shader RI: Clinical pharmacokinetics of anxiolytics and hypnotics in the elderly: therapeutic considerations (Part I). Clin Pharmacokinet 21(3):165–177, 1991 1684924

Halperin D, Reber G: Influence of antidepressants on hemostasis. Dialogues Clin Neurosci 9(1):47–59, 2007 17506225

Han BH, Palamar JJ: Trends in cannabis use among older adults in the United States, 2015–2018. JAMA Intern Med 180(4):609–611, 2020 32091531

Hawthorne JM, Caley CF: Extrapyramidal reactions associated with serotonergic antidepressants. Ann Pharmacother 49(10):1136–1152, 2015 26185277

Hedges D, Jeppson K, Whitehead P: Antipsychotic medication and seizures: a review. Drugs Today 39(7):551–557, 2003 12973403

Jacobson SA: Clinical Manual of Geriatric Psychopharmacology, Second Edition. Arlington, VA, American Psychiatric Publishing, 2014

Klotz U: Pharmacokinetics and drug metabolism in the elderly. Drug Metab Rev 41(2):67–76, 2009 19514965

Lu CK, Kuang TM, Chou JC: Methylphenidate (Ritalin)-associated cataract and glaucoma. J Chin Med Assoc 69(12):589–590, 2006 17182354

Mangoni AA, Jackson SH: Age-related changes in pharmacokinetics and pharmacodynamics: basic principles and practical applications. Br J Clin Pharmacol 57(1):6–14, 2004 14678335

Markota M, Rummans TA, Bostwick JM, et al: Benzodiazepine use in older adults: dangers, management, and alternative therapies. Mayo Clin Proc 91(11):1632–1639, 2016 27814838

Patel D, Bertz R, Ren S, et al: A systematic review of gastric acid-reducing agent-mediated drug-drug interactions with orally administered medications. Clin Pharmacokinet 59(4):447–462, 2020 31788764

Pinkhasov A, Xiong G, Bourgeois JA, et al: Management of SIADH-related hyponatremia due to psychotropic medications—an expert consensus from the Association of Medicine and Psychiatry. J Psychosom Res 151:110654, 2021 34739943

Pollock BG: Psychotropic drugs and the aging patient. Geriatrics 53(Suppl 1):S20–S24, 1998 9745631

Rottach KG, Schaner BM, Kirch MH, et al: Restless legs syndrome as side effect of second generation antidepressants. J Psychiatr Res 43(1):70–75, 2008 18468624

Ryba N, Rainess R: Z-drugs and falls: a focused review of the literature. Sr Care Pharm 35(12):549–554, 2020 33258763

Sassi KLM, Rocha NP, Colpo GD, et al: Amphetamine use in the elderly: a systematic review of the literature. Curr Neuropharmacol 18(2):126–135, 2020 31660835

Savitt D, Jankovic J: Tardive syndromes. J Neurol Sci 389:35–42, 2018 29506749

Schneeweiss S, Setoguchi S, Brookhart A, et al: Risk of death associated with the use of conventional versus atypical antipsychotic drugs among elderly patients. CMAJ 176(5):627–632, 2007 17325327

Schneider LS, Dagerman KS, Insel P: Risk of death with atypical antipsychotic drug treatment for dementia: meta-analysis of randomized placebo-controlled trials. JAMA 294(15):1934–1943, 2005 16234500

Seim L, Vijapura P, Pagali S, et al: Common substance use disorders in older adults. Hospital Pract 48(sup1):48–55, 2020 32073917

Solomon HV, Greenstein AP, DeLisi LE: Cannabis use in older adults: a perspective. Harv Rev Psychiatry 29(3):225–233, 2021 33660625

Sommer BR, Fenn HH: Review of topiramate for the treatment of epilepsy in elderly patients. Clin Interv Aging 5:89–99, 2010 20458347

Tampi RR, Chhatlani A, Ahmad H, et al: Substance use disorders among older adults: a review of randomized controlled pharmacotherapy trials. World J Psychiatry 9(5):78–82, 2019 31559148

U.S. Food and Drug Administration: Public Health Advisory: Deaths with Antipsychotics in Elderly Patients with Behavioral Disturbances. U.S.Food and Drug Administration, April 11, 2005. Available at: https://psychrights.org/drugs/FDAantipsychotics4elderlywarning.htm. Accessed March 11, 2024.

Valiengo L, Maia A, Cotovio G, et al: Repetitive transcranial magnetic stimulation for major depressive disorder in older adults: systematic review and meta-analysis. J Gerontol A Biol Sci Med Sci 77(4):851–860, 2022 34432865

van Assema DME, Lubberink M, Boellaard R, et al: P-glycoprotein function at the blood-brain barrier: effects of age and gender. Mol Imaging Biol 14(6):771–776, 2012 22476967

Wang PS, Schneeweiss S, Avorn J, et al: Risk of death in elderly users of conventional vs. atypical antipsychotic medications. N Engl J Med 353(22):2335–2341, 2005 16319382

Wang S, Linkletter C, Dore D, et al: Age, antipsychotics, and the risk of ischemic stroke in the Veterans Health Administration. Stroke 43(1):28–31, 2012 22033997

Yip AG, George MS, Tendler A, et al: 61% of unmedicated treatment resistant depression patients who did not respond to acute TMS treatment responded after four weeks of twice weekly deep TMS in the Brainsway pivotal trial. Brain Stimul 10(4):847–849, 2017 28330592

Abbreviations

ACE	angiotensin-converting enzyme
ACh	acetylcholine
AChE	acetylcholinesterase
AChEI	acetylcholinesterase inhibitor
ACOG	American College of Obstetricians and Gynecologists
ADHD	attention-deficit/hyperactivity disorder
AED	antiepileptic drug
AGS	American Geriatrics Society
AIMS	Abnormal Involuntary Movement Scale
ALT	alanine aminotransferase
AMPA	α-amino-3-hydroxy-5-methyl-4-isoxazolepropionic acid
ANC	absolute neutrophil count
ARIA	amyloid-related imaging abnormalities
ASD	autism spectrum disorder
AST	aspartate transaminase
AUC	area under the curve
AV	atrioventricular
BDNF	brain-derived neurotrophic factor
BEN	benign ethnic neutropenia
BID or bid	twice a day
BMI	body mass index
BMP	basic metabolic panel
BP	blood pressure
BUN	blood urea nitrogen
CBC	complete blood count
CBT	cognitive-behavioral therapy
CGI	Clinical Global Impressions [scale]
cGMP	cyclic guanosine monophosphate
CHF	congestive heart failure
CINV	chemotherapy-induced nausea and vomiting

Cmax	maximum concentration
CMP	comprehensive metabolic panel
CNS	central nervous system
COPD	chronic obstructive pulmonary disease
COWS	Clinical Opiate Withdrawal Scale
CPK	creatine phosphokinase
CR	controlled-release
CrCl	creatinine clearance
CRP	C-reactive protein
CYP	cytochrome P450
DAT	dopamine transporter
DBS	deep brain stimulation
DEA	U.S. Drug Enforcement Administration
dL	deciliter
DORA	dual orexin receptor antagonist
DRESS	drug reaction with eosinophilia and systemic symptoms
DRG	dorsal root ganglion
DSM-5	Diagnostic and Statistical Manual of Mental Disorders, 5th Edition
DSST	Digit Symbol Substitution Test
ECG	electrocardiogram
ECT	electroconvulsive therapy
EEG	electroencephalogram
eGFR	estimated glomerular filtration rate
EMG	electromyogram
EPS	extrapyramidal side effects
ER	extended-release
ESRD	end-stage renal disease
FDA	U.S. Food and Drug Administration
FGA	first-generation antipsychotic
GABA	gamma-aminobutyric acid
GAD	generalized anxiety disorder
GFR	glomerular filtration rate
GHB	gamma-hydroxybutyrate
GPCR	G protein–coupled receptor

GSK-3 glycogen synthase kinase 3

HbA1c hemoglobin A1C (test)
HDL high-density lipoprotein
hERG human Ether-à-go-go-Related Gene
HLA human leukocyte antigen
HR heart rate
HSDD hypoactive sexual desire disorder
5-HT 5-hydroxytryptamine (serotonin)

IBS irritable bowel syndrome
IM intramuscular
INR international normalized ratio
IR immediate-release
IV intravenous

Kd dissociation constant
Ki inhibition constant

LA long-acting
LAI long-acting injectable
LDL low-density lipoprotein
LFT liver function test

MAO monoamine oxidase
MAOI monoamine oxidase inhibitor
mCPP meta-chlorophenylpiperazine
MDD major depressive disorder
MDMA 3,4-methylenedioxymethamphetamine
MDR multidrug-resistant
MDRD modification of diet in renal disease (equation)
MDSI major depressive disorder with suicidal ideation
mg milligram
μg microgram
MI myocardial infarction
mL milliliter
mmHg millimeters of mercury
mPFC medial prefrontal cortex

MRI	magnetic resonance imaging
ms	millisecond
NAC	*N*-acetylcysteine
NAS	neonatal abstinence syndrome
NCD	neurocognitive disorder
NDRI	norepinephrine and dopamine reuptake inhibitor
NET	norepinephrine transporter
ng	nanogram
NICE	National Institute for Health and Care Excellence
nM	nanomolar
NMDA	*N*-methyl-D-aspartate
NMS	neuroleptic malignant syndrome
NNT	number needed to treat
NRT	nicotine replacement therapy
NSAID	nonsteroidal anti-inflammatory drug
NTD	neural tube defect
OB/GYN	obstetrics/gynecology
OCD	obsessive-compulsive disorder
OCP	oral contraceptive pill
ODF	orally disintegrating film
ODT	orally disintegrating tablet
ODV	*O*-desmethylvenlafaxine (metabolite)
OSA	obstructive sleep apnea
OTC	over the counter
PAM	positive allosteric modulator
PCP	phencyclidine
PDE	phosphodiesterase}
PEG	polyethylene glycol
PET	positron emission tomography
PKU	phenylketonuria
PLLR	Pregnancy and Lactation Labeling Rule
PMDD	premenstrual dysphoric disorder
PO	oral; by mouth
PPH	postpartum hemorrhage

PPHN	persistent pulmonary hypertension of the newborn
PRN	as needed
PT	prothrombin time
PTSD	posttraumatic stress disorder
QD or qd	every day
QHS or qhs	every night at bedtime
QPM or qpm	once daily after noon
QTc	corrected QT interval
RCT	randomized controlled trial
RDA	recommended dietary allowance
REM	rapid eye movement
REMS	Risk Evaluation and Mitigation Strategy
RID	relative infant dose
RIMA	reversible inhibitor of monoamine oxidase A
RPR	rapid plasma reagin
rTMS	repetitive transcranial magnetic stimulation
SAI	short-acting injectable
SERT	serotonin transporter
SGA	second-generation antipsychotic
SIADH	syndrome of inappropriate antidiuretic hormone secretion
SJS	Stevens-Johnson syndrome
SL	sublingual
SLE	systemic lupus erythematosus
SNRI	serotonin-norepinephrine reuptake inhibitor
SPECT	single photon emission computed tomography
SR	sustained-release
SSRI	selective serotonin reuptake inhibitor
STD/I	sexually transmitted disease/infection
SUD	substance use disorder
TCA	tricyclic antidepressant
TD	tardive dyskinesia
TDM	therapeutic drug monitoring
TRH	thyrotropin9-releasing hormone
TEN	toxic epidermal necrolysis

TID or tid	three times a day
Tmax	time to reach maximum concentration
TMS	transcranial magnetic stimulation
TSH	thyroid-stimulating hormone
TTS	transdermal therapeutic system
UDS	urine drug screen
UGT	human uridine 5′-diphospho-glucuronosyltransferase
V_D	volume of distribution
VMAT	vesicular monoamine transporter
VNS	vagal nerve stimulation
WHO	World Health Organization
XR	extended-release
Y-BOCS	Yale-Brown Obsessive-Compulsive Scale

Index

*Page numbers printed in **boldface** type refer to tables.*